Clinical Pharmacology

'Nature is not only odder than we think, but it is odder than we can think.'

J B S HALDANE 1893–1964

'Patients may recover in spite of drugs or because of them.'

J H GADDUM 1959

'But know also, man has an inborn craving for medicine ... the desire to take medicine is one feature which distinguishes man the animal, from his fellow creatures. It is really one of the most serious difficulties with which we have to contend ... the doctor's visit is not thought to be complete without a prescription.'

WILLIAM OSLER 1894

'Morals do not forbid making experiments on one's neighbour or on one's self ... among the experiments that may be tried on man, those that can only harm are forbidden, those that are innocent are permissible, and those that may do good are obligatory.' 'Men who have excessive faith in their theories or ideas are not only ill prepared for making discoveries; they make very poor observations ... they can see in [their] results only a confirmation of their theory ... This is what made us say that we must never make experiments to confirm our ideas, but simply to control them.'

'Empiricism is not the negation of science, as certain physicians seem to think; it is only its first stage.'

'Medicine is destined to get away from empiricism little by little; like all other sciences, it will get away by the scientific method.'

'Considered in itself, the experimental method is nothing but reasoning by whose help we methodically submit our ideas to experience — the experience of facts.'

CLAUDE BERNARD 1865

'I do not want two diseases — one nature-made, one doctor-made.'

NAPOLEON BONAPARTE 1820

'The ingenuity of man has ever been fond of exerting itself to varied forms and combinations of medicines.'

WILLIAM WITHERING 1785

'All things are poisons and there is nothing that is harmless, the dose alone decides that something is no poison.'

PARACELSUS 1493–1541

'First do no harm.'
'It is a good remedy sometimes to use nothing.'

HIPPOCRATES 460–355 B.C.

Clinical Pharmacology

D R Laurence MD FRCP

Professor Emeritus of Pharmacology and Therapeutics,
School of Medicine, University College London, London,
UK

P N Bennett MD FRCP

Consultant Physician, Royal United Hospital, Bath and
Reader in Clinical Pharmacology, University of Bath,
Bath, UK

SEVENTH EDITION

With illustrations by the late Peter Kneebone and others

CHURCHILL LIVINGSTONE
EDINBURGH LONDON MADRID MELBOURNE NEW YORK AND TOKYO 1992

CHURCHILL LIVINGSTONE
Medical Division of Longman Group UK Limited

Distributed in the United States of America by Churchill
Livingstone Inc., 650 Avenue of the Americas, New York,
N.Y. 10011, and by associated companies, branches and
representatives throughout the world.

First Edition 1960
Second Edition 1962
Third Edition 1966
Fourth Edition 1973
Fifth Edition 1980
Sixth Edition 1987
Seventh Edition 1992
   Reprinted 1993

TRANSLATIONS
Previous editions
translated into Italian, Chinese
Spanish, Serbo-Croat,
Russian and Japanese

ISBN 0-443-04388-4

British Library Cataloguing in Publication Data
Laurence, D. R.
   Clinical pharmacology. — 6th ed.
   1. Drugs 2. Pharmacology
   I. Title II. Bennett, P. N.
   615'.1 RM300

Library of Congress Cataloging in Publication Data
Laurence, D. R. (Desmond Roger)
   (Clinical pharmacology)
   Bibliography: p.
   Includes index.
   1. Pharmacology. 2. Chemotherapy. I. Bennett,
P. N. II. Title. [DNLM: 1. Pharmacology, Clinical. QV 38
L379c]
RM300.L349 1987 615.7 86–29871

for Churchill Livingstone
Publisher: Timothy Horne
Project Editor: Kathleen Orr
Production Controller: Lesley Small
Designer: Design Resources Unit
Sales Promotion Executive: Hilary Brown

The
publisher's
policy is to use
**paper manufactured
from sustainable forests**

Produced by Longman Singapore Publishers (Pte) Ltd
Printed in Singapore

Preface

'For your own satisfaction and for mine, please read this preface.'[1]

> This book is about the scientific basis and practice of drug therapy. It is particularly intended for **undergraduate and graduate students of medicine.**

The general aspects of the *how* and *why* of drugs are for students. The practical details are to help them when they begin to prescribe on their own responsibility after graduating, and the book is offered as a guide to this.

Plainly the book contains many more facts than a student either needs or should attempt to learn. Students should read selectively, and we hope it will not be too difficult for them to do so. We would particularly suggest that students should read Chapters 1 to 8 and those parts of other chapters covering general background, principles or mechanisms of action.

In addition we hope that the book may be of use to some more experienced doctors in reminding them of general progress and practice in fields with which, perhaps, they are no longer primarily concerned, but which have not lost interest or all importance for them.

Justification. We believe that doctors who understand something of how drugs get into the body, of how they produce their effects, of their fate and of how evidence of therapeutic effect is assessed, will choose drugs more skilfully and use them more successfully than those who do not.

This book represents an attempt to provide pharmacological knowledge that is both interesting[2] and useful to the physician.

Most books of moderate size either confine themselves to discussing pharmacology without giving enough information for drugs to be selected and used effectively, or else they confine themselves to practical therapeutics and ignore the pharmacological background. It is too much to expect the now heavily burdened student to consult and integrate two works, one not always clearly related to clinical practice and the other often as arbitrary and as empirical as a cookery book.

This book is offered as a reasonably brief solution to the problem of combining practical clinical utility with some account of the principles of pharmacology on which clinical practice rests.

How much practical technical detail to include has been difficult to decide. In general, more such detail is provided for therapeutic practices that are complex or potentially dangerous *and* urgent; where there may be no time for consultation

---

[1] St. Francis of Sales: preface to Introduction to the devout life (1609).

[2] An author, poet and critic (Philip Larkin: 1922–85) has told that he judged fiction thus: 'Could I read it? If I could read it, did I believe it? If I believed it, did I care about it? And if I cared about it, what was the quality of my caring, and did it last?' It would be presumptuous of authors of a textbook to aspire to satisfy the criteria for fiction, so we will only say that we have been mindful of them in writing this book.

with colleagues or search in libraries, e.g. cardiac dysrhythmias, and less, or even none, on therapy that is generally conducted only by specialists or that can wait on such consultation, e.g. anticancer drugs; i.v. oxytocin. But always, especially with modern drugs with which the prescriber may not be familiar, the manufacturer's current literature should be consulted.

Use of the book. Students, undergraduate and graduate, are, or should be, concerned to *understand*, to develop a rational, critical attitude to drug therapy and they should therefore chiefly concern themselves with how drugs act and interact in disease and with how evidence of therapeutic effect is obtained and evaluated. They should not allow this to be impeded by attempts to memorise lists of alternative drugs and minor differences between them, or arbitrary practical details, such as dosage or solution strength, which should never be required of them in examinations; the only way to fix these in the mind is by actual prescribing.

The decision to try to include sufficient practical details to enable some drugs to be correctly used has inevitably made parts of the book tedious. In addition, it has been thought necessary to mention numerous drugs of doubtful merit, and what have been aptly called 'me-tooers', in order to enable drugs to be recognised and a choice to be made from amongst the huge number of drugs and formulations of drugs thrust at the clinician by a vigorous pharmaceutical industry.

We hope that students will readily see which sections of the book they can, and indeed should, neglect in their general reading, and that are for use when the responsibility of choice and administration becomes theirs.

The 'authority' of a textbook. If a book is to be a useful guide to drug use it must offer clear conclusions and advice. If it is to be of reasonable size alternative acceptable courses of action will often have to be omitted. What is recommended should be based on sound evidence where this exists, and on an assessment of the opinions of the experienced where it does not. Exceptions to all advice will occur,[3] and part of the clinician's skill lies in knowing when to depart from an ac-

cepted course. Nor can a textbook take account of all possible modifying factors, e.g. personality, intercurrent disease, metabolic differences, in any individual case.

The status of a textbook as a practical guide has been expressed in a legal judgement where an accusation of negligent treatment made against a doctor was supported by showing that he had not followed the orthodox treatment as stated in various textbooks. The Judge said that textbook writers were writing of a subject in general and not of a particular patient. A doctor was entitled to use his common sense, his experience, and his judgement as far as they fitted into a particular case. 'It would be a sorry day for the medical profession if it were to be said that no doctor ought to depart one tittle from that which he saw written in a textbook.'[4] Statements in textbooks were no substitute for the judgement of the physician in charge of the case. 'His Lordship could not follow slavishly the views expressed in textbooks . . . .'[4]

The guide to further reading at the end of each chapter is comprised of a few references to original papers, to referenced editorials and review articles from a small number of English language journals that are likely to be available in even the most modest hospital library in order to enable anyone, anywhere, to gain access to the original literature and to informed opinion, and also to provide interest and sometimes amusement. We urge students to select a title that looks interesting and to read the article. We do not attempt to document all the statements we make, which would be impossible in a book of this size.

The *general references* at the end of the book are to specialist reference books and journals that cover the whole field.

---

[3] Control of therapeutic claims is properly exercised by government regulatory authority, but limitation of doctors' freedom to prescribe what they have reason to believe best for the patients should be resisted on principle (although cost is increasingly regarded as overriding principle). The solution to bad doctoring is education, not the imposition of limitations on conscientious doctors. But if doctors will prescribe carelessly then society will take away their freedom. See isotretinoin, clozapine.

[4] Lancet 1960; 1:593.

It is assumed that the reader will possess a formulary and so the text has not been encumbered with exhaustive lists of preparations although it is hoped that enough have been mentioned to cover much routine prescribing, and many drugs have been included solely for identification.

London and Bath, 1992

D. R. L.
P. N. B.

Acknowledgements

- It is not possible for two individuals to cover the whole field of drug therapy from their own knowledge and experience, and we are deeply grateful to all those who have with such good grace given us their time and energy to supply valuable facts and opinions, they principally include:

Dr E S K Assem
Dr N B Bennett
Dr M Davis
Dr Sheila Gore
Dr J Guillebaud
Dr W N Hubbard
Prof D H Jenkinson
Dr D A Lewis
Prof P J Maddison
Prof Sir William Paton
Prof B N C Prichard
Dr J P D Reckless
Dr D A F Robertson
Dr Gillian Robinson
Dr C R J Singer
Dr J A Vale
Dr C Ward
Prof O Wrong

- Other acknowledgements are made in the appropriate places.
- Much of any merit this book may have is due to the generosity of those named above as well as others too numerous to mention who have put their knowledge and practical experience of the use of drugs at our disposal. Responsibility for any errors rests with us.
- In addition, permission to quote directly from the writings of some authorities has been generously granted and we thank the authors and their publishers who have given it.
- The late Peter Kneebone's illustrations speak for themselves.
- Particular thanks are due to Kathleen Orr (publisher's project editor) for able, calm and tactful support and improvements.

Contents

Topics in drug therapy and clinical pharmacology

SYNOPSIS

Drug therapy involves many considerations beyond the strictly scientific pharmacological aspects of medicines. It includes numerous considerations relating to prescribers themselves and to patients.

- The therapeutic situation
- Benefits and risks
- The public view of drugs and prescribers
- Criticisms of modern drugs
- Complementary and traditional medicine
- Responsibility for drug-caused injury
- Chronic pharmacology
- Warnings to patients and consent to treatment
- Why drug therapy carries unavoidable risk
- Reasons for taking a drug history from patients
- Placebos
- Prescribing and drug consumption
- Economics: cost-benefit, cost-effectiveness and quality of life
- Patient compliance
- Doctor compliance
- Self-medication and medicines in the home

THE THERAPEUTIC SITUATION

Poisons in small doses are the best medicines; and useful medicines in too large doses are poisonous. (William Withering, 'discoverer' of digitalis, 1789)

The use of drugs[1] to increase human happiness by elimination or suppression of diseases and symptoms and to improve the quality of life in other ways is a serious matter and involves not only technical but psychosocial considerations. We therefore begin this book with a series of essays on what we think are important topics.

Medicines are part of our way of life from birth, when we enter the world with the aid of drugs, to death where drugs assist (most of) us to depart with minimal distress and perhaps even with a remnant of dignity. In between these events we regulate our fertility, often, with drugs. We tend to take such usages for granted.

But during the intervals remaining, an average family experiences illness on one day in four and between the ages of 20 and 45 years a lower-middle-class man experiences approxi-

---

[1] A World Health Organization Scientific Group has defined a drug as 'any substance or product that is used or intended to be used to modify or explore physiological systems or pathological states for the benefit of the recipient'. WHO Tech Rep Ser 1966; no. 341: 7.

A *drug* is a single chemical substance that forms the active ingredient of a *medicine*, which latter may contain many other substances to deliver the drug in a stable form, acceptable and convenient to the patient. The terms will be used more or less interchangeably in this book. To use the word 'drug' intending only a harmful, dangerous or addictive substance is to abuse a respectable and useful word.

mately one life-endangering illness, 20 disabling (temporarily) illnesses, 200 non-disabling illnesses and 1000 symptomatic episodes,[2] and medicines play a major role in these.

Before treating any patient with drugs,[1] doctors should have made up their minds on 8 points:

1. Whether they should interfere with the patient at all and if so —
2. What alteration in the patient's condition they hope to achieve.
3. That the drug they intend to use is best capable of bringing this about.
4. How they will know when it has been brought about.
5. That they can administer the drug in such a way that the right concentration will be attained in the right place at the right time and for the right duration.
6. What other effects the drug may have and whether these may be harmful.
7. How they will decide to stop the drug.
8. Whether the likelihood of benefit, and its importance, outweighs the likelihood of damage, and its importance, i.e. to consider *benefit versus risk*, or *efficacy in relation to safety*.

It is clear that drug therapy involves a great deal more than matching the name of the drug to the name of a disease; it requires knowledge, judgement, skill and wisdom, but above all a sense of responsibility. A book can provide knowledge and can contribute to the formation of judgement, but it can do little to impart skill and wisdom, which are the products of experience and innate and acquired capacities.

Everybody knows that drugs can do good

Medically this good may sometimes seem trivial, as in the avoidance of a sleepless night in a noisy hotel or of social embarrassment from a profusely running nose due to seasonal pollen allergy (hay-fever). Such benefits, however, are not necessarily

trivial to recipients, concerned to be at their best in important matters, whether of business, of pleasure or of passion, i.e. with quality of life.

Or the good may be literally life-saving, as in serious acute infections (pneumonia, septicaemia) or in the prevention of life-devastating disability from severe asthma, from epilepsy or from blindness due to glaucoma.

Everybody knows that drugs can do harm

This harm may be relatively trivial, as in hangover from a hypnotic or sleepiness from an H_1-receptor antihistamine used for hay-fever (though these effects may be a cause of serious road accidents).

The harm may also be life-destroying, as in the rare sudden death following an injection of penicillin, rightly regarded as one of the safest of antibiotics, or the destruction of the quality of life that occasionally attends the use of drugs that are effective in asthma and rheumatoid arthritis (adrenocortical steroids, penicillamine).

There are risks in taking medicines just as there are risks in food and transport. There are also risks in not taking medicines when they are needed, just as there are risks in not taking food or in not using transport when they are needed.

Efficacy and safety do not lie solely in the chemical nature of the drug. Doctors must choose which drugs to use and must apply them correctly in relation not only to their properties, but also to those of the patients and their disease. Then patients must use the prescribed medicine correctly.

Use of drugs

Drugs are used in three principal ways:

1. **Curative**, as primary therapy (as in bacterial and parasitic infections) or as auxiliary therapy (as with anaesthetics, and ergometrine and oxytocin in obstetrics).

2. **Suppressive** of diseases or symptoms, used continuously or intermittently to maintain health without attaining cure, as in hypertension, diabetes, epilepsy, asthma or to control symptoms

---

[2] Quoted in: Anderson J A D, ed. Self medication. Lancaster: MTP Press, 1979.

such as pain and cough, whilst awaiting recovery from the causative disease.

3. **Preventive** (prophylactic), as when a non-immune person enters a malarial area, or contraception.

BENEFITS AND RISKS

Benefits of drugs are manifest to doctor and patient and also, it might be thought, obvious to even the most unimaginative healthy people who find themselves dismayed by some aspects of modern technology.

Modern technological medicine has been criticised, justly, for following the tradition of centuries by waiting for disease to occur and then trying to cure it rather than seeking to prevent it from occurring in the first place. It has also been criticised for failure, as judged by population health statistics. It is pointed out, e.g. that improved living conditions rather than medical treatment have played the major role in the enormous decline in the death rate from infectious diseases over the past 150 years; although latterly vaccines have made, and continue to make, a massive contribution. It is true that the biggest changes in some important areas of health result from social and economic development rather than from the application of technical medicine; that 'prevention is better than cure' is a familiar saying because it is true.

But people still frequently fall sick and will continue to do so, although the pattern of disease in the community changes, infectious disease in the young giving place to degenerative disease in the old. We must look at population statistics; but we must also, in a humane society, look to the individual sufferers and to their quality of life.

It is good to prevent tuberculosis; but those who are unfortunate enough to contract the disease will be grateful for drugs.

It is good to prevent cancer, and ways of doing so for some cancers, e.g. stopping smoking, are known, though too seldom adopted; but those who fall sick will be grateful for drugs, surgery and radiation, whether these cure or whether they only ease the passage through the last phase of life.

It is better to prevent some heart disease, by moderate and sensible living, including moderation in eating, though such measures are all too little adopted; but those who fall sick will be grateful for drugs.

It would be better, if we only knew how, to prevent rheumatoid arthritis, epilepsy, pernicious anaemia, many cancers and diabetes, but we do not know how and sufferers are grateful for drugs. In any case we all have eventually to die of something, and the likelihood that the mode of death for most of us, even after practising all the excesses of advice on how to live a healthy life, will be free from pain, anxiety, cough, diarrhoea, paralysis (the list is endless) seems so small that it can be disregarded. Drugs already provide immeasurable solace in these situations, but better drugs are needed and their development should be encouraged.

Doctors know the sick are thankful for drugs just as a dedicated pedestrian struck down by a passing car is thankful for a motor ambulance to take him to hospital.

Benefits of drugs in individual diseases are discussed throughout this book and will not be further expanded here. But a general discussion of risk is appropriate.

The two dimensions of risk

1. the likelihood or probability of an adverse event
2. its severity

Whenever a drug is given a risk is taken

The risk is made up of the properties of the drug, of the prescriber, of the patient and of the environment; it is often so small that second thoughts are hardly necessary, but sometimes it is substantial. The doctor must weigh the likelihood of gain for the patient against the likelihood of loss. There are often insufficient data for a rational decision to be reached, but a decision must yet be made and this is one of the greatest difficulties of clinical practice. Its effect on the attitudes of doctors is often not appreciated by those who have never been in this situation. The patients' protection lies in the doctors' knowledge of the drug and of the disease, and experience of both, together with knowledge of the patient. For instance, in typhoid fever the risk of aplastic anaemia due to the chloramphenicol used to treat it is far less than the risk of the patient dying from untreated disease. In less dangerous infections the decision is less easy.

In some diseases in which drugs will ultimately be needed they may not benefit the patient in the early stages. For example, victims of early parkinsonism or hypertension may be but little inconvenienced by the disease, and the premature use of drugs, whilst reducing parkinsonian symptoms and blood pressure, can exact such a price in side-effects (including fatigue, which may be unrecognised as a side-effect and which is common with β-adrenoceptor blockers) that patients prefer the untreated state; what patients will tolerate depends on their personality, their attitude to disease, their occupation, mode of life and relationship with their doctor.

Physician-induced (iatrogenic) disease

The most shameful act in therapeutics, apart from killing the patient, is to injure a patient who is but little disabled or who is suffering from a self-limiting disorder. Such iatrogenic disease,[3] induced by misguided treatment, is far from rare.

Doctors who are temperamentally extremist will do less harm by therapeutic nihilism than by optimistically overwhelming patients with well-intentioned polypharmacy. The latter course is the easier to follow because it gives more immediate satisfaction to the patients (though this is changing), to their families and indeed to the doctors themselves. All are able to feel cosily that it is clear that the doctors are doing all they can, which is liable to mean a great deal more than is wise. Habitual prescribing in response to any complaint from a patient, and in particular habitual polypharmacy, is sure to blur the process

of rational thought that should precede the use of any drug, and both doctors and patients will be the worse for this.

If in doubt whether or not to give a drug to a person who will soon get better without it, don't.

In 1917, Sollmann felt able to write

Pharmacology comprises some broad conceptions and generalisations, and some detailed conclusions, of such great and practical importance that every student and practitioner should be absolutely familiar with them. It comprises also a large mass of minute details, which would constitute too great a tax on human memory, but which cannot safely be neglected.[4,5]

If the last sentence was true when it was written, it is much more true now. The selection of useful drugs from the multitude, not only offered to, but thrust upon the doctor by skilful and sometimes misleading advertising, is a matter of great importance. The doctor's aim must be not merely to give the patient what will do good, but to give *only* what will do good, or at least more good than harm.

The three major grades of risk: unacceptable, acceptable and negligible

In the presence of serious disease and with sufficient information on both the disease and the drug, then decisions in the first two categories, though they may be painful, present relatively obvious problems. But where the disease risk is remote, e.g. mild hypertension, or where drugs are to be used to increase comfort or to suppress symptoms that are, in fact, bearable, or for con-

---

[3] *Iatrogenic* means 'physician-caused', i.e. disease consequent on following medical advice or intervention.

[4] Sollman T A. Manual of pharmacology. Philadelphia: Saunders, 1917.
[5] The *information explosion* of recent decades will one day be brought under control when prescribers can, from their desktop computer terminals, enter the facts about their patient, e.g. age, sex, weight, principal and secondary diagnoses, and receive suggestions for which drugs should be considered with proposed doses and precautions. The limitations on such a service are financial and logistic; the technology exists now. In the meantime, prescribers *must* ensure that they are aware of the basic information contained in manufacturers' data sheets and standard Formularies.

venience rather than need, then the issues of risk acceptance are less obvious.

Risks should not be considered without reference to benefits any more than benefits should be considered without reference to risks.

Risks are among the facts of life. In whatever we do and in whatever we refrain from doing, we are accepting risk. Some risks are obvious, some are unsuspected and some we conceal from ourselves. But risks are universally accepted, whether willingly or unwillingly, whether consciously or not.[6]

The two broad categories of risk

First are those that we accept by deliberate, choice, even if we do not exactly know their magnitude, or we know but wish they were smaller, or, especially where the likelihood of harm is remote though the consequences may be grave, we do not even think about the matter. Such risks include transport and sports, both of which are inescapably subject to potent physical laws such as gravity and momentum, and surgery to rectify disorders that could either be tolerated or treated in other ways, e.g. hernia, much cosmetic surgery.

Second are those risks that are imposed on us in the sense that they cannot be significantly altered by individual action. Risks such as those of food additives, e.g. preservatives, colouring, air pollution and some environmental radioactivity are imposed by man. But there are also risks, imposed by nature such as skin cancer due to excess ultraviolet radiation in sunny climes, as well as some radioactivity.

The motives for accepting risk are various and numerous and include the general attitudes of individuals to life, to work and to pleasure.

It seems an obvious truth that unnecessary risks should be avoided, but there is disagreement on what risks are truly unnecessary and, on looking closely at the matter, it is plain that many people habitually take risks in their daily life that it would be a misuse of words to describe as necessary.

It is also the case that some risks, though known to exist, are, in practice, ignored other than by conforming to ordinary prudent conduct, e.g. the employment of competent electricians and gas fitters in the home, looking before crossing the road, not accepting a lift in a friend's car if he is drunk. There can be few passengers who seek out the figures for individual airlines and take them into account before making a booking. The reason for this is that the risks of flying by any reasonably reputable airline are so small as to be ignored by ordinary people, i.e. *the risks are negligible in the sense that they do not influence behaviour.*

In general it has been suggested that, in medical cases, concern ceases when risks fall below about 1 in 100 000 so that then the procedure becomes regarded as 'safe'. In such cases, when disaster occurs, it can be difficult indeed for individuals to accept that they 'deliberately' took a risk; they feel 'it should not have happened to me' and in their distress they may seek to lay blame on others where there is no fault or negligence, only misfortune.

The benefits of chemicals used to colour food verge on or even attain negligibility, and some are known to cause allergy in man. Yet our society permits their use.

The benefits of oral contraceptives and of penicillin are undoubted and the risks are equally undoubted and have been measured, and their use continues and expands because the perceived benefits outweigh the risks.

In no countries are the risks of heroin dependence acceptable, but in all countries the risks of tobacco are acceptable or, at least, accepted. Deaths from tobacco and alcohol use far exceed those of therapeutic agents and road transport.

The risks of drugs have become a major topic of public and medical concern over the last 20 years, and this concern, often amounting to alarm, has accelerated since the thalidomide disaster of 1960–61 (p. 65), which provided an exceptionally dramatic demonstration of the worst that drugs can do.

There is general agreement that drugs prescribed for disease are themselves the cause of a significant amount of disease (adverse reactions), of death, of permanent disability, of recoverable illness and of minor inconvenience.

---

[6] Pochin E E. Br Med Bull 1975; 31: 184.

THE PUBLIC VIEW OF DRUGS AND PRESCRIBERS

Until recently, when discussing drugs used in medicine it was not generally thought necessary to take serious account of the public view, and indeed the public view was one of innocent acceptance; it did not significantly affect the practice of doctors and their relations with patients. But this has changed; increasingly doctors are criticised not only by individual patients, but by associations of patients formed for that purpose, amongst others; the mass media have found that drugs provide an unfailing topic for sensational entertainment, and that drugs and doctors separately and together provide the media people with occasions when 'It becomes more than a moral duty to speak one's mind. It becomes a pleasure.'[7]

Doctors can no longer behave as though all their prescribing decisions are a matter for themselves alone, with little or no involvement of the patient. Hence the following discussion.

The current public view of modern medicines, ably fuelled by the mass media, is a compound of vague expectation of 'miracle' cures with outrage when anything goes wrong. Successes soon become a routine taken for granted without thankfulness; failures, the drug accidents, are remembered and resented perpetually. But this state of affairs is a manifestation of normal human nature, and doctors who rail against it are wasting their time. The public is fickle, demanding, prone to make snap judgements and to righteous indignation. It is quite unrealistic to expect the public to have balanced, well-thought-out views on any complex topic: there are far too many of these anyway. It is also unreasonable to expect the public to trust the medical profession to the extent of leaving to it all drug matters. Just as 'War is much too serious a thing to be left to the military',[8] so drugs are much too serious a thing to be left to the medical profession and to the pharmaceutical industry.

It has long been a source of wonder to doctors that a public, if the mass media are to be believed, that seems to fear and hate drugs, actually consists of individuals who when met in the clinic seem to have an insatiable appetite for drugs; 'Surely there is something you can give me, doctor?'

It is endlessly reiterated that the public does not understand that virtually all drug use carries risk and that it cannot be otherwise. If the public does not understand this, it is not for want of telling. But such apparently invincible ignorance, if it exists, must have a deeper cause than mere deafness. When a drug is suspected of causing harm, then any good it may have done is discounted in the public mind by rage against doctors, drug developers, regulatory authorities, and indeed rage against technology and science itself.

The reasons for this are many and complex.

Industrially developed societies have been encouraged to believe that technology based on science would solve most, if not all their problems, including the problems of attaining happiness. Expectations have been raised and now, at the end of the 20th century with the manifest achievement of technology all around us, the naive belief that happiness can be a part of the technological package is increasingly seen to be false.

The public, fickle as always, turns on science and technology in disappointed resentment. The oft-repeated public warnings of the medical profession that drugs unavoidably carry risks despite skilful development and use are treated as though they have never been. A drug accident occurs and scapegoats[9] must be found whether or not someone is at fault.

The public wants benefits without risks and without having to alter its unhealthy ways of living; a deeply irrational position. But it is easy to understand that a person who has taken into his body a chemical with intent to relieve suffering, whether or not it is self-induced, or to prevent

---

[7] O Wilde (1854–1900). The importance of being Earnest: Act II.
[8] Attributed both to C-M de Talleyrand (1754–1838) and to Georges Clemenceau (1841–1929), French statesmen.

---

[9] An animal symbolically laden with human sins by humans and, by extension, a person blamed for what should fall on others.

disease, can feel a profound resentment when harm follows. Patients do not understand what has happened, all they know is that a doctor has prescribed a product of a profitable multinational industry; all they did was to swallow it and now they are injured. They are not interested in being told that they voluntarily took a risk, even in the event that this was explained and that they truly understood it; and they are not interested in being told that the doctor took a risk on their behalf, for it is the patient and not the doctor who is hurt. They are also not interested in being told (should this happen to be the case) that as no one is at fault they must regard their misfortune as an accident and simply accept it. If it is added that the injury is a likely consequence of the patients' own genetic make-up, then insult is added to the injury. Whether or not this attitude is reasonable is irrelevant; that is how people feel, and they will not easily change.

Patients are increasingly aware that there is justified criticism of the standards of medical prescribing, indeed doctors are in the forefront of this; as well as justified criticism of promotional practices of the profitably rich, aggressive, international pharmaceutical industry.

The present situation, a mix of resentment, mistrust and misunderstanding, must at least not be allowed to get worse. There are obvious areas where some remedial action is possible.

- Improvement of **prescribing** by doctors, including better communication with patients, i.e. doctors must learn to feel that introduction of foreign chemicals into their patients' bodies is a serious matter, which the vast majority do not feel at present.
- Introduction of no-fault **compensation** schemes for serious drug injury (some countries already have these; see p. 13).
- Free public discussion of the issues between the medical profession, industrial drug developers, politicians and other 'opinion-formers' in society, and patients (the public). Doctors should not hesitate to take part in such exchanges if they have any talent for exposition and can remain calm (this is essential) under provocation.
- **Restraint** in promotion by the pharmaceu-

tical industry including self-control by both industry and doctors in their necessarily close relationship. The medical and scientific departments of pharmaceutical companies generally do not have control over the marketing department and over advertising; they should.

If restraint is not forthcoming then both doctor and industry can expect more control to be exercised over them by politicians responding to public demand. If doctors do not want their prescribing to be restricted, they should prescribe better.

CRITICISMS OF MODERN DRUGS

Some critics have attracted public attention for their view that modern drug therapy, indeed modern medicine in general, does more harm than good; others, whilst admitting some benefits from drugs, insist that this is medically marginal. These opinions rest on the undisputed fact that favourable trends in many diseases preceded the introduction of modern drugs and were due to economic and environmental changes, sanitation, nutrition, housing. They also rest on the claim that drugs have not changed expectation of life or mortality (as measured by national mortality statistics) and that drugs can cause illness (adverse reactions).

If something is to be measured then the correct standards must be chosen. Overall mortality figures are an extremely crude and often an irrelevant measure of the effects of drugs whose major benefits are so often on *quality* of life rather than on its *quantity*.

Two examples of inappropriate measurements will suffice:

1. In the case of infections it is not disputed that environmental changes have had a greater beneficial effect on health than the subsequently introduced antimicrobials. But this does not mean that environmental improvements alone are sufficient in the fight against infections. When comparisons of illnesses in the pre- and post-antibiotic eras are made, like is not compared with like. Environmental changes achieved their results when mortality from infections was high and

antimicrobials were not available; antimicrobials were introduced later against a background of low mortality as well as of environmental change; decades separate the two parts of the comparison, and observers, diagnostic criteria and data recording changed during this long period.[10] It is evident that determining the value of antimicrobials is not simply a matter of looking at mortality rates.

2. About 1% of the UK population has *diabetes mellitus* and about 1% of death certificates mention diabetes. This is no surprise because all must die and insulin is no cure[11] for this lifelong disease. A standard medical textbook of 1907 stated that juvenile-onset 'diabetes is in all cases a grave disease, and the subjects are regarded by all assurance companies as uninsurable lives: life seems to hang by a thread, a thread often cut by a very trifling accident.' The modern young diabetic is accepted by most, if not all, life insurance companies with no or only modest financial penalty, the premium of a person 5–10 years older. Before insulin replacement therapy was available few survived beyond 3 years[12] after diagnosis; they died for lack of insulin. It is unjustified to assert that a treatment is worthless just because its mention on death certificates (whether as a prime or as a contributory cause) has not changed. The relevant criteria for juvenile-onset diabetes are *change in the age* at which the subjects die and the *quality of life* between diagnosis and death, and both of these have changed enormously.

Critics naturally also point to the areas where drug benefits are controversial or absent, and there are plenty of these; but they simply tell us that medical and biological sciences, like all sciences, have a lot of unsolved problems before them. They tell nothing about what can be achieved with the tools we now have. Similarly, inappropriate medical use of drugs and their social abuse are regrettable and tell us of human inadequacies, but do not diminish the successes of scientific medicine.

The critics assert that modern drugs are a failure, that therapeutic claims are false, and that adverse effects are too frequent (indeed they are), and are commonly concealed or ignored. They also assert that there is a 'conspiracy' between the medical profession and the pharmaceutical industry to exploit the community for mutual benefit. Both industry and profession would be well advised to review their close association with a more critical eye than heretofore, and doctors should think less of their bellies ('there is no such thing as a free lunch') and their pockets and more of the fact that their first duty lies, and must be seen to lie, with their *patients.*

Finally, critics attack the low standards of prescribing and a prime objective of this book is to enable doctors to prescribe better. But no book can inculcate the *sense of responsibility* that all prescribers should have as with their pens they flood their patients' bodies with foreign chemicals.

It is heartening, however, to know that there is not a polarisation of views, with assailants of drugs all outside the medical profession and champions solely within. Awareness and criticism of shortcomings of drugs and drug use is a day-to-day constituent of medical literature and meetings and there are innumerable patients with serious disease, e.g. epilepsy, glaucoma and those who have benefited from surgical anaesthesia, who know their lives and happiness are or have been transformed by drugs and who are fittingly thankful.

Doubtless doctors are as liable to be arrogant, complacent and ignorant as are all human beings, including their critics, but heat without light is generated by the angry recrimination about drugs that is so customary today.

COMPLEMENTARY AND TRADITIONAL MEDICINE

Because practitioners of complementary[13] and traditional medicine are severely critical of mod-

---

[10] Lever A F. Lancet 1977; 1: 352.

[11] A *cure eliminates* a disease and may be withdrawn when this is achieved.

[12] Even if given the best treatment. 'Opium alone stands the test of experience as a remedy capable of limiting the progress of the disease', wrote the great Sir William Osler, successively Professor of Medicine in Pennsylvania, McGill, Johns Hopkins and Oxford University, in 1918, only three years before the discovery of insulin.

ern drugs, because they use drugs according to their own special beliefs, and because they are currently attracting more attention than previously (in so-called developed societies), it is appropriate to discuss drug use in complementary or alternative medical systems here.

Public disappointment that scientific medicine can neither guarantee happiness nor wholly eliminate the disabilities of degenerative diseases in long-lived populations, as well as the fact that drugs used in modern medicine can cause serious harm, naturally leads to a revival of interest in alternatives that promise efficacy with safety. These range from revival of traditional medicine to adoption of the more modern cults,[14] e.g.

homoeopathy, which are described as *complementary*, *alternative* or *fringe* medicine.

These terms are apt because when any practice, whatever its source, is shown to be effective by testing according to rational (scientific) criteria it will become accepted by conventional medicine and so cease to be an alternative, fringe or complementary practice. Willingness to follow where the evidence leads is a distinctive feature of conventional scientific medicine.

Note. A scientific approach does not mean a patient must be treated as a mere biochemical machine. It does not mean the exclusion of spiritual, psychological and social dimensions of human beings. But it does mean treating these in a rational manner.

Traditional or indigenous medicinal therapeutics has developed since before history in all societies. It comprises a mass of practices varying from the worthless to highly effective remedies, e.g. digitalis (England), quinine (South America), reserpine (India), atropine (various countries). It is the task of science to find the gems and to discard the dross,[15] and at the same time to leave intact socially valuable supportive aspects of traditional medicine.

Complementary medicine caters, in general, for people whom scientific medicine cannot or does not help: it does not compete with the successful mainstream of scientific medicine, but offers comfort especially to two classes of patient, (a) those with a bad prognosis or severe organic functional disability, and (b) those whose disorder has a major psychological component.

Features common to complementary medicine cults are absence of scientific thinking, naive acceptance of hypotheses, uncritical

---

[13] The term *complementary* seems to make a less ambitious claim than *alternative* medicine, and is preferred.

[14] A *cult* is a practice that follows a dogma, tenet or principle based on theories or beliefs of its promulgator to the exclusion of demonstrable scientific experience (definition of the American Medical Association).

The profusion of medical cults tells its own story. Scientific medicine changes in accord with evidence obtained by scientific enquiry applied with such intellectual rigour as is humanly possible. But this is not the case with cults, the claims for which are characterised by absence of rigorous intellectual evaluation. Medical cults and practices listed in a publication of the World Health Organization (Bannerman R H et al, eds. Traditional medicine and health care coverage. Geneva, 1983) include: homoeopathy, anthroposophical medicine, applied kinesiology, kirlian photography, reflexology, osteopathy, chiropractic, rolfing, breathing, radiesthesia, radionics, orgone therapy, pyramid therapy, naturopathy, dianetics, interferential therapy, aromatherapy, biochemics, orthomolecular medicine, bioenergetics, enlightenment intensive. The list speaks for itself, and leaves the question why, if each cult has the efficacy claimed by its exponents, orthodox medicine and indeed the other cults are not swept away. Some practitioners use orthodox medicine and, where it fails, turn to cult practices. Where such complementary practices give comfort they are not to be despised, but their role and validity should be clearly defined. No community can afford to take these cults at their own valuation; they must be tested, and tested with at least the rigour required to justify a therapeutic claim for a new drug. It is sometimes urged in extenuation that traditional and cult practices do no harm to patients, unlike synthetic drugs. But even if that were true (which it is not), investment of scarce resources in delivering what may be ineffective, though sometimes pleasing, experiences, e.g. dance therapy, exaltation of flowers, and the admittedly inexpensive urine therapy, means that these resources are not available for other desirable social objectives, e.g. housing, art subsidies, medicine. We do not apologise for this diversion to consider medical cults and practices, for the world cannot afford unreason, and the antidote to unreason is reason and the rigorous pursuit of knowledge.

[15] Traditional medicine is being fostered particularly in countries where scientific medicine is not accessible to large populations for economic reasons, and destruction of traditional medicine would leave unhappy and sick people with nothing. For this reason governments are supporting traditional medicine and at the same time initiating scientific clinical evaluations of the numerous plants and other items employed, many of which contain biologically active substances. The World Health Organization encourages these programmes.

acceptance of causation, e.g. reliance on anecdote, and assumption that if recovery follows treatment it is due to the treatment (the *post hoc ergo propter hoc*[16] fallacy), and close attention to the patient's personal feelings. Lack of understanding of how therapeutic effects may be measured is also a prominent feature. Exponents often state that comparative controlled trials of their medicines versus orthodox medicines are impracticable because the more rigid double-blind randomised controlled designs are inappropriate and in particular do not allow for the individual approach characteristic of complementary medicine. But modern therapeutic trial designs can cope with this. A few, generally unsatisfactory, trials comparing homoeopathic with orthodox medicines have been done (some with an outcome favourable to homoeopathy), but a lot more study is needed if either advocates or critics are to change their attitudes.

One difficulty of doing definitive trials (which are tedious and expensive) is that so weak is the evidence for the medical cults, with regard to both empirical evidence of efficacy and theoretical basis, that those competent to do valid studies, and having a duty to use resources wisely, are liable to put the scientific evaluation of complementary medicine low on their list of priorities, at least until the complementary practitioners understand the scientific approach and are willing to accept its application. But there remain extremists who contend that they understand scientific method, and reject it as invalid for what they do and believe, i.e. their beliefs are not, in principle, refutable. This is the position taken up by magic and religion where subordination of reason to faith is a virtue.

This book is not an appropriate place to attempt a broad discussion of complementary medicine. But it is useful to list some common beliefs of its practitioners and then to consider homoeopathy, a cult that particularly relies on drugs used in an unconventional or unscientific way.

Beliefs commonly met, which seem to be characteristic of complementary medicine

- *That synthetic modern drugs are toxic, but products obtained in nature are not*; the former statement is true, but the latter is false; there is a profusion of toxic substances in nature — animal, vegetable and mineral — e.g. venoms, toxins, digitalis, laetrile, arsenic.[17]
- *That traditional (pre-scientific) medicines have special virtue*; this belief seems to be based on a vague nostalgia for a past 'golden age' which never existed and on the grounds that natural products are used.
- *That scientific medicine will only accept evidence that remedies are effective where the mechanism is also understood.* This is so plainly untrue that it is difficult to understand how the belief has gained currency; empirical evidence ('suck it and see') of efficacy has always been sufficient to justify use, e.g. penicillin, morphine, which were in use long before their mechanisms of action were understood. But knowledge of mechanisms is plainly desirable because it contributes to safer and more effective use and also allows the prospect of deliberate development of improvements.
- Linked to the above is the false belief *that scientific medicine recognises no form of evaluation other than the strict randomised controlled trial* of single medicines, and that complementary medicine cannot be scientifically evaluated because

---

[16] Latin: after this, therefore on account of this.

[17] Herbal teas containing pyrrolidizine alkaloids (*Senecio, Crotalaria, Heliotropium*) cause serious hepatic veno-occlusive disease. *Comfrey* (*Symphitum*) is similar but also causes hepatocellular tumours and haemangiomas. *Sassafras* (carminative, antirheumatic) is hepatotoxic. *Mistletoe* (*Viscum*) contains cytotoxic alkaloids. *Ginseng* contains oestrogenic substances which have caused gynaecomastia: long-term users may show 'ginseng abuse syndrome' comprising CNS excitation: arterial hypotension can occur. *Liquorice* (*Glycyrrhiza*) has mineralcorticoid action: see carbenoxolone. An amateur 'health food enthusiast' made himself a tea from 'an unfamiliar (to him) plant' in his garden: unfortunately this was the familiar foxglove (*Digitalis purpurea*): happily he recovered. Other toxic natural remedies include lily of the valley (*Convallaria*) and horse chestnut (*Aesculus*). 'The medical herbalist is at fault for clinging to outworn historical authority and for not assessing his drugs in terms of today's knowledge, and the orthodox physician is at fault for a cynical scepticism with regard to any healing discipline other than his own.' (Penn R G. 1983. Adv Dr React Bull; no. 102).

patients receive different treatment according to their individuality.[18]

- *That scientific medicine rests on acceptance of rigid and unalterable dogmas*; it is plainly hard for practitioners of complementary medicine to understand that in scientific medicine any belief can be and is modified or abandoned when evidence is produced that justifies this; science-based medicine is flexible (though some of the practitioners may not be) and that is the reason for its successes, which are generally not denied by practitioners of complementary medicine; scientific medicine follows, sometimes stumbling, where the evidence leads. Thus, when the claims of alternative cults have been subject to tests as intellectually rigorous as those nowadays required to justify therapeutic claims, any practice that passes will become generally accepted regardless of its source.

- *That if a patient gets better when treated in accordance with certain beliefs, this provides evidence for the truth of these beliefs.*

- *That because conventional medicine and particularly the drugs it uses can cause substantial harm (iatrogenic disease) this is evidence for the therapeutic validity of alternative approaches*, and for the (unwarranted) assumption that complementary medicine is not also a source of iatrogenic disease.

- *Complementary medicine charges that orthodox medicine seriously neglects the patient as a whole integrated human being* (body, mind, spirit) and treats him too much as a machine. Orthodox practitioners may well feel uneasily that there has been and still is truth in this, that some doctors have been seduced by the enormous successes of medical science and technology and have become liable to look too narrowly at their patients and too easily to rely on a prescription where a much broader response is required.

The management of the patient as a whole being (holistic medicine) should be the hall-mark of good medicine, however and whenever practised; but the humane application of technology does present enormous challenges, e.g. intensive therapy units, radiotherapy, cancer chemotherapy. The management of the patient as a whole being of body, mind and spirit is a strong point of complementary medicine. Homoeopathic management, for example, involves 'what might be called a short psychoanalysis, using relatively stereotyped questions',[19] it attaches importance to patients' cravings and interests, their responses to hot and cold, motion, rest, moistness, dryness; 'for it is only when hidden feelings and fears are brought to the surface that the homoeopath can select a remedy that will stimulate the defence mechanism and bring about a cure'.[20] It is evident that such an approach is likely to give particular satisfaction in psychological and psychosomatic conditions for which orthodox doctors in a hurry have been all too ready to think that a prescription meets all the patients' needs.[21] Much of the recent increased interest in complementary medicine stems from the inadequacies of overbusy and, let us admit it, sometimes bored conventional doctors compared with the attentiveness of practitioners of complementary medicine, as well as from the disappointment caused by inevitable failure to meet patients' over-optimistic expectations.

Homoeopathy

The following will suffice to give the flavour of one complementary medicine cult and the kind of criticism that it has to contend with.

Homoeopathy[22] is a system of medicine founded by Samuel Hahnemann (German physician: 1755–1843) and expounded by him in the *Organon of the rational art of healing*.[23]

---

[18] This view seems to assert that benefit, e.g. in arthritis, is measurable or not measurable according to the system of medical practice that has delivered it. There is neither intellectual nor factual basis for such belief.

[19] Hickman A D. Br Med J 1963; 1: 523.
[20] Vithoulkas G. World Health Forum (WHO Geneva) 1983; 4: 99. But yet homoeopathic medicines are sold directly to the public from self-selection stands, i.e. in circumstances where such exploration and counselling cannot be provided.
[21] A randomised controlled trial in irritable bowel syndrome of routine medical treatment versus the same management plus individual psychotherapy has shown that the psychotherapy was beneficial in both short- and long-term progress. Svendlund J et al. Lancet 1983; 2: 589.
[22] Greek: *homos*: same; *patheia*: suffering.
[23] 1810: trans. Wheeler C E. London: Dent, 1913.

Hahnemann described his position:

After I had discovered the weakness and errors of my teachers and books I sank into a state of sorrowful indignation, which had nearly disgusted me with the study of medicine. I was on the point of concluding that the whole art was vain and incapable of improvement. I gave myself up to solitary reflection, and resolved not to terminate my train of thought until I had arrived at a definite conclusion on the subject.[24]

By understandable revulsion at the medicine of his time, by experimentation on himself (a large dose of quinine made him feel as though he had a malarial attack) and by search of records he 'discovered' a 'law' that is central to homoeopathy (and from which the name is derived):[25]

Similar symptoms in the remedy remove similar symptoms in the disease. The eternal, universal law of Nature, that every disease is destroyed and cured through the similar artificial disease which the appropriate remedy has the tendency to excite, rests on the following proposition: that *only one disease can exist in the body at any one time.*

In addition to the above, he 'discovered' that *the effect of drugs is potentiated by dilution (provided the dilution is shaken correctly)* even to the extent that an effective dose may not contain a single molecule of the drug. It has been pointed out[25] that the 'thirtieth potency' (1 in 10^{60}), recommended by Hahnemann, provided a solution in which there would be one molecule of drug in a volume of a sphere of literally astronomical circumference. That a dose in which no drug is present (including such preparations of sodium chloride) can be therapeutically effective is explained by the belief that there is a spiritual energy diffused throughout the medicine by the particular way in which the dilutions are shaken (succussion) during preparation or that the active molecules leave behind some sort of 'imprint' on solvent or excipient.[26]

Thus, writes a critic 'We are asked to put aside the whole edifice of evidence concerning the physical nature of materials and the normal concentration-response relationships of biologically active substances in order to accommodate homoeopathic potency.'[27] But no hard evidence that tests the hypothesis is supplied to justify this, and we are invited, for instance, to accept that sodium chloride merely diluted is no remedy, but that 'it raises itself to the most wonderful power through a well-prepared dynamisation process' and stimulates the defensive powers of the body against the disease.

The dogmas of homoeopathy have incurred ridicule, which is resented by its practitioners who insist that they are misunderstood and who tartly observe that critics have generally not made a serious study of homoeopathy, and that patients treated according to homoeopathic principles commonly recover, which is certainly true, but true of all forms of medicine including other cults. Pharmacologists generally feel that in the absence of conclusive evidence from empirical therapeutic trials conducted according to modern standards, there is no point in discussing the hypotheses of homoeopathy. But it is always necessary to bear in mind that useful discoveries may be made in pursuing unsubstantiated hypotheses, and empirical studies can be made without accepting any particular theory.

Conclusion regarding complementary medicine

There is a single fundamental issue between conventional scientific medicine and traditional and complementary medicine (though it is often obscured by detailed debates on individual practices); the issue is, *what constitutes acceptable evidence,* i.e. the nature, quality, and interpretation of evidence, that can justify general adoption of modes of treatment and acceptance of hypotheses.

[24] Hahnemann S. Aesculapius in the balance. Leipsic: 1805.
[25] Clark A J. General pharmacology, Heffter's Handbuch, Berlin: Springer. 1937.
[26] Homoeopathic practitioners repeatedly express their irritation that critics give so much attention to dilution. They should not be surprised considering the enormous implications of their claim.

[27] Cuthbert A W. Pharmaceut J; 15 May 1982: 547.

RESPONSIBILITY FOR DRUG-CAUSED INJURY

This topic raises important issues affecting medical practice and development of needed new drugs, as well as of law and of social justice.

Negligence and liability

All civilised legal systems provide for compensation to be paid to a person injured as a result of using a product that is defective due to negligence (failure to exercise reasonable care).[28] But there is a growing opinion that special compensation for personal injury, beyond what any available social security system provides, should be automatic and not dependent on fault and proof of fault of the producer, i.e. there should be 'liability irrespective of fault', 'no-fault liability' or 'strict liability'.[29] After all, victims need assistance (compensation) regardless of the cause of injury and whether or not the producer, and, in the case of drugs, the prescriber, deserves punishment.

Many countries are now revising their laws on liability for personal injury due to manufactured products, and are legislating Consumer Protection Acts (Statutes) which include medicines, for 'drugs represent the class of product in respect of which there has been the greatest pressure for surer compensation in cases of injury'.[30]

Issues that are central to the debate include:

● *Capacity to cause harm* is inherent in drugs[31] in a way that sets them apart from other manufactured products; harm often occurs in the absence of fault.

● *Safety*, i.e. the degree of safety that a person is entitled to expect, and adverse effects that should be accepted without complaint, must often be a matter of opinion, and will vary with the disease being treated.

● *Causation*, i.e. proof that the drug in fact caused the injury, is often impossible, particularly where it increases the incidence of a disease that occurs naturally.

● *Contributory negligence*. Should compensation be reduced in smokers and drinkers where there is evidence that these pleasure-drugs increase liability to adverse reactions to therapeutic drugs?

● *The concept of defect*,[31] i.e. whether the drug or the prescriber or indeed the patient can be said to be 'defective' so as to attract liability, is a highly complex matter and indeed is a curious concept as applied to medicine.

● *A solution* to the problem of injury caused by medicines. Despite all the above there is a class of drug injury that can be identified as particularly disturbing to the public mind, its sense of justice, and as being deserving of compassion. This is the *rare serious injury* that is totally disproportionate to the significance normally attached to the treatment, and that was not taken into account (because it was so rare) when deciding to use the drug, so that it was treated as a negligible risk, e.g. fatal blood dyscrasia from indomethacin used for dysmenorrhoea (a licensed indication) in a woman with three dependent children. But in advocating this we must remember to spare a thought for the family of a similar person who has died of similar natural disease and who are not offered any special compensation.

Nowhere has a scheme that meets all the major difficulties yet been implemented. This is not because there has been too little thought, it is because the subject is so difficult.

---

[28] A plaintiff seeking to obtain compensation from a defendant (via the law of negligence) must prove three things: 1, that the defendant owed a duty of care to the plaintiff; 2, that the defendant failed to exercise reasonable care; and 3, that the plaintiff has suffered actual injury as a result.

[29] The following distinction is made in some discussions of product liability:
1. *strict* liability: compensation is provided by the producer/manufacturer.
2. *no fault* liability or scheme: compensation is provided by a central fund.

[30] Royal Commission on Civil Liability and Compensation for Personal Injury. 1978. London: HMSO. Cmnd. 7054. Although the Commission considered compensation for death and personal injury suffered by any person through manufacture, supply or use of products, i.e. all goods whether natural or manufactured, and included drugs and even human blood and organs, it made no mention of tobacco and alcohol.

[31] This discussion is about drugs that have been properly manufactured and meet proper standards, e.g. of purity, stability, as laid down by regulatory bodies or pharmacopoeias. A *manufacturing defect* would be dealt with in a way no different from manufacturing errors in other products.

An outline for a workable scheme

- *New unlicensed drugs undergoing early trial in small numbers of subjects* (healthy or patient volunteers): the producer should be strictly liable for all adverse effects.
- *New unlicensed drugs undergoing extensive trials* in patients who may reasonably expect benefit: the producer should be strictly liable for any serious effect.
- *New drugs after licensing by an official regulatory body*: liability for serious injury should now be shared with the community, which is expecting to benefit from new drugs.
- *Standard drugs in day-to-day therapeutics*:
  1. there should be a *no-fault scheme*, operated by or with the assent of government, that has authority, through tribunals, *quickly* to decide cases and to make awards. This body would have authority to reimburse itself from others — manufacturer, supplier, prescriber — wherever that was appropriate. An award must not have to wait on the determination of prolonged, vexatious and expensive court proceedings.
  2. *Patients would be compensated* where:
     a. causation is proved on 'balance of probability'[32]
     b. the injury was serious
     c. the event was rare and remote and not reasonably taken into account in making the decision to treat.

CHRONIC PHARMACOLOGY: the consequences of prolonged administration of drugs and their withdrawal

The proportion of the population taking drugs continuously for large portions of their lives increases as tolerable suppressive and prophylactic remedies for chronic or recurrent conditions are developed, e.g. for arterial hypertension, diabetes, mental diseases, epilepsies, gout, collagen diseases, thrombosis, allergies and various infections. In some cases the treatment introduces significant hazard into patients' lives and the cure can be worse than the disease if it is not skilfully managed. In general the dangers of a

drug are not markedly increased if therapy lasts years rather than months; exceptions include renal damage due to analgesic mixtures, and carcinogenicity.

Chronic drug use interferes with self-regulating systems

When self-regulating physiological systems, (generally controlled by negative feedback systems, e.g. endocrine, cardiovascular) are subject to interference, their control mechanisms respond to minimise the effects of the interference and to restore the previous steady state or rhythm: this is *homeostasis*. The previous state may be a normal function, e.g. ovulation (a rare example of a positive feedback mechanism), or an abnormal function, e.g. high blood pressure. If the body successfully restores the previous steady state or rhythm then the subject has become *tolerant* to the drug, i.e. a higher dose is needed to produce the desired previous effect.

In the case of hormonal contraceptives, persistence of effect on ovulation occurs and is desired, but persistence of other effects, e.g. on blood coagulation and metabolism, is not desired.

In the case of arterial hypertension, tolerance to a single drug commonly occurs, e.g. reduction of peripheral resistance by a vasodilator is compensated by an increase in blood volume that restores the blood pressure; this is why a diuretic is commonly used together with a vasodilator in therapy.

Feedback systems. The endocrine system serves fluctuating body needs. Glands are therefore capable of either increasing or decreasing their output by means of negative (usually) feedback systems. An administered hormone or hormone analogue activates the receptors of the feedback system so that high doses cause suppression of natural production of the hormone. On withdrawal of the administered hormone the control mechanism takes time, months in the case of the hypothalamus/pituitary/adrenal cortex, to recover completely, and sudden withdrawal of administered corticosteroid can result in an acute deficiency state that may be life-endangering.

Regulation of receptors. The number (den-

---

[32] This is the criterion for civil law, rather than 'beyond reasonable doubt', which is the criterion of criminal law.

sity) of receptors on cells (for hormones, autacoids and drugs), the number occupied (affinity), and the fit of the molecule (sensitivity) can change in response to the concentration of the specific binding molecule or ligand (Latin: *ligare*, to bind), whether this be agonist or antagonist (blocker), always tending to restore cell function to its normal or usual state. Prolonged high concentrations of agonist (whether administered as a drug or overproduced in the body by a tumour) cause a reduction in the number of receptors available for activation (*down-regulation*); and changes in receptor affinity and sensitivity and the prolonged occupation of receptors by inert molecules (antagonists) leads to an increase in the number of receptors (*up-regulation*). At least some of this may be achieved by receptors moving inside the cell and out again (*internalisation* and *externalisation*).

Down-regulation and accompanying receptor changes may explain the tolerant or refractory state seen in severe asthmatics who no longer respond to β-adrenoceptor agonists.

The occasional exacerbation of ischaemic cardiac disease on sudden withdrawal of a β-adrenoceptor blocker may be explained by *up-regulation* during its administration, so that on withdrawal an above-normal number of receptors suddenly becomes accessible to the normal chemotransmitter (noradrenaline). Up-regulation with rebound sympathomimetic effects may be innocuous to a moderately healthy cardiovascular system, but the increased oxygen demand of these effects can have serious consequences where ischaemic disease is present and increased oxygen need cannot be met (angina pectoris, dysrhythmia, infarction). Unmasking of a disease process that has worsened during prolonged suppressive use of the drug, i.e. *resurgence*, may also contribute to such exacerbations.

The rebound phenomenon is plainly a potential hazard and the use of a β-adrenoceptor blocker in the presence of ischaemic heart disease would be safer if rebound could be eliminated. Now, some β-adrenoceptor blockers are not pure blockers (antagonists); they also have some agonist (sympathomimetic) activity, i.e. they are *partial agonists*; it seems possible that the presence of some agonist action along with the principal blocking effect might prevent the generation of additional adrenoceptors (up-regulation), and indeed there is evidence that rebound is less or is absent with partial agonist β-adrenoceptor blockers, e.g. pindolol.

Sometimes a distinction is made between *rebound* (recurrence at intensified degree of the symptoms for which the drug was given) and *withdrawal syndrome* (appearance of new additional symptoms). The distinction is quantitative and does not imply different mechanisms.

Rebound and withdrawal phenomena occur erratically. In general, they are more likely with drugs having a short half-life (abrupt drop in plasma concentration) and pure agonist or antagonist action. They are less likely to occur with drugs having a long half-life and (probably) with those having a mixed agonist/antagonist (partial agonist) action on receptors.

Clinically important consequences of abrupt withdrawal of drugs are known to occur with the following:

Cardiovascular system: antihypertensives (especially clonidine), β-adrenoceptor blockers.
Nervous system: all depressants (hypnotics, sedatives, alcohol, opioids), antiepileptics, antiparkinsonian agents: tricyclic antidepressants.
Endocrine system: adrenal steroids.
Immune inflammation: adrenal steroids.

Resurgence of chronic disease which has progressed in severity although its consequences have been wholly or partly suppressed, i.e. a catching-up phenomenon is an obvious possible consequence of withdrawal of effective therapy, e.g. warfarin withdrawal in ischaemic heart disease; in corticosteroid withdrawal in autoimmune disease there may be both resurgence and rebound.

Rebound, withdrawal and resurgence (defined above) are phenomena that are to be expected. In many cases the exact mechanisms remain obscure but clinicians have no reason to be amazed when they occur, and in the case of rebound they may particularly wish to use gradual withdrawal wherever drugs have been used to modify complex self-adjusting systems, and to suppress (without cure) chronic diseases.

Other aspects of chronic drug use

Metabolic changes over a long period may induce disease, e.g. thiazide diuretics (diabetes mellitus), adrenocortical hormones (osteoporosis), phenytoin (osteomalacia). Drugs may also enhance metabolism of the primary drug and other drugs (enzyme induction).

Specific cell injury or *cell functional disorder* occur with individual drugs or drug classes, e.g. tardive dyskinesia (dopamine receptor blockers), retinal damage (chloroquine, phenothiazines), retroperitoneal fibrosis (methysergide). Cancer may occur, e.g. with oestrogens (endometrium), and with immunosuppressive (anticancer) drugs.

Dangers of intercurrent illness — these are particularly notable with anticoagulants, adrenal steroids and immunosuppressives.

Dangers of interactions with other drugs or diet — monoamine oxidase inhibitor antidepressants (pethidine, sympathomimetics, cheese), antihypertensives (sympathomimetics, including appetite suppressants, tricyclic antidepressants), digoxin (diuretics), hypnotics and tranquillisers (alcohol), and interactions due to enzyme induction and inhibition (see Interactions).

Summary. The objective of the above account of some consequences of prolonged drug administration is to remind the user that drugs do not only induce their known listed primary actions, but they:

- evoke compensatory responses in the complex inter-related physiological systems that they perturb, and that these systems need time to recover on withdrawal of the drug (gradual withdrawal can give this time; it is sometimes mandatory and never harmful);
- induce metabolic changes that may be trivial in the short term, but serious if they persist for a long time;
- may produce localised effects in specially susceptible tissues and induce serious cell damage or malfunction;
- increase susceptibility to intercurrent illness and to interaction with other drugs that may be taken for new indications.

That such consequences will occur with prolonged drug use is to be expected, and, with a moderate knowledge of physiology, pathology and pharmacology, combined with an awareness that the unexpected is to be expected ('There are more things in heaven and earth, Horatio, than are dreamt of in your philosophy'[33]) patients requiring long-term therapy may be managed safely, or at least with minimum risk of harm, and enabled to live happy lives.

WARNINGS TO PATIENTS AND CONSENT TO TREATMENT

Just as engineers say that the only safe aeroplane is the one that stays on the ground in still air on a disused airfield or in a locked hangar, so the only safe drug is one that stays in its original package. If drugs are not safe then plainly patients are entitled to be warned of their hazards.

It is self-evident to patients that when doctors propose treatment it is because they think it will do good. It is not equally self-evident to patients that there is a possibility of harm, and it certainly would be wrong that the onus to enquire about risk should be put on them; the doctor manifestly has a general duty to offer relevant information. Patients may opt to leave to the doctor the decision to use or not to use the treatment, making use of the doctor's training, knowledge of the treatment and knowledge of the patient, as it is their right to choose to do. Alternatively, patients may wish to hear a detailed explanation and decide for themselves, as is equally their right. In any case the doctor has some duty to warn.

Warnings to patients may be divided into two classes:

1. Warnings that will affect the patient's decision to accept or reject the treatment.
2. Warnings that will affect the safety of the treatment once it has begun, e.g. risk of stopping treatment, occurrence of drug toxicity.

There is no formal legal or ethical obligation on doctors to warn all patients of *all* possible adverse consequences of treatment. It is their duty

---

[33] W Shakespeare (1564–1616) Hamlet: I.V.166.

to adapt the information they give so that the best interest of each patient is served. In one court case a judge declared that there was no obligation on doctors to go over with their patients anything more than the inherent implication of the particular treatment proposed. If there was a real risk inherent in a procedure of some misfortune occurring, then doctors should certainly warn patients of the possibility that the misfortune might arise, however well the treatment was performed. Doctors should take into account the personality of the patient, the likelihood of any misfortune arising, and what warning was necessary for each particular patient's welfare.[34]

It is part of the professionalism of doctors to tell what is appropriate in their patients' interest. But this must be deliberate. If things go wrong they must be prepared to defend what they did, or, more important in the case of warnings, what they did not do, as being in their patient's best interest.

There has been public concern that doctors deliberately and arrogantly withhold information from patients. If public pressure that doctors should really try to tell *all*, or even most, were really to become so strong and persistent that the profession felt obliged to acquiesce, there can be no doubt the practice of medicine, for not only the doctor but also the patient, would change in a way that neither party, particularly not the patient, would like. The plain impossibility of meeting the requirement orally must result in extensive lists being printed (for all forms of treatment, including surgery). Some think this would frighten some patients, and maybe it would, but it would confuse more.

In conclusion. Doctors have a duty to warn and inform patients who undergo medical treatment or participate in research:

* so that they can make an informed decision whether to accept treatment
* to render continuing treatment safer
* to allow medical research to be conducted to the highest ethical standard.

---

[34] Legal correspondent. Br Med J 1980; 280: 575.

WHY DRUG THERAPY CARRIES UNAVOIDABLE RISK

A risk-free drug would be one for which:

* the physician knew exactly what action was required and used the drug correctly
* the drug did that and nothing else, either by true biological selectivity or by selective targeted delivery
* exactly the right amount of action, not too little, not too much, was easily achieved.

These criteria may be completely fulfilled, e.g. in a streptococcal infection sensitive to penicillin in a patient whose genetic constitution does not render him liable to an allergic reaction to penicillin.

These criteria are partially fulfilled in insulin-deficient diabetes. But the natural controls of insulin secretion in response to need (food, exercise) are lacking and even sophisticated technology cannot yet exactly mimic the normal physiological responses. The criteria are still farther from realisation in, e.g. hyperlipidaemias and schizophrenia.

Why criteria for a risk-free drug are not met

1. *Drugs are insufficiently selective.* As the concentration rises, a drug that is highly selective at low concentrations will begin to affect other target sites (receptors, enzymes); a disease process (cancer) is so close to normal cellular mechanisms that totally selective cell kill is impossible (though cure of some cancers is attainable at an acceptable price in toxicity).

2. *Drugs are selective*, but the mechanism affected has widespread functions and interference with it cannot be limited to one site only, e.g. monoamine oxidase inhibitors, propranolol, aspirin.

3. *Prolonged modification of cellular mechanisms* can lead to permanent change in structure and function, e.g. carcinogenicity.

4. *Insufficient knowledge of disease processes* (atherosclerosis) and of drug action (hypolipidaemics) can lead to interventions that, though undertaken with the best intentions, are harmful.

5. *Patients are genetically heterogeneous* to an

enormous degree and may have an unpredictable immunological response to drugs.

6. *Dosage adjustment according to need is unavoidably imprecise* (diabetes mellitus, depression).

7. *Ignorant and casual prescribing.*

Reduction of drug risk

This can be achieved by:

- *Better knowledge of disease* (research); as much as 40% of useful medical advances derive from basic research that was not funded with the practical outcome in view.
- *Site-specific delivery: drug targeting*
  — by topical (local) application
  — by target-selective carriers (see p. 77).
- *Site-specific effect*: by molecular manipulation.
- Informed, careful and responsible prescribing.

REASONS FOR TAKING A DRUG HISTORY FROM PATIENTS

- Drugs are a cause of disease. Withdrawal of drugs can cause disease, e.g. adrenal steroid, antiepileptic.
- Drugs can conceal disease, e.g. adrenal steroid.
- Drugs can interact causing positive adverse effect or negative adverse effect, i.e. therapeutic failure.
- Drugs can give diagnostic clues, e.g. ampicillin in infectious mononucleosis, a diagnostic side-effect, not a diagnostic test.
- Drugs can cause false results in clinical chemistry tests, e.g. plasma cortisol, urinary catecholamine, urinary glucose.
- Drug history can assist choice of drugs in the future.
- Drugs can leave residual effects after administration has ceased, e.g. chloroquine, digoxin, adrenal steroid.

The therapeutic situation

It is evident that patients are not treated in a vacuum and that they respond to a variety of subtle forces around them in addition to the specific therapeutic agent under investigation.[35]

When a patient is given a drug his responses are the resultant of numerous factors:

- The pharmacodynamic effect of the drug and interactions with any other drugs the patient may be taking
- The pharmacokinetics of the drug and its modification in the individual due to genetic influences, disease, other drugs
- The physiological state of the end-organ, whether, for instance, it is over- or underactive
- The act of medication, including the route of administration and the presence or absence of the doctor
- The doctor's mood, personality, attitudes and beliefs
- The patient's mood, personality, attitudes
- What the doctor has told the patient
- The patient's past experience of doctors
- The patient's estimate of what has been received and of what ought to happen as a result
- The social environment, e.g. whether supportive or disheartening.

The relative importance of these factors varies according to the circumstances — an unconscious patient with meningococcal meningitis does not have a personal relationship with the doctor, but patients sleepless with anxiety because they cannot cope with their family responsibilities may be affected as much by the interaction of their own personalities with that of the doctor as by the diazepam prescribed by the latter, and the same applies to appetite suppressants in food addicts.

The physician may consciously use all of the factors listed above in therapeutic practice. But it is still not enough that patients get better, it is essential to know *why* they do so. This is because potent drugs should only be given if their pharmacodynamic effects are needed. If other factors are the effective agents, then any drug given will be a placebo and placebos should be harmless. The double-blind technique in therapeutic trials used with placebo (or dummy) medication

---

[35] Sherman L J. Am J Psychiatry 1959; 116: 208.

represents an attempt to discriminate true pharmacodynamic effects from the other aspects of the therapeutic situation.

PLACEBOS[36]

All treatments have a psychological component, whether to please (true placebo effect) or, occasionally, to vex (negative placebo effect).

Placebos are used for two purposes:

1. as a **control** in scientific evaluation of drugs (see Therapeutic trials)
2. to **benefit** or please a patient not by any pharmacological actions, but by psychological means.

A placebo is a vehicle for cure by suggestion, and is surprisingly often successful, if only temporarily. *All treatments carry placebo effect* — physiotherapy, psychotherapy, surgery — but it is most easily investigated with drugs, for the active and the inert can often be made to appear identical so that comparisons can be made.

The deliberate use of drugs as placebos is a confession of failure by the doctor. Failures however are sometimes inevitable and an absolute condemnation of the use of placebos on all occasions would be unrealistic.

Placebos are usually given to patients with mild psychological disorders who attribute their symptoms to physical disease. There is no doubt that alleviation can sometimes be achieved but it is usually only temporary, and may make any subsequent attempt to face reality more difficult.

Deliberate use of placebo therapy

The principal objection to deliberate use of placebo therapy is that the patient, reasonably, interprets the advice to take medicine as meaning that the doctor admits a physical basis for the symptoms; so that when, later, an attempt is made to attribute a psychological cause this will not be accepted. Placebos may also be used in patients with chronic incurable diseases when they need a prop to sustain their courage. Apart

from this compassionate use, placebos should only be prescribed after a serious attempt to avoid using them has failed, and then only briefly; the placebo should consist of a substance innocuous and cheap (vitamin mineral supplements can be used), unless patients pay for it themselves, when high cost greatly potentiates its effect.

In addition to the psychological suggestion inevitable in any act of medication, deliberate verbal suggestion has been shown to raise the threshold for pain and indeed to reverse pharmacodynamic effects at least temporarily. Such psychological effects are operative in any enthusiastically pursued therapeutic regimen.

It is of great importance that all who administer drugs should be aware that their attitudes to the treatment may greatly influence the result. Undue scepticism may prevent a drug from achieving its effect and enthusiasm or confidence may potentiate the actions of drugs.

A **placebo-reactor** is an individual who reports changes of physical or mental state after taking a pharmacologically inert substance. Such suggestible people are likely to respond favourably to *any* treatment. They have deceived doctors into making false therapeutic claims and have provided the basis for many therapeutic reputations.

Negative reactors, who develop adverse effects when given a placebo, exist but, fortunately, are fewer.

Some 35% of the physically ill and 40% or more of the mentally ill respond to placebos. Placebo reaction is an inconstant attribute — a person may respond at one time in one situation and not at another time under different conditions. However, there is some consistency in the type of person who specially tends to react to placebos. In one study on medical students, psychological tests revealed that those who reacted to a placebo tended to be extraverted, sociable, less dominant, less self-confident, more appreciative of their teaching, more aware of their autonomic functions and more neurotic than their colleagues who did not react to a placebo under the particular conditions of the experiment.

Tonics are placebos. They may be defined as substances with which it is hoped to strengthen

---

[36] Latin: *placebo*, I shall be pleasing or acceptable.

those so weakened by disease, misery, overindulgence in play or work, or by physical or mental inadequacy, that they cannot face the stresses of life. The essential feature of this weakness is the absence of any definite recognisable defect for which there is a known remedy. There can be very few doctors who believe that there is any pharmacological basis for tonics. Benefits are attributable to placebo effects and it is to be hoped that explanation and reassurance will eventually take the place of 'tablets'. Many people still expect a tonic from their doctor following an illness and they are sceptical and shocked if told that the benefits that they feel are not the result of pharmacological action.

If either the doctor or the patient believes in tonics to such a degree that one must be prescribed, a mineral and vitamin supplement such as those promoted specially for the aged will suffice. There are innumerable proprietary tonics, some of which contain highly active drugs including CNS stimulants; these should be avoided. The indiscriminate use of vitamins as tonics is widely advocated by pharmaceutical companies and practised by the gullible. Vitamins A and D can cause serious toxic effects.

There is every reason for doctors to cultivate techniques for the psychological potentiation of drugs, for their aim is to help patients, but it is essential that they should be aware of what they are doing and not deceive themselves about the physical power of their remedies. Some doctors can be accurately described as having placebo personalities.

PRESCRIBING AND DRUG CONSUMPTION

Choice of drugs. There are national differences in prescribing that are the result of differing therapeutic approach between doctors in different countries, e.g. in hypertension, diabetes and mental disorders.

Cost and range. Pharmaceutical Services have comprised about 8–10% of the UK National Health Service expenditure over the past 30 years.

A National Health Service offers opportunities to get information on prescribing habits and costs not previously available, because general practitioner prescriptions are all sent to a pricing office that arranges to pay the supplying pharmacist. It has been found that prescription frequency and cost per prescription is lower for older than for younger doctors. There is no reason to think that the patients of older doctors are worse off as a result.

Despite enormous individual variation it seems that most doctors do about 75% of their prescribing from about 100 preparations (not 100 different drugs), but the maximum number of preparations used by an individual doctor can be as high as 500.[37]

Antimicrobials head the list of prescribed drugs, followed by diuretics, analgesics, tranquillisers, gastrointestinal medicines, adrenal steroid topical preparations, bronchodilators and cough medicines.

Total consumption (self-prescribed plus doctor-prescribed) of drugs is headed by analgesics, cough and cold medicines and vitamins and tonics (50%) with antibiotics a close fourth, followed by drugs for skin diseases, cardiovascular diseases, hormones, tranquillisers and sedatives, antirheumatic drugs and antacids.

Amount. Consumption of drugs has become a normal aspect of daily life in modern society.

In the UK on average the 57 million population (patients) consult their doctors three times a year and receive a prescription averaging 1.6 items at two of these consultations. Nearly as many prescription items again are issued without direct contact between doctor and patient.

In a study of prescriptions issued by general practitioners to a sample population of about 40 000 in the UK[38] in one year it was found that 54% of men and 66% of women had at least one drug dispensed. Psychotropic drugs (affecting

---

[37] The World Health Organization publishes an updated series of reports on *The use of essential drugs*, which gives guidance for establishing national programmes for supply of drugs; about 290 products are listed. The pharmaceutical industry dislikes the concept that some drugs may be classed as *essential* and therefore others, presumably, as *inessential*. But the WHO programme has attracted much interest and approval. See WHO Tech Rep Ser current edition.

[38] Skegg D C G et al. Br Med J 1977; 1: 1561.

behaviour) were prescribed to 10% of men and 21% of women. Of women aged 45–59 years, 33% received a psychotropic drug and 11% were given an antidepressant. One psychotropic drug, diazepam (Valium), generally prescribed as a sedative against anxiety and insomnia, was given to 6% of the population.

A survey in 9 Western European countries disclosed that the proportion of all people using a tranquilliser or sedative drug was 17% in Belgium and France, 14% in the UK and 10% in Spain. The proportion of women was twice that of men and use increased with age.

In Denmark it is calculated that every person is prescribed a dose of a tranquilliser every second or third day and an analgesic every eighth day per annum.

So, for a sizeable proportion of people, medicine taking has become a habit often encouraged, or at least supported by their doctors.[39]

The consumption of both self- and doctor-prescribed drugs has increased rapidly in Australia, the USA and the UK.

It is evident that people have an increasing desire for medicines and that this is well catered for by manufacturers and doctors. The question arises whether this desire is solely the result of a true medical need, i.e. whether the drugs are curing or preventing disease. We do not think it is. Drug consumption in our societies is unnecessarily high and it causes a significant burden of drug-induced disease; current levels of drug use are probably symptomatic of underlying stresses and pressures in urban societies together with a cultural background that accepts the social use of medicines and encourages unduly high expectations in relation to health, with a low threshold of what constitutes illness.

Repeat prescriptions

About two-thirds of general (family) practice prescriptions are for repeat medication (half issued by the doctor at a consultation and half via the receptionist without contact with the doctor):

95% of patients' requests are acceded to without further discussion;

25% of patients who receive repeat prescriptions have had 40 or more repeats;

55% of patients aged over 75 years are on repeat medication.

An analysis of patients who received the same preparation for above 6 months, and often for years — 'long-repeat patients' — concluded that the patients are unhappy and their unhappiness manifests itself as unpleasant bodily sensations. The doctor can find no definite disease but he goes on trying and makes multiple diagnoses, often psychiatric. However, since no satisfactory diagnosis is established, no rational therapy can be provided. The patient continues to complain and the doctor continues to try unsuccessfully. Eventually doctor and patient take refuge uneasily in 'long-repeat prescriptions'. Of course, many patients taking the same drug for years are doing so for the best reason, i.e. firm diagnosis for which effective therapy is available, such as epilepsy, diabetes, hypertension; but many are not.

Summary

Repeat prescriptions can be classified[40] thus:

- For the *specific pharmacodynamic (therapeutic) effect* of the drug.
- As a way of *maintaining a relationship* (by both doctor and patient); the prescription provides contact, but it can be kept impersonal; anxious phobic patients use this relationship to escape the pain of trying to eliminate their phobia, and the doctor may collude with them in this.
- As *a gift* — a symbol of a wish to do something when the prescriber cannot think of anything better.
- To fulfil *socially motivated patient demands*, e.g. weight reduction.
- As a way of *getting rid of the patient*.

[39] Dunnell K, Cartwright A. Medicine takers prescribers and hoarders. London: Routledge & Kegan Paul, 1972. A classic study.

[40] Harris C M. Br Med J 1980; 281: 57.

ECONOMICS: COST-BENEFIT, COST-EFFECTIVENESS AND QUALITY OF LIFE

The appetite of citizens for health care based on their real needs, on their wants and on their (often unrealistic) expectations exceeds the capacity of even the richest societies to deliver. Health care resources are therefore rationed in one way or another, whether according to national social policies or to individual wealth. The debate on supply is not about whether there should be rationing, but about what form rationing should take.

Drugs comprise a significant element in the cost of health services (about 10% of expenditure in the UK National Health Service). In the UK family doctors (general practitioners) prescribe drugs to an annual value of well above their earnings, i.e. collectively family doctors dispose of enormous resources and are visibly the objects of assiduous courtship by a hospitable pharmaceutical industry. Traditionally doctors think only of their individual patients' needs. But the individual patient also wants a good general service, which cannot be provided if resources are squandered in any one area, e.g. overprescribing.

Increasing attention, therefore, is now being given to economics in health care, including drug use.

Economics is the science of the distribution of resources

Three economic concepts have particular importance to the thinking of every doctor who takes up a pen to prescribe, i.e. to distribute resources.

1. *Opportunity cost* means that which has to be sacrificed in order to carry out a certain course of action, i.e. costs are benefits foregone elsewhere — if money is spent on prescribing, that money is not available for another purpose; wasteful prescribing can be seen as an affront to those who are in serious need, e.g. institutionalised mentally handicapped citizens who everywhere would benefit from increased resources.

2. *Cost-effectiveness analysis* is concerned with how to attain a given objective at minimum cost, e.g. prevention of postsurgical venous thromboembolism by heparin, warfarin, aspirin, external pneumatic compression; analysis includes cost of materials, of adverse effects, of any tests, of nursing and doctor time.

3. *Cost-benefit analysis* is concerned with issues of whether (and to what extent) to pursue objectives and policies; it is thus a broader activity than cost-effectiveness analysis and has to concern itself with the quality as well as the quantity (duration) of life.

Some doctors in richer societies, unfamiliar with these concepts and feeling uneasily or resentfully that material values (prices) cannot or should not be placed on life and its quality, refuse to agree that economics can have a role in the practice of medicine, declaring that doctors must do their best for each individual patient regardless of cost. We all wish this could be so, but it cannot be, and there are two replies to those who take up that position:

- There is no society in the world where all can have all the medical care they want or need regardless of cost and
- By their daily intuitive decision-taking doctors in health services are directing resources to selected individuals and therefore necessarily depriving others of the opportunity to use these same resources for what may be their greater need.

The economists' objective

This is to ensure that needs are defined and that available resources are deployed according to priorities set by society, which has an interest in fairness between its members. The question is whether resources are to be distributed in accordance with an unregulated power struggle between professionals and associations of patients and public pressure groups, all, no doubt, warmhearted towards deserving cases of one kind or another, but none able to view the whole scene; or whether there is to be a planned evaluation that allows division of the resources on the basis of some visible attempt at fairness.

But the enemies of cost-benefit appraisal have a valid point when they challenge the economists to show that *quality* of life can be measured. This challenge is now being met.

Quality of life

Everyone is familiar with the measurement of the benefit of treatment in saving or extending life, i.e. life expectancy: the measure is the quantity of life (in years). But it is evident that life may be extended and yet have a low quality, even to the point that it is not worth having. It is therefore useful to have a unit of health measurement that combines the quantity of life with its quality to allow individual and social decisions to be made on a sounder basis than mere intuition.

To meet this need there has been developed the *quality-adjusted-life-year* (QALY); estimations of years of life expectancy are modified according to estimations of quality of life.

Quality of life has four dimensions[41]

1. physical mobility
2. freedom from pain and distress
3. capacity for self-care
4. ability to engage in normal social interactions

The approach to measure quality of life has been developed into a questionnaire *measure of what the subject perceives as personal health*. This explores the *six areas* that best reflect problems with health: sleep, physical mobility, energy, pain, emotional reactions, and social isolation. It also investigates the *seven areas* of daily life most often affected by health or its diminution: paid employment, looking after the house, social life, home life, sex life, hobbies and interests, and holidays.

Already studies in which quality-of-life measures are included have been done in drug therapy of peptic ulcer and rheumatism, and the assessments are being refined to provide improved assessment of the benefits and risks to the individual and to society of medicines.

---

[41] Williams A. In Smith G T, ed. Measuring the social benefits of medicine. London: Office of Health Economics, 1983.

PATIENT COMPLIANCE[42]

It might seem reasonable to assume that a patient given a prescription will obtain the medicine and actually consume it. The assumption would be wrong. The rate of non-presentation of prescriptions has been estimated as 1–5%. Where patients have to pay this can have a simple economic explanation.

But further, having obtained the medicine, some 40–50% of patients do not accurately follow the prescriber's instructions or do not take it at all.

There are two major aspects of patient compliance:

1. *non-comprehension* of instructions, so that the patient *cannot* comply; due to inadequacy of the doctor or of the patient.

2. *comprehension* of instructions, but failure to carry them out.

Major factors established as associated with non-compliance

- *Education*: low level
- *Anxiety*: a barrier to both comprehension and retention of information
- *Disease*: psychiatric diagnosis
- *Regimen*: complexity (more than two administrations per day)
- *Source of medicine*: time-wasting or inconvenient clinics
- *Doctor/patient relation*: inadequate supervision; patient dissatisfaction with doctor, including the feeling he or she does not know the doctor well
- *Patient*: inappropriate health beliefs, including the idea that medicine can be stopped as soon as the patient feels better; failure of memory; family instability
- *Adverse drug reactions*

---

[42] The term *compliance* has been objected to as having overtones of obsolete, arrogant attitudes, implying 'obedience' to doctors' 'orders'. But this seems oversensitive and the suggested alternatives, *adherence* and *cooperation* do not have quite the right meaning. We retain *compliance*, pointing out that it applies also to doctors who do not follow prescribing instructions, e.g. in official Data Sheets. *Doctor compliance* must, of course, precede *patient compliance* (see below).

Level of intelligence within the normal range is not an important factor, nor is duration of therapy.

The wide range of factors to be taken into account in special cases is illustrated by the use of a single dose of radioactive iodine to treat hyperthyroidism in patients likely to be non-compliant with continuous antithyroid medication (carbimazole). Since patients will inevitably become hypothyroid years hence due to the radioactive iodine, and will then have to take thyroxine daily for the rest of their lives, the problem of compliance is postponed rather than eliminated.

Patients should not be blamed for non-compliance where the prescriber has failed to give adequate instructions. *Written information* increases patient satisfaction and benefits compliance if it is easy to read and accompanied by oral advice. The fears of conservative, paternalistic doctors that information will scare patients so as to reduce compliance have been shown rarely to be justified. Compliance is also benefited by engaging the patient as an understanding participant in the management of the disease, e.g. diabetes, hypertension, rather than as a simple recipient who is subject only to exhortation to do as told, with threats of displeasure or disaster for disobedience.

Studies of what patients remember of what the doctor has told them give results that will occasion no surprise. About one-third of patients have been found unable to recount instructions immediately on leaving the doctor's consulting room; brevity, clarity and repetition by the doctor improve patient recall. Proper labelling of the container supplied to the patient or special packaging (calendar packs for oral contraceptives) naturally also helps, as may pamphlets of standard written advice on management of chronic diseases, e.g. diabetes, hypertension.

> It is unlikely that any patient will reliably take more than three drugs without special supervision.

What every patient needs to know[43]

- The *name* of the medicine.

- The *objective*
    to treat the *disease*
    to relieve *symptoms*
    i.e. how important the medicine is, whether the patient can judge its efficacy and *when* benefit can be expected to occur.
- How and when to *take* the medicine.
- Whether it matters if a dose is *missed* and what, if anything, to do about it.
- How *long* the medicine is likely to be needed.
- How to recognise *side-effects* and any action that should be taken, including effects on car driving.
- Any *interaction* with alcohol or other medicines.

Note: It is plain that all this cannot be told to the patient briefly with any hope that it will be remembered; directions on the container, special packaging and other written matter will be useful in addition to oral instructions from doctor and pharmacist.

A remarkable instance of non-compliance with hoarding was that of a 71-year-old man who attempted suicide and was found to have in his home 46 bottles containing 10 685 tablets. Analysis of his prescriptions showed that over a period of 17 months he had been expected to take 27 tablets of several different kinds daily.[44]

From time to time there are campaigns to collect all unwanted drugs from homes in an area. Usually the public are asked to deliver the drugs to their local pharmacies. In one UK city of 600 000 population, 500 000 'solid dose units' (tablets, capsules, etc.) were handed in (see Opportunity cost).

Obviously small children, the old and mentally incapacitated patients cannot comply with instructions and family aid must be enlisted. But evidence suggests that any psychiatric diagnosis (except presumably an obsessional state) is likely to be associated with low compliance. Anecdotes circulate concerning the effect of discarded psychotropic drugs on the vegetation in the grounds

[43] From Drug Ther. Bull. 1981; 19: 73.
[44] Smith S E et al. Lancet 1974; 1: 937.

of psychiatric hospitals, and on the adverse effect of discarded drugs on the aerodynamic capacities of seagulls visiting a hospital in the UK.

Evaluation of compliance

Merely asking patients whether they have taken the drug as directed is not likely to provide reliable evidence.[45] The figures for non-compliance are based on studies that include interview, counting tablets that remain when the patient attends the doctor, blood or urine testing for the drug or a marker included in the tablet, e.g. riboflavin, phenol red, and measuring pharmacodynamic effect.

Of course undiscovered non-compliance can invalidate therapeutic trials.

Major aspects are illustrated in one study of 674 children with acute otitis media prescribed an oral antibiotic and a nasal decongestant for 10 days.[46] The first major non-compliance was the failure of 374 patients to return for review. Of the 300 who did return, the following was found:

- 86% of parents thought their child's illness moderate or severe
- 7% of children received the full course
- treatment had stopped by the fourth day in over one-third, especially in children of poorly educated or single mothers
- 3% had spilled the medicine or broken the bottle
- Some container labels were illegible or legible but incorrect
- Doctors gave poorly memorable information, did not provide medicine for immediate use to cover the period until the prescription could be dispensed, and they prescribed in fractions of a spoonful (see Doctor compliance below).

Successful drug therapy comprises a great deal more than choosing the right drug.

---

[45] The way the patient is questioned may be all-important, e.g. 'Were you able to take the tablets?' may get a truthful reply where, 'Did you take the tablets?' may not, because the latter question may be understood by the patient as implying personal criticism. (Pearson R M. Br. Med J 1982; 285: 757.)
[46] Mattar M E et al. J Pediatr 1975; 87: 137.

DOCTOR COMPLIANCE

Errors of prescribing

It would be inappropriate to discuss the failings of patients to take prescribed drugs, without reference to the errors of doctors in prescribing, and other staff in administering drugs in hospital. Compliance is not a concept for patients alone; doctors have a *duty* to comply, i.e. not to be ignorant, to refrain from inappropriate prescribing, to tell patients what they need to know, to warn (p. 16), and quite simply to recognise the importance of what they are doing; if doctors wrote bank cheques as badly as they commonly write prescriptions, they would soon be in trouble.

In one study in a university hospital, where standards might be expected to be high, there was an error of drug use (dose, frequency, route) in 3% of prescriptions and an error of prescription writing (in relation to standard hospital instructions) in 30%. In 79% of patients there was at least one error in prescription writing. Many errors were trivial, but many could have resulted in overdose, serious interaction or undertreatment.

In other hospital studies error rates in drug administration of 15–25% have been found, rates rising rapidly where 4 or more drugs are being given concurrently, as is often the case; studies on hospital in-patients show that each receives about 6 drugs, and up to 20 during a stay is not rare.

It has been found that merely providing information (on antimicrobials) did not influence prescribing, but gently asking physicians to justify their prescriptions caused a marked fall in inappropriate prescribing.

SELF-MEDICATION AND MEDICINES IN THE HOME

To feel unwell is common, though the frequency varies with social and cultural circumstances, and it is both natural and desirable that people should care for themselves as far as is practicable.

People commonly experience symptoms or complaints and commonly want to take remedial action. In one study of adults randomly selected from a large population, 9 out of 10 had one or more complaints in the 2 weeks before interview; in another of premenopausal women a symptom occurred as often as one day in 3; in both studies a medicine was taken for more than half these occurrences.

About one in 30–40 symptoms is taken to a doctor. Self-medication is not a substitute for visiting the doctor (though this has been commonly supposed and frequently asserted) and purchasers of these 'home medicines' visit their doctors as often as does the rest of the population. It seems that the public is sensible enough to realise that doctors have little to contribute to many minor ills and, taking into account the natural reluctance to visit a doctor that sensible people feel, as well as the inconvenience, it is easily understandable that patients prefer 'do it yourself', i.e. self-medication. The commonest symptoms experienced are 'undue' tiredness, pain (headache, backache), indigestion, 'nerves' and depression, and cough; medication is taken in anything from 40–70% of incidents.

The medicines most commonly purchased from pharmacies are analgesics, antacids, laxatives,[47] antitussives and expectorants. About 20% of purchases are for long-term use. Experience of adverse effects is as low (8%), as is knowledge of them (8–20%). When purchasers are asked their reason for choosing a medicine they give first the user's own assessment of need, closely followed by advice from pharmacist and doctor; promotion via the mass media is thought least influential (though advertisers might well claim that their skills are so subtle as to account for users thinking they are making their own judgement when they are not).

Half the purchasers of home medicines are aged above 65 years; some studies have found a marked preponderance ($\times$ 4) of women purchasers; women experience more symptoms than men, but they may also more often be making purchases for others — spouses, old parents or children.

---

[47] Extensive use of laxatives indicates that patients/the public do *not* know best, and need advice.

Self-medication is appropriate

- for short-term relief of symptoms where accurate diagnosis is unnecessary
- for the relief of mild cases of some chronic or recurrent diseases, e.g. eczema
- when the drug has a large margin of safety.

In general modern drugs will only be deemed suitable for self-medication by direct sale to the public after prolonged and safe use as prescription-only medicines.

In the UK, a survey[39] has shown that 99% of a sample of homes contained one or more medicines. The average number of items was 10.3 (3 doctor-prescribed, 7.3 non-prescribed); nearly all had some kind of analgesic and skin cream; one-fifth had sedatives, tranquillisers or sleeping tablets and two-fifths had one or more items that the informant could not identify. In only two of 686 homes were any medicines locked up; medicines were most commonly kept in the kitchen.

GUIDE TO FURTHER READING

Bagenal F S et al 1990 Survival of patients with breast cancer attending Bristol Cancer Help Centre. Lancet 336: 606 [A scientific study of conventional and complementary medicine]: also subsequent correspondence

Cohen E P 1988 Direct-to-the-public advertisements of prescription drugs. New England Journal of Medicine 318: 373

Drummond M G et al 1982 Assessing the costs and benefits of treatment alternatives. British Medical Journal 285: 1561, 1638

Editorial 1979 The real world of drug prescribing. Lancet 2: 781

Editorial 1988 When to believe the unbelievable. Nature 333: 787 (A report of an investigation into experiments with antibodies in solutions that contained no antibody molecules (as in some homoeopathic medicines). The editor of *Nature* took a three-person team (one of whom was a professional magician, included to detect any trickery) on a week-long visit to the laboratory that claimed positive results. Despite the scientific seriousness of the operation it developed comical aspects (codes of the contents of test tubes were taped to the laboratory ceiling); the Nature team, having reached an unfavourable view of the experiments 'sped past the [laboratory] common room filled with champagne bottles destined now not to be opened'). Full reports in this issue of Nature (28 July 1988), including an acrimonious response by the original scientist, are *highly recommended reading*, both for scientific logic and entertainment

Feely J et al 1990 Hospital formularies: need for continuous intervention. British Medical Journal 300: 28

Herxheimer H 1987 Basic information that prescribers are not getting about drugs. Lancet 1: 31

Herxheimer A 1991 How much drug in a tablet? Lancet 337: 346, also p. 846

Kleinjen J et al 1991 Clinical trials in homoeopathy. British Medical Journal 302: 316, also subsequent correspondence 529, 727, 960

Laporte J-R et al 1983 Drug utilisation studies: a tool for determining the effectiveness of drug use. British Journal of Clinical Pharmacology 16: 301

Melmon K L et al 1983 The undereducated physician's therapeutic decisions. New England Journal of Medicine 308: 1473

Michel J-M 1985 Why do people like medicines? A perspective from Africa. Lancet 1: 210

Mullan K 1988 Writing a wrong [a legal action against a doctor and a pharmacist for negligence in prescribing and dispensing]. British Medical Journal 297: 470

Pullar T et al 1989 Time to stop counting the tablets? Clinical Pharmacology and Therapeutics 46: 163

Schaffner W et al 1983 Improving antibiotic prescribing in office practice. A controlled trial of three educational methods. Journal of the American Medical Association 250: 1728

Steel K et al 1981 Iatrogenic illness on a general medical service at university hospital. New England Journal of Medicine 304: 638

2

Clinical pharmacology

SYNOPSIS

- Clinical pharmacology is the scientific study of drugs in man
- It is concerned with the optimisation of drug therapy

DRUGS IN MAN

The development of pharmacological science in the early 20th century coupled with the technological advances of organic synthetic chemistry has been followed in mid-century by what has aptly been called the drug explosion of the past 50 years.[1] The eruption into therapeutics of thousands of new drugs, as well as a general information explosion in medicine, has called into being workers specialising in the scientific study of drugs in man or clinical pharmacology. The subject is increasingly recognised as both a health care and an academic specialty, indeed no medical school can be considered complete without a department or sub-department of Clinical Pharmacology.

The clinical pharmacologist's work is to provide facts and opinions that are useful for optimising the treatment of patients, and therapeutic success with drugs is becoming more and more dependent on the user having a technical knowledge of both pharmacodynamics and pharmacokinetics; a humane and caring doctor cannot dispense with technical skill.

Clinical pharmacology comprises two major parts:

1. Pharmacology
   - *pharmacodynamics*: how drugs, alone and in combination, affect the body (young, old, well, sick)

---

[1] Modell W. Clin Pharmacol Ther 1961; 2: 1.

29

- *pharmacokinetics*: absorption, distribution, metabolism, excretion or, how the body, well or sick, affects drugs.
2. Therapeutic evaluation
  - whether a drug is of value
  - how it may best be used
  - formal therapeutic trials
  - surveillance studies for both efficacy and adverse effects: pharmacoepidemiology and pharmacovigilance (p. 119).

Clinical pharmacologists also engage in various other activities related to these two main areas, e.g.

- prescribing systems
- cost-benefit analysis
- official drug regulation.

Work in these categories has long been done well by clinical scientists and physicians, but has largely resulted from the chance availability of a drug having particular interest for them; it has not been systematic. The magnitude of the need for clinical pharmacology, as shown by the disagreements on when and how to use many drugs (tranquillisers, adrenal steroids) and their safety in relation to their benefits (drugs in pregnancy, antidepressants) now demands the full-time attention of clinical workers, whether or not they care to call themselves clinical pharmacologists. All that is needed in addition to training in medicine and pharmacology is 'enthusiasm, stemming from the knowledge that through the study of drugs, medicine can be changed even more in the next fifty years than it has been in the past fifty' (H F Dowling).

If it is desired to single out a pioneer clinical pharmacologist it would surely be Harry Gold (1899–1972) of Cornell University, USA, whose influential studies in the 1930s showed us how to be clinical pharmacologists. In 1952 he wrote a seminal article, '*The proper study of mankind is man*',[2] which deserves re-reading. He writes,

a special kind of investigator is required, one whose training has equipped him not only with the principles and technics of laboratory pharmacology but also with knowledge of clinical medicine . . .

Clinical scientists of all kinds do not differ fundamentally from other biologists; they are set apart only to the extent that there are special difficulties and limitations, ethical and practical, in seeking knowledge from man.[3] Many clinical problems can best be tackled by using animals to fill the inevitable gaps resulting from the exigencies of clinical practice.

Pharmacology is the same science whether it is animal or man that is investigated. The need for it grows rapidly as not only scientists, but now the whole community, can see its promise of release from distress and death over yet wider fields. The concomitant dangers of drugs (fetal deformities, adverse reactions, dependence) only add to the need for the effective and ethical application of science to drug invention, evaluation, and use, i.e. clinical pharmacology.

---

[2] Gold H. 1952 American Journal of Medicine 12: 619. The title is taken from *An Essay on Man* by Alexander Pope (1688–1744); the whole passage is relevant to modern clinical pharmacology and drug therapy.

Know then thyself, presume not God to scan,
The proper study of mankind is man,
Placed on this isthmus of a middle state,
A being darkly wise, and rudely great:
With too much knowledge for the sceptic side,
With too much weakness for the stoic's pride,
He hangs between; in doubt to act or rest;
In doubt to deem himself a god or beast;
In doubt his mind or body to prefer;
Born but to die, and reas'ning but to err;
Alike in ignorance, his reason such,
Whether he thinks too little or too much;
Chaos of thought and passion, all confused;
Still by himself abused, or disabused;
Created half to rise, and half to fall;
Great lord of all things, yet a prey to all;
Sole judge of truth, in endless error hurled;
The Glory, jest and riddle of the world!

[3] *Self-experimentation* has always been a feature of clinical pharmacology. A survey of 250 members of the Dutch Society of Clinical Pharmacology evoked 102 responders of whom 55 had done experiments on themselves (largerly for convenience) (van Everdingen et al Lancet 1990; 336: 1448). A spectacular example occurred at the 1983 meeting of the American Urological Association at Las Vegas, during a lecture on pharmacological penile erection, when the lecturer stepped out from behind the lectern to demonstrate personally the efficacy of the technique (Zorgniotti A W Lancet 1990; 336: 1200).

GUIDE TO FURTHER READING

Alvan G et al 1983 Problem-oriented drug information: a clinical pharmacological service. Lancet 2: 1410.

Anglo-American Workshop on Clinical Pharmacology 1986 Present status and future direction of clinical pharmacology. Clinical Pharmacology and Therapeutics 39: 435

Atkinson A J et al 1984 University and pharmaceutical industry co-operation: the need to plan for the future. Clinical Pharmacology and Therapeutics 35: 431

Crooks J 1983 Drug epidemiology and clinical pharmacology. Their contribution to patient care. British Journal of Clinical Pharmacology 16: 351

Dollery C T 1987 The future of clinical pharmacology and therapeutics. Clinical Pharmacology and Therapeutics 41: 1

Dukes G 1990 Clinical pharmacology and primary health care in Europe. European Journal of Clinical Pharmacology 38: 315

Gold H 1961 The proper study of mankind is man. American Journal of Medicine 12: 619

Modell W 1961 The drug explosion. Clinical Pharmacology and Therapeutics 2: 1

Orme M et al 1990 The teaching and organisation of clinical pharmacology in European medical schools. European Journal of Clinical Pharmacology 38: 101

Prichard B N C et al 1971 Clinical pharmacology: function, organisation, and training. Lancet 2: 653

Vesell E S 1985 Clinical pharmacology: a personal perspective. Clinical Pharmacology and Therapeutics 38: 603

World Health Organization 1970 Clinical pharmacology, scope, organisation, and training. WHO Tech Rep Ser 446

3

Discovery and development of drugs

SYNOPSIS

New drugs enter medical practice continuously. Their development is an exercise in prediction, from laboratory studies in animals, what effect they will have in man.

- Approaches to drug discovery
- Pharmacology in drug development
- The process of new drug development
- Prediction: pharmacology, toxicology
- Drug quality
- Conclusion on pre-clinical testing
- Orphan drugs

APPROACHES TO DRUG DISCOVERY

More and more doctors are playing a role in evaluation of new drugs; those that are not are faced with the problems of whether to prescribe them, or they meet patients taking them. It is, therefore, not only of interest, but also important that doctors should have a general knowledge of the process of drug discovery in an industry that actively seeks to influence what they do, that delivers enormous benefits, but which is also subject to rising criticism of its role in medicine and society. When making criticisms it should be borne in mind that the pharmaceutical industry is also heavily regulated by governments acting on behalf of society and that the official regulators play a decisive role in determining what shall and what shall not be made available for general prescribing and the therapeutic claims that a manufacturer may make.

It will be obvious from the account that follows that drug development is an extremely arduous, highly technical and enormously expensive operation. Successful developments (<1% of compounds that go into test eventually become licensed medicines) must carry the cost of the failures (>99%).[1] It is also obvious that such programmes are likely to be carried to completion only when the organisations and the individuals within them are motivated overall by the challenge to succeed, to serve society and to make money.

There are innumerable complex and potentially useful, as well as harmful, substances found in nature, made by animals, plants, bacteria and fungi. Some are themselves useful medicines, others can be used as a starting point by the synthetic chemist, but most new drugs are now synthetic chemicals.

Until the end of the 19th century the discovery of drugs was entirely a matter of chance and serendipity.[2] Paul Ehrlich (1854–1915) put an end to this by developing the idea and the scientific basis for *selective toxicity*.

The whole business of drug development rests on biological *selectivity* and *prediction* of this in man.

PHARMACOLOGY IN DRUG DEVELOPMENT

Most new drugs are developed in industrial rather than in academic laboratories. These two kinds of laboratory are complementary, having important, though different, approaches, the 'organised opportunism' of the industrial and the 'knowledge for its own sake' of the academic laboratory. The academic workers are often fired with interest to use the discoveries of the industrial scientists as tools to explore fundamental mechanisms and indeed industrial discoveries make a major contribution to basic pharmacology as their mechanism of action is probed and defined, e.g. aspirin, cimetidine. The rational development of new drugs by industry is easier when the fundamental biochemical nature of normal and

diseased processes is understood: e.g. the development of histamine receptor blockers depended on knowledge that histamine was released in the body and was a mediator in urticaria, hay fever and normal gastric acid secretion; the efficacy of allopurinol in gout could be predicted from knowledge of the path of synthesis of uric acid in the body. Cures for human cancer are more likely to be found if details of the biochemistry of malignant and normal cells are understood than by empirically testing tens of thousands of chemicals selected at random or because they are related to existing relatively unselective and inefficient anticancer drugs.

The most frequent purpose of research in the drug industry can be stated simply; it is to discover profitable drugs. For a drug to be profitable it should be both useful and safe, properties that are evaluated eventually by the clinician. The task of the pharmacologist is to predict these properties from animal experiments, within the limitations imposed by availability of facilities and staff. This must be done in such a way that the possibility of missing a useful drug is minimised; in other words, the 'screening' programme must be efficient.[3]

The greatest difficulties for the laboratory pharmacologist lie in designing animal experiments to yield the maximum information from a relatively few animals, and to be relevant to human physiology and disease. It is, for example, particularly difficult to design animal experiments to test drugs for their possible efficacy in human mental disorders, but relatively easy to test them for anticoagulant effects because animal and human blood clots by similar mechanisms and because measurement of clotting is easy.

At long last the scientific study of molecular structure and pharmacological action allows the claim that drugs may actually be *designed* and *purpose-made* reasonably frequently.

The principal approaches to drug discovery

1. *Synthesis of analogues, agonists or antagonists*, of natural hormone, autacoid or transmitter

---

[1] One substantial research-based compass (Janssen) made, over 32 years (1953–85), approximately 70 000 new molecules of which, in 1985, 50 were in use as human and 14 as veterinary medicines; 5 as antimycotics for plants; and one for wood protection. The company's biological screening system was capable of making 'go or no-go' decisions at a rate of 25 new molecules per working day, i.e. up to 5000 per year (Dr Paul Janssen, personal communication, 1985).
  Medicinal drugs produced by this company include, diphenoxylate, loperamide, domperidone, ketanserin, haloperidol, dextromoramide, cinnarizine, miconazole and mebendazole.
[2] Serendipity is the faculty of making fortunate discoveries by general sagacity or by accident: the word derives from a fairy tale about three princes of Serendip (Sri Lanka) who had this happy faculty.

---

[3] Vane J R. In: Laurence D R, Bacharach A L, eds. Evaluation of drug activities. London: Academic Press, 1963.

substances, or of molecules that modify understood biochemical process, may create real novelty in therapeutics, e.g. histamine H_2-receptor blocking drugs, dopamine agonists and antagonists, calcium channel blockers, and prostaglandins. The successes of this approach provide strong arguments for society to support research in the basic medical sciences, for to know how the body works normally and how it goes wrong (disease) allows rationally planned interference that may enhance the health and happiness of mankind (the fact that well-meant attempts can go badly wrong provides an argument for more and better science, not for giving up and stopping research).

2. *Modification of the structures of known drugs* is obviously likely to produce more agents with similar properties or only minor differences, and this is much complained of ('*me-too*' or '*me-again*' drugs). But molecular design, aided by computer modelling, is now so sophisticated that it is possible to take a molecule and eliminate one or more actions and enhance another to produce novel, selective results. Sulphonamides (antimicrobials), sulphonylureas (antidiabetics), thiazides (diuretics), acetazolamide (carbonic anhydrase inhibition for glaucoma), are all derived from the first sulphonamides synthesised in the early 1930s.

3. *Random screening*. When completely novel chemicals are made and unfamiliar substances isolated from natural sources there is a case for screening them in a battery of animal tests designed to detect 'interesting' effects. Such screening is now highly sophisticated.

4. *Discovery of new uses for drugs already in general use* as a result of intelligent observation and serendipity, e.g. β-adrenoceptor block for hypertension, aspirin for antithrombotic effect.

THE PROCESS OF NEW DRUG DEVELOPMENT

The process of new drug development may be summarised as follows:

- Idea or hypothesis
- Synthesis of substances
- Studies in animals[4]

Studies in animals

1. Pharmacodynamics
   The actions relevant to the proposed therapeutic use, and other effects at that dose.
2. Pharmacokinetics
   How the drug is distributed in and disposed of by the body.
3. Toxicology
   Whether and how the drug causes injury.
   (a) Single dose studies (acute toxicity).
   (b) Repeated dose studies (subacute, intermediate and chronic or long-term toxicology).
   (c) Duration of repeated-dose studies:

INTENDED DURATION OF USE IN MAN	DURATION OF STUDIES IN ANIMALS
Single dose (or several doses on one day)	14 days
up to 10 days	28 days
up to 30 days	90 days
beyond 30 days	180 days

4. Special toxicology
   Interaction of drug with genetic material.
   (a) Mutagenicity. A bacterial mutagenicity test which demonstrates the induction of point mutations (base-pair changes and frame-shift mutations) is always required. Some mutations result in the development of cancer.
   (b) Definitive carcinogenicity (oncogenicity) tests are not required prior to the early studies in man unless there is serious reason to be suspicious of the drugs, e.g. the mutagenicity test is unsatisfactory; the structure, including likely metabolites in man, gives rise to suspicion; or the histopathology in repeated-dose animal studies is suspicious.

Full scale (most of the animals' life) carcinogenicity tests will generally only be required if the drug is to be given to man for above one year.

It has been pointed out that the strongest ev-

---

[4] Mouse, rat, hamster, guinea pig, rabbit, cat, dog, monkey. Not all are used for any one drug.

idence that a compound is a carcinogenic hazard for man is epidemiological; that although most known human carcinogens are also carcinogenic for experimental animals, there are many substances that are carcinogenic for animals but which have not been found to be carcinogenic for man; and that extrapolation to man is a difficult, sometimes arbitrary procedure.

It may be asked why any novel compound should be given to man before full-scale formal carcinogenicity studies are completed. The answers are that animal tests are uncertain predictors (above), that such a requirement would make socially desirable drug development expensive to a seriously damaging degree, or might even cause novel ventures to cease. This would be caused by both delay and the cost of the greatly increased number of tests that would have to be done on compounds that are eventually abandoned for other reasons. This may seem right or wrong, but it is how things are at present.

(c) Reproduction studies are conducted to detect:

- damage to male and female gametes
- effects on intrauterine homeostasis
- embryogenesis
- toxic effect on the fetus
- effects on maternal metabolism damaging to the fetus
- effects on uterine growth and development
- effects on parturition
- effects on postnatal development, suckling of the young and maternal lactation
- late effects on the progeny, e.g. behaviour, fertility
- second generation effects.

It is plain that this is a major laboratory exercise.

Ethics of using animals in drug development[5]

No one will read the above scheme with satisfac-

tion and some will read it with disgust. Many tests in drug development are done on anaesthetised animals and many on isolated organs of animals killed 'humanely', and increasingly on tissue cultures. But it is not yet possible to replace the whole animal with its intact integrated physiological systems.

All this would be totally unjustified if results useful to man could not be obtained. In many known respects animals are similar to man, but in many respects they are not.

As knowledge of basic mechanisms advances, in vitro biochemical preparations and tissue cultures may one day allow prediction of what effect a drug will have in intact man, and tests on whole animals will not be required. This time is a long way off, for cells in tissue culture develop characteristics, e.g. new receptors, that they did not have when subject to the control mechanisms of the body. However, we welcome research designed to reduce the need to use animals.

PREDICTION: PHARMACOLOGY, TOXICOLOGY

It is frequently pointed out that regulatory guidelines are not rigid requirements to be universally applied. But whatever the intention, they do tend to be treated as minimum requirements if only because research directors fear to risk holding up their expensive coordinated programmes with disagreements that result in their having to go back to the laboratory, with consequent delay and financial loss.

Knowledge of the *mode of action* of a potential new drug obviously greatly enhances prediction from animal studies of what will happen in man. Whenever practicable such knowledge should be obtained; sometimes this is quite easy, but sometimes it is impossible. Many drugs have been introduced safely without such knowledge, the later acquisition of which has not always made an important difference to their use, e.g. antibiotics. The mechanisms of therapeutic action of drugs in many areas remains obscure, e.g. psychiatry, and any requirement that it be defined before exploratory clinical use could delay valuable therapeutic advance.

---

[5] An admirable discussion of the issues will be found in Paton W. Man and mouse. London: Oxford, 1984 and in Zbinden G. Alternatives to animal experimentation. Trends in Pharmacological Sciences 1990; 11: 104.

But in many areas, a lot that is relevant to prediction of effects in man can be discovered, and so should be required before clinical trial, e.g. antihypertensives, anticoagulants, β-adrenoceptor blocking drugs. In the development of new drugs, there can be no immutable rule. But failure to take this matter seriously can lead to disaster, e.g. a drug may lower the plasma lipids, but if this is at a late stage of lipid synthesis, it may be at the cost of accumulation of precursors that may themselves be damaging. On the other hand, to refuse to allow clinical investigation of a potential antiepileptic, antipsychotic, anaesthetic or antibiotic where the developer had found himself unable to define the precise mode of action would be perverse.

The pharmacological studies are integrated with those of the toxicologist to build up a picture of the undesired as well as of the desired drug effects.

Generally, in *pharmacological testing* the investigators know what they are looking for and choose the experiments to gain their objectives.

But in *toxicological testing* the investigators have less clear ideas of what they are looking for; they are screening for risk, unexpected as well as expected, and certain major routines must be done. Toxicity testing is therefore liable to become mindless routine to meet regulatory requirements to a greater extent than are the pharmacological studies.

All drugs are poisons if enough is given and the task of the toxicologist is to find out whether, where and how a compound acts as a poison to animals, and to give an opinion on the significance of the data in relation to risks likely to be run by human beings. This will remain a nearly impossible task until biochemical explanations of all effects can be provided. The toxicologist is in an unenviable position. When a useful drug is safely introduced he is considered to have done no more than his duty. When an accident occurs he is invited to explain how this failure of prediction came about. When he predicts that a chemical is unsafe in a major way for man, his prediction is never tested.

Acute toxicity tests are performed to determine the adverse effects of increasing single doses and how death is caused. They are also used to establish what is unsuitably called the *therapeutic index* or ratio. This concept was devised by Ehrlich as: maximum tolerated dose ÷ minimum curative dose (see p. 78). In a drug development laboratory practical use can be made of a modification of this concept provided it is recognised that, as with all animal data, it cannot be arbitrarily transferred to man. The *therapeutic index for animals* is nowadays calculated as: plasma concentration causing adverse effect ÷ plasma concentration causing therapeutic effect. The objective is to get some notion of benefit : risk ratio.

But it is more important to discover *how* the compound acts as a poison and this may need microscopical and biochemical studies with repeated or chronic administration.

Species differences between animals, and between animals and man, are a source of problems of interpretation. A famous species difference is the lethal bleeding from the intestine of guinea pigs following penicillin administration (due to an effect on the gut bacteria on which obligatory vegetarian species rely to break down cellulose) and its almost negligible toxicity to non-herbivores, including man.

Fortunately such differences of the effect of a drug on the body (pharmacodynamics) are less common than are differences in the effect of the body on a drug (pharmacokinetics), but gross differences in rate or path of metabolism may make nonsense of *chronic toxicity studies* undertaken to predict toxicity to man, as may unanticipated environmental influences, e.g. drug metabolising enzyme induction due to insecticide used routinely in an animal house for pest control.

It is clear that many common unwanted effects that limit the use of a drug in man cannot be predicted from animals, e.g. malaise and many cardiovascular and central nervous system symptoms. Nor, at present, can allergic reactions, e.g. some blood disorders and urticaria.

Special toxicology testing (above) involves three areas in which a drug accident might occur on a substantial scale. All are concerned with the interaction of the drug with genetic material or its expression in cell division (reproduction, mutagenesis, oncogenesis).

In all three areas there is particular concern because the effect may be delayed and hard to recognise at an early stage and may be the same as natural disease so that it is particularly difficult reliably to identify its cause.

1. Reproduction, including fertility and teratogenesis (Greek: *teratos* = monster; *genesis* = production) (see p. 130). Extensive testing of new drugs in pregnant animals has been mandatory since the thalidomide disaster. At first, administration of the drug in early pregnancy in two animal species was thought sufficient. But now animal tests are much more extensive. How far such tests, especially when giving positive results only at high dose, provide genuine prediction and so protection for humanity remains uncertain. But as a consequence of thalidomide regulatory authorities closely control this area.

This problem of predicting from animal experiments what new substances will cause fetal damage in man, when there is not even a reliable list of existing drugs that have the effect in man to provide a guide to devising animal tests, will be neither easily nor soon solved. Two illustrations suffice — it has been found that salicylates are teratogenic in rats. There is no reason to believe salicylates to be seriously teratogenic in man at present, though aspirin is not clear of suspicion. Some adrenal steroids are highly teratogenic in rabbits, but do not appear to be so in man.

2. Mutagenesis. Drugs may cause abnormalities of genetic material (genes, chromosomes) of cells so that a permanent change in the hereditary constitution (mutation) occurs.

When a mutation occurs in reproductive cells (spermatozoa, ova) then a hereditary defect occurs. This defect may appear in the first generation progeny of the individual, or it may be of a recessive kind that will only become evident if two individuals affected by the chemical mutagen mate. Thus the effect of a mutagenic drug might not appear for months or even years or might even go unrecognised. The longer the interval the more difficult attribution of the true cause is likely to be.

Where a mutation occurs in somatic (non-reproductive) cells, then these tissues, e.g. bone marrow cells, may develop abnormal characteristics and become malignant; in the case of the bone marrow this is leukaemia. In this area of risk too, it can be difficult to establish a causal association with the drug, which may have been taken and then stopped a long time previously; there is some hope of doing so where an effect is dramatic in frequency or in kind, but where there is merely a moderate increase in the incidence of a common condition then there is little prospect of detecting it and finding the cause.

Epidemiological rather than experimental laboratory techniques are required to determine what *is* happening in man rather than what *might* be happening. Medical record-linkage schemes are being developed so that it will become possible to examine, e.g. the drug history of all patients having a particular disease; also prescription monitoring so that the medical history of those taking a particular drug can be studied.

It is known that in appropriate experimental situations anticancer drugs, nitrite ion (used as a food preservative, or produced in the body), caffeine (coffee) and ionising radiation can be mutagenic, as also may be habitual tobacco smoking.

What is not known is how much hazard, if any, these pose to man in the actual conditions of ordinary life. At present no systematic monitoring of populations for mutations is taking place, except insofar as birth defect and cancer registries may be recording effects of mutation.

3. Carcinogenesis. Malignant and benign tumours occur spontaneously and can also be induced by drugs and other chemicals, sometimes as a result of mutation. The possibility of malignant tumours being caused by drugs (carcinogenesis) is a major concern.

The topic is extremely complex and controversial.

There are two important stages in carcinogenesis — initiation and promotion. Thus two substances may be necessary to cause cancer, an initiator and a promoter. But virtually any irritant substance seems to be carcinogenic in animals

---

[6] Moore G E et al. JAMA 1977; 238: 397. The authors advised the government to consider banning money as unsafe.

under the right experimental conditions. Glass, platinum foil, plastics (credit cards), American dimes[6] and strong glucose solutions have been found to be carcinogenic in animals.

Cytotoxic anticancer drugs are carcinogenic in both animals and man; they are usually also teratogenic and mutagenic.

Carcinogens may act directly on cells or secondarily through changes in the hormone balance of the body.

Where a drug is under suspicion then *case control studies* (see index) become practicable.

It might be thought reasonable that a drug should be banned if it comes under the slightest suspicion of carcinogenicity or mutagenicity. But slight suspicions are easy to arouse and hard to verify. Possibly definitive investigations are so enormously time-consuming and expensive that, when suspicion is only slight, it becomes impossible to assert that 'where safety is concerned expense is no object'. Precipitate action on only slight suspicion (especially that aroused by limited laboratory experiments in animals) is likely to do more harm than good in disrupting medical practice without corresponding benefit to patients. When a useful drug is under consideration to be banned it is necessary to consider the alternatives that replace it and whether there is adequate knowledge of them; commonly there is not. This may at first sight seem a callous attitude but a blind 'safety at all costs' approach, in these as in many other areas of life, may in fact incur costs in deprivation of benefits, costs that are excessive even in these important and emotionally charged areas (see isotretinoin).

Until the science is more developed it should probably remain the case that carcinogenicity testing is sometimes demanded and sometimes not, and that a simple mutagenicity test is always required.

DRUG QUALITY

It is easy for an investigator or prescriber, interested in pharmacology, toxicology and therapeutics, to forget the fundamental importance of chemical and pharmaceutical aspects. An impure, unstable drug is useless. Pure drugs that remain pure drugs after 5 years of storage in hot, damp climates are vital to therapeutics. The record of manufacturers in providing this is impressive.

CONCLUSION ON PRE-CLINICAL TESTING

As drugs are developed and promoted for long-term use in more and relatively trivial conditions, e.g. minor anxiety or slight high blood pressure, and affluent societies become less and less willing to tolerate small physical or mental discomforts, demanding relief without even minor inconvenience, drug therapy will continue to increase and the problem of predicting not only the efficacy, but also the safety of drugs, will grow. Only profound knowledge of biochemical mechanisms will eliminate risk in the introduction of new drugs, and this is a long way off. In the meantime failures of prediction will continue to occur.

Limited resources of scientific manpower and money will not be used to the best advantage if the public shock over thalidomide (p. 65) and subsequent events is allowed to express itself in governmental regulations requiring a plethora of expensive tests (and toxicity testing is very expensive), many of them of dubious meaning for anything other than the animal concerned. Such a policy would prevent industrial laboratories from devoting resources to investigation of fundamental mechanisms of drug action, in the knowledge of which alone lies health with safety.

This account of pre-clinical drug development, largely stressing the difficulties and the imponderables, may be put into perspective (before we proceed to evaluation in man) by the following figures on the general safety of drugs in relation to *fatal accidents* and to *smoking* (per annum) in recent times in the UK (pop. 57 million).

DEATHS DUE TO:	
therapeutic use of drugs (named on death certificate)	40–50
accident in the home	6000
motor vehicle accidents	5500
malignant pulmonary neoplasms	28 000

When the pre-clinical testing has been completed to the satisfaction of the developer, of the national regulatory agency, and of the clinical investigator who will carry the programme forward, the time has come to administer the drug to man and so to launch the experimental programme that will decide whether the drug is only a drug or whether it is also a medicine. This is the subject of the next chapter.

ORPHAN DRUGS

A free market economy is liable to leave untreated, rare diseases, e.g. some cancers (in all countries) and some common diseases, e.g. parasitic infections (in poor countries).

Where a drug is not developed into a usable medicine because the costs will not be recovered by the developer then it is known as an *orphan drug*, and the disease is an *orphan disease*; the sufferer is a *health orphan*.

The remedy for these situations lies in government itself undertaking drug development (which is liable to be inefficient) or in government-offered incentives, e.g. tax relief, exclusive marketing rights, to pharmaceutical companies; and in the case of poor countries, international aid programmes; such programmes are being implemented.

GUIDE TO FURTHER READING

Black J W 1986 Pharmacology: analysis and exploration. British Medical Journal 293: 252

Brodie B B 1972 Difficulties in extrapolating data on metabolism of drugs from animal to man. Clinical Pharmacology and Therapeutics 3: 374

Editorial 1983 Doctors and the drug industry. British Medical Journal 286: 579

Hillman A L et al 1991 Avoiding bias in the conduct and reporting of cost-effectiveness: research sponsored by pharmaceutical companies. New England Journal of Medicine 324: 1362

Lasagna L 1982 Will all new drugs become orphans? Clinical Pharmacology and Therapeutics 31: 285

Lasagna L 1987 On assuring pharmacotherapeutic progress in the 21st century. British Journal of Clinical Pharmacology 23: 659

Lis Y et al 1989 Novel medicines marketed in the UK (1960–87). British Journal of Clinical Pharmacology 28: 333

Mattison N et al 1988 New drug development in the United States, 1963 through 1984. Clinical Pharmacology and Therapeutics 43: 290

Melmon K L 1976 The clinical pharmacologist and scientifically unsound regulations for drug development. Clinical Pharmacology and Therapeutics 20: 125

Orme M et al 1989 Healthy volunteer studies in Great Britain: the results of a survey into 12 months activity in this field. British Journal of Clinical Pharmacology 27: 125

Schrogie J J et al 1977 Evaluation of the prison inmate as a subject in drug assessment. Clinical Pharmacology and Therapeutics 21: 1

Tishler M 1973 Drug discovery — background and foreground. Clinical Pharmacology and Therapeutics 14: 479

Weatherall M 1982 An end to the search for new drugs? Nature 296: 387

4

Evaluation of drugs in man: therapeutic trials

SYNOPSIS

New drugs are gradually introduced via clinical pharmacological studies in rising numbers of healthy and/or patient volunteers until enough information has been gained to justify a formal therapeutic study. This is usually a randomised controlled trial where a precisely framed question is posed and answered by treating equivalent groups of patients in different ways.

The key to the ethics of such studies is informed consent by patients, efficient scientific design and review by an independent Research Ethics Committee. The key interpretative factors in the analysis of trial results are calculations of confidence intervals and of statistical significance.

Finally, surveillance studies detect rare adverse effects and allow accurate comparisons of safety; they also define patterns of drug use in the community.

- Rational introduction of a new drug to man
- Experimental therapeutics
- The need for statistics
- Therapeutic trial design
- Ethics of research in man
- Interpretative factors: Statistical significance, Confidence intervals, Types of error
- The size of a therapeutic trial
- What difference can be measured?
- Double-blind and single-blind techniques
- Placebo medication as a control
- Within- and between-patient studies
- Some mortal sins of clinical assessment
- Pharmacoepidemiology
- Reliability of published therapeutic trials

INTRODUCTION

When studies in animals predict that a new chemical may be a useful medicine, i.e. effective and safe in relation to its benefits, then the time has come to put it to the test in man.

We devote substantial space to clinical evaluation of drugs for the reasons given at the start of Chapter 3 and because the topic provides an exercise in logical thinking that must benefit all who have to choose therapy for patients.

When the new chemical entity offers a possibility of doing something that has not been done before or of doing something familiar in a different way, it can be seen to be worth testing. But where it is a new member of a familiar class of drug, potential advantage may be harder to see. Yet these 'me-too' drugs are often worth testing. Prediction from animal studies of modest but useful clinical advantage is uncertain and therefore if the new drug seems reasonably effective and safe in animals it is also reasonable to test it in man. The point has been put cogently: 'it is possible to waste too much time in animal studies before testing a drug in man'.[1] Though satisfactory both qualitatively and quantitatively in animals, it may be useless in man solely because its duration of action is too short or too long, so that

the practice of studying the physiologic disposition of a drug in man only after it is clearly the drug of choice in animals not only may prove short-sighted

---

[1] Brodie B B. Clin Pharmacol Ther 1962; 3: 374.

and time consuming, but also may result in relegating the best drug for man to the shelf for evermore.[1]

RATIONAL INTRODUCTION OF A NEW DRUG TO MAN

This proceeds in a commonsense manner that is conventionally divided into four phases.

These phases are divisions of convenience in what is a continuous extending process beginning with a single subject closely observed in the laboratory and proceeding to tens of subjects (healthy subjects and volunteer patients) through hundreds of patients, to thousands before the drug is agreed to be a medicine by a national or regional regulatory authority and is licensed for general prescribing. The process may be abandoned at any stage. The phases may be defined as follows:

Phase 1 Clinical pharmacology (20–50 subjects)

— Healthy volunteers or patients, according to class of drug and its safety
— Pharmacokinetics (absorption, distribution, metabolism, excretion)
— Pharmacodynamics (biological effects) where practicable; tolerance; safety; efficacy.

Phase 2 Clinical investigation (50–300)

— Patients
— Pharmacokinetics; pharmacodynamics, dose-ranging in expanding, carefully controlled studies for efficacy and safety.

Phase 3 Formal therapeutic trials
(randomised controlled trials; 250–1000+)

— Efficacy on a substantial scale; safety; comparison with other drugs.

Phase 4 Post-licensing (marketing) studies (2000–10 000+)

— Surveillance for safety and efficacy: further formal therapeutic trials, including comparisons with other drugs.

Official regulatory guidelines for studies in man

These ordinarily include:

● Studies of *pharmacokinetics* and (when other manufacturers have similar products) of *bioequivalence* (equal bioavailability between products used for the same purpose is plainly important).

● *Therapeutic trials* (reported in detail) that substantiate the safety and efficacy of the drug under likely conditions of use, e.g. a drug for long-term use in a common condition will require a total of at least 100 patients (preferably more) treated continuously for about one year as well as hundreds more treated for shorter periods. At least three independent trials are likely to be required.

● *Special groups.* If the drug will be used in, e.g. the *elderly*, then elderly people should be studied if there are reasons for thinking they may react to or handle the drug differently.

● *Fixed-dose combination* products will require explicit justification (see p. 102).

● *Interaction studies* with other drugs likely to be taken simultaneously (plainly all possible combinations cannot be evaluated; an intelligent choice, based on knowledge of pharmacodynamics and pharmacokinetics, is made).

● The application for a licence for general use (Product Licence) should include a draft *Data (information) Sheet*[2] for prescribers and sometimes for patients. This should include information on the form of the product (tablet, capsule, sustained release, liquid form, etc), its uses, dosage (adults, children, elderly where appropriate), contraindications (strong recommendation), warnings and precautions (less strong), side-effects/adverse reactions, overdose and how to treat it.

EXPERIMENTAL THERAPEUTICS

As the number of potential medicines produced increases, the problem of who to test them on grows. Clearly there are two main groups, healthy

---

[2] Medicines need instruction manuals just as do domestic appliances.

volunteers, volunteer patients (and, very rarely, non-volunteer patients); it is evident that some drug actions can be demonstrated on healthy people (anticoagulant, anaesthetic) whereas others cannot (antiparkinsonian, antimicrobial) so that to try the latter on healthy volunteers to obtain pharmacokinetic and safety data is to treat man formally as an experimental animal, risking toxicity, however remotely, to obtain information of no benefit to the subject; this is increasingly often done; it poses ethical problems (see p. 46).

Doctors cannot afford to ignore the principles of therapeutic evaluation, for such studies provide the basis of choice of drugs for individual patients, and enable prediction of the outcome of treatment with less uncertainty. It is useful to know a good therapeutic study from a bad, for the latter are common, and both good and bad are thrust at doctors by vested interests. More difficult, some bad studies, previously easily detectable, are now replete with the jargon of the formal therapeutic trial; the terms random allocation, double-blind, statistically significant, and probability, are draped around what on close inspection is seen to be, scientifically, a fraud.

Throughout this book, lists of alternative drugs are given, often without any serious attempt to discriminate between them. The reason for this is that useful discrimination is impossible because it is not easy to find people prepared to carry out detailed comparative trials on closely similar drugs; therefore, non-experimental surveillance techniques that evaluate drugs under conditions of ordinary use are an increasingly important development.

Therapeutic investigations

These employ two classes of endpoint or outcome:

1. *The therapeutic effect itself*, e.g. sleep, eradication of infection, and
2. *A factor related to the therapeutic effect, or surrogate effect* (with varying degrees of certainty), e.g. blood lipids or glucose, or blood pressure; in diseases in which surrogate effects are employed, true therapeutic effect, i.e. healthy life free from

complications, can only be measured by studying large numbers of patients over years. Such long-term studies are indeed necessary, but are impracticable on organisational and financial grounds prior to releasing all new drugs for general prescription. It is in such areas as these that techniques of large-scale surveillance for efficacy, as well as for safety, under conditions of ordinary use, are needed to supplement the necessarily smaller and shorter formal therapeutic trials employing surrogate effects.

Therapeutic evaluation

This is conducted in two principal ways:

- *Formal therapeutic trials* (experimental cohort studies)
- *Surveillance programmes*, e.g. case-control studies, and observational cohort studies (large-scale monitoring for efficacy and/or adverse reactions).

When a new drug is being developed, the first therapeutic trials are devised to find out the best the drug can do under conditions ideal for showing efficacy, e.g. uncomplicated disease of mild-to-moderate severity in patients taking no other drugs, with carefully supervised administration by specialist doctors. Interest lies particularly in patients who complete a full course of treatment. If the drug is ineffective in these circumstances there is no point in proceeding with an expensive development programme. Such studies are sometimes called, a little inappropriately, 'explanatory' trials.

If the drug is found useful in these trials, then it becomes desirable next to find out whether it can be successful and safe in the rough and tumble of routine medical practice, in patients of all ages, at all stages of disease, with complications, taking other drugs and relatively unsupervised. Interest continues in all patients from the moment they are entered into the trial and it is maintained if they fail to complete, or even to start, the treatment, for what is wanted is to know the outcome in all patients deemed suitable for therapy, not only in those who successfully complete it. The reasons some drop out may be related to aspects of the treatment. Such trials are therefore analysed on *intention to treat* rather than on completion of treatment; i.e. the investigator is not allowed to risk introducing bias by exercising his own judgement as to who should or should not be excluded from the analysis.[3] In these real life, or naturalistic, conditions the drug may not perform so well, e.g. minor adverse effects may now cause patient non-compliance which had been avoided by supervision and enthusiasm in the early trials. These naturalistic studies are sometimes called 'pragmatic' trials.

Formal therapeutic trials are expensive and are hard to administer. Surveillance studies are less precise but compensate for this by their convenience and/or large size and closeness to the realities of ordinary medical practice.

Formal therapeutic trials are unlikely to reveal:

- *adverse effects that are uncommon or occur only after prolonged use*, e.g. oral contraceptives and vascular disease; renal damage due to analgesics
- *effects in special population groups*, e.g. pregnancy, renal or hepatic disease, since these are generally excluded, reasonably, from formal therapeutic trials
- *unexpected therapeutic effects*, i.e. potential new uses
- *interactions* between drugs.

Conclusion

Drug evaluation comprises formal therapeutic trials followed by surveillance studies.

Pickering wrote,

... therapeutics is the branch of medicine that, by its very nature, should be experimental. For if we take a patient afflicted with a malady and we alter his conditions of life ... we are performing an experiment. And if we are scientifically minded we should record the results. Before concluding that the change for better or for worse in the patient is due to the specific treatment employed, we must ascertain ... whether the result was merely due to

the natural history of the disease ... or whether it was due to some other factor which was necessarily associated with the therapeutic measure in question. And if, as a result of these procedures we learn that the therapeutic measure employed produces a significant, though not very pronounced improvement, we would experiment with the method, altering dosage or other detail to see if it can be improved. This would seem the procedure to be expected of men with six years of scientific training behind them.

But it has not been followed. Had it been done we should have gained a fairly precise knowledge of the place of individual methods of therapy in disease, and our efficiency as doctors would have been enormously enhanced.[4]

There are some who dislike or reject the notion of deliberate experimentation on the sick, feeling that a scientific approach implies an unsympathetic or even a malevolent disposition. They forget that in the past positively harmful treatments have been widely used for many years (e.g. bleeding for pneumonia) because of the lack of recognition of the need, as well as lack of knowledge of the techniques, of scientific evaluation of therapy. It has been pointed out that where the worth of a treatment, new or old, is in doubt, there may be a greater obligation to test it critically than to go on prescribing it supported only by habit or wishful thinking.

> The choice before doctors is not whether they should experiment on their patients, but whether they should do so in a planned or in a haphazard fashion.

The choice is whether they should try to organise their experience so that it is of value to themselves and to others or to follow the notoriously unreliable 'clinical impression'. The latter is the less ethical course.

Doctors who think they can assess the value of a treatment by using it on patients in an uncontrolled fashion have the whole history of therapeutics against them. It is given to only a few to test a treatment that dramatically alters disease and whose efficacy is obvious with casual use, and even then details of its application will

---

[3] Analysis excluding patients who have failed to complete may also be presented provided the full 'intention to treat' analysis is also displayed.

[4] Pickering G W. Proc Roy Soc Med. 1949; 42: 229.

generally need carefully planned studies, e.g. adrenal steroids in rheumatoid arthritis and asthma, where wrong use may be more dangerous than no use.

Modern scientific techniques uncover the most effective treatments whilst exposing the smallest numbers to the less effective or positively harmful; they save lives, time and money. They are not unethical for they are only properly used when the relative merits of treatments are genuinely uncertain.

Some patients find it hard to put their confidence in a doctor who, openly admitting uncertainty, is using two treatments concurrently in order to achieve a true measure of their relative values. They need the emotional security that is provided by doctors who behave as though they know, indeed, who sometimes themselves believe they know, even though patients may rightly suspect that there are others of equal authority who take an opposite view.

Though the 'statistical therapeutic comparison' or 'formal therapeutic trial' or 'randomised controlled trial,' discussed below, is a powerful tool for advancing therapy, it does not suit every occasion. Sometimes, as in malaria or diabetes, there are clinical or laboratory tests that will rapidly tell whether a treatment is effective, though they may not provide evidence of a marginal difference between effective drugs, and in tuberculous meningitis a single recovery was considered adequate evidence of therapeutic efficacy.

THE NEED FOR STATISTICS

In order to decide whether patients treated in one way are benefited more than those treated in another, there is no possibility of avoiding the use of numbers. The mere statement by a clinician that patients do better with this or that treatment is due to his having formed an opinion that more patients are helped by the treatment advocated than by other treatments. The opinion is based on numbers, but having omitted to record exactly how many patients have been treated by different methods and having omitted to ensure that the only variable factor affecting the patient was the treatment in question, only a 'clinical impression', instead of facts, can be stated. This is a pity, for progress is delayed when convinced opinions are offered in place of convincing facts.

Statistics may be defined as 'a body of methods for making wise decisions in the face of uncertainty'.[5] Used properly, it is a tool of great value for promoting efficient therapy.

Over 100 years ago Francis Galton saw this clearly.

In our general impressions far too great weight is attached to what is marvellous. . . . Experience warns us against it, and the scientific man takes care to base his conclusions upon actual numbers. The human mind is . . . a most imperfect apparatus for the elaboration of general ideas. . . . General impressions are never to be trusted. Unfortunately when they are of long standing they become fixed rules of life, and assume a prescriptive right not to be questioned. Consequently, those who are not accustomed to original enquiry entertain a hatred and a horror of statistics. They cannot endure the idea of submitting their sacred impressions to cold-blooded verification. But it is the triumph of scientific men to rise superior to such superstitions, to devise tests by which the value of beliefs may be ascertained, and to feel sufficiently masters of themselves to discard contemptuously whatever may be found untrue . . . the frequent incorrectness of notions derived from general impressions may be assumed. . . .[6]

THERAPEUTIC TRIAL DESIGN (the randomised controlled trial: general aspects)

The aims of a therapeutic trial, not all of which can be attempted on any one occasion, are to decide the following:

- whether a treatment is of value
- how great its value is (compared with other remedies, if such exist)
- in what types of patients it is of value
- what is the best method of applying the treatment; how often, and in what dosage if it is a drug
- what are the disadvantages and dangers of the treatment.

---

[5] Wallis W A et al. Statistics, a new approach. London: Methuen, 1957.
[6] Galton F. Generic images. Proceedings of the Royal Institution, 1879.

Bradford Hill[7] defines the therapeutic trial as a carefully, and ethically, designed experiment with the aim of answering some *precisely framed question*. In its most rigorous form it demands *equivalent groups* of patients *concurrently treated* in different ways. These groups are constructed by the *random allocation* of patients to one or other treatment. . . . In principle the method is applicable with any disease and any treatment. It may also be applied on any scale; it does not necessarily demand large numbers of patients.

This is the classic randomised controlled trial.

Three important points in the above definition may be stressed.

Equivalent groups of patients

If the treatment groups differ significantly in age, sex, race, duration of disease, severity of disease or in any other possibly relevant factor, it will not be possible to attribute differences in outcome to the treatment under investigation, unless there is some way of eliminating the bias that has entered. The best way of getting equivalent groups is by allotting patients to them by *random allocation*.[8]

The function of randomisation is to eliminate systematic biases, known (personal judgements of clinicians or patients) or unknown, that could affect assignment to treatment.

To allot patients alternately or otherwise systematically is not satisfactory as investigators almost inevitably know into what treatment group a patient will go whilst engaged in deciding whether the patient should enter the trial, and may be unconsciously influenced by this if they have strong feelings about either the patient or the value of the respective treatments. With random allocations in sealed envelopes the treatment groups into which the patients go are only discovered after it has been decided to enter them into the trial.

[7] Bradford Hill A. Principles of medical statistics. London: Hodder and Stoughton, 1977.
[8] It is not necessary to have equal numbers in each group, especially if the natural history of the disease is well known, when a 2:1 ratio can be used instead of the usual 1:1. Random number series can be adapted to provide unequal groups or allocation may be devised to change during the trial so that more patients are progressively allocated to the most successful treatment — 'play the winner' allocation.

Time and place of treatments

Treatments must be carried out concurrently (at the same time) and concomitantly (at the same place) for the reasons given above and because diseases may vary in severity with time and place.

Thus controls from the past (*historical controls*) are nearly always unacceptable.

Precisely framed question

Before commencing any therapeutic trial it is essential to formulate exactly the question that is to be answered. For example: 'Is drug X capable of relieving the pain of osteoarthrosis more or less completely, with greater or fewer side-effects and for a shorter or longer time than is drug Y?' The question should be as simple as possible, for to try to discover too much can be a cause of failure, and it should be kept in mind throughout the whole process of designing the trial. Neglect to set down at the start exactly what is the objective of the study invites failure.

ETHICS OF RESEARCH IN MAN (and particularly of the randomised controlled trial)

Modern medicine is accused of callous application of science to human problems. Official regulatory bodies rightly require scientific evaluation of drugs. Drug developers need to satisfy the regulators and they also seek to persuade an increasingly sophisticated medical profession to prescribe their products. For these reasons scientific drug evaluation as described here is likely to increase in volume and more and more doctors will be personally involved.

Therefore we provide discussion of the ethics of medical research in man.

Research involving human subjects

This may be:
- **therapeutic**: that which may actually have a therapeutic effect or provide information that can be used to help the participating subjects;
- **non-therapeutic**: that which provides information that cannot be of direct use to them,

e.g. healthy volunteers always and patients sometimes.

The right to choose

Potential research subjects have the right to choose for themselves whether or not they will participate in research, i.e. they have the right to autonomy. They should be given whatever information is necessary for making an informed choice (consent). The issue of *consent* bulks large in discussions of the ethics of human experimentation and is a principal concern of the Research Ethics Committees that are now the norm in medical research.

Some dislike the word 'experiment' in relation to man, thinking that its mere use implies a degree of impropriety in what is done. It is better, however, that all should recognise the true meaning of the word, 'to ascertain or establish by trial',[9] that the benefits of modern medicine derive wholly from experimentation and that some risk, however slight, is inseparable from medical advance. The duty of all doctors lies in ensuring that in their desire to help patients in general they should never allow themselves to put the individual who has sought their aid at any disadvantage, for 'the scientist or physician has no right to choose martyrs for society',[10] i.e. the ethical principle of *non-maleficence*.

Physicians deal with individuals and have sometimes argued against the statistical therapeutic trial that it does not tell what will happen to any one individual who consults them. This is obviously true, but the knowledge gained from such studies that, with a treatment, $x\%$ recover, $y\%$ improve and $z\%$ are unchanged, with details of unwanted effects, provides a better basis for the choice of therapy for individuals than the often divergent clinical impressions of doctors.

It is, of course, only proper to perform a therapeutic trial when the doctors genuinely do not know which treatment is best, and if they are prepared to withdraw individual patients or to stop the whole trial if at any time they become convinced that it is in the patients' interest to do so.

If it is not known whether one treatment is better than another, then nothing is lost by allotting patients at random to those treatments under test, and it is in everybody's interest that good treatments should be adopted and bad treatments abandoned as soon as possible. It is, of course, more difficult to justify testing a new treatment when existing treatments are good than when they are bad, and this difficulty is likely to grow. It involves weighing the needs of future patients who may benefit from the results of a study against those of the patients who are taking part, some of whom will receive new (and possibly less effective) treatment, i.e. the principle of *justice*.

The randomised controlled trial, particularly, has been subject to ethical criticism. Objections have always, often justly, been raised to the conduct of individual randomised controlled trials, but of recent years these have been extended to the principles on which such trials are based.

The interaction of ethical and scientific issues

This has been well summarised in a Report:[11]

An analysis of the ethical problems of therapeutic trials might begin with a question long familiar to moral philosophy: what is the nature and degree of certitude required for an ethical decision? More precisely, *is there any ethically relevant difference between the use of statistical methods and the use of other ways of knowing, such as experience, common sense, guessing, etc? When decisions are to be made in uncertainty, is it more or less ethical to choose and abide by statistical methods of defining 'certitude' than to be guided by one's hunch or striking experience?* These questions are raised by the assertion that it is ethically imperative to conclude a clinical trial when a 'trend' appears. . . . . . . the choice of statistical methods can constitute in many circumstances an acceptable ethical approach to the problem of decision in uncertainty.

As physician-investigators seek knowledge about safety and efficacy of medicines, which is a social good, the dignity of individuals must not be overridden. The therapeutic trial is both ethically required for the social good of more effective

---

[9] Oxford English Dictionary.
[10] Kety S. Quoted by Beecher H K. JAMA 1959; 169: 461.

[11] Eur J Clin Pharmacol 1980; 18: 129.

medical care and is capable of being designed in ways which respect the wellbeing and rights of individual participants.

Conclusion

The objective must be that no patient should be worse off than he might have been in the hands of a reasonable and competent physician.

INTERPRETATIVE FACTORS

Hypothesis of no difference

When it is suspected that treatment A may be superior to treatment B and it is wished to find out the truth it is convenient, and only seemingly eccentric, to set about it by testing the hypothesis that the treatments are equally effective, or ineffective, as the case may be — the 'no difference' hypothesis (*null hypothesis*). Thus, when two groups of patients have been treated (between patient comparison) or each patient has had a course of each drug (within-patient comparison) and it has been found that improvement has occurred more often with one treatment than with the other, it is necessary to decide how likely it is that this difference is due to a real superiority of one treatment over the other.

Statistical significance

A statistical significance test[12] will tell how often a difference of the observed size would occur due to chance (random influences) if there is, in reality, no difference between the treatments. If the result of the test is that the observed difference is unlikely where there is truly no difference between treatments, then we need to know what degree of assurance, or confidence, we may have in the precision or power of this estimate, i.e. we need to know the confidence interval.

Confidence intervals

Confidence intervals are expressed as a range of values within which we may be 95% (or other chosen %) certain that the true value lies. The range may be broad, indicating uncertainty, or narrow, indicating (relative) certainty.

Confidence intervals reveal the precision of an estimate. A wide confidence interval points to a lack of information, whether the difference is statistically significant or not, and is a warning (against placing much weight on, or confidence in, the results of small studies.) Confidence intervals are extremely helpful in interpretation, particularly of small studies, as they show *the degree of uncertainty related to a result* — such as the difference between two means — whether or not it was statistically significant. Their use in conjunction with non-significant results may be especially enlightening.[12]

A finding of *not statistically significant* can only be interpreted as meaning there is no clinically useful difference if the *confidence interval* of the result is also stated in the report and is narrow. If the confidence interval is wide a real difference may have been missed in a trial of the size performed. Small numbers of patients inevitably give low precision.

Types of error

Confidence intervals provide us with information on the likelihood of falling into one of the two kinds of error of therapeutic experiments:

- *Type I error*, i.e. finding a difference between treatments when in reality they do not differ.
- *Type II error*, i.e. finding no difference between treatments when in reality they do differ to an extent doctors would want to know about — the *target* difference.

It is up to the clinician to decide the *target difference* and what probability level (for either type of error) he will accept if he is to use the result as a guide to action; this the statistical significance test alone cannot tell him.

The statistical tests do not prove that a difference is due to one treatment being better than another or not better than another, as the case may be, they merely provide probabilities.

[12] Altman D et al. Br Med J 1983; 286: 1489.

A difference may be statistically significant and have a narrow confidence interval but may be clinically unimportant.

Some detail further explaining the above

Statistical significance. In clinical practice most agree that if the statistical significance test shows that, the no-difference hypothesis being true, a difference as large as that observed would only occur five times if the experiment were repeated 100 times, then this is acceptable as sufficient evidence that the null hypothesis is unlikely to be true (but not impossible), i.e. that there is a real difference between the treatments. This level of probability is generally expressed in therapeutic trials as, the difference was 'statistically significant' 'significant at the 5% level' or 'P[13] = 0.05'. Statistical significance simply means, unlikely result if there is no genuine treatment difference.

If the analysis reveals that, the no-difference hypothesis being true, the observed difference, or greater, would only occur *once* if the experiment were repeated 100 times, the results are generally said to be 'statistically highly significant', 'significant at the 1% level' or '$P = 0.01$'.

Confidence intervals. Plainly trials should be devised to have adequate *precision* or *power*, i.e. an at least 80% chance of detecting the defined useful target effect within narrow confidence limits, at 5% statistical significance ($P = 0.05$). It is not worth starting a trial that has less than a 50% chance of achieving the set objective, because the power of the trial is too low; but such small trials are frequently done and published without any statement of power or confidence interval, which would reveal their inadequacy. What is required in trial reports are statements such as the following:

1. the observed difference between the treatment groups is not *statistically significant* ($P > 0.05$) but this result is compatible (95% confidence interval) with there being a real difference between the treatments with a range as wide as + 30% to − 20%, i.e. almost as large in the opposite direction, which wide range means the trial is useless as a guide to action; not only is the range wide, but it spans zero.

2. the observed difference between the treatment groups is *statistically significant* ($P < 0.05$), but this result is compatible with there being a real difference with a range of 2–35% (same direction). With such a wide range the trial may be thought inadequate, e.g. the target (useful) difference may have been set at 20%.

But where the range is narrow, 30–38%, it is above the target difference (20%) and so is clinically important as well as statistically significant; then the trial will be thought to give reliable information that may (provided it is independently confirmed) provide a basis for action.

THE SIZE OF A THERAPEUTIC TRIAL

Before starting a therapeutic trial it is necessary to decide when it should stop.

The number of patients required for a therapeutic trial depends on what difference the investigator regards as clinically important and the number of patients likely to be available.

A clinician will turn to a statistician to help him. An estimate can only be provided if he will tell the statistician what magnitude of difference he is interested in detecting[14] *and* the risks he will tolerate of errors of Types I and II, i.e. of accepting a difference where it does not exist and of missing a difference that does exist. The result of this calculation is commonly a shock to the clinician who may have, a little vaguely, and full of therapeutic enthusiasm, begun by saying that he wants to detect 'any' difference, however small, and to be 'quite certain' that it is real.

A trial that offers a better than even chance of detecting a difference of 2:3, i.e. 2 deaths (or other event) in one treatment group against 3

---

[13] P = percentage divided by 100 (chance proportion).

[14] The *target difference.* Differences fall into three grades: (1) that the doctor will ignore, (2) that will make the doctor wonder what to do (more research needed), and (3) that will make the doctor act, i.e. change prescribing practice.

deaths in the other, which can well be a clinically important difference, will require numbers of patients that provide for about 100 deaths (or other event) in the trial. But such a probability (better than even chance) may be thought insufficient, and to become reasonably sure that a difference of this magnitude (2 : 3) will be detected, a trial involving about 200 deaths will be needed. If the death rate is 20%, then the trial should be planned to include about 1000 patients — a daunting prospect.

A trial that would detect (with statistical significance at 5% level, see above) a treatment that raised a cure rate from 75% to 85% would require 500 patients for 80% power. Obviously larger differences require fewer patients, and smaller differences require more patients (these figures make it clear why surveillance techniques of therapeutic evaluation are attracting increasing interest).

Fixed-sample trials

It is therefore necessary, after deciding in consultation with a statistician what difference it is realistic to seek and with what precision, having regard to the time, energy and number of patients available, to agree on the number of patients to be treated, to treat them and then to test the results.[14] Then there is less likelihood of hitting on a falsely 'significant' difference. This is a fixed-sample trial and at the end there may be disappointment if, when the results are examined, they just miss the agreed acceptable level of statistical significance. Here, having presented their results, clinicians are entitled to express their opinion on their meaning, and the size of the confidence interval will be of great assistance (see above). It is here too that the results of independent workers are helpful; *confirmation by others is an essential process in therapeutic advance* as in all science. It is *not* legitimate, having just failed (say, $P = 0.06$) to reach the agreed level (say, $P = 0.05$) to take in a few more patients in the hope that they will bring P down to 0.05 or less, for this is deliberately not allowing chance and the treatment to be the sole factors involved in the outcome, as they should be. At least this

is the theory, but 'only an investigator with superhuman will power or completely chaotic records could supervise a clinical trial for months or years without ever looking to see which way the results were drifting'[15] and being influenced by them in deciding when to stop the trial. Strictly this is not in accordance with statistical principles (see below), but it will doubtless continue to be done. It has been suggested that 'the simplest solution is to continue as at present, where most published P-values need to be mentally doubled. The only completely ethical and valid alternative is for every clinical trial to have a professional statistician, using weekly computerised analyses to administer a sequential design'.[15]

Variable number trials

Designs in which the number of subjects is not decided in advance have been developed in response to the evident need for a design that allows *continuous or intermittent* assessment as the trial proceeds and stops it *either* as soon as a statistically significant result is reached *or* when such a result becomes unlikely. The essential feature has to be that the trial is terminated when a *pre*-determined result is attained and not when the investigator, looking at the results to date, thinks it appropriate; (few investigators would be able to resist picking out the moment when the difference was statistically significant, which inevitably would mean a high rate of false-positive results). Truly continuous monitoring (*sequential analysis*) imposes severe restrictions and a compromise has been attained; it allows a formal analysis to be conducted at several *pre-determined* intervals and a decision made to stop or to continue. Such interim analyses reduce the statistical significance of the trial, but not to a serious degree if they are done, say, less than four times in a big trial. Such *modified sequential designs* recognise the realities of medical practice and provide a reasonable trade-off between statistical, medical and ethical needs. It is virtually a necessity to

[15] Peto R et al. Br J Cancer 1976; 34: 585; 35: 1.

have expert statistical advice when undertaking such trials.

If an experiment is ill-designed or ill-conducted it cannot be salvaged by statistics and statisticians are justifiably annoyed if they are invited to attempt such an operation.

WHAT DIFFERENCE CAN BE MEASURED?

The sensitivity of therapeutic trials. Definitive therapeutic trials are expensive and tedious and may be so prolonged that aspects of treatment have been superseded by the time a result is obtained. Of studies in cancer it is said:

The practical conclusion is that clinical trials can easily monitor death rate ratios between two treatments which are 1:3 or better, but that detection of anything less extreme than 2:3 is very difficult. These summary ratios are very important, and should be written on the shirt-cuffs of all trial organisers, as attempting to study a difference which could not plausibly be as extreme as 2:3 by a clinical trial is a common mistake.[16]

It is plain that a single trial will seldom give a conclusive answer to a therapeutic question. Confirmatory trials by other people in other centres play a major role in reaching reasonable certainty in therapeutics.

Meta-analysis. But where numerous trials have been done and the outcomes vary, it is tempting to collect them all together and analyse the accumulated results using appropriate statistical methods (it is *not* acceptable to do a simple addition of groups). This meta- (or overall) analysis can be enlightening, but the trials selected must meet the criteria of a good scientific study and the final result must be treated with caution.

DOUBLE-BLIND AND SINGLE-BLIND TECHNIQUES

The fact that both doctors and patients are subject to bias due to their beliefs and feelings has led to the invention of the double-blind technique. This is a

control device to prevent bias from influencing results. On the one hand it rules out the effects of hopes and anxieties of the patient by giving both the drug under investigation and a placebo (dummy) of identical appearance in such a way that the subject (the first 'blind' man) does not know which he is receiving. On the other hand, it also rules out the influence of preconceived hopes of, and unconscious communication by, the investigator or observer by keeping him (the second 'blind' man) ignorant of whether he is prescribing a placebo or an active drug. At the same time, the technique provides another control, a means of comparison with the magnitude of placebo effects.
The device is both philosophically and practically sound.[17]

A non-blind trial is called an 'open' trial.

The double-blind technique should be used if possible whenever evaluation depends on other than strictly objective measurements. There are occasions when it might at first sight seem that criteria of clinical improvement are objective when in fact they are not, e.g. the range of voluntary joint movement in rheumatoid arthritis has been shown to be greatly influenced by psychological factors, and a moment's thought shows why, for the amount of pain a patient will put up with is influenced by his mental state.

Sometimes the double-blind technique is not possible because, e.g. side-effects of an active drug reveal which patients are taking it or tablets look or taste different; but it never carries a disadvantage, 'only protection against spurious data'. It is not, of course, used with drugs fresh from the animal laboratory, whose dose and effects in man are unknown, although the subject may legitimately be kept in ignorance (single-blind) of the time of administration. Single-blind technique has little use in therapeutics research as it is equally important that the observer also be blind.

Ophthalmologists are understandably disinclined to refer to the double-blind technique; they call it double-masked.

---

[16] Peto M et al. Br J Cancer 1976; 34: 585.

[17] Modell W. JAMA 1958; 167: 2190.

PLACEBO MEDICATION AS A CONTROL (see also p. 19)

Dummy or placebo treatment is used in conjunction with the double-blind technique.

Its use is not invariably necessary nor indeed ethical, for it is not permissible to deprive patients of seriously effective therapy. In drug trials in, say, epilepsy or tuberculosis, the control groups comprise patients receiving the best available therapy.

The inert placebo or dummy is useful to:

● Distinguish the pharmacodynamic effects of a drug from the psychological effects of the act of medication and circumstances surrounding it, e.g. increased interest by the doctor, more frequent visits, etc.
● Distinguish drug effects from fluctuations in disease that occur with time and other external factors, provided active treatment, if any, can be ethically witheld.
● Avoid false negative conclusions. For example, a therapeutic trial of a new analgesic should consist of comparison of the new drug with a dummy[18] as well as with a proved active analgesic. If all three treatments give the same result, a likely explanation is that the method used (including trial size) is incapable of distinguishing between an active and an inactive drug and so should be modified; whereas if only the new drug and the dummy are used and give identical results, there are two possible explanations, first that the method used is insensitive and second that the new drug has only placebo-effect, i.e. is pharmacologically inactive at the dose used.

The use of a placebo or dummy treatment poses ethical problems but is often preferable to the continued use of treatments of unproven efficacy or safety. It is not inherently unethical. Investigators who propose to use a placebo or otherwise withhold effective treatment should specifically justify their intention. Frequently, consent can be obtained to the use of a placebo without impairing the scientific validity of the procedure if the patient is invited to agree that an inert preparation will (or may) be used (and why it will be used) at some time during the course of treatment, but without specifying exactly when. Generally, patients easily understand the concept of distinguishing between the imagined effects of treatment and those due to a direct action on the body.

WITHIN- AND BETWEEN-PATIENT (PARALLEL GROUP) STUDIES

Sometimes in chronic stable disease that cannot be cured but can be alleviated it is possible to give each of the treatments under test, including placebo, to each patient, thus conveniently using them as their own controls (a cross-over study), e.g. in parkinsonism or hypertension. When this is done it is important to ensure in a small series that each drug both precedes and follows each other drug the same number of times, to avoid the risk of systematic bias due to changes with time and 'carry-over' effect, i.e. interaction of the drug given first with that given second. If in an analgesic trial a less effective drug always follows a more effective, the weaker drug may be dismissed as ineffective because the patient's judgement has become influenced by the high degree of relief provided by the more effective drug. The less effective drug must precede as well as follow both the more effective drug and the dummy (if any) if error is to be avoided. In addition, persistence of a drug or metabolites, and enzyme induction, may influence the response to a subsequent drug.[19] For these reasons between-patient studies are preferred, but they require more subjects.

In acute self-limiting diseases it is plainly impossible to give more than one treatment to one patient and the controls must be other patients, i.e. between-patient or parallel groups.

Naturally there is a temptation simply to give a new treatment to all patients and to compare the results with the past, i.e. *historical controls.*

---

[18] Careful design allows a patient unrelieved by a placebo, or by an ineffective new drug, to be quickly given a known active drug.

[19] 'Carry-over' can be minimised by inserting 'washout' periods between active treatments, but these are not always ethically acceptable.

Unfortunately this is almost always[20] unacceptable, even with a disease such as leukaemia, for standards of diagnosis and treatment change with time, severity of disease (infections) fluctuates. The provision stands that controls must be concurrent and concomitant (p. 46).

Some mortal sins of clinical assessment[21]

- *Enthusiasm and scepticism*:
  'A marvellous/useless drug, this.'
- *Change of assessor*:
  'Do the measurements for me Jim/Miss Jones/darling.'
- *Change of time*:
  'Don't worry about the assessment. Go ahead with lunch/X-rays/physiotherapy/your bath.'
- *Squeezing*:
  'You're much better, aren't you, Miss B?'
  'Any indigestion yet, Miss B?'
- *Pride*:
  '*I'm honest. No need for placebo in my trials.*'
- *Impurity*:
  'We're short of cases: she'll have to do.' 'A few aspirins won't make much difference.'
- *Imbalance*:
  'Sex/severity/treatment order, doesn't matter.'
- *Error*:
  'Not quite significant. Let's try sequential analysis.'

PHARMACOEPIDEMIOLOGY

Three important epidemiological approaches are used to determine how the results of controlled therapeutic trials are translated into performance in the looser conditions of use in the community, and especially to the detection of uncommon adverse reactions. They are not experimental (as is the randomised trial where entry and allocation of treatment are strictly controlled). They are *observational* in that the groups to be compared have been assembled from subjects who already are,

or who are not (the controls), taking the treatment in the ordinary way of medical care.

1. The observational cohort[22] study

Patients receiving the drug are collected and followed up to determine the outcomes (therapeutic and adverse). This is forward-looking (prospective) research. *Prescription event monitoring* (p. 119) is an example, and there is an increasing tendency to recognise that many new drugs should be monitored in this way when prescribing becomes general. Major difficulties include selection of an appropriate control group, the need for large numbers of subjects and for prolonged surveillance. This sort of study is scientifically inferior to the experimental cohort study (randomised controlled trial) and is cumbersome for research on drugs. Happily, clever epidemiologists have devised an alternative, the case-control study.

2. The case-control study

This reverses the direction of scientific logic from forward-looking (prospective) to backward-looking (retrospective)[23] investigation. The investigator assembles a group of patients who have the condition it is desired to investigate, e.g. women who have had an episode of thromboembolism. A control group of women who have not had an episode of thromboembolism is then assembled, e.g. similar age, parity and smoking habits, from hospital admissions for other reasons, or primary care records, and a complete drug history is taken from each group, i.e. the two groups are 'followed up' backwards to determine the proportion in each group that has taken the suspect agent, in this case the oral contraceptive pill.

To solve the question of thromboembolism and the combined oestrogen-progestogen contraceptive pill by means of an observational cohort study required enormous numbers of sub-

---

[20] Criteria for cautiously but usefully employing historical controls are suggested by Bailar J C et al. Studies without internal controls. N Engl J Med 1984; 311: 156.
[21] Hart F D et al 1972 Measurement in rheumatoid arthritis. Lancet 2: 28.

[22] Used here for a group of people having a common attribute, e.g. they have all taken the same drug.
[23] For this reason Feinstein has named these *trohoc* (*cohort* spelled backwards) studies.

jects[24] (the adverse effect is, happily, uncommon) followed over years. An investigation into cancer and the contraceptive pill by an observational cohort would require follow-up for 10–15 years. This approach is evidently cumbersome and expensive, and cannot satisfy the urgent need for an answer once a suspicion is raised.

But a case-control study can be done quickly; it has the advantage that it begins with a much smaller (compared with the cohort) number of cases (hundreds or less) of disease, though it has the disadvantage that it follows up subjects backwards and there is always suspicion of the intrusion of unknown and so unavoidable biases in selection of both patients and controls. Here again, independent repetition of the studies, if the results are the same, greatly enhances confidence in the outcome.

A major disadvantage of the case-control study is that it requires a definite hypothesis or suspicion of causality. A cohort study on the other hand does not; subjects can be followed 'to see what happens' (event recording).

Case-control studies do not prove causation.[25] They reveal associations and it is up to investigators and critical readers to decide what is the most plausible explanation of the associations revealed.

Feinstein has pointed out that the validity of case-control studies can be increased if the standards of entry and evaluation are raised to those applied to experimental studies in the same field (randomised controlled trials). He concludes that

Epidemiologic research has become increasingly important because it offers a substitute for the unattainable scientific "gold standard" of a randomised experimental trial . . . An insistence on high scientific quality can help epidemiologic studies

achieve the standards and rigor of research in other branches of modern science.[26]

3. Record linkage by computer

This allows correlation in a population of life and health events with history of drug use. It is being developed as far as resources permit. It includes prescription event monitoring, see 1. above.

RELIABILITY OF PUBLISHED THERAPEUTIC TRIALS

From time to time people experienced in therapeutic evaluation study published therapeutic trials and report their conclusions.

In one study it was concluded that about 66% of published papers are acceptable and 33% unacceptable according to what are now generally agreed criteria.

In another study 50% of papers were found to have statistical errors of which half were serious, and in 8% of papers a claim was made that was unsupportable on re-examination of the data.

IN CONCLUSION

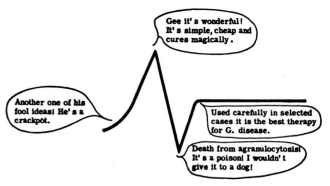

Fig. 4.1 Oscillations in the development of a drug[27]

---

[24] The Royal College of General Practitioners (UK) recruited 23 000 women takers of the pill and 23 000 controls in 1968 and issued a report in 1973. It found an approximate doubled incidence of venous thrombosis in combined-pill takers (the dose of oestrogen has been reduced since this study).

[25] Experimental cohort studies (randomised controlled trials) are on firmer ground with regard to causation. In the experimental cohort study there should be only *one* systematic difference between the groups (i.e. the treatment being studied). In case-control studies the groups may differ systematically in several ways.

[26] Feinstein A et al N Engl J Med 1982; 307: 1611.

[27] By courtesy of Dr. Robert H. Williams and the Editor of JAMA.

GUIDE TO FURTHER READING

Angell M 1989 Negative studies. New England Journal of Medicine 321: 464

Brewin C R et al 1989 Patient preferences and randomised trials. British Medical Journal 299: 313

Byar D P 1990 Design considerations for AIDS trials. New England Journal of Medicine 323: 1343

Cook C H C et al 1988 Another trial that failed. Lancet 1: 524

Editorial 1987 Drop-outs from clinical trials. Lancet 2: 892

Editorial 1990 Should we case-control? Lancet 1: 1127

Hellman S et al 1991 Of mice but not men — problems of the randomized clinical trial. New England Journal of Medicine 324: 1585

Herxheimer A 1988 The rights of the patient in clinical research. Lancet 2: 1128

Laupacis A et al 1988 An assessment of clinically useful measures of the consequences of treatment.

New England Journal of Medicine 318: 1728

Mainland D 1984 Statistical ritual in clinical journals: is there a cure? British Medical Journal 288: 841, 920

Merigan T C 1990 How AIDS trials are pioneering new strategies. New England Journal of Medicine 323: 1341

Moscucci M et al 1987 Blinding, unblinding, and the placebo effect. Clinical Pharmacology and Therapeutics 41: 259

Passamani E 1991 Clinical trials — are they ethical? New England Journal of Medicine 324: 1589

Rothman D J 1987 Ethics and human experimentation. New England Journal of Medicine 317: 1195

Shapiro S 1989 The role of automated record linkage in the postmarketing surveillance of drug safety: a critique. Clinical Pharmacology and Therapeutics 46: 371; (responses to the article) 387, 391, 478, 479

Tunkel V 1989 Drug trials: who takes the risk? Lancet 2: 609

5

Official regulation of medicines

SYNOPSIS

Governments undertake to regulate
medicines/drugs because prescribers and users
cannot determine for themselves the quality, safety,
efficacy and supply of all medicines. Official
regulation carries risks and is prone to protect itself
from criticism by raising safety standards to such a
level that drug developers are discouraged from
investing the enormous resources required.

THE BASIS

Neither patients nor doctors are in a position to
decide for themselves across the range of
medicines that they use, which ones are pure and
stable and effective and safe. They need some
assurance that the medicines they are offered
fulfil these requirements and are supported
with information that permits optimal use. Only
governments can provide such assurance, insofar
as it can be provided.

Official or statutory regulation of medicines provides a perfect example of the role
of governments:

1. To enable citizens to undertake jointly tasks
   that they cannot undertake individually
2. To protect individual citizens from the
   actions of others.

The objective of official regulation is to ensure
a supply of effective and safe (for their purpose)
medicines, whether by selection from amongst
those used in traditional systems or by modern
invention. Insufficiently safe or ineffective
medicines should be identified and eliminated.
An unduly rigorous approach may both result in
wrong judgements and unnecessarily deprive the
community of comforts that are harmless but
which provide psychological support. In respect
of these latter it is the function of official drug
regulation to ensure that any such placebo
medicines are known for what they are and that
unjustified therapeutic claims are not made.

OFFICIAL (STATUTORY) DRUG REGULATION

This is concerned with:

- **quality**, i.e. purity, stability (shelf-life)
- **safety**
- **efficacy**
- **supply**, i.e. whether the drug is to be unrestrictedly available to the public or confined to sales through pharmacies or to doctors' prescriptions.

A basic requirement of any control system is that no medicine may be sold or supplied without prior licensing or registration by government. If there is no licensing system there is no control.

Plainly, manufacturers and developers need to be told what kinds of data and in what amount are likely to persuade the regulatory authority to grant a licence. Therefore the authority issues 'guidelines', generally stating that these will be interpreted and applied 'flexibly'. But, almost inevitably, flexible guidelines tend to become minimal requirements in the day-to-day operation of a legislative act by government servants.

Some history

The beginning of substantial government intervention in the field of medicines paralleled the proliferation of synthetic drugs in the early 20th century when the traditional and familiar pharmacopoeia[1] expanded slowly and then, in mid-century, with enormous rapidity; intervention was initially confined to safety aspects and was developed piecemeal as issues arose, until the thalidomide disaster of 1961 (see p. 65) caused governments all over the world to rationalise, formalise and extend their control of medicines in single, though often complicated, laws.

Governmental controls developed approximately as follows.

Safety came first, with restrictions on supply of 'dangerous drugs' especially drugs of addiction.

Then followed controls on **quality** in manufacture which were evoked by the introduction of preparations of substances occurring naturally in the body, e.g. insulin (1922) on accurate dose of which the life of large numbers of diabetics depends. Inefficient or incompetent manufacture (impurity, inefficacy, instability) will cause deaths, and since consumers are not able to determine for themselves whether the preparation offered is reliable, they require protection against defective products. Therefore government control is essential in the public interest.

Efficacy received less attention. In the first half of this century drug therapy was relatively uncritical, though in the UK a law was passed forbidding advertising to the public of 'cures' for veneral disease, tuberculosis and epilepsy. Drug therapy was based on assertions derived from the impressions of physicians. In mid-century, methods of formal therapeutic evaluation, though foreshadowed by isolated individuals in the previous 200 years, became established, and scientific comparisons of the efficacy of new and old medicines became commonplace.

But governments did not act to extend control of medicines to include efficacy as well as safety; there was no public pressure for them to do so. The most effective pressure that persuades politicians that they should act radically and quickly is a public scandal where failure to respond will make them so unpopular that they fail to achieve re-election.

The first comparatively comprehensive drug regulatory law prior to thalidomide was passed in the USA in 1938, following the death of about 107 people due to the use of diethylene glycol (a constituent of antifreezes) as a solvent for a liquid formulation of sulphanilamide for treating common infections.[2] The sulphonamides, introduced in 1935, were the first major therapeutic advance against common bacterial infections.

In early 1937, in the USA, tablets and capsules of sulphanilamide were marketed by a number of firms including the S. E. Massengill Company of Tennessee. In June 1937 the firm's salesmen

---

[1] *Pharmacopoeia*: a book (often official) listing drugs, their uses, standards of purity etc.

[2] Report of the Secretary of Agriculture submitted in response to resolutions in the House Representatives and Senate (USA): JAMA 1937; 109: 1985, the principal source of this story.

reported a demand for the drug in liquid form (easier for children to take). Since sulphanilamide is relatively insoluble in the usual vehicles, a number of other solvents used in industry were tried. Diethylene glycol was effective and an 'elixir' was made of drug, solvent, flavouring and water. No tests in animals were made to determine the toxicity either of the ingredients separately or of the finished product, or to determine whether the mixture was stable, i.e. whether the drug decomposed in the solvent when stored. The company's laboratory merely checked the mixture for appearance, flavour and fragrance. No special studies were conducted in man. This procedure was compatible with the then existing law in the USA.

In October 1937, news of deaths in Oklahoma was telephoned to the US Food & Drug Administration (FDA) by a physician. Eight children with sore throats and one adult with gonorrhoea had died after taking the 'elixir'. When the Massengill Company heard of the deaths it sent out 1100 telegrams to its customers and salesmen asking for recovery of all 'elixir' that had been sold. Since these requests seemed unlikely to impress receivers with the true urgency of the situation, the investigating FDA inspectors insisted, on October 19, that a more cogent telegram be sent:

Imperative you take up immediately all elixir sulphanilamide you dispensed. Product may be dangerous to life. Return our expense.

Large amounts were sent back, but it was essential that *all* be recovered. Almost all the 239 FDA inspectors and chemists were assigned to this task. Warnings were broadcast by radio and newspaper. Individual prescriptions were identified and pursued.

Massengill Company travelling salesmen were pursued from hotel to hotel and interviewed. One salesman was uncooperative, but changed his mind when jailed. Most doctors and pharmacists cooperated. But one doctor who had admitted dispensing to five patients refused their names though claiming they were all alive. Enquiry revealed he had supplied seven patients and four were dead.

Typical effects occurred 24–48 hours after taking the elixir, with nausea, vomiting, malaise,

severe abdominal pain, sometimes diarrhoea, and anuria, the patient became unconscious and either died after 2–7 days or recovered over 7–21 days. Autopsy disclosed renal and hepatic damage.

On October 23, Dr. Massengill issued a press statement:

My chemists and I deeply regret the fatal results, but *there was no error in manufacture of the product*. We have been supplying legitimate professional demand and *not once could have foreseen the unlooked-for results*. I do not feel that there was any responsibility on our part.

Evidence of toxicity of ethylene glycol in man was available prior to marketing this 'elixir'. The effects are easily shown in animals.

'Federal officials were miserably handicapped by the weak law'.[3]

The USA Congress now acted quickly and passed a bill providing that no new drug or any modifications of old drugs should be placed on the market until the entire formula had been submitted to the government's Food and Drug Administration.

All this took place nine years after a pharmacologist speaking before the Section of Pharmacology and Therapeutics of the American Medical Association (1929) said: 'There is no short cut from chemical laboratory to clinic, except one that passes too close to the morgue.'

Other countries did not learn the lesson provided by the USA and it took the thalidomide disaster of 1960–61 to make governments all over the world initiate comprehensive control over all aspects of drug introduction, prescribing and supply. Those governments that already had some control system extended it.

But no regulatory system can guarantee complete safety. Therefore it is interesting to consider whether the thalidomide disaster (p. 65) might have been prevented in Europe by a control system such as was then in force in the USA.

Thalidomide was developed in West Germany and introduced thence into other countries.

The USA and the UK have similar attitudes to technical medicine. The former had a com-

---

[3] JAMA 1938; 111: 583, 919.

prehensive regulatory body (FDA) in 1960 and the latter did not. It might be thought that this would provide a field test of the usefulness of official drug regulation. But it did not.

Thalidomide was marketed in the UK, according to accepted practice at that time (which did not include routine testing on pregnant animals), without official review or hindrance, but it was delayed in the USA by the routine administrative machinery. During this delay period it was discovered and published in the UK that thalidomide could cause peripheral neuritis in man. Naturally this led to further cautious delay in the USA and during this further period the harmful effect on the fetus was revealed in other countries.

Mere delay protects, provided others are using the drugs concerned. But it can also deprive populations of valuable drugs.

REQUIREMENTS OF MODERN DRUG REGULATION

A modern drug regulatory authority requires the following:

- **Pre-clinical tests**
  1. Tests carried out in animals to allow some prediction of potential efficacy and safety in man (see Ch. 3).
  2. Chemical and pharmaceutical quality (purity, stability, formulation, etc.)

- **Clinical (human) tests.** Phases 1, 2, 3 (p. 42), to determine whether the drug deserves to be licensed or registered for general prescription (the drug being supplied for these trials by the developers generally without payment, for it is not yet a medicine).

Regulatory review

The authority formally reviews both pre-clinical and clinical data and decides whether the drug can be granted a licence for general prescribing (Product Licence), i.e. it is deemed to be a medicine and it can be marketed with therapeutic claims.[4] The regulatory authority decides what therapeutic claims can be made and also must be satisfied of the adequacy of the information to be provided to prescribers (Data Sheet) and also, where appropriate, any Patient Information Leaflet (which is particularly important with preparations for long-term use such as oral contraceptives). Where a drug has special advantage, but also has special risk, restrictions on its promotion and use can be imposed, e.g. see isotretinoin and clozapine.

When a novel drug is granted a Product Licence it is recognised as a medicine by independent critics and there is rejoicing amongst those who have spent many years developing it. But the testing is not over, the most stringent test of all is about to begin. It will be used in all sorts of people of all ages and sizes and having all sort of other conditions. Its use can no longer be so closely supervised as hitherto. Doctors will prescribe it and patients will use it correctly and incorrectly. It will have effects that have not been anticipated. It will be taken in overdose. It has to find its place in therapeutics.

Post-licensing/marketing surveillance (Phase 4) has thus become an essential stage of drug evaluation. It is neither easy nor cheap to accomplish.

The important objective is to obtain information on very large numbers of patients, 10 000–20 000, in observational cohort studies, e.g. prescription event monitoring (p. 119) and case-control studies where appropriate; spontaneous reporting of suspected adverse reactions is also encouraged, e.g. by marking the drug with a special symbol, ▼ in formularies (in the UK).

Further randomised controlled trials (experimental cohort studies) especially comparing the new drug with those already available will continue, for a long time in the case of really novel advances.

DISCUSSION

It may be wondered why post-licensing/marketing surveillance should be necessary. Commonsense would seem to dictate that safety and efficacy of

---

[4] A Product Licence should be granted for a limited period only, e.g. 5 years.

a drug should be fully defined before it is granted a Product Licence (marketed). Pre-licensing trials with very close supervision are commonly limited to hundreds of patients and this is unavoidable, chiefly because this close supervision is impracticable on a large scale for a very long time.

Closely supervised pre-marketing trials (particularly when no exciting result is anticipated but merely a possibility of modest advance) constitute a tremendous burden on both investigators and patients. Interest of the doctor flags, willingness of patients to accept the inconvenience of close supervision declines, precise records become imprecise, patients drop out. Even if mammoth controlled trials are done, and they have been done and are very expensive, there is no assurance of useful result.

An 8-year study of treatment of diabetes,[5] which started in 1961, cost US$7.7 million (at then current rates) and did not answer the problems of long-term management of maturity-onset diabetes.

Multicentre and international studies of drug treatment of mild high blood pressure have taken years to complete and cost the equivalent of many millions of US$.

Definitive therapeutic studies in such diseases, which are essential for individual, social and economic reasons, require large-scale production of drugs and their use in many thousands of patients over years. In medical and social terms it seems irrelevant whether the drug is 'marketed' or not; in any case it must be paid for by somebody, and, in fact, always ultimately by the public.

Medicines must be allowed to be sold at a reasonably early stage of development if research-based industry is to continue to operate. Of course there will be no question of granting a licence to sell until there is evidence that the majority of patients will benefit. But the rarer risks cannot be accurately determined until as many as 100 000 or even one million patients have used the drug and their experience has been recorded. Such experience may take years. The only way in which this experience can be financed

is by selling the drug. Selling the drug need not mean its use is not being closely supervised. It is the supervision and evaluation that is important to patients rather than whether it is supplied 'free' or for money. But a flow of money is essential to industry to support manufacture, distribution and research into further new drugs.

It is for these reasons that post-licensing schemes are increasingly regarded as essential to complete the definitive evaluation of drugs under conditions of ordinary use on a large scale, these programmes being preferable to attempts to enlarge and prolong formal therapeutic trials.

The regulatory organisation has the power to control the claims and to ensure that necessary information is provided to prescribers and patients so they will not be misled. But allowing sale and general prescribing no longer means the end of the period of formal evaluation.

It is now recognised that full evaluation of medicines commonly takes extensive use over many years[6] and techniques are being adapted to this fact and devised to reduce the period to a minimum.

Oral contraceptives, antidiabetic agents and hormone replacement therapy for post-menopausal women are examples where benefit: risk evaluation proceeds over decades. Major tranquillisers are still controversial after more than 25 years of widespread use.

The requirements of regulatory authorities increase as unexpected events occur amidst public outcry against both developers and the authorities.

For example, before thalidomide (1961) it was not a routine practice to test new drugs on pregnant animals. After thalidomide it became the routine to test all new drugs during early pregnancy in animals, at which stage the major organ forming processes take place. Now testing has expanded to cover risk at all stages of the

---

[5]JAMA 1975; 231: 583.

[6] For these reasons the UK and many other countries having a research-based industry do not require that a drug or medicine (formulation) be shown to be better than others as a condition for marketing. But Norway approaches this by requiring that medical 'need' be shown as a condition for marketing. Norway has available about 1900 formulations (chemical entities plus dose forms) and the UK has about 6000.

reproductive process. Thus it is hoped to avoid future accident. In fact, little is known of the predictive value of such tests. But there is no doubt whatever as to their cost in money and scientific resources.

Increasingly drugs are also tested for carcinogenicity and mutagenicity.

And so it goes on; the labour and cost of drug testing prior to administration to man steadily increases. This could be justified if there were good assurance that the increase really gave extensive protection to man. But there are grounds for believing that such tests have a limited and uncertain value *except* where precise mechanisms have been determined.

We are not saying that tests in animals are of no use. They are essential within their limitations. We would regard the use in man of chemicals on which there was no information on their effects in animals in these special areas as quite unacceptable.

We consider that the pursuit, by public demand and by the natural desire of drug scientists and official regulatory bodies, of virtually absolute safety, or 'safety at any cost', even when lip service is sometimes paid to the inevitability of hazard, is now reaching a point where it may, paradoxically, act against the public interest. It may stop the development of new drugs for serious and untreatable (especially for rare) disease by rendering research programmes prohibitively costly, and by causing the withdrawal of drugs before their risks have been quantified and calmly reviewed in relation to the risks of disease and of daily life in general.

Already an oral contraceptive must undergo research and safety testing for about 8 years before trial in woman (or man), and there is then no substantial certainly that it will not then fail the necessarily large and rigorous human testing programme.

Whether drugs are developed by private or state enterprise, considerations of investment of the now enormous resources demanded are liable to turn those responsible to seek other outlets for their skills and for their investment.

Always it must be remembered that though there are risks in taking drugs, there are also risks is not taking drugs, and there are risks in not developing new drugs.

DECISION TAKING: UNCERTAINTY, RISK AND REGRET AVOIDANCE

Official regulation has risks as well as benefits. Wrong or hasty decisions may often affect only individual drugs, but wrong policies may have widespread adverse effects on socially desirable drug development and use.

It has been pointed out that in medicine, 'The trend of greater risks for greater gain is likely to continue'.[7] The fact that society wants the benefits of medical advance but pays only lipservice to the proposition that risks are inescapable puts a heavy psychological burden on drug regulators. Regulators are in the business of taking risks on behalf of society, and, through their political masters, are answerable to society.

The principal theme of regulation is, inevitably, *risk avoidance*. Those who engage in statutory regulation are to some extent prisoners of its post-thalidomide origin and of the enormous labour of the operation. Drug developers, whilst they accept the principle of official regulation, resent its rigidities and what they see as excessive requirements, believing many of them to be harmful, but they also need to know where they stand and so they encourage, whether consciously or not, the development of the very regulations they so often deplore. This applies particularly to arbitrary safety requirements, when a research director cannot afford to be told that an expensive programme is deemed insufficient for reasons that are no more than a matter of opinion or that a clinical trial that was terminated after 10 months should have lasted one year, and it must be started anew.

It is difficult to stand back and view the general scene. But anyone who does this is likely to agree that we are operating a system that is based on unproved predictive assumptions. This was unavoidable in the immediate aftermath of thalidomide when, understandably, the pressures

---

[7] Royal Commission on civil liability and compensation for personal injury. London: HMSO, CMND. 7054–1, 1978.

to get something started quickly were irresistible. But there has been no comprehensive scientific monitoring of the performance of regulation (not an easy task) *with* provision for change in the light of the results.[8] Thirty years after thalidomide the operation remains essentially unchanged. A perceptive comment on one drug withdrawal was, 'The present system is too slow at detecting risk as well as unduly apt to slam the brakes on hard once it is detected.'[9]

In *taking decisions*, it has been pointed out,[10] there are three kinds of uncertainty:

- of the *facts*
- of the *public reaction to the facts*
- of the *future consequences of decisions*.

Regulators are influenced not only to avoid risk but to avoid regret later and this latter consideration has a profound effect whether or not the decision taker is conscious of it.

Therefore there are two important subjective human factors, *uncertainty* and *regret avoidance* and it is easy to agree that, 'Balancing the benefits against the risks belongs not in the domain of science but to society. The judgement is a value judgement — a social rather than a scientific decision.'[11] All this tends to promote defensive regulation.

The kind of risk-taking that is in the interest of society requires high-quality data at the licensing stage plus a sound plan of post-licensing (marketing) investigation. If this latter is not done, any adverse events or scandal will almost unavoidably result in the condemnation of the drug. No regulatory body can face the prospect of being in the position of ignoring bad data until good data can be obtained and then later finding that the good data confirm the earlier condemnation already demanded by the mass media. For this reason alone we must give priority to raising the standard of data at all stages of drug development and ensuring that its collection continues after a product licence has been granted. This is

in the interest of the pharmaceutical industry. In a crisis, a company that has not good data can expect no help from the regulatory body; indeed it can only expect a negative decision.

Collective decision-making by advisory groups (as in UK)[12] of people of different disciplines who comparatively seldom meet, who are in uncertainty as described above and who are subject to considerable pressure of regret avoidance must tend to defensive policies and to discourage innovatory thinking.

The practical situation is that there is virtually always an insufficiency of knowledge on which to make rational and reliable judgements and there are always more investigations that might be done; and there is no prospect of this situation changing. We all know this, but we behave much of the time as though it were not so.

Advisory committees know from experience that society as a whole (or as represented by politicians and the mass media), though it may 'know' that 'there is no such thing as a safe drug' will not behave as if it really understood this when an unpredicted risk eventuates; blame will be allocated and a scapegoat will be sought, and protestations by developers and regulators are vain because data are always inadequate.

It is self-evident that it is much harder to detect and quantitate a *good* that is *not* done, than it is to detect and quantitate a *harm* that *is* done. Therefore, although it is part of the decision-taker's job to facilitate the doing of good, the avoidance of harm looms larger. The risk of a decision that results in harm being done and detected dominates the mind in a way that the risk of possible failure to do good, even if it is detected, cannot do. Attempts to convict regulators of failing to do good (e.g. the delay in introducing valuable new drugs in the USA due to regulatory procrastination, the 'drug lag') do not induce the same feelings of horror in regulators that are induced by the prospect of finding they have approved a drug that has, or

---

[8] A start has been made. Lunde I, Dukes M N G. On regulating regulation. Eur J Clin Pharmacol 1981; 19: 1.
[9] The Times, 24 August 1982.
[10] Lord Ashby. Proc Roy Soc Med 1976; 69: 721.
[11] B. Commoner 1977.

[12] In the UK, the Committee on Safety of Medicines and the Medicines Commission. These are QUANGOS (*quasi-autonomous non-government organisations*); their membership, appointed by government to give independent advice, is sarcastically said to consist of 'the good and the great'.

may have, caused serious injury and that the victims are about to appear on television.[13]

This is not to ridicule the regulators and their advisers. They are doing their best, and commonly make good and sensible decisions that receive no congratulations. But we do not often think of the human aspects of their work.

THE FUTURE

Specialists in the study of risk management do not agree that current approaches to drug regulation can be effective, and think that as long as they continue to be used the future is bleak.

'We are, sadly but simply, hooked on a risk control policy which gives us little but which we can no longer do without.' This is shown by the behaviour of regulators and the public with each new drug accident (or presumed drug accident). On each occasion they re-fight the old battles. They seem wedded to belief in

Prospective, knowledge-presuming notions of rationality in which optimal or best-possible decisions and rules are derived from existing available information and are implemented by virtue of their assumed rationality. Subsequent performance is assumed to be optimal if these rules are rigorously enforced. Success is deemed to be within our grasp if we persist in this course.[14]

This quote is a little difficult to follow at first reading, but it is worth trying again and reflecting on it.

We are faced with 'risk assessors' sincere knowledge-seeking efforts to identify potential dangers' and to construct a rigid or near-rigid framework for detecting dangers. The regulator in fact agrees he always has too little knowledge but he behaves as though the unknown is a 'wrinkle to be ironed out of a fabric.' In this he is wrong and the history of risk management shows the inadequacy of the approach. Our

ignorance will always remain greater than our knowledge.

It is pointed out that the practical mainstay of man and beast in daily life may be a better model, i.e. the acceptance of the inevitability of incomplete knowledge as central, to be lived with and accommodated rather than overcome. 'The fundamental question is not how to calculate, control, or even reduce risk', which is what we currently attempt, 'it is how to increase our risk-taking abilities'; to develop rational coping systems, i.e. institutions that can continuously respond to and learn from the inevitable surprises awaiting us; our future may depend on our ability to design such institutions for 'adaptive risk management'. This would also include a user-friendly system for compensating the victims of drug accidents.

For drug regulation this means continuous evaluation of the efficacy of regulations, the kinds of risks detected and the kinds that go undetected (we are just beginning to do this), so that armed with such knowledge we can decide what are the tasks that post-licensing surveillance schemes can fulfil and the kinds of situations best solved by intensive pre-licensing studies.

Only when we begin to blend the results of such studies in the careful design of integrated risk management strategies will we be able to move much beyond the present unsatisfactory state of management by polemic.

We should seriously try to understand that salvation does not lie in lists of requirements modified intermittently and almost always upwards, and indeed it is not to be found in a traditional scientific approach. Risk-management, which is what we are talking about, belongs, it is suggested, in the realm of 'trans-science' and not science. Trans-science treats questions that transcend science, i.e. 'questions that can be asked of science and yet which cannot be answered by science', e.g. How safe is safe enough? Plainly scientists have a role but it is a role different from that in which questions can be unambiguously answered by science. We see what is meant by this when we read that Congress of the USA:

---

[13] The very last thing a drug regulator wishes to be able to say is, 'I awoke one morning and found myself famous': (Lord Byron (1788–1824) on the publication of his poem Childe Harold's Pilgrimage).
[14] William C. Clark of the International Institute for Applied Systems Analysis (Austria) to whom we are grateful for permission to quote: Clark W C. In: Schwing R C, Albers W A eds. Societal risk assessment. New York: Plenum Press, 1980.

has failed repeatedly to meet FDA's (Food and Drug Administration) own requests for an unambiguous legislative mandate specifying what balance of risks and benefits *does* constitute the public good, how this is to be democratically determined and achieved.

The FDA will have known that Congress could not answer, yet Congress repeatedly intervenes in the functioning of the FDA, interventions that have been described as resembling 'nothing so much as Keystone Cops Scenarios.'[15]

The most important lesson of both experience and analysis is that societies' abilities to cope with the unknown depend on the flexibility of their institutions and individuals, and on their capability to experiment freely with alternative forms of adaptation to the risks which threaten them.

Neither the witch hunting hysterics nor the mindlessly rigid regulations characterizing so much of our present chapter in the history of risk management say much for our ability to learn from the past.[14]

THE WORLD HEALTH ORGANIZATION (WHO) ESSENTIAL DRUGS PROGRAMME

Essential drugs are those that satisfy the health care needs of the majority of the population; they should therefore be available at all times in adequate amounts and in the appropriate dosage forms.[16]

WHO provides a model list of drugs and classes of drugs (with model prescribing information) which countries needing such advice can use as a basis for their own choices.

The list is updated every few years and contains about 290 items (including a few non-drug products, i.e. barrier contraceptives).

APPENDIX
A TALE TO REMEMBER: THE THALIDOMIDE DISASTER

Thalidomide has provided a terrible lesson to the world in regard to drug development, testing, naming, prescribing and consumption. It deserves to be remembered as follows:

Until 1961 the public took a largely romantic interest in the development and introduction of new drugs and its attention was only turned to the subject when it learned from the press, generally incorrectly, and several times a year, that a 'miracle drug' had been discovered. In 1961 a major breakthrough did occur — man discovered that drug introduction was more hazardous than he had previously believed. The thalidomide disaster aroused public opinion, forced governments to regulate drug introduction and therapeutic claims and all concerned with this process got a salutary shock. Our attitude to casual use of drugs can never be and should never be the same since thalidomide, and therefore the story is given in detail here.

In 1960–61 in West Germany an outbreak of phocomelia occurred. Phocomelia means 'seal extremities'; it is a congenital deformity in which the long bones of the limbs are defective and substantially normal or rudimentary hands and feet arise on, or nearly on, the trunk, like the flippers of a seal; other abnormalities may occur simultaneously. Phocomelia is ordinarily exceedingly rare.

Most West German clinics had no cases during the 10 years up to 1959. In 1959, in 10 clinics, 17 were seen; in 1960, 126; in 1961, 477. The European outbreak seemed confined to West Germany (though a similar but smaller occurrence was simultaneously noted in Australia), and this, with the steady increase, made a virus infection, such as rubella, seem unlikely as a cause. Radioactive fall-out was considered and so were X-ray exposure of the mother, hormones, foods, food preservatives and contraceptives. One doctor, investigating his patients retrospectively with a questionnaire, found that 20% reported taking Contergan in early pregnancy. He questioned the patients again and 50% then admitted taking it; *many said they had thought the drug too obviously innocent to be worth mentioning initially*.[17]

In November 1961, the suggestion that a drug,

---

[15] Early Hollywood silent slapstick comedy films.
[16] The use of essential drugs. Geneva. WHO, 1990.

[17] Illustrating the problems of retrospective research, e.g. case-control studies; enquiries of patients are unreliable.

unnamed, was the cause of the outbreak was publicly made by the same doctor at a paediatric meeting, following a report on 34 cases of phocomelia. 'That night a physician came up to him and said, "Will you tell me confidentially, is the drug Contergan? I ask because we have such a child and my wife took Contergan."' Several letters followed, asking the same question, and it soon became widely known that thalidomide (Contergan, Distaval, Kevadon, Talimol, Softenon) was probably the cause. It was withdrawn from the West German market in November 1961 and from the British market in December 1961. By that time reports had also come from other countries.

Thalidomide was recommended for use in pregnant women. It had not been tested on pregnant animals. When it was eventually tested it was at first difficult to induce fetal deformity (until it was used on New Zealand White Rabbits).

A *case-control study* showed that of 46 cases of phocomelia 41 mothers had taken thalidomide and of 300 mothers with normal babies none had taken thalidomide, between the fourth and ninth week of pregnancy.

Soon more reports were forthcoming and despite the fact that such retrospective studies do not provide conclusive evidence of cause and effect, judgement could no longer be suspended on such an important matter, for the drug was not a vital one. But prospective observational cohort studies were quickly made in antenatal clinics where women had yet to give birth — though few, they provided evidence incriminating thalidomide. The worst had happened, a trivial new drug was the cause of the most grisly disaster in the short history of modern scientific drug therapy. Many thalidomide babies died, but many live on with deformed limbs,[18] eyes, ears, heart and alimentary and urinary tracts.

The West German Health Ministry estimated that thalidomide caused about 10 000 birth deformities is babies, 5000 of whom survived and 1600 of whom would eventually need artificial

limbs. In Britain there were probably at least 600 live births of malformed children of whom about 400 survived. The world total of survivors was probably about 10 000.

Thalidomide had been marketed in West Germany in 1956 and in Britain in 1958, as a sedative and hypnotic. Its chief merit seemed to be that overdose did not cause coma, probably because, with suitable particle size, elimination balanced absorption; given orally to animals a lethal dose could not be reached. Suicides were disappointed by thalidomide. Liquid formulations introduced later did not have this advantage and serious overdose could occur.

Thalidomide seemed a safe and pleasant hypnotic, and no doubt some patients found it preferable to others, but in the context of all drug therapy any advantages were trivial, and there were reasonable alternatives.

Despite the absence of any other notable properties, thalidomide, skilfully promoted and credulously prescribed and taken by the public — it was also sold without prescription — achieved huge popularity, it 'became West Germany's baby-sitter'. It was a routine hypnotic in hospitals and was even recommended to help children adapt themselves to a convalescent home atmosphere and was sold mixed with other drugs for symptomatic relief of pain, cough and fever.

In 1960–61 it had become evident that prolonged use of thalidomide could cause hypothyroidism and peripheral neuritis. The latter effect was the principal reason why approval for marketing in the USA, as Kevadon, had been delayed by the US Food and Drug Administration. Approval had still not been given when the fetal effects were discovered and so general distribution was avoided. Nonetheless some 'thalidomide babies' were born in the USA following indiscriminate pre-marketing clinical trials by 1270 doctors who gave the drug to 20 771 patients, of whom at least 207 were pregnant. Other countries in which cases of thalidomide phocomelia occurred include Australia, Belgium, Brazil, Canada, East Germany, Egypt, Israel, Lebanon, Peru, Spain, Sweden and Switzerland, although the drug was not marketed in all these.

Thalidomide has anti-inflammatory and im-

---

[18] For pictures of thalidomide deformities, see Br Med J 1962; 2: 646, 647, and JAMA 1962, 180: 1106.

munosuppressant actions and retains a limited specialist use in special cases, e.g. lepromatous leprosy.

The question whether the company was liable *in law* for the consequences of thalidomide was not tested in the courts since it paid compensation, having admitted 'moral' but not 'legal' liability. The law on 'product liability' ('strict' liability, 'no fault' liability) is developing in many countries, including the European Community, partly, indeed, as a result of the thalidomide disaster.

So rapidly did the news of the thalidomide disaster spread that some mothers who had taken it knew of the risk weeks before their babies were born. Of course, not all who took thalidomide during the crucial period (37th to 54th days from the first day of the last menstruation) had abnormal babies, perhaps no more than 20%; there is no reliable figure.

The thalidomide disaster provided the impetus for the introduction of national drug regulatory authorities worldwide.

GUIDE TO FURTHER READING

Editorial 1990 WHO's essential drugs concept. Lancet 1: 1003

Herxheimer A 1984 Immortality for old drugs. Lancet 2: 1460 and subsequent correspondence.

Hvidberg E F 1989 Good clinical practice: a way to better drugs. British Medical Journal 299: 580

Kaithin K I et al 1989 The drug lag: An update of new drug introductions in the United States and in the United Kingdom, 1977 through 1987. Clinical Pharmacology and Therapeutics 46: 121 and allied articles 139, 146

Kessler D A 1989 The regulation of investigational drugs. New England Journal of Medicine 320: 281

Litvack J I et al 1989 Setting the price for essential drugs: necessity and affordability. Lancet 2: 376

Richard B W et al 1987 Drug regulation in the United States and the United Kingdom: the Depo-Provera story. Annals of Internal Medicine 106: 886. An anlysis of how drug regulators in the USA and the UK came to opposite conclusions on the same data.

On thalidomide

Chamberlain G 1989 The obstetric problems of the thalidomide children. British Medical Journal 298: 6

Editorial 1981 Thalidomide: 20 years on. Lancet 2: 510

Mellin G W et al 1962 The saga of thalidomide. New England Journal of Medicine 267: 1184, 1238

6

Classification of drugs: names of drugs

SYNOPSIS

- Classification: drugs cannot be classified and named according to a single rational system because the requirements of pharmacologists, chemists and doctors differ.
- Nomenclature: nor is it practicable always to present each drug (medicine) under a single name because the formulations in which they are presented as prescribable medicines vary widely and commercial considerations are too often paramount.
  Generic (non-proprietary) names should be used as far as possible except where pharmaceutical bioavailability problems have overriding importance.

In any science there are two basic requirements, classification and nomenclature (names).

CLASSIFICATION

It is evident from the way this book is organised that there is no homogeneous system for classifying drugs that suits all purposes. Drugs are commonly categorised according to the convenience of who is discussing them — clinicians, pharmacologists or medicinal chemists.

Drugs may be classified by:

1. *Therapeutic use*, e.g. antimicrobial, antidiabetic, antihypertensive, analgesic
2. *Mode* or *site of action*
   a. *molecular interaction*, e.g. receptor blockers, enzyme inhibitors
   b. *cellular site*, e.g. loop diuretic, catecholamine uptake inhibitor (imipramine)
   c. *physiological system*, e.g. vasodilator, lipid-lowering, anticoagulant.
3. *Molecular structure*, e.g. barbiturate, glycoside, alkaloid, steroid.

NOMENCLATURE (names)

Any drug may have names in all three of the following classes:

1. the *full chemical* name

2. *a non-proprietary*[1] (official, approved, generic) name used in pharmacopoeias and chosen by official bodies
3. a *proprietary* name or names that are the commercial property of a pharmaceutical company/ies.

Example:

1. 3-(10,11-dihydro-5H-dibenz [*b,f*]-azepin-5-yl) propyldimethylamine
2. imipramine
3. Tofranil (UK), Prodepress, Surplix, Deprinol, etc. (various countries)

In this book proprietary names are distinguished by a capital letter.

The principal features of names

- The *full chemical name* describes the compound for chemists. It is obviously unsuitable for prescribing.
- The *non-proprietary (generic) name.*

  Three principles remain supreme and unchallenged in importance: the need for distinction in sound and spelling, especially when the name is handwritten; the need for freedom from confusion with existing names, both non-proprietary and proprietary, and the desirability of indicating relationships between similar substances,[2]

  e.g. di*azepam*, nitr*azepam*, flur*azepam* are all benzodiazepines.

- The *proprietary name* is a trade mark applied to a particular formulation(s) of a particular substance by a particular manufacturer. It is designed to maximise the differences with the names of the same drugs marketed by rivals, and with other drugs of the same class for obvious commercial reasons. Thus the three drugs

named above are Valium, Mogadon and Dalmane.

The use of non-proprietary names

The principal reasons for advocating the habitual use of non-proprietary (*generic*) names in prescribing are:

Clarity: because it gives information of the class of drug, e.g. nortriptyline and amitriptyline are plainly related, but their proprietary names are Allegron and Lentizol.

There have been cases of prescribers, when one drug had failed, unwittingly changing to another drug of the same group or even to the same drug, thinking that such different names must mean different drugs. Multiple names for the same drug are commonly totally uninformative, see the example in the previous column (imipramine). Such occurrences are a criticism of the prescriber, but they are also a criticism of the system that allows such confusion.

Economy: drugs sold under non-proprietary names are usually, but not always, cheaper than those sold under proprietary names.

Convenience: the pharmacist can supply whatever he stocks[3] whereas if a proprietary name is used he is usually obliged to supply that preparation alone. He may have to send for the preparation named although he has an equivalent in stock. But hospitals commonly allow substitution so that drugs can be bought in bulk. Mixtures of drugs are sometimes given non-proprietary names, often having the prefix *co-* to indicate more than one active ingredient, e.g. co-trimoxazole for Bactrim and Septrin, but many are not because they exist for commercial advantage rather than for therapeutic need. No prescriber can be expected to write out the ingredients, so proprietary names are used in many cases, there being no alternative.

International travellers with chronic illnesses will be grateful for international non-proprietary names[4] (proprietary names often differ from

---

[1] This is not strictly the same as a 'generic' name. 'Sulphonamide', 'barbiturate' are generic names, i.e. refer to a class or genus of compounds. But 'generic' is often misused to mean 'non-proprietary'. Unfortunately this misuse has become standard practice and so will be used in this sense in this book.
[2] Trigg R B. 1978; Pharmaceutical Journal 220: 181.

[3] This can result in supply of a formulation of appearance different from that previously used. Patients naturally find this disturbing.
[4] Selected by the World Health Organization.

country to country: the reasons are linguistic as well as commercial).

The use of proprietary names

The principal non-commercial reason for advocating the use of proprietary names in prescribing is consistency of the product, so that problems of quality, especially bioavailability, are reduced. There is substance in this argument, though it is sometimes exaggerated.

It is reasonable to use proprietary names when dosage, and therefore pharmaceutical bioavailability, are critical so that small variations in the amount of drug available for absorption can have big effects on the patient, e.g. drugs with low therapeutic ratio, digoxin, hormone replacement therapy, adrenocortical steroids (all uses), antiepileptics, cardiac antidysrhythmics, warfarin. Also, with the introduction of complex formulations, e.g. sustained release, it is important clearly to identify these, and use of proprietary names has a role.

The pharmaceutical industry regards freedom to market under brand names and to advertise or, as it calls the latter, to 'effectively (bring) to the notice of the medical profession', as two of the essentials of the 'process of discovery in a vigorous competitive environment'.[5]

The present situation is that industry spends an enormous amount of money promoting its many names for the same article; and the community, as represented by the UK Department of Health, spends a small sum trying to persuade doctors to forget the brand names and to use non-proprietary names. The ordinary doctor who prescribes for his ordinary patients is the target of both sides.

Whatever the theoretical pros and cons, one thing is plain, that until non-proprietary names approach in brevity and euphony those coined by pharmaceutical companies, the fight for their general use is a losing one. If one of the chief purposes of a drug name is that it should be used by doctors when prescribing, then provision of

such non-proprietary names as ceftazidime for Fortum, or even benzathine penicillin for Penidural defeats this purpose.

The search for proprietary names is a 'major problem' for pharmaceutical companies, increasing, as they are, their output of new preparations. A company may *average* 30 new preparations a year, another warning of the urgent necessity for the doctor to cultivate eclecticism, which can be done only on a foundation of knowledge of drugs and of criteria for their clinical assessment. The bleak outlook for prescribers is shown by the following.

One firm (in the USA) 'commissioned an IBM machine to produce a dictionary of forty-two thousand nonsense words of an appropriate scientific look and sound'. An official said,

Thinking up names has been driving us cuckoo around here . . . proper chemical names are hopeless for trade purposes, of course . . . Doctors are the market we shoot for. A good trade name carries a lot of weight with doctors . . . they're more apt to write a prescription for a drug whose name is short, and easy to spell and pronounce, but has an impressive medical ring . . . . We believe there are enough brand new words in this dictionary to keep us going for years. . . . We don't yet know what proportion of names is unpronounceable . . . how many are obscene, either in English or in other languages, and how many are objectionable on grounds of good taste: 'Godamycin' would be a mild example.

The names which 'look and sound medically seductive' are being picked out. 'Words that survive scrutiny will go into a stock-pile and await the inexorable proliferation of new drugs.'[6]

Perhaps the doctors have themselves to blame for this prospect which is made more appalling by the news that no other industry has a faster rate of innovation and product obsolescence.

About names of drugs, the medical profession is irritated by the pharmaceutical industry and the pharmaceutical industry is irritated by the medical profession.

In practical terms, most doctors have a British National Formulary on their desks, which includes a reasonably comprehensive glossary of proprietary

---

[5] Annual Report, 1963–1964. Association of British Pharmaceutical Industries.

[6] New Yorker, 14 July 1956.

drugs with their approved names. *The range of drugs prescribed by any individual is remarkably narrow, and once the decision is taken to 'think generic' surely the effort required is small*[7]

and, we would add, worthwhile.

Confusing names

The need for both clear thought and clear handwriting is shown by the frequency with which medicines of totally different class have closely similar names, both proprietary and non-proprietary, e.g. Asilone/Ilosone, atropine/Intropin, chlorpromazine/chlorpropamide, co-trimoxazole/clotrimazole, Daonil/De-Nol/Danol,

---

[7] Editorial Br Med J 1977; 4: 980, see also subsequent correspondence (our italics, DRL, PNB).

etc. Serious injury has occurred due to confusion of names and the dispensing of the wrong drug.

GUIDE TO FURTHER READING

Controversies in therapeutics 1988 The cases for and against prescribing generic drugs. British Medical Journal 297: (Collier J Generic prescribing benefits patients) 1596 (Cruickshank J M Don't take innovative research based pharmaceutical companies for granted) 1597

Editorial 1968 Brand names. 1: 781

Taussig H B 1963 The evils of camouflage as illustrated by thalidomide. New England Journal of Medicine 180: 92, Editorial, p. 108

7

General pharmacology

SYNOPSIS

How drugs act and interact, how they enter the body, what happens to them inside the body, how they are eliminated from it; the effects of genetics, age, and disease on drug action — these topics are important for, although they will generally not be in the front of the conscious mind of the prescriber, an understanding of them will enhance rational decision taking.

Knowledge of the requirements for success and the explanations for failure and for adverse events will enable the doctor to maximise the benefits and minimise the risks of drug therapy.

Pharmacodynamics
• Qualitative aspects of drug action
    Receptors, Enzymes, Selectivity
• Quantitative aspects of drug action
    Dose response, Potency, Therapeutic efficacy, Tolerance

Pharmacokinetics
• Time course of drug concentration: Order of reaction; Plasma half-life and steady-state concentration; Plasma concentration and pharmacological effect: therapeutic drug monitoring
• Individual processes: Drug passage across cell membranes, Absorption, Distribution, Metabolism, Elimination
• Drug dosage: Dosing schedules
• Individual or biological variation: Variability due to inherited influences, environmental and host influences
• Drug interactions: outside the body, at site of absorption, during distribution, directly on receptors, during metabolism, during excretion

Pharmacodynamics is what drugs do to the body: pharmacokinetics is what the body does to drugs.

It is self-evident that knowledge of pharmacodynamics is essential to the choice of drug therapy. But the well-chosen drug may fail to produce benefit or may be poisonous because too little or too much is present at the site of action for too short or too long a time. Drug therapy can fail for pharmacokinetic as well as for pharmacodynamic reasons. Those who try to practise drug therapy by remembering an apparently arbitrary list of actions or indications cannot provide the standard of care that patients have a right to expect.

Technical incompetence in the modern doctor is inexcusable and technical competence and a humane approach are not incompatibles as is sometimes suggested.

PHARMACODYNAMICS

Understanding the mechanisms of drug action is not only an objective of the pharmacologist who seeks to develop new and better drugs, it also a basis of the intelligent use of medicines.

QUALITATIVE ASPECTS OF DRUG ACTION

It is appropriate to begin by considering what drugs do and how they do it, i.e. the nature of drug action. Body functions are mediated through control systems that involve receptors, enzymes, carrier molecules and other specialised macromolecules such as DNA. Most drugs act by altering the body's control systems. Some do so unselectively, e.g. general anaesthetic agents and alcohol, and such substances tend to interfere with multiple systems thereby causing unwanted as well as wanted effects. The majority of medicinal drugs act by binding to some specialised constituent of the cell selectively to alter its function and consequently that of the physiological or pathological system to which it contributes. Such drugs are biologically selective and structurally specific in that small modifications to their chemical structure may profoundly alter their effect.

Mechanisms of drug action

An overview of the mechanisms of drug action shows that drugs act on:

the cell membrane by

- action on *specific receptors,*[1] e.g. agonists and antagonists on adrenoceptors, histamine receptors, acetylcholine receptors
- interference with selective *passage of ions across membranes,* e.g. calcium entry (or channel) blockers
- *inhibition of membrane bound enzymes and pumps,* e.g. membrane bound ATPase by cardiac glycoside; tricyclic antidepressants block the pump by which amines are actively taken up from the exterior to the interior of nerve cells
- *physicochemical interaction,* e.g. general and local anaesthetics and alcohol appear to act on the lipid, protein or water constituents of nerve cell membranes

---

[1] A *receptor* mediates a biological effect, e.g. adrenoceptor; a *binding site*, e.g. plasma albumin, does not.

metabolic processes within the cell by

- *enzyme inhibition,* e.g. monoamine oxidase by phenelzine, cholinesterase by pyridostigmine, xanthine oxidase by allopurinol
- *inhibition of transport processes* that carry substances across cells, e.g. blockade of anion transport in the renal tubule cell by probenecid can be used to delay excretion of penicillin, and to enhance elimination of urate
- *incorporation into larger molecules,* e.g. 5-fluorouracil, an anticancer drug, is incorporated into messenger-RNA in place of uracil
- in the case of successful *antimicrobial agents,* by altering metabolic processes unique to microorganisms, e.g. penicillin interferes with formation of the bacterial cell wall, *or* by showing enormous quantitative differences in affecting a process common to both humans and microbes e.g. inhibition of folic acid synthesis by trimethoprim

outside the cell by

- *direct chemical interaction,* e.g. chelating agents, antacids
- *osmosis,* as with purgatives, e.g. magnesium sulphate, and diuretics, e.g. mannitol which are active because neither they nor the water in which they are dissolved are absorbed by the cells lining the gut and kidney tubules respectively.

The more important mechanisms

Receptors

Most receptors are protein molecules. When the agonist binds to the receptor, the proteins undergo an alteration in conformation which induces changes in systems within the cell that in turn bring about the response to the drug. For example, activation of β-adrenoceptors by a catecholamine (the *first messenger*) increases the activity of adenylate cyclase which raises the rate of formation of cyclic AMP (the *second messenger*), a modulator of the activity of several enzyme systems that cause the cell to act. Other drug-receptor effects are mediated through control of membrane ion channels closely associated with the receptor, e.g. calcium entry blockers.

Radioligand binding studies[2] have shown that the receptor numbers do not remain constant but change according to circumstances. When tissues are continuously exposed to an agonist, the number of receptors decreases (*down-regulation*) and this may be a cause of tachyphylaxis (loss of efficacy with frequently repeated doses), e.g. in asthmatics who use adrenoceptor agonist bronchodilators excessively. Prolonged contact with an antagonist leads to formation of new receptors (*up-regulation*). Indeed, one explanation for the worsening of angina pectoris or cardiac ventricular dysrhythmia in some patients following abrupt withdrawal of a β-adrenoceptor blocker is that normal concentrations of circulating catecholamines now have access to an increased (*up-regulated*) population of β-adrenoceptors.

Agonists. Drugs that activate receptors do so because they resemble the natural transmitter or hormone, but their value in clinical practice often rests on their greater capacity to resist degradation and so to act for longer than the natural substances they mimic; for this reason bronchodilation produced by salbutamol lasts longer than that induced by adrenaline.

Antagonists (blockers) of receptors are sufficiently similar to the natural agonist to be 'recognised' by the receptor and to occupy without activating it, thereby preventing (blocking) the natural agonist from exerting its effect. Drugs that have no activating effect whatever on the receptor are termed *pure antagonists*.

Partial agonists. Some drugs in addition to blocking access of the natural agonist to the receptor are capable of a low degree of activation, i.e. they have both antagonist and agonist action. Such substances are said to show *partial agonist activity* (PAA). The β-adrenoceptor antagonists pindolol and oxprenolol have partial agonist activity (in their case it is often called *intrinsic sympathomimetic activity*) (ISA), whilst propranolol is devoid of agonist activity, i.e. it is a pure antagonist. A patient may be as extensively 'β-blocked' by propranolol as by pindolol, i.e. exercise tachycardia is abolished but the resting heart rate is lower on propranolol; such differences have clinical importance.

Inverse agonists. Some substances produce effects that are specifically *opposite* to those of the agonist. The agonist action of benzodiazepines on the benzodiazepine receptor in the CNS produces sedation, anxiolysis, muscle relaxation and controls convulsions; substances called β-carbolines which also bind to this receptor cause stimulation, anxiety, increased muscle tone and convulsions; they are inverse agonists. Both types of drug act by modulating the effects of the neurotransmitter gamma-aminobutyric acid (GABA).

Receptor binding (and vice versa). If the forces that bind drug to receptor are weak (hydrogen bonds, van der Waals bonds, electrostatic bonds), the binding will be reversible; if the forces involved are strong (covalent bonds), then binding will be effectively irreversible. An antagonist that binds *reversibly* to a receptor can by definition be displaced from the receptor by mass action (see p. 80) of the agonist (and vice versa). If the concentration of agonist increases sufficiently above that of the antagonist the response is restored. This phenomenon is commonly seen in clinical practice — the patient who is taking a β-adrenoceptor blocker, and whose low resting heart rate can be increased by exercise, is showing that he can raise his sympathetic drive to release enough noradrenaline (agonist) to diminish the prevailing degree of receptor blockade. Increasing the dose of β-adrenoceptor blocker will limit or abolish exercise-induced tachycardia, showing that the degree of blockade is enhanced as more drug becomes available to compete with the endogenous transmitter. Since agonist and antagonist *compete* to occupy the receptor according to the law of mass action, this type of drug action is termed *competitive antagonism*. When receptor-mediated responses are studied either in isolated

---

[2] The extraordinary discrimination of this technique is shown by the calculation that the total β-adrenoceptor protein in a large cow amounts to 1 mg. Maguire M E et al. 1977 In: Greengard P, Robison G A, eds Adv Cycl Nucleotide Res. New York: Raven Press, 8: 1.

tissues or in intact man, a graph of the logarithm of the dose given (horizontal axis), plotted against the response obtained (vertical axis), commonly gives an S-shaped (sigmoid) curve, the central part of which is a straight line. If the measurements are repeated in the presence of an antagonist, and the curve obtained is parallel to the original, but displaced to the right, then antagonism is said to be competitive and the agonist to be *surmountable.*

Drugs that bind *irreversibly* to receptors include phenoxybenzamine (to the α-adrenoceptor). Since such a drug cannot be displaced from the receptor, increasing the concentration of agonist does not fully restore the response and antagonism of this type is said to be *unsurmountable.*

The log-dose-response curves for the agonist in the absence of and in the presence of a *non-competitive* antagonist are not parallel. Some toxins act in this way, e.g. α-bungarotoxin, a constituent of some snake and spider venoms, binds irreversibly to the acetylcholine receptor and is used as a tool to study it. Restoration of the response after irreversible binding requires elimination of the drug from the body and synthesis of new receptor, and for this reason the effect may persist long after drug administration has ceased. Naturally irreversible agents find little place in clinical practice.

Enzymes

Interaction between drug and enzyme is in many respects similar to that between drug and receptor. Drugs may alter enzyme activity because they resemble a natural substrate and hence compete with it for the enzyme. For example, enalapril is effective in hypertension because it is structurally similar to that part of angiotensin I which is attacked by angiotensin-converting enzyme (ACE); by occupying the active site of the enzyme and so inhibiting its action enalapril prevents formation of the pressor angiotensin II. Carbidopa competes with levodopa for dopa decarboxylase and the resulting reduction in metabolism of levodopa in the blood (but not in the brain to which carbidopa does not penetrate) is the basis for the use of this combination in

Parkinson's disease. Ethanol prevents metabolism of methanol to its toxic metabolite, formic acid, by competing for occupancy of the enzyme alcohol dehydrogenase; this is the rationale for using ethanol in methanol poisoning. The above are examples of competitive (*reversible*) inhibition of enzyme activity. *Irreversible* inhibition occurs with organophosphorus insecticides which combine covalently with the active site of acetyl cholinesterase; recovery of cholinesterase activity depends on the formation of new enzyme. Covalent binding of aspirin to cyclo-oxygenase inhibits the enzyme in platelets for their entire lifespan because platelets have no system for synthesising new protein and this is why low doses of aspirin are sufficient for antiplatelet action.

Physiological (functional) antagonism

An action on the same receptor is not the only mechanism by which one drug may oppose the effect of another. Extreme bradycardia following overdose of a β-adrenoceptor blocker can be relieved by atropine which accelerates the heart by blockade of the parasympathetic branch of the autonomic nervous system, the cholinergic tone of which (vagal tone) operates continuously to slow it. Bronchoconstriction produced by histamine released from mast cells in anaphylactic shock can be counteracted by adrenaline which relaxes bronchial smooth muscle (β$_2$-adrenoceptor effect). In both cases, a pharmacological effect is overcome by a second drug which acts via a different physiological mechanism, i.e. there is *physiological* or *functional* antagonism.

Selectivity of drug action

The pharmacologist who produces a new drug and the doctor who gives it to a patient share the desire that it should possess a selective action so that management of the patient is not complicated by additional and unwanted (adverse) effects.

There are in general two approaches to obtaining selectivity of drug action:

1. By modification of drug structure

Many drugs are designed to have a structural similarity to some natural constituent of the body, e.g. a neurotransmitter, a hormone, a substrate for an enzyme, and achieve selectivity of action by replacing or competing with that natural constituent. Enormous scientific effort and expertise go into the synthesis and testing of analogues of natural substances in order to create drugs capable of obtaining a specified effect and that alone. The approach is the basis of modern drug design and it has led to the production of adrenoceptor antagonists, histamine-receptor antagonists and many other important medicines. But there are biological constraints to selectivity. Anticancer drugs that act against rapidly dividing cells lack selectivity because they also damage other tissues with a high cell replication rate, such as bone marrow and gut epithelium.

2. By selective delivery to the desired site of action (drug targeting)

The objective of target tissue selectivity can sometimes be achieved by simple topical application, e.g. skin, eye and special drug delivery systems, as by intrabronchial administration of β_2-adrenoceptor agonists or corticosteroids (inhaled pressurised metered aerosol for asthma). Selective targeting of drugs to less accessible sites of disease offers considerable scope for therapy as technology develops, e.g. attaching drugs to antibodies selective for cancer cells.

Stereoselectivity. Drug molecules are three-dimensional and many drugs contain one or more *asymmetric* or *chiral* centres in their structures, i.e. a single drug can be in effect a mixture of two non-identical mirror images (like a mixture of left- and right-hand gloves). The two forms which are known as *enantiomorphs* can exhibit very different biological activity, e.g. the S(−) form of warfarin is four times more active than the R(+) form.

QUANTITATIVE ASPECTS OF DRUG ACTION

That a drug has a desired *qualitative* action is obviously all-important, but it is not by itself enough. There are also *quantitative* aspects, i.e. the right *amount* of action is required and with some drugs the dose has to be very precisely adjusted to deliver this, neither too little nor too much, to escape both inefficacy and toxicity, e.g. digoxin, lithium, gentamicin. Whilst the general correlation between dose and response may evoke no surprise, certain characteristics of the relation are fundamental to the way drugs are used. These are:

The extent to which the desired response alters as the dose is changed

Change in response with alteration of dose is defined by the shape of the dose-response curve which conventionally has dose plotted on the horizontal and response on the vertical axis. A steep-rising and prolonged curve indicates that a small change in dose produces a large change in drug effect, e.g. loop diuretics. By contrast the dose-response curve for the thiazide diuretics soon reaches a plateau; e.g. the clinically useful dose range for bendrofluazide is between 2.5 and 10 mg and increasing the dose beyond this produces no added diuretic effect though it adds to toxicity. The wanted and unwanted effects of drugs have their own dose-response curves (see below). Toxicity is commonest with drugs that have steep dose response curves for both the wanted and unwanted effects.

Potency

The terms *potency* and *efficacy* are often used imprecisely and so confusingly. It is pertinent to make a clear distinction between them, particularly in relation to claims made for usefulness in therapeutics. *Potency* is the amount (weight) of drug in relation to its effect, e.g. if weight-for-weight drug A has a greater effect than drug B, then drug A is more potent than drug B, but the maximum therapeutic effect obtainable may be similar with both drugs. The diuretic effect of bumetanide 1 mg is equivalent to frusemide 50 mg, thus bumetanide is more potent than frusemide but both drugs achieve about the same maximum effect. The difference in weight of drug that has to be administered is of no clinical significance unless it is great.

Therapeutic efficacy

Therapeutic efficacy is the capacity of a drug to produce an effect and refers to the maximum such effect, e.g. if drug A can produce a therapeutic effect that cannot be obtained with drug B, however much of drug B is given, then drug A has the higher therapeutic efficacy. Differences in therapeutic efficacy are of great clinical importance. Amiloride (low efficacy) can at best cause no more than 5% of the filtered sodium load to be excreted and there is no point in increasing the dose beyond that which achieves this for no greater diuretic effect can be attained; bendrofluazide (moderate efficacy) can cause no more than 10% of the filtered sodium load to be excreted no matter how much drug is administered; frusemide (high efficacy) can cause 25% and more of filtered sodium to be excreted, hence it is called a high efficacy diuretic.

The therapeutic index

When the dose of a drug is increased progressively, the desired response in the patient usually rises to a maximum beyond which further increases in dose elicit no greater benefit but induce only unwanted effects. This is because a drug does not have a *single dose-response curve, but a different curve for each action,* so that new and unwanted actions are recruited if dose is increased after the maximum therapeutic effect has been achieved. Thus a sympathomimetic bronchodilator might exhibit one dose-response relation for decreasing airways resistance and another for increase in heart rate. Clearly the usefulness of any drug is intimately related to the extent to which such dose-response relations can be separated. Ehrlich introduced the concept of the *therapeutic index* as the maximum tolerated dose divided by the minimum curative dose, but since such single doses cannot be determined accurately, the index is never calculated in

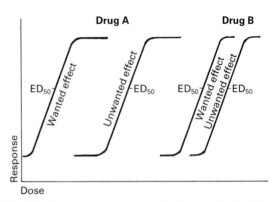

Fig. 7.1 Dose response curves for two hypothetical drugs Drug A: the dose that causes maximum wanted effect causes no unwanted effect. The ratio ED_{50} (unwanted effect)/ED_{50} (wanted effect)[3] indicates that it has a large therapeutic ratio: it is thus highly *selective* in its action. Drug B causes unwanted effects at doses well below that which produces its maximum benefit. The ratio ED_{50} (unwanted effect)/ED_{50} (wanted effect) indicates that it has a small therapeutic ratio: it is thus *non-selective*

this way in man. A dose that has some unwanted effect in 50% of humans, e.g. a specified increase in heart rate, in the case of an adrenoceptor agonist bronchodilator can be related to that which is therapeutic in 50%, e.g. a specified decrease in airways resistance, although in practice such information is not available for many drugs. Nevertheless the therapeutic index does embody a concept that is fundamental in comparing the usefulness of one drug with another, namely, safety in relation to efficacy. The concept is expressed diagrammatically in Figure 7.1.

Acquired and natural tolerance

Tolerance is said to have developed when it becomes necessary to increase the dose of a drug to obtain an effect previously obtained with a smaller dose. *Acquired tolerance* is familiar especially with opioids and is due to reduced efficacy at receptor sites. It can also be due to increased metabolism as a result of enzyme induction. There is commonly cross-tolerance between drugs of similar structure and sometimes between those of dissimilar structure. There is

[3] ED_{50} = effective dose in 50% of subjects.

also *natural tolerance* which is not induced by the drug but is due to inherent factors (see Pharmacogenetics, p. 104).

Biological assay (bioassay) and standardisation

Biological assay is the process by which the activity of a substance (identified or unidentified) is measured on living material, e.g. contraction of bronchial, uterine or vascular muscle. It is only used when chemical or physical methods are not practicable as in the case of a mixture of active substances, or of an incompletely purified preparation, or where no chemical method has been developed. The activity of a preparation is expressed relative to that of a standard preparation of the same substance. The controlled therapeutic trial is a special form of bioassay.

Biological standardisation is a specialised form of bioassay. It involves matching of material of unknown potency with an International or National Standard with the objective of providing a preparation for use in therapeutics and research. The results are expressed as units of a substance rather than its weight, e.g. insulin.

PHARMACOKINETICS

To initiate the action of a drug that is desired is a *qualitative* choice but, when the qualitative choice is made considerations of *quantity* inevitably arise; it is possible to have too much or too little of a good thing. To obtain the right effect at the right intensity, at the right time, for the right duration, with minimum risk of unpleasantness or harm, is what pharmacokinetics is about.

Dosage regimens of long-established drugs were devised by trial and error. Doctors learned by experience the dose, the frequency of dosing, and the route of administration that was most likely to give a beneficial effect and least likely to be toxic. Apart from being laborious and putting patients at risk, this empirical ('suck it and see') approach left some questions unanswered. It did not explain, for example, why digoxin is effective in a once-daily dose, whereas aspirin may need to be given 4 times daily; why a dose of morphine is more effective if it is given intramuscularly than if the same amount is taken by mouth; why insulin is useless unless it is injected. The answers to these questions lie in understanding how drugs cross membranes to enter the body, how they are distributed round it in the blood and other body fluids, how they are bound to plasma proteins and tissues (which act as stores) and how they are eliminated from the body. These processes can now be quantified and allow efficient development of dosing regimens.

Pharmacokinetics[4] is concerned with the *rate* at which drug molecules cross cell membranes to enter the body, to distribute within it and to leave the body, as well as with the structural changes (metabolism) to which they are subject within it.

The subject will be discussed under the following headings:

- The time course of drug concentration and effect
  The order of reaction (whether processes are first- or zero-order)
  Plasma half-life and steady-state concentration
  Plasma concentration and pharmacological effect
- The individual processes
  Absorption
  Distribution
  Metabolism
  Elimination

THE TIME COURSE OF DRUG CONCENTRATION AND EFFECT

A number of important topics are fundamental to the understanding of this process.

THE ORDER OF REACTION
First-order processes

Drugs taken into the body are subject to the pro-

---

[4] Greek: *pharmakon* drug, *kinein* to move.

cesses of absorption, distribution, metabolism and excretion. In the majority of instances, the rates at which these processes occur are proportional to the concentration of the drug. In other words, transfer of drug across a cell membrane or formation of a metabolite is *high at high* concentrations and falls in proportion to be *low at low* concentrations. This is because the processes follow the *Law of Mass Action*, which states that the rate of reaction is directly proportional to the active masses of reacting substances. In other words, at high concentrations, there are more opportunities for crowded molecules to interact with each other or to cross cell membranes than at low, uncrowded concentrations. Processes for which rate is proportional to concentration are called first-order.

In doses used clinically, most drugs are subject to first-order processes of absorption, distribution, metabolism and elimination and the knowledge that a drug exhibits first-order kinetics is useful; e.g. it can be predicted that a 50% or 100% increase in dose will lead to an increase in steady-state plasma concentration by the same percentage. The converse will also be true: since rate and concentration are in proportion, when dosing is discontinued, the rate of elimination from plasma falls as the plasma concentration falls and the time for *any* plasma concentration to fall by 50% ($t_{\frac{1}{2}}$, the plasma half-life) will always be the same; thus it is possible to quote a single figure for the $t_{\frac{1}{2}}$ of the drug. In this book $t_{\frac{1}{2}}$ means plasma $t_{\frac{1}{2}}$ unless otherwise stated.

Zero-order processes

As the amount of drug in the body rises, those processes that have limited capacity become saturated, i.e. the rate of the process reaches a maximum at which it stays constant, e.g. due to limited amount of an enzyme, and further increase in rate is impossible despite an increase in the dose of drug. Clearly, these are circumstances in which the rate of reaction is *not* proportional to dose, and processes that exhibit this type of kinetics are described as *rate-limited* or *dose-dependent* or *zero-order* or as showing *saturation kinetics*. In practice enzyme mediated metabolic reactions are the most likely to show rate-limitation because the amount of enzyme present is finite and can become saturated. Passive diffusion does not become saturated. There are some important consequences of zero-order kinetics.

Alcohol (ethanol) is a drug whose kinetics have considerable implications for society as well as for the individual, as follows.

Alcohol is subject to first-order kinetics with a $t_{\frac{1}{2}}$ of about one hour at plasma concentrations below 10 mg/dl (attained after drinking about two-thirds of a glass of wine or beer). Above this concentration the enzyme (alcohol dehydrogenase) that converts the alcohol into acetaldehyde approaches and then reaches saturation, at which point alcohol metabolism cannot proceed any faster. Thus if the subject continues to drink, the blood alcohol concentration rises disproportionately, for the rate of metabolism remains the same (at about 10 ml or 8 g/h for a 70 kg man), and alcohol shows zero-order kinetics.

Consider a man of average size whose life is unhappy to a degree where he drinks about half (375 ml) a standard bottle of whisky (40% alcohol), i.e. 150 ml of alcohol, over a short period, absorbs it and goes very drunk to bed at midnight with a blood alcohol concentration of about 250 mg/dl.

If alcohol metabolism were subject to *first-order* kinetics, with a $t_{\frac{1}{2}}$ of one hour throughout the whole range of social consumption, the subject would halve his blood alcohol concentration each hour and, when he drove his car to work at 08.00 hr the next morning, it is easy to calculate that he would have a negligible blood alcohol concentration (less than 1 mg/dl) though, no doubt, a severe hangover which might reduce his driving skill.

But alcohol is subject, at these high concentrations, to *zero-order* kinetics and so, metabolising about 10 ml of alcohol per hour, after 8 h the subject will have eliminated 80 ml, leaving 70 ml in his body and giving a blood concentration of about 120 mg/dl. The legal limit for car driving in UK is a generous 80 mg/dl and at 120 mg/dl a serious accident is likely. The subject will be convicted of drunk driving on his way to work despite his indignant protests that the blood or breath alcohol determination must be faulty since he has not touched a drop since midnight. He will, deservedly, be banned from the road, and will thus have leisure to reflect on the difference between *first-order* and *zero-order* kinetics.

This is an example thought up for this occasion, although no doubt something close to it happens in real life often enough, but an example important in therapeutics is provided by **phenytoin**. At low doses the elimination of phenytoin proceeds as a first-order process, i.e. as dose is increased there is a *proportional* increase in the steady-state plasma concentration because elimination increases to match the increase in dose. But gradually, the enzymatic elimination process approaches and reaches saturation, attaining a maximum rate beyond which it cannot increase; the process has become constant and zero-order. Since further increases in dose cannot be matched by increase in the rate of metabolism the plasma concentration rises steeply and *disproportionately*, with danger of toxicity. No doubt many drugs could exhibit saturation kinetics if a high enough dose were taken. The distinction between first-order and zero-order kinetics becomes a clinically important issue when the change from one to the other occurs within the range of therapeutic dosing. This is the case with alcohol, phenytoin and salicylate (at high therapeutic doses). Clearly saturation kinetics is a significant factor in delay in recovery from drug overdose with, e.g. phenytoin or aspirin.

When a drug is subject to first-order kinetics and by definition the rate of elimination is proportional to plasma concentration, then the $t_{\frac{1}{2}}$ is a constant characteristic, i.e. a single value can be quoted throughout the plasma concentration range, and this is convenient. If the rate of a process, e.g. removal from the plasma by metabolism, is not directly proportional to plasma concentration, then the $t_{\frac{1}{2}}$ cannot be constant. Consequently, when a drug exhibits zero-order elimination kinetics no single value for its $t_{\frac{1}{2}}$ can be quoted for, in fact, $t_{\frac{1}{2}}$ decreases as plasma concentration falls. Certain simple and valuable calculations are dependent on knowing the $t_{\frac{1}{2}}$: estimation of time to eliminate a drug; construction of dosing schedules; prediction of the time to achieve steady-state plasma concentration. These become too complicated to be of much practical use when elimination kinetics approach zero order.

PLASMA HALF-LIFE AND STEADY-STATE CONCENTRATION

The manner in which plasma drug concentration rises or falls when dosing is begun, altered or ceased follows certain simple rules which provide a means for rational control of drug effect. Central to understanding these is the concept of half-life. Consider the time course of a drug in the blood after an i.v. bolus injection, i.e. a single dose injected in a period of seconds as distinct from a continuous infusion. Plasma concentration will rise quickly as drug enters the blood to reach a peak; there will then be a sharp drop as the drug distributes round the body (*distribution phase*) which will be followed by a steady decline as drug is removed from the blood by the liver or kidneys (*elimination phase*). If the elimination processes are first-order, the time taken for any concentration point in the elimination phase to fall to half its value is always the same; in other words, the **half-life** or half-time ($t_{\frac{1}{2}}$), which is the time taken for the plasma concentration to fall by half, is a constant, as is illustrated in Figure 7.2.

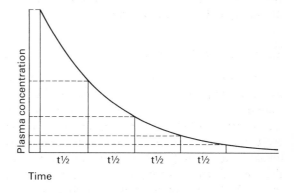

Fig. 7.2 Changes in plasma concentration following an i.v. bolus injection of a drug, in the elimination phase (the distribution phase, see text, is not shown); as elimination is a first-order process, the time taken for any concentration to fall by 50% ($t_{\frac{1}{2}}$) is the same

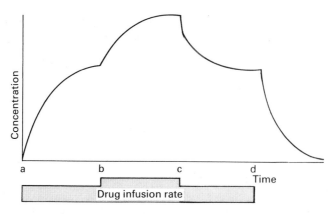

Fig. 7.3 Changes in drug plasma concentration during the course of a constant-rate i.v. infusion.
a: the infusion commences and plasma concentration rises to reach a steady state (plateau) in about $5 \times t\frac{1}{2}$.
b: the infusion rate is increased by 50% and the plasma concentration rises further to reach a new steady state in another $5 \times t\frac{1}{2}$; this new steady state is 50% greater than the original steady state.
c: the infusion is decreased to the original rate and the plasma concentration returns to the original steady state in $5 \times t\frac{1}{2}$.
d: the infusion is discontinued and the plasma concentration falls to virtually zero in $5 \times t\frac{1}{2}$

The $t\frac{1}{2}$ is the single pharmacokinetic characteristic of a drug that it is most useful to know for it may be used to predict the manner in which plasma concentration alters in response to starting, altering or ceasing drug administration. These events are illustrated in Figure 7.3 and the subsequent text.

Consider how plasma concentration increases after dosing begins

When a drug is given at a constant rate the amount in the body and with it the plasma concentration rise until a state is reached at which the rate of administration of drug to the body is exactly equal to the rate of elimination. This is called the *steady state* and when it is attained the amount of drug in the body remains constant; the plasma concentration is on a *plateau*. Figure 7.3 depicts the smooth changes in plasma concentration that result from a constant i.v. infusion. Clearly if a drug is given by intermittent oral or intravenous dose, the plasma concentration will fluctuate between peaks and troughs, but in time all the peaks will be of equal height and all the troughs will be of equal depth; this is also called a steady-state concentration, since the mean concentration is constant.[5] It is important to know *when* steady state has been reached, for maintaining the same dosing schedule will ensure a constant amount of drug action and the patient will experience neither toxicity nor decline of effect. The $t\frac{1}{2}$ provides the answer: with the passage of each $t\frac{1}{2}$ period of time, the plasma concentration rises by *half the difference between the current concentration and the ultimate steady-state (100%) concentration.*

Rise in plasma concentration of a drug administered by constant-rate i.v. infusion

in $1 \times t\frac{1}{2}$ the concentration will reach $100/2 = 50\%$

---

[5] The peaks and troughs can be of practical importance with drugs of low therapeutic index, e.g. aminoglycoside antibiotics, and it is often necessary to monitor both for safe therapy.

in $2 \times t\frac{1}{2}$ the concentration will reach
50 + 50/2 = 75%
in $3 \times t\frac{1}{2}$ the concentration will reach
75 + 25/2 = 87.5%
in $4 \times t\frac{1}{2}$ the concentration will reach
87.5 + 12.5/2 = 93.75%
in $5 \times t\frac{1}{2}$ the concentration will reach
93.75 + 6.25/2 = 96.875% of the ultimate
steady state.

The significant fact is that when a drug is given at a constant rate the *time to reach steady state* depends only on the $t\frac{1}{2}$ and, for all practical purposes, after 5 $t\frac{1}{2}$s the amount of drug in the body will be constant and the plasma concentration will be at a plateau.

Consider how plasma concentration alters when dosing alters

The same principle holds for change from any steady-state plasma concentration to a new steady state brought about by increase or decrease in the rate of drug administration, provided the kinetics remain first-order. Thus when the rate of administration is altered to cause either a rise or a fall in plasma concentration, a new steady-state concentration will eventually be reached and it will take a time equal to five $\times t\frac{1}{2}$ to reach the new steady state.

Note that the actual level of any steady-state plasma concentration (as opposed to the time taken to reach it) is determined only by the difference between the rate of drug administration (input) and the rate of elimination (output). If drug elimination remains constant and administration is increased by 50%, in time a new steady-state concentration will be reached which will be 50% greater than the original.

Consider how plasma concentration declines from steady state after dosing ceases

Since $t\frac{1}{2}$ is the time taken for any plasma concentration to decline by one-half, starting at any steady-state (100%) plasma concentration:

Fall in plasma concentration when drug administration ceases

in $1 \times t\frac{1}{2}$ the plasma concentration will fall to 50%
in $2 \times t\frac{1}{2}$ the plasma concentration will fall to 25%
in $3 \times t\frac{1}{2}$ the plasma concentration will fall to 12.5%
in $4 \times t\frac{1}{2}$ the plasma concentration will fall to 6.25%
in $5 \times t\frac{1}{2}$ the plasma concentration will fall to 3.125% of the steady-state concentration.

Hence the $t\frac{1}{2}$ can predict the extent of decline in plasma concentration at various times after dosing is discontinued, including the time in which elimination from plasma is almost complete i.e. a time equal to $5 \times t\frac{1}{2}$.

The relation between $t\frac{1}{2}$ and time to reach steady-state plasma concentration applies to all drugs that obey first-order kinetics, as much to dobutamine ($t\frac{1}{2}$ 2 min) when it is useful to know that an alteration of infusion rate will reach a plateau within 10 min, as to digoxin ($t\frac{1}{2}$ 36 h) when a constant dose will give a steady plasma concentration only after 7.5 days.

Plasma $t\frac{1}{2}$ values are given in the text where they seem particularly relevant. Inevitably, natural variation within the population produces a range in $t\frac{1}{2}$ values for any drug. For clarity only single average $t\frac{1}{2}$ values are given while recognising that

Table 7.1 Plasma $t\frac{1}{2}$ of some drugs

Drug	$t\frac{1}{2}$
dobutamine	2 min
benzylpenicillin	30 min
amoxycillin	1 h
paracetamol	2 h
midazolam	3 h
tolbutamide	6 h
atenolol	7 h
chlorpropamide	40 h
diazepam	40 h
warfarin	44 h
ethosuximide	54 h

the population range may be as much as 50% from the stated figure in either direction.

A few $t_{\frac{1}{2}}$ values are listed in Table 7.1 so that they can be pondered upon in relation to clinical practice.

The biological effect $t_{\frac{1}{2}}$ is the time in which the biological effect of a drug declines by one-half. With drugs that act competitively on receptors (α- and β-adrenoceptor agonists and antagonists) the biological effect $t_{\frac{1}{2}}$ can be provided with reasonable accuracy. Sometimes the biological effect $t_{\frac{1}{2}}$ cannot be provided; e.g. with antimicrobials when the number of infecting organisms and their sensitivity determine the outcome.

PLASMA CONCENTRATION AND PHARMACOLOGICAL EFFECT: THERAPEUTIC DRUG MONITORING

The issues that concern the practising doctor are not primarily those of changing drug plasma concentration but relate to drug effect: to the onset, magnitude and duration of action of individual doses. Because accurate information about the time course of drug action is more difficult to obtain and is therefore scarce, the plasma $t_{\frac{1}{2}}$ is often taken as a general guide to duration of drug action (although it is not necessarily synonymous with the latter). This immediately raises implications about the relation between drug plasma concentration and effect. Experience shows that patients differ greatly in the amount of drug required to achieve the same response.

The dose of warfarin that maintains a therapeutic concentration may vary as much as 5-fold between individuals, and there are many other examples. This is hardly surprising considering known variation in rates of drug metabolism, in disposition and in tissue responsiveness, and it raises the question of how optimal drug effect can be achieved quickly in each patient, i.e. can drug therapy be individualised? A logical approach is to assume that effect is related to drug concentration at the receptor site in the tissues and that in turn the plasma concentration is likely to be related to, though not necessarily the same as, tissue concentration. Indeed, for many drugs,

correlation between plasma concentration and clinical effect is better than that between dose and effect. Yet monitoring therapy by measuring drug in plasma is of practical use only in selected instances. The reasons for this repay some thought.

Plasma concentration may be obviously not worth measuring

This is the case where dose can be titrated against a quickly and easily measured effect such as blood pressure (antihypertensives), weight (diuretics), prothrombin time (oral anticoagulants) or blood sugar (hypoglycaemics).

Plasma concentration may have no correlation with effect

This is the case with drugs that act irreversibly and these have been named 'hit and run drugs' because their effect persists long after the drug has left the plasma. Such drugs destroy or inactivate target tissue (enzyme, receptor) and restoration of effect occurs only after days or weeks, when resynthesis takes place, e.g. monoamine oxidase inhibitors, aspirin (on platelets), some anticholinesterases and anticancer drugs.

Plasma concentration may correlate poorly with effect

• Inflammatory states may cause misleading results if only total drug concentration is measured. Many basic drugs, e.g. lignocaine, disopyramide, bind to acute phase proteins, e.g. α_1-acid glycoprotein, which are present in greatly elevated concentration in inflammatory states. The consequent rise in total drug concentration is due to increase in *bound* (inactive) but not in the *free* (active) concentration and correlation with effect will be poor if only total drug is measured. The best correlation is likely to be achieved by measurement of free (active) drug in plasma water but this is technically more difficult and total drug in plasma is usually monitored in routine clinical practice.

• Sometimes the effect of a drug declines as dose is increased beyond an optimum point. Nortriptyline is most effective in a range 50–150 µg/l of plasma. The lack of benefit below 50 µg/l is expected, and presumably represents concentrations too low to inhibit the amine pump; loss of effect at concentrations in excess of 150 µg/l is unexpected, and may be due to the α-adrenoceptor blocking effect of nortriptyline which becomes important only at higher concentration. The phenomenon arises because drugs may have more than one action (and so more than one dose-response curve) depending on the dose used. An intermediate range in which effective action is obtained is called a *therapeutic window*.

- The assay procedure may not measure metabolites of a drug that are pharmacologically active, e.g. some benzodiazepines, or may measure metabolites that are pharmacologically inactive; in either event correlation between plasma concentration and effect is weakened.

Plasma concentration may correlate well with effect

When this is the case, and when the effect is inconvenient to measure, dosage may best be monitored according to the plasma drug concentration (in relation to a previously defined optimum range).

Plasma concentration monitoring has proved useful in the following situations:

- When the desired effect is suppression of infrequent sporadic events such as epileptic seizures or episodes of cardiac dysrhythmia.
- When there is no quick and reliable assessment of effect, e.g. mood changes in a depressed patient, and where social environment plays a role as great or even greater than that of the drug.
- When lack of therapeutic effect and toxicity may be difficult to distinguish. Digoxin is both a treatment for, and sometimes the cause of cardiac supraventricular dysrhythmia; a plasma digoxin measurement will help to distinguish whether a dysrhythmia is due to too little or too much digoxin.
- To reduce the risk of adverse drug effects, e.g. otic damage with aminoglycoside

antibiotics or adverse CNS effects of lithium, when therapeutic doses are close to toxic doses (low therapeutic index).

- To check patient compliance on a drug regimen, e.g. when there is failure of therapeutic effect at a dose that is expected to be effective.
- To treat drug overdose.

The interpretation of drug concentration measurements

- A target therapeutic concentration range quoted for a drug should be regarded only as a guide to help to optimise dosing and should be evaluated with other clinical indicators of progress.
- Consider whether a patient has been taking a drug for a sufficient time to reach steady-state conditions, i.e. whether 5 $t_\frac{1}{2}$ periods have elapsed since dosing commenced or since the last change in dose. In the case of drugs that alter their own rates of metabolism by enzyme induction, e.g. carbamazepine and phenytoin, it is best to allow 2–4 weeks to elapse between change in dose and plasma concentration measurement. Sampling when plasma concentrations are still rising or falling towards a steady state is likely to be misleading.
- Consider whether *peak* or *trough* concentration should be measured. As a general rule when a drug has a short $t_\frac{1}{2}$ it is desirable to know both; monitoring peak (15 min after an i.v. dose) and trough (just before the next dose) concentrations of gentamicin ($t_\frac{1}{2}$ 2.5 h) helps to provide efficacy without toxicity. For a drug with a long $t_\frac{1}{2}$, it is usually best to sample just before a dose is due, i.e. trough concentration, or as near it as possible.

Recommended plasma concentrations for drugs appear throughout this book where these are relevant.[6]

---

[6] Concentrations of drugs in biological fluids are currently expressed in a dangerously confusing variety of notations, e.g. mg/100 ml, mg/l, micromol/l. Standardisation is desirable and the convention is likely to become molar unit per litre, i.e. SI (Système International) units.

INDIVIDUAL PHARMACOKINETIC PROCESSES

The following section considers the processes whereby drugs are absorbed into, distributed around, metabolised by and excreted from the body. Common to all these is the necessity for drugs to pass across cell membranes.

DRUG PASSAGE ACROSS CELL MEMBRANES

Our bodies are labyrinths of fluid-filled spaces. Some, such as the lumina of the kidney tubules or intestine, are connected to the outside world; the blood, lymph and cerebrospinal fluid are enclosed. These spaces are lined by sheets of cells and the extent to which a drug can cross epithelia or endothelia is fundamental to its clinical use. It is the major factor that determines whether a drug can be taken orally for systemic effect and whether within the glomerular filtrate it will be reabsorbed or excreted in the urine.

Cell membranes are essentially bilayers of lipid molecules with 'islands' of protein and they preserve and regulate the internal environment. Lipid-soluble substances diffuse readily into cells and therefore throughout body tissues. Adjacent epithelial or endothelial cells are joined by so-called tight junctions, some of which are believed to contain water-filled channels through which water-soluble substances of small molecular size may filter. The jejunum and proximal renal tubule contain many such channels and are called *leaky* epithelia, whereas the tight junctions in the stomach and urinary bladder do not have these channels and water cannot pass; they are termed *tight* epithelia. Special protein molecules within the lipid bilayer allow specific substances to enter or leave the cell preferentially (carrier proteins).

> The passage of drugs across membranes is determined by the natural processes of filtration, carrier-mediated transport and diffusion.

Filtration

Aqueous channels in the tight junctions between adjacent epithelial cells allow the passage of some water-soluble substances. Neutral or uncharged, i.e. non-polar, molecules pass most readily since the pores are believed to be electrically charged. Within the alimentary tract, pores are largest and most numerous in jejunal epithelium and filtration allows for rapid equilibration of concentrations and consequently of osmotic pressures across the mucosa. Ions such as sodium enter the body through the aqueous channels and pore size probably limits passage to substances of low molecular weight, e.g. methanol (mol. wt. 32) or glycerol (mol. wt. 92). Filtration seems to play at most a minor role in drug transfer within the body except for glomerular filtration, which is an important mechanism of drug excretion.

Carrier-mediated transport

Some drugs move into or out of cells against a concentration gradient, i.e. by *active transport*. These processes involve endogenous molecules, expend cellular energy and are more rapid than transfer by diffusion. The mechanisms show a high degree of specificity for particular compounds because they have evolved from biological needs for the uptake of essential nutrients or elimination of metabolic products. Thus, drugs that are subject to them bear some structural resemblance to natural constituents of the body. Examples of active transport systems are the absorption of iron by the gut, levodopa across the blood–brain barrier and the secretion of many organic acids and bases by renal tubular and biliary duct cells. Carrier-mediated transport that does not require energy is called *facilitated diffusion*, e.g. vitamin B_{12} absorption; carrier-mediated diffusion is subject to saturation and can be inhibited.

Diffusion

This is the most important means by which a drug enters the tissues and is distributed through them. It refers simply to the natural tendency of any substance to move from an area of high concentration to one of low concentration. In the context of an individual cell, the drug moves passively at a rate proportional to the concentration difference across the cell membrane, i.e. it shows first-order kinetics; cellular energy is not required, which means that the process does not become saturated and is not inhibited by other substances.

The dominating importance of lipid solubility to drug transfer across membranes is clear. Drugs exhibit greater or lesser degrees of lipid solubility according to environmental pH and the structural properties of the molecule. Broadly speaking, water solubility is favoured by the possession of alcoholic (–OH), amide (–CO.NH$_2$) or carboxylic (–COOH) groups, and the formation of glucuronide and sulphate conjugates. Presence of a benzene ring, a hydrocarbon chain, a steroid nucleus or halogen (–Br, –Cl, –F) groups favours lipid solubility.

It is useful to classify drugs in a physicochemical sense into:

1. Those that are variably ionised according to environmental pH (electrolytes) (lipid-soluble or water-soluble).
2. Those that are incapable of becoming ionised whatever the environmental pH (un-ionised, non-polar substances) (lipid-soluble).
3. Those that are permanently ionised whatever the environmental pH (ionised, polar substances) (water-soluble).

Drugs that are variably ionised according to environmental pH

Many drugs are weak electrolytes, i.e. their structural groups ionise to a greater or lesser extent, according to environmental pH. Most such molecules are present partly in the ionised and partly in the un-ionised state. The degree of ionisation influences lipid solubility (and hence diffusibility) and so affects absorption, distribution and elimination.

Ionisable groups in a drug molecule tend either to lose a hydrogen ion (acidic groups) or to add a hydrogen ion (basic groups). The extent to which a molecule has this tendency to ionise is given by the dissociation (or ionisation) constant (Ka). This is usually expressed as the pKa, i.e.

the negative logarithm of the Ka (just as pH is the negative logarithm of the hydrogen ion concentration). In an acidic environment, i.e. one already containing many hydrogen ions, an acidic group tends not to lose a hydrogen ion and remains un-ionised; a relative deficit of hydrogen ions, i.e. a basic environment, favours dissociation of the hydrogen ion from an acidic group which thus becomes ionised. The opposite is the case for a base. The issue may be summarised:

- acidic groups become less ionised in an acidic environment
- basic groups become less ionised in a basic (alkaline) environment
- and vice versa.

This in turn influences diffusibility since:

- un-ionised drug is lipid-soluble and diffusible and
- ionised drug is lipid-insoluble non-diffusible.

The profound effect of environmental pH on the *degree* of ionisation is best shown when the relation between these is quantified. It is convenient to remember that when the pH of the environment is the same as the pKa of a drug within it, then the ratio of un-ionised to ionised molecules is 1:1. But for every unit by which pH is changed, the un-ionised:ionised ratio changes 10-fold, as Table 7.2 shows.

Table 7.2 pH and ionisation

pH	acid un-ionised:ionised	base un-ionised:ionised
= pKa –2 units	100:1	1:100
= pKa –1 unit	10:1	1:10
= pKa	1:1	1:1
= pKa + 1 unit	1:10	10:1
= pKa + 2 units	1:100	100:1

pH variation and drug kinetics. Studies of the partitioning of a drug across a lipid membrane according to differences in pH have been developed as the *pH partition hypothesis*. There is a wide range of pH in the gut (pH 1.5 in the stomach; 6.8 in the upper and 7.6 in the lower intestine). But the pH inside the body is maintained within a limited range, (pH 7.4 ± 0.04) so that only drugs that are substantially un-ionised at this pH will be lipid-soluble, diffuse across tissue boundaries and so be widely distributed, e.g. into the CNS. Urine pH varies between the extremes of 4.6 and 8.2; thus the amount of drug reabsorbed from the renal tubular lumen by passive diffusion can be very much affected by the prevailing urine pH.

Consider the effect of pH changes on the disposition of aspirin (acid, pKa 3.5). In the stomach aspirin is un-ionised and thus lipid-soluble and diffusible. When aspirin enters the gastric epithelial cells (pH 7.4) it will ionise, become less diffusible and so will localise there. This *ion trapping* is one mechanism whereby aspirin is concentrated in, and so harms, the gastric mucosa. In the body aspirin is metabolised to salicylic acid (pKa 3.0) which at pH 7.4 is predominantly ionised and thus remains in the extracellular fluid. Eventually the molecules of salicylic acid in the plasma are filtered by the glomeruli and pass into the tubular fluid which is generally more acidic than plasma and causes a proportion of salicylic acid to become un-ionised and lipid-soluble so that it diffuses back into the tubular cells. Alkalinising the urine with sodium bicarbonate causes more salicylic acid to become ionised and lipid-insoluble so that it remains in the tubular fluid, and is eliminated in the urine. This effect is sufficiently great for alkalinising the urine to be effective treatment for salicylate (aspirin) overdose.

Conversely, acidifying the urine by i.v. infusion of arginine or lysine hydrochloride increases the elimination of the base amphetamine (pKa 9.9).

Drugs that are incapable of becoming ionised include digoxin and chloramphenicol. Having no ionisable groups, they are unaffected by environmental pH, are lipid-soluble and so diffuse readily across tissue boundaries. These drugs are also referred to as *non-polar*.

Drugs that are permanently ionised carry groups which dissociate so strongly that they remain ionised at all values of the body pH. Such compounds are termed *polar*, for their groups are either negatively charged (acidic, e.g. heparin) or positively charged (basic, e.g. ipratropium, tubo-curarine, suxamethonium) and all have a very limited capacity to cross cell membranes. This is a disadvantage in the case of heparin which is not absorbed by the gut and must be given parenterally. Conversely, heparin is a useful anticoagulant in pregnancy because it does not cross the placenta (which the orally effective warfarin does and is liable to cause fetal haemorrhage as well as being teratogenic).

The clinical relevance of drug passage across membranes may be illustrated with reference to the following:

Brain and cerebrospinal fluid (CSF). The capillaries of the cerebral circulation differ from those in most other parts of the body in that they lack the channels between endothelial cells through which substances in the blood normally gain access to the extracellular fluid. There are tight junctions between adjacent capillary endothelial cells which together with their basement membrane and a thin covering from the processes of astrocytes, separate the blood from the brain tissue. This barrier places constraints on the passage of substances from the blood to the brain and CSF. Compounds that are lipid-insoluble do not cross it readily, e.g. atenolol, compared with propranolol (lipid-soluble), and CNS side-effects are more prominent with the latter. Therapy with methotrexate (lipid-insoluble) may have no effect on leukaemic deposits in the CNS. Conversely lipid-soluble substances enter brain tissue with ease; thus diazepam (lipid-soluble) given intravenously is effective within one minute for status epilepticus; the level of general anaesthesia can be controlled closely by altering the concentration of inhaled anaesthetic gas (lipid-soluble).

Placenta. Chorionic villi, consisting of a layer of trophoblastic cells that enclose fetal capillaries, are bathed in maternal blood. The large surface area and blood flow (500 ml/min) are essential for gas exchange, uptake of nutrients and elimination of waste products. The fetal and maternal bloodstreams are therefore separated by a lipid barrier that readily allows the passage of lipid-soluble substances but excludes water soluble compounds, especially those with molecular weight exceeding 600.[7]

This exclusion is of particular importance with short-term use, e.g. tubocurarine (lipid-insoluble) given as a muscle relaxant during Caesarian section does not affect the infant; with long-term use, however, all compounds will eventually enter the fetus to some extent (see Drugs and the embryo and fetus, p. 130).

ABSORPTION

Commonsense considerations of anatomy, physiology, pathology, pharmacology, therapeutics and convenience determine the routes by which drugs are administered. Usually these are:

- *Enteral* by mouth (swallowed) or by sublingual or buccal absorption, rectum
- *Parenteral* by intravenous injection or infusion, intramuscular injection, subcutaneous injection or infusion, inhalation, topical application for local or for systemic (transdermal) effect
- *Other routes*, e.g. intrathecal, intradermal, intranasal, intratracheal, intrapleural, are used when appropriate.

The features of the various routes, their advantages and disadvantages are now considered.

Drug absorption from the gastrointestinal tract

The *small intestine* is the principal site for absorption of nutrients and it is also where most orally administered drugs enter the body. This part of the gut has two important attributes, an enormous surface area (estimated to be 4500 m^2 or about half the size of a football pitch), and an epithelium through which fluid readily passes in response to osmotic differences caused by the presence of food. It follows that drug access to the small intestinal mucosa is important and disturbed alimentary motility can reduce absorption, i.e. if gastric emptying is slowed by food, or intestinal transit is accelerated by gut infection. The

colon is capable of absorbing drugs and many sustained-release formulations probably depend on absorption at this site.

Absorption of ionisable drugs from the *buccal mucosa* is influenced by the prevailing pH which is 6.2–7.2. Lipid-soluble drugs are rapidly effective by this route because blood flow through the mucosa is abundant and entry is directly into the systemic circulation, avoiding the possibility of first-pass inactivation in the liver (see below). The stomach does not play a major role in absorbing drugs, even those that are acidic and thus un-ionised and lipid soluble at gastric pH, because its area is much smaller than that of the small intestine and gastric emptying is speedy ($t_{\frac{1}{2}}$ 30 min).

Enterohepatic circulation

This system is illustrated by the bile salts, which are conserved by circulating between liver and intestine about eight times a day. A number of drugs form conjugates with glucuronic acid in the liver and are excreted in the bile. These glucuronides are too polar (ionised) to be reabsorbed; they therefore remain in the gut where they are hydrolysed by enzymes and bacteria to release the parent drug which is then reabsorbed and reconjugated in the liver. Enterohepatic recycling appears to help maintain the effect of sulindac, pentaerythritol tetranitrate and ethinyloestradiol.

Systemic availability and bioavailability

When a drug is injected intravenously it enters the systemic circulation and thence gains access to the tissues and to receptors, i.e. 100% is available to exert its therapeutic effect. If the same quantity of the drug is swallowed, it does not follow that the entire amount will reach first the portal blood and then the systemic blood, i.e. its availability for therapeutic effect via the systemic circulation may be less than 100%. The anticipated response to a drug may not be achieved unless biological availability is taken into account. In a strict sense, considerations of reduced availability apply whenever any drug

---

[7] Most drugs have a molecular weight of less than 600 (e.g. diazepam 284, morphine 303) but some have more (erythromycin 733, digoxin 780) (gallamine 891, which is relevant to Caesarian section).

intended for systemic effect is given by any route other than the intravenous, but in practice the issue concerns enteral administration. This may be thought of in three main ways:

1. Pharmaceutical factors[8]

The amount of drug that is released from a dose form is highly dependent on its formulation. With tablets, for example, particle size (surface area exposed to solution), diluting substances, tablet size and pressure used in the tabletting machine can affect *disintegration* and *dissolution* and so the *bioavailability* of the drug. Manufacturers are expected to produce a formulation with an unvarying bioavailability so that the same amount of drug is released with the same speed from whatever manufactured batch or brand the patient may be taking. Substantial differences in bioavailability of digoxin tablets from one manufacturer occurred when the technique and machinery for making the tablets were changed; also tablets containing the same amount of digoxin but made by different companies, were shown to produce different plasma concentrations and therefore different effects, i.e. there was not *therapeutic equivalence*. Physicians tend to ignore pharmaceutical formulation as a factor in variable or unexpected responses, because they do not understand it and feel entitled to rely on reputable manufacturers and official regulatory authorities to ensure provision of reliable formulations. Good pharmaceutical companies reasonably point out that, having a reputation to lose, they take much trouble to make their preparations consistently reliable. This is a matter of great importance when dosage requires to be precise (anticoagulants, antidiabetics, adrenal steroids). The following account by Lauder Brunton in 1897 indicates that the phenomenon of variable bioavailability is not recent.

A very unfortunate case occurred some time ago in a doctor who had prescribed aconitine to a patient and gradually increased the dose. *He thought he was quite certain that he knew what he was doing.* The druggist's supply of aconitine ran out, and he procured some new aconitine from a different maker. This turned out to be many times stronger than the other, and the patient unfortunately became very ill. *The doctor said, 'It cannot be the medicine',* and to show that this was true, he drank off a dose himself with the result that he died. So you must remember the difference in the different preparations of aconitine,[9]

i.e. they had different bioavailability and so lacked therapeutic equivalence.

2. Biological factors

Those related to the gut include destruction of drug by gastric acid, e.g. benzylpencillin, and impaired absorption due to intestinal hurry which is important for all drugs that are slowly absorbed. Drugs may also bind to food constituents, e.g. tetracyclines to calcium and to iron, or to other drugs, e.g. acidic drugs to cholestyramine, and the resulting complex is not absorbed.

3. Presystemic (first-pass) elimination

Despite the fact that they readily enter gut mucosal cells, some drugs appear in low concentration in the *systemic* circulation. The reason lies in the considerable extent to which such drugs are metabolised in a single passage through the gut wall and (principally) liver, an important feature of the oral route. As little as 10–20% of the parent drug may reach the systemic circulation unchanged but the degree of presystemic

---

[8] Some definitions of enteral dose-forms: *Tablet*: a solid dose form in which the drug is compressed or moulded with pharmacologically inert substances (excipients); variants include sustained release and coated tablets. *Capsule*: the drug is provided in a gelatin shell or container. *Mixture*: a liquid formulation of a drug for oral administration. *Suppository*: a solid dose-form shaped for insertion into rectum (or vagina, when it may be called a *pessary*); it may be designed to dissolve or it may melt at body temperature (in which case there is a storage problem in countries where the environmental temperature may exceed 37°); the vehicle in which the drug is carried may be fat, glycerol with gelatin, or macrogols (polycondensation products of ethylene oxide) with gelatin. *Syrup*: the drug is provided in a concentrated sugar (fructose or other) solution. *Linctus*: a viscous liquid formulation, traditional for cough.

[9] The doctor died of cardiac dysrhythmia and/or cerebral depression. Aconitine is a plant alkaloid and has no place in medicine.

elimination differs much between drugs and between individuals. Hence the phenomenon of first-pass elimination adds, in some cases significantly, to variation in systemic plasma concentrations, and thus in response to the drugs that are subject to this process. By contrast, if the same dose is given intravenously, 100% becomes systemically available and the patient is exposed to higher concentrations with greater, but more predictable, effect. Once a drug is in the systemic circulation, irrespective of which route is used, about 20% is subject to the hepatic metabolic processes in each circulation because that is the proportion of cardiac output that passes to the liver.

Drugs for which presystemic elimination is significant include:

ANALGESICS	ADRENOCEPTOR BLOCKERS	OTHERS
dextro-propoxyphene	labetalol	chlormethiazole
morphine	metoprolol	chlorpromazine
pentazocine	oxprenolol	isosorbide dintrate
pethidine	propranolol	nortriptyline

If the reader cares to list the *enteral* and *parenteral* doses of the above drugs that achieve comparable effects, the difference introduced by presystemic elimination will be apparent. Note that if a drug produces active metabolites, differences in dose may not be as great as those anticipated on the basis of differences in plasma concentration of the parent drug after intravenous and oral administration.

In severe hepatic cirrhosis with both impaired liver cell function and well developed channels shunting blood into the systemic circulation without passing through the liver, first-pass elimination is reduced and systemic availability is increased. The result of these changes is an increased likelihood of exaggerated response to normal doses of drugs having high hepatic clearance and, on occasion, frank toxicity.

Drugs that exhibit the hepatic first-pass phenomenon do so because of the rapidity with which they are metabolised. The rate at which drug is delivered to the liver, i.e. blood flow, is then the main determinant of its metabolism. Many other drugs are completely metabolised by the liver but at a slower rate and consequently loss in the first pass through the liver is unimportant. The parenteral dose of these drugs does not need to be reduced to account for presystemic elimination. Such drugs include: chloramphenicol, diazepam, phenytoin, theophylline, warfarin.

Advantages and disadvantages of enteral administration

By swallowing

1. For systemic effect

Advantages are convenience and acceptability.

Disadvantages are that absorption may be delayed, reduced or even enhanced after food or slow or irregular after drugs that inhibit gut motility (antimuscarinic). Differences in presystemic elimination may introduce variation in drug effect between patients. Some drugs are not absorbed (gentamicin) and some drugs are destroyed in the gut (insulin, oxytocin, some pencillins). Tablets taken with too small a quantity of liquid and in the supine position, can lodge in the oesophagus with delayed absorption and may even cause ulceration (sustained release potassium chloride and doxycycline tablets), especially in the feeble elderly and those with an enlarged left atrium which impinges on the oesophagus.[10]

2. For effect in the gut

Advantages are that the drug is placed at the site of action (neomycin, anthelminthics), and with non-absorbed drugs the local concentration can be higher than would be safe in the blood.

Disadvantages are that drug distribution may be uneven, and in some diseases of the gut the whole thickness of the wall is affected (severe bacillary dysentery, typhoid) and effective blood concen-

---

[10] Ideally solid-dose forms should be taken standing up and washed down with 150 ml (tea cup) of water; even sitting (higher intra-abdominal pressure) impairs passage. At least patients should be told to sit and take 3 or 4 mouthfuls of water (a mouthful = 30 ml) or a cupful. Some patients do not even know they should take water.

trations (as well as luminal concentrations) may be needed.

Sublingual or buccal sulcus for systemic effect

Advantages are that quick effect is obtained (glyceryl trinitrate, nifedipine and ergotamine are given thus), especially if the tablet is chewed giving greater surface area for solution. The effect can be terminated by spitting out the tablet.

Disadvantages are the inconvenience if use has to be frequent, irritation of the mucous membrane and excessive salivation which promotes swallowing, so losing the advantages of this route.

Rectal administration

1. For systemic effect (suppositories or solutions). The rectal mucosa has a rich blood and lymph supply and, in general, dose requirements are either the same or slightly greater than those needed for oral use. Drugs chiefly enter the portal system, but those that are subject to hepatic first-pass elimination may escape this if they are absorbed from the lower rectum which drains directly to the systemic circulation. The degree of presystemic elimination thus depends on distribution within the rectum and this is somewhat unpredictable.

Advantages are that a drug that is irritant to the stomach can be given by suppository (aminophylline, indomethacin), the route is suitable in vomiting, motion sickness, migraine or when a patient cannot swallow, and when cooperation is lacking (sedation in children).

Disadvantages are psychological in that the patient may be embarrassed or may like the route too much, that rectal inflammation may occur with repeated use and that absorption can be unreliable, especially if the rectum is full of faeces.

2. For local effect, e.g. in proctitis or colitis; an obvious use.

A survey in the UK showed that a substantial proportion of patients did not remove the wrapper before inserting the suppository.

Parenteral administration (for systemic and local effect)

Intravenous (bolus or infusion). An i.v. bolus,

i.e. rapid injection, passes round the circulation being progressively diluted each time; it is delivered principally to the organs with high blood flow (brain, liver, heart, lung, kidneys).

Advantages are that the i.v. route gives swift, effective and highly predictable blood concentration and allows rapid modification of dose, i.e. immediate cessation of administration is possible if unwanted effects occur during administration. The route is suitable for administration of drugs that are not absorbed from the gut or are too irritant (anticancer agents) to be given by other routes.

Disadvantages are the hazard if a drug is given too quickly, as plasma concentration may rise at such a rate that normal mechanisms of distribution and elimination are outpaced. (Some drugs will act within one arm-to-tongue circulation time which is 13 ± 3 s; with most drugs an injection given over 4 or 5 circulation times seems sufficient to avoid excessive plasma concentrations.) Local venous thrombosis is liable to occur with prolonged infusion and with bolus doses of irritant formulations, e.g. diazepam, or microparticulate components of infusion fluids especially if small veins are used. Infection of the intravenous catheter and the small thrombi on its tip are also a risk during prolonged infusions.

Intramuscular injection. Blood flow is greater in the muscles of the upper arm than in the gluteal mass and thigh, and also increases with physical exercise. (Usually these influences are unimportant but one football-playing patient who was given an intramuscular injection of a sustained release phenothiazine had to be substituted towards the end of the game when he developed an extrapyramidal disorder, presumably due to too rapid absorption of the drug.)

Advantages are that the route is reliable, is suitable for irritant drugs, and depot preparations (pencillins, neuroleptics, medroxyprogesterone) can be used at monthly or longer intervals. Absorption is more rapid than following subcutaneous injection (soluble preparations are absorbed within 10–30 min).

Disadvantages are that the route is not acceptable for self-administration, and it may be painful.

Subcutaneous injection

Advantages are that the route is reliable and is acceptable for self-administration.

Disadvantages are poor absorption in peripheral circulatory failure. Repeated injections at one site can cause lipoatrophy, resulting in erratic absorption (see insulin).

Inhalation

1. As a *gas*, e.g. volatile anaesthetics.

2. As an *aerosol*, e.g. β_2-adrenoceptor agonist bronchodilators. Aerosols are particles dispersed in a gas, the particles being small enough to remain in suspension for a long time instead of sedimenting rapidly under the influence of gravity; the particles may be liquid (fog) or solid (smoke).

3. As a *powder*, e.g. sodium cromoglycate. Particle size and air flow velocity are important. Most particles above 5 µm in diameter impact in the upper respiratory areas; particles of about 2 µm reach the terminal bronchioles; a large proportion of particles less than 1 µm will be exhaled. Air flow velocity diminishes considerably as the bronchi progressively divide, promoting drug deposition peripherally.

Advantages are that drugs as gases can be rapidly taken up or eliminated, giving the close control that has marked the use of this route in general anaesthesia from its earliest days. Self-administration is practicable. Aerosols and powders provide high local concentration for action on bronchi, minimising systemic effects; aerosols can also be used for systemic effect, e.g. ergotamine for migraine.

Disadvantages are that special apparatus is needed (some patients find pressurised aerosols difficult to use to best effect) and a drug must be non-irritant if the patient is conscious. Obstructed bronchi (mucus plugs in asthma) may cause therapy to fail.

Topical application

1. For local effect, e.g. to skin, eye, anal canal and rectum, vagina.

Advantage is the provision of high local concentration without systemic effect (usually[11]).

Disadvantage is that absorption can occur, especially when there is tissue destruction so that systemic effects result, e.g. adrenal steroids and neomycin to the skin, atropine to the eye. Ocular administration of a β-adrenoceptor blocker may cause sytemic effects and such eye drops are contraindicated for patients with asthma or chronic lung disease. There is extensive literature on this subject characterstised by expressions of astonishment that serious effects can occur.

2. For systemic effect. Transdermal delivery systems (TDS) release drug through a rate-controlling membrane into the skin and so into the systemic circulation. Fluctuations in plasma concentration associated with other routes of administration are largely avoided, as is first-pass elimination in the liver. Glyceryl trinitrate and postmenopausal hormone replacement therapy may be given this way, in the form of a sticking plaster attached to the skin[12] or as an ointment (glyceryl trinitrate).

DISTRIBUTION

If a drug is required to act throughout the body or to reach an organ inaccessible to topical administration, it must be got into the blood and

---

[11] A cautionary tale. A 70-year-old man reported left breast enlargement and underwent mastectomy; histological examination revealed benign gynaecomastia. Ten months later the right breast enlarged. Tests of endocrine function were normal but the patient himself was struck by the fact that his wife had been using a vaginal cream (containing 0.01% dienestrol) initially for atrophic vaginitis but latterly the cream had been used to facilitate sexual intercourse which took place two to three times a week. On the assumption that penile absorption of oestrogen was responsible for the disorder, exposure to the cream was terminated. The gynaecomastia in the remaining breast then resolved (Di Raimondo CV et al. N Engl J Med 1980; 302: 1089).

[12] But TDS may have an unexpected outcome, for not only may the sticking plaster drop off unnoticed, it may find its way onto another person. An hypertensive father rose one morning and noticed that his clonidine plaster was missing from his upper arm. He could not find it and applied a new plaster. His nine-month-old child, who had been taken into the paternal bed during the night because he needed comforting, spent an irritable and hypoactive day, refused food but drank and passed more urine than usual. The missing clonidine patch was discovered on his back when he was being prepared for his bath. No doubt this was accidental, but children also enjoy stick-on decoration and the possibility of poisoning from misused, discarded or new drug plasters means that these should be kept and disposed of as carefully as oral formulation (Reed M T et al. N Engl J Med 1986; 314: 1120).

into other body compartments. Most drugs distribute widely — in part dissolved in body water, in part bound to plasma proteins, in part to tissues. Distribution is often uneven, for drugs may bind selectively to plasma or tissue proteins or be localised within particular organs. Clearly, the site of localisation of a drug is likely to influence its action, e.g. whether it crosses the blood–brain barrier to enter the brain; the *extent* (amount) and *strength* (tenacity) of protein or tissue binding will affect the time it spends in the body and thereby its duration of action.

Drug distribution, its quantification and its clinical implications are now discussed.

Distribution volume

The distribution volume of a drug is the volume in which it appears to distribute (or which it would require) if the concentration throughout the body were equal to that in plasma, i.e. as if the body were a single compartment. An explanation follows.

The pattern of distribution from plasma to other body fluids and tissues is a characteristic of each drug that enters the circulation and it varies between drugs. Precise information on the concentration attained by a drug in various tissues and fluids requires biopsy samples and for understandable reasons this is usually not available for humans. What can be sampled readily in humans is *blood plasma*, the drug concentration in which, taking account of the dose given, is a measure of whether a drug tends to remain in the circulation or to distribute from the plasma into the tissues. If a drug remains mostly in the plasma, its distribution volume will be small; if it is present mainly in other tissues the distribution volume will be large.

Such information is clinically useful. Consider drug overdose. Removing a drug by haemodialysis is likely to be a beneficial exercise only if a major proportion of the total body load is in the plasma, e.g. with salicylate which has a small distribution volume; but haemodialysis is an inappropriate treatment for overdose with pethidine which has a large distribution volume. These however, are generalisations and if the knowledge

of distribution volume is to be of practical value it must be *quantified* more precisely.

The *principle* for establishing the distribution volume is essentially that of using a dye to find the volume of a container filled with liquid. The weight of dye that is added divided by the concentration of dye once mixing is complete gives the distribution volume of the dye, which is the volume of the container. Similarly, the distribution volume of a drug in the body may be determined after a single intravenous bolus dose by dividing the amount of drug given by the concentration achieved in plasma.[13]

The result of this calculation, the *distribution volume*, in fact only rarely corresponds with a physiological body space such as extracellular water or total body water, for it is a measure of volume a drug would *apparently* occupy knowing the dose given and the plasma concentration achieved and assuming the entire volume is at that concentration. For this reason, it is often referred to as the *apparent distribution volume*. Indeed, for some drugs that bind extensively to extravascular tissues, the apparent distribution volume, which is based on the resulting low plasma concentration, is many times total body volume (see list below).

Thus the distribution volume may be defined as *the volume of fluid in which the drug appears to distribute with a concentration equal to that in plasma.*

The list in Table 7.3 illustrates a range of apparent distribution volumes. The names of those substances that distribute within (and have been used to measure) physiological spaces are in italics.

Selective distribution within the body occurs

---

[13] Clearly a problem arises in that the plasma concentration is not constant but falls after the bolus has been injected. To get round this, use is made of the fact that the relation between the *logarithm* of plasma concentration and the time after a single intravenous dose is a straight line. The log concentration-time line extended back to zero time gives the theoretical plasma concentration at the time the drug was given. In effect, the assumption is made that drug distributes instantaneously and uniformly through a single compartment, the distribution volume. This mechanism, although seeming artificial, does usefully characterise drugs according to the extent to which they remain in or distribute out from the circulation.

Table 7.3 Apparent distribution volume of some drugs
(Figures are in litres for a 70 kg person who would displace about 70 l)[14]

Drug	Distribution volume	Drug	Distribution volume
Evans blue	3 (plasma volume)	atenolol	77
heparin	5	diazepam	140
aspirin	11	pethidine	280
inulin	15 (extracellular water)	digoxin	420
gentamicin	18	nortriptyline	1000
frusemide	21	dothiepin	4900
amoxycillin	28	chloroquine	13 000
antipyrine	43 (total body water)		

because of special affinity between particular drugs and particular body constituents. Many drugs bind to proteins in the plasma; in the tissues, phenothiazines and chloroquine bind to melanin-containing tissues, including the retina, which may explain the occurrence of retinopathy. Drugs may also concentrate selectively in a particular tissue because of specialised transport mechanisms, e.g. iodine in the thyroid.

Plasma protein and tissue binding

Many natural substances circulate around the body partly free in plasma water and partly bound to plasma proteins; these include cortisol, thyroxine, iron, copper and, in hepatic or renal failure, by-products of metabolism. Drugs, too, circulate in the protein-bound and free states, and the significance is that the *free fraction* is pharmacologically active whereas the *protein bound* component is a reservoir of drug that is inactive because of this binding. Free and bound fractions are in equilibrium and free drug removed from the plasma by metabolism, dialysis or excretion is replaced by drug released from the bound fraction. Association and dissociation between drug and plasma protein are usually rapid.

Albumin is the main binding protein for many natural substances and drugs. Each albumin molecule consists of a chain of 584 amino acids held in a series of loops by bridging disulphide bonds. This complex structure has a net negative charge at blood pH and a high *capacity* but low (weak) *affinity* for many basic drugs, i.e. a lot is bound but it is readily released. Two particular sites on the albumin molecule bind acidic drugs with high affinity (strongly) but these sites have low capacity. Saturation of binding sites on plasma proteins in general is unlikely in the doses in which most drugs are used. Other binding proteins in the blood include lipoprotein and α_1-acid glycoprotein, both of which carry basic drugs such as quinidine, chlorpromazine and imipramine. Such binding may have implications for therapeutic drug monitoring according to plasma concentration (see p. 84). Thyroxine and sex hormones are bound in the plasma to specific globulins.

Disease may modify protein binding of drugs to an extent that is clinically relevant as Table 7.4 shows. In *chronic renal failure*, hypoalbuminaemia and retention of (as yet unidentified) products of metabolism that compete for binding sites on protein, are both responsible for the decrease in protein binding of drugs. Most affected are acidic drugs that are highly protein bound, e.g. phenytoin, and special care is needed when initiating and modifying the dose of such drugs for patients with renal failure (see also Drugs and renal disease, p. 470).

Chronic liver disease also leads to hypoalbuminaemia and increase of endogenous substances such as bilirubin that may compete for binding sites on protein. Drugs that are nor-

---

[14] Litres per kg are commonly used, but give a less vivid image of the implication of the term 'apparent', e.g. chloroquine.

mally extensively protein bound should be used with special caution, for increased free concentration of diazepam, tolbutamide and phenytoin have been demonstrated in patients with this condition (see also Drugs and liver disease p. 543).

The free, unbound and therefore pharmacologically active percentages of some drugs are listed in Table 7.4 to illustrate the range and, in some cases, the changes caused by disease.

Table 7.4 Examples of plasma protein binding of drugs and effects of disease

Drug	% unbound (free)	
warfarin	1	
diazepam	2	(6% in liver disease)
frusemide	2	(6% in nephrotic syndrome)
tolbutamide	2	
clofibrate	4	(11% in nephrotic syndrome)
amitriptyline	5	
phenytoin	9	(19% in renal disease)
triamterene	19	(40% in renal disease)
trimethoprim	30	
theophylline	35	(71% in liver disease)
morphine	65	
digoxin	75	(82% in renal disease)
amoxycillin	82	
ethosuximide	100	

Drugs may *interact* at plasma protein binding sites as is discussed on p. 113.

Some drugs distribute readily to regions of the body other than plasma, as a glance at Table 7.3 will show. These include many lipid-soluble drugs which may enter fat stores, e.g. most benzodiazepines, verapamil and lignocaine. Less is known about *tissue*, e.g. muscle, binding than about plasma protein binding because solid tissue samples can be obtained only by invasive biopsy, but extensive binding to tissues delays elimination from the body and accounts for the long $t\frac{1}{2}$ of chloroquine and amiodarone. Displacement from tissue binding sites may be a mechanism for drug interaction (see p. 113).

METABOLISM

Most drugs are treated by the body as foreign substances (xenobiotics) and become subject to its various mechanisms for ridding itself of chemical intruders.

Metabolism is a general term for chemical transformations that occur within the body and its processes change drugs in two major ways:

- by reducing lipid solubility
- by reducing biological activity.

Reducing lipid solubility

Metabolic reactions tend to make a drug molecule progressively more water-soluble and so favour its elimination in the urine. Consider the situation if there were no drug metabolising enzymes.

For simplicity let us assume that a drug is evenly distributed throughout body water. If the compound has a low lipid solubility, about five hours would elapse before half the substance is lost from the body; if the drug is also secreted by the (renal) tubules, this time will be shortened to as little as one hour. However, if the drug is lipid-soluble, the excretion rate will be drastically reduced by back diffusion into the plasma from the tubular segment where the urine is concentrated. About thirty days would elapse before half the drug leaves the body. This extended duration might be an advantage with an antibacterial agent but would be of doubtful value with an anaesthetic agent. If a drug . . . is also reversibly localised in tissues its half-life would be about 100 years — considerably longer than those of the physician and patient combined![15]

Some environmental chemicals may persist indefinitely in our fat deposits, e.g. dicophane (DDT), with consequences that are as yet unknown.

Drug metabolising enzymes were developed during evolution to enable the body to dispose of lipid-soluble substances such as hydrocarbons, sterols and alkaloids, that are ingested with food.[16]

---

[15] Brodie BB, 1964 In: Binns TB (ed) Absorption and distribution of drugs. London: Livingstone.
[16] Fish lose lipid-soluble substances through the gills. They do not need such effective metabolising enzymes and they have not got them.

Altered biological activity

The end result of metabolism usually is the abolition of biological activity but various steps in between may have the following consequences:

1. Conversion of a pharmacologically active to an inactive substance: most drugs

2. Conversion of a pharmacologically active to another active substance:

ACTIVE DRUG	ACTIVE METABOLITE
amitriptyline	nortriptyline
codeine	morphine
chloroquine	hydroxychloroquine
diazepam	oxazepam
spironolactone	canrenone

3. Conversion of a pharmacologically inactive to an active substance, i.e. *prodrugs*:

INACTIVE SUBSTANCE	ACTIVE METABOLITE(S)
azathioprine	mercaptopurine
benorylate	salicylic acid and paracetamol
cholecalciferol	1-α-hydroxycholecalciferol
cyclophosphamide	4-ketocyclophosphamide
enalapril	enalaprilat
sulindac	sulindac sulphide
sulphasalazine	5-aminosalicylic acid
talampicillin	ampicillin

The metabolic processes

The liver is by far the most important drug metabolising organ although a number of tissues, including the kidney, gut mucosa, lung and skin also contribute. It is useful to think of drug metabolism in two broad phases:

Phase 1 metabolism brings about a change in the drug molecule by oxidation, reduction or hydrolysis and often introduces a chemically active site into it. The new metabolite may retain biological activity but have different pharmacokinetic properties, e.g. a shorter $t_\frac{1}{2}$. The most important single group of reactions is the oxidations, in particular those undertaken by the so-called mixed-function oxidases which, as the name indicates, are capable of metabolising a variety of compounds, i.e. because of mixed-function oxidases we do not need to possess new enzymes for every existing or yet-to-be-synthesised drug.

Phase I oxidation of some drugs results in the formation of *epoxides* which are short-lived and highly reactive metabolites. Epoxides are important because they can bind irreversibly through covalent bonds to cell constituents; indeed, this is one of the principal ways in which drugs are toxic to body tissues. Glutathione is a tripeptide that combines with epoxides, rendering them inactive and its presence in the liver is part of an important defence mechanism against hepatic damage by halothane and paracetamol.

Phase II metabolism involves union of the drug with one of several polar (water soluble) endogenous molecules that are products of intermediary metabolism, to form a water-soluble conjugate which is readily eliminated by the kidney or, if the molecular weight exceeds 300, in the bile. Thus morphine, paracetamol and salicylates form conjugates with glucuronic acid (derived from glucose); oral contraceptive steroids form sulphates; isoniazid, phenelzine and dapsone are acetylated. Conjugation with a more polar molecule is also a mechanism by which natural substances are eliminated, e.g. bilirubin as glucuronide, oestrogens as sulphates. Phase II metabolism almost invariably *terminates* biological activity.

Enzyme induction

The mechanisms that the body evolved over millions of years to metabolise foreign substances now enable it to meet the modern environmental challenges of tobacco smoke, hydrocarbon pollutants, insecticides, and drugs. Thus, at times of high exposure, our enzyme systems respond by increasing in amount and so in activity, i.e. they are *induced*; when exposure falls off, enzyme production lessens. For example, a first alcoholic drink taken after a period of abstinence from alcohol may have quite a significant effect on behaviour but the same drink taken at the end of two weeks' regular imbibing may pass almost unnoticed because the individual's liver enzyme activity is increased so that alcohol is metabolised more rapidly and has less effect, i.e. *tolerance* has been acquired.

Inducing substances in general share some important properties; they tend to be lipid-soluble, they are substrates though sometimes only minor ones, e.g. DDT, for the enzymes they induce and they generally have long t_2^1s. The time for onset and offset of induction depends on enzyme t_2^1, but significant induction generally occurs within a few days and it passes off over 2 or 3 weeks following withdrawal of the inducer.

It follows that the capacity of the body to metabolise drugs can be altered by certain medicinal drugs themselves and by other substances; clearly this phenomenon has implications for drug therapy. More than 200 substances have been shown to induce enzymes in animals but the list of *proven enzyme inducers in man* is much more restricted.

Substances that cause enzyme induction in man

barbecued meats	griseofulvin
Brussels sprouts	meprobamate
barbiturates	phenytoin
carbamazepine	primidone
DDT (dicophane	phenobarbitone
and other	rifampicin
insecticides)	sulphinpyrazone
ethanol (chronic)	tobacco smoke
glutethimide	

Enzyme induction is relevant to drug therapy for the following reasons:

- *Clinically important drug interactions may result*, e.g. in failure of oral contraceptives or loss of anticoagulant control.
- *Disease may result*. Antiepilepsy drugs increase the breakdown of dietary and endogenously formed vitamin D, producing an inactive metabolite — in effect a vitamin D deficiency state, which can result in osteomalacia. The accompanying

hypocalcaemia can increase the tendency to fits and a convulsion may lead to fracture of the demineralised bones.

- *Tolerance to drug therapy may result* and provide an explanation for suboptimal treatment, e.g. with an antiepilepsy drug.
- *Variability in response to drugs is increased.* Enzyme induction caused by heavy drinking or heavy smoking may be an unrecognised cause for failure of an individual to achieve the expected response to a normal dose of a drug.
- *Drug toxicity* may be more likely. Regular heavy drinkers of alcohol are probably more likely to develop liver toxicity after paracetamol overdose by increased production of an hepatotoxic metabolite.

Enzyme inhibition

Consequences of inhibiting drug metabolism can be more profound than those of enzyme induction. Effects of enzyme inhibition by drugs also tend to be more selective than those of enzyme induction. Consequently, enzyme inhibition offers more scope for therapy (see Table 7.5).

Table 7.5:   Drugs that act by enzyme inhibition

Drug	Enzyme inhibited	Treatment of
acetazolamide	carbonic andhydrase	glaucoma
allopurinol	xanthine oxidase	gout
aspirin	platelet cyclo-oxygenase	transient ischaemic attacks
benserazide	DOPA decarboxylase	Parkinson's disease
disulfiram	aldehyde dehydrogenase	alcoholism
enalapril	angiotensin converting enzyme	hypertension cardiac failure
nonsteroidal anti-inflammatory drugs	prostaglandin synthase	pain, inflammation premature labour
phenelzine	MAO A type	depression
selegiline	MAO B type	Parkinson's disease

Enzyme inhibition by drugs is also the basis of a number of *clinically important drug interactions* (see p. 115).

ELIMINATION

Drugs are eliminated from the body after being partly or wholly converted to water-soluble metabolites or, in some cases, without being metabolised. The physiological processes by which drugs and metabolites leave the body are now considered. To avoid repetition the account refers to *drug* whereas the processes deal with both drug *and its metabolites*.

Renal elimination

The following mechanisms are involved.

Glomerular filtration. The rate at which a drug enters the glomerular filtrate depends on the concentration of free drug in plasma water and on its molecular weight. Substances that have a molecular weight in excess of 50 000 are excluded from the glomerular filtrate while those of molecular weight less than 10 000 (which includes almost all drugs)[17] pass easily through the pores of the glomerular membrane.

Renal tubular excretion. Cells of the proximal renal tubule actively transfer strongly charged molecules from the plasma to the tubular fluid. There are two such systems, one for *acids*, e.g. penicillin, frusemide, and one for *bases*, e.g. amiloride, amphetamine.

Renal tubular reabsorption. The glomerular filtrate contains drug at the same concentration as it is free in the plasma, but the fluid is concentrated progressively as it flows down the nephron so that a gradient develops, drug in the tubular fluid becoming more concentrated than in the blood perfusing the nephron. Since the tubular epithelium has the properties of a lipid membrane, the extent to which a drug diffuses back into the blood will depend on its lipid solubility, i.e. on its pKa and on the pH of tubular fluid. If the fluid becomes more alkaline, an acidic drug ionises, becomes less lipid soluble and

its reabsorption diminishes, but a basic drug becomes un-ionised (and therefore more lipid soluble) and its reabsorption increases. Manipulation of urine pH is given useful expression when sodium bicarbonate is given to treat overdose with aspirin.

Faecal elimination

When a drug intended for systemic effect is taken by mouth, a proportion may remain in the bowel and be excreted in the faeces. Sometimes the objective of therapy is that drug be not absorbed from the gut, e.g. neomycin. Drug in the blood may also diffuse passively into the gut lumen, depending on its pKa and the pH difference between blood and gut contents. The effectiveness of activated charcoal by mouth for drug overdose depends partly on its adsorption of such diffused drug, which is then eliminated in the faeces (p. 137, 141).

Biliary excretion. In the liver there is one active transport system for acids and one for bases, similar to those in the proximal renal tubule, and in addition, there is a system that transports un-ionised molecules, e.g. digoxin, into the bile. Small molecules tend to be reabsorbed by the bile canaliculi and in general only compounds that have a molecular weight greater than 300 are excreted in bile.

Pulmonary elimination

The lungs are the main route of elimination (and of uptake) of volatile anaesthetics. Apart from this, they play only a trivial role in drug elimination. The route however, acquires notable medico-legal significance when ethanol concentration is measured in the air expired by vehicle drivers and pedestrians involved in road traffic accidents (breathalyser).

Clearance

Clearance of drug may be calculated for an organ or for the whole body. The term has the same meaning as the familiar *renal creatinine clearance*, which is a measure of removal of endogenous cre-

---

[17] Most drugs have a molecular weight less than 1000.

atinine from the plasma. Clearance values can provide useful information about the biological fate of a drug. Renal clearance of a drug that is eliminated only by filtration by the kidney obviously cannot exceed the glomerular filtration rate (127 ml/min in the adult male). If a drug is found to have a renal clearance in excess of this, then it must in addition be actively secreted by the kidney tubules, e.g. benzylpenicillin (renal clearance 480 ml/min).

Breast milk

Most drugs that are present in a mother's plasma appear to some extent in her milk though the amounts are so small that loss of drug in milk is of no significance as a mechanism of elimination.[18] Even small amounts, however, may sometimes be of significance for the suckling child whose drug metabolic and eliminating mechanisms are immature.

Whilst most drugs taken by the mother pose no hazard to the child, there are exceptions, as follows:

Drugs and breast feeding[19]

Alimentary tract. Sulphasalazine may cause adverse effects and mesalazine appears preferable.

Anti-asthma. Theophylline, diprophylline are eliminated slowly by the neonate: observe the infant for irritability or disturbed sleep.

Anticancer. Regard as unsafe because of inherent toxicity.

Antidepressants. Avoid doxepin, a metabolite of which may cause respiratory depression.

Antidysrhythmics (cardiac). Amiodarone is present in high and disopyramide in moderate amounts but effects in the infant have not been reported.

Antiepilepsy. General note of caution: observe the infant for sedation and poor suckling. Primidone, ethosuximide and phenobarbitone are

present in milk in high amounts, phenytoin and sodium valproate less so.

Anti-inflammatory. Regard salicylates as unsafe (possible association with Reye's syndrome).

Antimicrobials. Metronidazole is present in milk in moderate amounts, avoid prolonged exposure. Nalidixic acid and nitrofurantoin should be avoided where glucose-6-phosphate dehydrogenase deficiency is prevalent. Avoid clindamycin, dapsone, lincomycin, sulphonamides. Regard chloramphenicol as unsafe.

Antipsychotics. Phenothiazines, butyrophenones and thioxanthenes are best avoided unless the indications are compelling: amounts in milk are small but animal studies suggest adverse effects on the developing nervous system. In particular, moderate amounts of sulpiride enter milk. Lithium is probably best avoided.

Anxiolytics and sedatives. Benzodiazepines are safe if use is brief but prolonged use may cause somnolence or poor suckling.

Beta-adrenoceptor blockers. Neonatal hypoglycaemia is possible. Sotalol and atenolol are present in the highest amounts.

Hormones. Oestrogens, progestogens and androgens suppress lactation in high dose. Oestrogen/progesterone oral contraceptives are present in amounts too small to be harmful but may suppress lactation if it is not well established.

Miscellaneous. Bromocriptine suppresses lactation. Caffeine may cause infant irritability in high doses.

DRUG DOSAGE

Drug dosage can be of five main kinds:

1. *Fixed dose.* The effect that is desired can be obtained at well below the toxic dose (many mydriatics, diuretics, analgesics, oral contraceptives, antimicrobials) and enough drug can be given to render individual variation clinically insignificant.

2. *Variable dose with crude adjustments.* Here fine adjustments make comparatively insignificant differences and the therapeutic end-point may be hard to measure (depression, anxiety), may change only slowly (thyrotoxicosis), or may vary because of pathophysiological factors (analgesics, adrenal steroids for suppressing disease).

---

[18] But after mercury poisoning breast milk is a major route of elimination.

[19] Bennett PN (ed) 1988 Drugs and human lactation. Amsterdam: Elsevier.

3. *Variable dose with fine adjustments.* Here a vital function (blood pressure, blood sugar), that often changes rapidly in response to dose changes and can easily be measured repeatedly, provides the end-point. Adjustment of dose must be accurate. Adrenocortical replacement therapy falls into this group, whereas adrenocortical pharmacotherapy falls into (2) above.

4. *Maximum tolerated dose* is used when the ideal therapeutic effect cannot be achieved because of the occurrence of unwanted effects (anticancer drugs; some antimicrobials). The usual way of finding this is to increase the dose until unwanted effects begin to appear and then to reduce it slightly, or to monitor the plasma concentration.

5. *Minimum tolerated dose.* This concept is not so common as (4), above, but it applies to long-term adrenocortical steroid therapy against inflammatory or immunological conditions, e.g. in asthma and rheumatoid arthritis, when the dose that provides symptomatic relief may be so high that serious adverse effects are inevitable if it is continued indefinitely. The patient must be persuaded to accept incomplete relief on the grounds of safety. This can be difficult to achieve.

DOSING SCHEDULES

Whatever their type, dosing schedules are simply schemes aimed at achieving a desired effect whilst avoiding toxicity. In the discussion that follows it is assumed that drug effect relates closely to plasma concentration, which in turn relates closely to the amount of drug in the body.

The *objectives* of a dosing regimen where *continuing effect* is required are:

● To specify an *initial* dose that attains the desired effect rapidly without causing toxicity. Often the dose that is capable of *initiating* drug effect is the same as that which maintains it. On repeated dosing however, it takes $5 \ t_{\frac{1}{2}}$ periods to reach steady-state concentration in the plasma and this lapse of time may be undesirable. The effect may be achieved earlier by giving an initial dose that is larger than the maintenance dose; the initial dose is then called the *priming* or *load-ing* dose, i.e. the priming dose is that dose which will achieve a therapeutic effect in an individual whose body does not already contain the drug.

● To specify a dose which, repeated, maintains the effect, i.e. the *maintenance* dose; how much drug, and how often. Intuitively, the solution might be to give half the initial dose at intervals equal to its plasma $t_{\frac{1}{2}}$, for this by definition is the time in which the plasma concentration that achieves the desired effect declines by half. Whether or not this approach is satisfactory or practicable, however, depends very much on the half-life itself, as is illustrated by the following cases:

Case examples

1. *The half-life is 6–12 h.* In this, instance, replacing half the initial dose at intervals equal to the $t_{\frac{1}{2}}$ can indeed be a statisfactory solution because dosing every 6–12 h is acceptable.

2. *The half-life is greater than 24 h.* With once-daily dosing (which is desirable for compliance) giving half the priming dose every $t_{\frac{1}{2}}$ means that more drug is entering the body than is leaving it each day, and the drug will accumulate indefinitely. The solution is to replace only that amount of drug that leaves the body in 24 h. This quantity can be calculated once the initial dose and dose interval have been decided and the $t_{\frac{1}{2}}$ is known.

3. *The half-life is less than 3 h.* Dosing at intervals equal to the $t_{\frac{1}{2}}$ would be so frequent as to be unacceptable, and the answer is to use *continuous intravenous infusion* if the $t_{\frac{1}{2}}$ is very short, e.g. dopamine ($t_{\frac{1}{2}}$ 2 min, thus steady state plasma concentration will be reached in $5 \times t_{\frac{1}{2}} = 10$ min), or, if the $t_{\frac{1}{2}}$ is longer, e.g. lignocaine ($t_{\frac{1}{2}}$ 90 min) to use a priming dose as an intravenous bolus followed by a constant intravenous infusion. Intermittent adminstration of a drug with short half-life is nevertheless reasonable provided large fluctuations in plasma concentration are acceptable, i.e. that the drug has a large therapeutic index. Benzylpenicillin has a $t_{\frac{1}{2}}$ of 30 min but is effective in a 6-hourly regimen because the drug is so non-toxic that it is possible to give a dose safely that achieves a plasma concentration many times in excess of the minimum inhibitory concentration for sensitive organisms.

Prolongation of drug action

- *A larger dose* is the most obvious way to prolong a drug action. As this is not always feasible, other mechanisms are used.
- *Vasoconstriction* will reduce local blood flow so that distribution of drug away from an injection site is retarded, e.g. local anaesthetic action is prolonged by combination with adrenaline.
- *Slowing of metabolism* may usefully extend drug action, as when a dopa decarboxylase inhibitor, e.g. carbidopa, is combined with levodopa (as Sinemet) for parkinsonism.
- *Delayed excretion* is seldom practicable, the only important example being the use of probenecid to block renal tubular excretion of penicillin, e.g. when the latter is used in single dose to treat gonorrhoea.
- *Molecular structure* may be altered to prolong effect, e.g. the various benzodiazepines.
- *Pharmaceutical formulation.* The objective of an *even* as well as a *prolonged* effect is more often achieved by manipulating the formulation in which a drug is presented.

Sustained-release (oral) preparations can reduce the frequency of medication to once a day, and compliance is made easier for the patient. Most long-term medication for the elderly can now be given as a single morning dose. In addition sustained-release preparations may avoid local bowel toxicity due to high local concentrations, e.g ulceration of the small intestine with KCl tablets, and may also avoid the toxic peak plasma concentrations that can occur when dissolution of the formulation and so absorption of the drug are rapid.

Depot (injectable) preparations are more reliable because the environment in which they are deposited is more constant than can ever be the case in the alimentary tract and medication can be given at longer intervals, even weeks. In general such preparations are pharmaceutical variants, e.g. microcrystals, or the original drug in oil, wax, gelatin or synthetic media. They include phenothiazine tranquillisers, the various insulins and penicillins, preparations of vasopressin, benzathine penicillin and medroxy-progesterone. Solid tablets of hormones are sometimes implanted subcutaneously. The advantages of infrequent administration and better patient compliance in a variety of situations are obvious.

Reduction of absorption time

This can be achieved by making a soluble salt of the drug which is rapidly absorbed from the site of administration. In the case of s.c. or i.m. injections the same objective may be obtained with *hyaluronidase*, an enzyme which depolymerises hyaluronic acid, a constituent of connective tissue that prevents the spread of foreign substances, e.g. bacteria, drugs. By combining an injection with hyaluronidase, a drug spreads rapidly over a wide area and so is absorbed more quickly. Ergometrine may be given thus by nurses who are not trained to give i.v. injections.

Dose, body weight and body surface area

When a fixed dose is inappropriate, it is usual to adjust the dose according to *body weight*. Adjustment according to *body surface area* may be more appropriate, for this is *directly related to metabolic rate* (the same result is obtained by taking the body weight to the power of 0.7). Figure 7.4 relates body weight to percentage of adult dose on this basis, and its use is recommended where a calculation has to be made, e.g. for infants, and only the adult dose is known.

Fixed-dose drug combinations

This section refers to *combinations of drugs in a single pharmaceutical formulation*. It does not refer to concomitant drug therapy, e.g. in infections, hypertension and in cancer, when several drugs are given separately.

Fixed-dose drug combinations are *appropriate* for:

- *convenience, with improved patient compliance.* This is particularly appropriate when two drugs are used at constant dose, long-term, for an

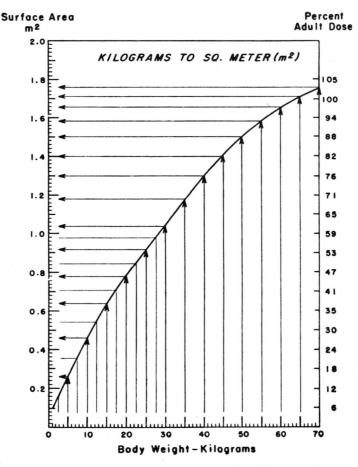

Fig. 7.4 Chart for estimation of dose from body weight and surface area. The figures on the right show what per cent of the adult dose should be given (by courtesy of the authors and publishers; Talbot N B, Richie R H, Crawford J D Metabolic homeostasis: a syllabus for those concerned with the care of patients. Cambridge, Mass: Harvard University Press, 1959)

asymptomatic condition, e.g. a thiazide plus a β-adrenoceptor blocker in mild or moderate hypertension. The fewer tablets the patients have to take, the more reliably will they use them, especially the elderly who as a group receive more drugs because they have multiple pathology.

● *enhanced effect*. Single drug treatment of tuberculosis leads to the emergence of resistant mycobacteria; this effect is prevented or delayed by using two or more drugs simultaneously. Combining isoniazid with rifampicin (Rifinah, Rimactazid) ensures that single drug treatment cannot occur; treatment has to be two drugs or no drug at all. Oral contraception (with an oes-

trogen and progestogen combination) is given for the same reason.

● *minimisation of unwanted effects*. Combining levodopa with benserazide (Madopar) or with carbidopa (Sinemet) slows its metabolism outside the central nervous system so that smaller amounts of levodopa can be used; this reduces side-effects.

Fixed-dose drug combinations are *inappropriate*:

● *when the dose of one or more of the component drugs may need to be adjusted independently*. A drug with a wide dose-range that must be adjusted to suit the patient's response is unsuitable for combination with a drug that has a narrow dose range;

- *if the time-course of drug action* demands different intervals between administration of the components;
- *if irregularity of administration*, e.g. in response to a symptom such as pain or cough, is desirable for some ingredients but not for others.

Conclusions

Therapeutic aims should be clear. Combinations should not be prescribed unless there is good reason to consider that the patient needs *all* the drugs in the formulation and that the doses are appropriate and will not need to be adjusted separately. Rational combinations can provide advantage, just as inappropriate combinations may be dangerous (and identification of a drug causing an adverse effect may be difficult when a combination is used). Thus combinations of iron with folic acid and cyanocobalamin are hazardous if they delay diagnosis of pernicious anaemia. But the fact that iron plus a little folic acid is properly used in pregnancy for routine anaemia prophylaxis simply confirms that combinations can be rationally devised to meet particular needs.

INDIVIDUAL OR BIOLOGICAL VARIATION

That individuals respond differently to drugs, both from time to time and from other individuals is a matter of everyday experience. Doctors need to accommodate for individual variation, for it may explain both adverse response to a drug and failure of therapy. Sometimes there are obvious physical characteristics such as age, race (genetics) or disease that warn the prescriber to adjust drug dose but there are no external features that signify, e.g., pseudocholinesterase deficiency, which causes prolonged paralysis after suxamethonium. An understanding of the reasons for individual variation in response to drugs is relevant to all who prescribe. Both pharmacodynamic and pharmacokinetic effects are involved

and the issues fall in two general categories: inherited influences and environmental and host influences.

VARIABILITY DUE TO INHERITED INFLUENCES: PHARMACOGENETICS

Consider how individuals in a population might be expected to respond to a fixed dose of a drug; some would show less than the usual response, most would show the usual response and some would show more than the usual response. This type of variation is described as *continuous* and in a graph the result would appear as a normal or Gaussian distribution curve, similar to the type of curve that describes the distribution of height, weight or metabolic rate in a population. The curve is the result of a multitude of factors, some *genetic* (multiple genes), some *environmental,* that contribute collectively to the response of the individual to the drug; they include race, sex, diet, weight, environmental and body temperature, circadian rhythm, absorption, distribution, metabolism, excretion and receptor density, but *no single factor* has a predominant effect. Less commonly, variation is *discontinuous* when differences in response: (a) reveal a discrete subgroup who respond differently from the general population, e.g. poor drug oxidisers or (b) separate the general population into quantitative groups, e.g. fast and slow acetylators of isoniazid. Discontinuous variation most commonly occurs when response to a drug is controlled by a single gene.

Pharmacogenetics is concerned with drug responses that are governed by heredity. Inherited factors causing different responses to drugs are commonly biochemical because single genes govern the production of enzymes.

Inherited abnormal responses to drugs mediated by single genes are called *idiosyncrasy* and cause *increased, decreased* and *bizarre* responses to drugs.

Heritable conditions causing increased or toxic drug responses

Acetylator status

Acetylation is an important route of metabolism

Table 7.6 Acetylator status

Ethnic group	Rapid acetylators (%)
Inuit (Canadian eskimos)	95
Japanese	88
Thais	72
Latin Americans	70
Black Americans	52
White Americans	48
Britons	38
Swedes	32
Egyptians	18

for many drugs that possess an $-NH_2$ group. Population studies have shown that individuals are either rapid or slow acetylators but the proportion of each varies greatly between races as shown in Table 7.6.

The importance of acetylator status to therapy is illustrated by the following examples:

Isoniazid may cause peripheral neuropathy in slow acetylators on standard doses (to prevent this in practice, it is simpler routinely to add pyridoxine to the antituberculosis regimen than to establish every patient's acetylator status). Acute hepatocellular necrosis with isoniazid is more common in rapid acetylators, perhaps because they more readily form an hepatotoxic metabolite. *Hydralazine* and *procainamide* may cause antinuclear antibodies to develop in the plasma of slow acetylators, and some proceed to systemic lupus erythematosus. *Sulphasalazine* (salicylazosulphapyridine; used for ulcerative colitis) causes adverse effects more frequently in slow acetylators, probably because of the sulphapyridine component which is inactivated by acetylation. *Dapsone* appears to cause more red cell haemolysis in slow acetylators; rapid acetylators may need higher doses to control dermatitis herpetiformis and leprosy.

Defective carbon oxidation

Variation in response to some drugs can be attributed to genetic polymorphisms of oxidation of their carbon-centres. Individuals may be classed as extensive or poor oxidisers and the latter are at special risk of adverse effects with standard doses of drugs that include debrisoquine (hypotension), metoprolol, bufuralol, timolol (in-

creased beta-blockade), nortriptyline (postural hypotension), nifedipine (prolonged cardiovascular action).[20] There are over 5 million slow oxidisers in the UK population.

Glucose-6-phosphate dehydrogenase (G-6-PD) deficiency

G-6-PD activity is important to the integrity of the red blood cell through a chain of reactions:

1. It is an important source of reduced nicotinamide-adenine dinucleotide phosphate (NADPH) which maintains erythrocyte glutathione in its reduced form.

2. Reduced glutathione is necessary to keep haemoglobin in the reduced (ferrous), rather than in its ferric state (methaemoglobin) which is useless for oxygen carriage.

3. Build-up of methaemoglobin in erythrocytes impairs the function of sulphydryl groups, especially those associated with the stability of the cell membrane.

Individuals who are G-6-PD deficient may suffer acute haemolysis if they are exposed to certain *oxidant* substances, including drugs. Characteristically there is an acute haemolytic episode 2–3 days after starting the drug. The haemolysis is self-limiting, only older cells with least enzyme being affected. The condition is common in African, Mediterranean, Middle East and South East Asian races and in their descendants and, throughout the world, affects some 100 million people. As deficiency may result from inheritance

---

[20] The poor oxidiser state was first revealed in rather dramatic circumstances in the laboratory of R L Smith, Professor of Biochemical Pharmacology, St Mary's Hospital Medical School, London, who was investigating the variable dose requirements of patients receiving the two antihypertensive drugs debrisoquine and bethanidine. He writes: 'I took 40 mg of debrisoquine sulphate; within two hours my blood pressure crashed to 70/50 mm Hg and I was unable to stand for four hours due to incapacitating postural hypotension . . . . it was two days until the blood pressure returned to normal. Analysis of my urine revealed that nearly all the dose was excreted as unchanged drug, whereas other subjects who showed little if any cardiovascular response to the same dose of debrisoquine, converted it to the 4-hydroxy metabolite. However the drama of the clinical response to a single dose of debrisoquine catalysed a search for its explanation and culminated in the uncovering of the first example of a genetic polymorphism of drug oxidation.'

of any one of numerous variants of G-6-PD, affected individuals exhibit differing susceptibility to haemolysis, i.e. a substance which affects one G-6-PD deficient subject adversely may be harmless in another. The following guidelines apply:[21]

Drugs that carry a definite risk of haemolysis in most G-6-PD deficient subjects include:
Dapsone (and other sulphones), methylene blue, niridazole, nitrofurantoin, pamaquin, primaquine, quinolones, some sulphonamides.
Drugs that carry a lesser risk of haemolysis in some G-6-PD deficient subjects include:
aspirin, chloroquine[22] menadione, probenecid, quinidine, quinine.[22]

Affected individuals are also susceptible to exposure to nitrates, anilines and naphthalenes (found in moth balls). Some individuals experience haemolysis after eating the broad bean, *Vicia fava*, and hence the term *favism*. Curiously, this genetic defect may confer a biological advantage for G-6-PD deficient individuals appear to resist carriage of falciparum malaria, presumably because their red cells do not survive well in the circulation.

Pseudocholinesterase deficiency

The neuromuscular blocking action of suxamethonium is terminated by plasma pseudocholinesterase. 'True' cholinesterase (acetylcholinesterase) hydrolyses acetylcholine released by nerve endings, whereas various tissues and plasma contain other non-specific, hence 'pseudo', esterases. Affected individuals form so little plasma pseudocholinesterase that metabolism of suxamethonium is seriously reduced. The deficiency characteristically comes to light when a patient fails to breathe spontaneously after a surgical operation and assisted ventilation may have to be undertaken for hours. Relatives of an affected individual, for this as for other inherited abnormalities carrying avoidable risk, should be sought out, checked to assess their own risk, and told of the result. The prevalence of pseudocho-

linesterase deficiency in the UK population is about 1 in 2500.
Malignant hyperthermia (p. 378).
Porphyria (p. 122).

Heritable conditions causing decreased drug responses

● *Resistance to coumarin anticoagulants.* Subjects of this rare inherited abnormality possess a variant of the enzyme that converts vitamin K to its reduced and active form, which enzyme the coumarins normally inhibit; patients require 20 times or more of the usual dose to obtain an adequate clinical response. A similar condition also occurs in rats and has practical importance as warfarin, a coumarin, is used as a rat poison (rats with the gene are dubbed 'super-rats' by the mass media).

● *Resistance to suxamethonium.* This rare condition is characterised by increased pseudocholinesterase activity and failure of normal doses of suxamethonium to cause muscular relaxation (*cf* cholinesterase deficiency, above).

● *Resistance to vitamin D.* Individuals develop rickets which responds only to huge doses of vitamin D, i.e. × 1000 the standard dose.

● *Bacterial resistance* to drugs is genetically determined and is of great clinical importance.

Conclusion

It is likely that many clinically important single gene differences in response to drugs remain to be discovered. Once a genetic difference, e.g. a metabolic reaction, is understood, it will be possible to predict what will happen when drugs of particular molecular structures are administered. But whether patients should be screened routinely for such differences in drug response is a matter of clinical importance as well as economics and logistics.

VARIABILITY DUE TO ENVIRONMENTAL AND HOST INFLUENCES

A multitude of factors related both to the in-

---

[21] Data from British National Formulary, 1991, with permission which is gratefully acknowledged.
[22] Acceptable in acute malaria.

dividual and his or her environment contribute to differences in drug response. In general, their precise role is less well documented than is the case with genetic factors but their range and complexity are illustrated by the following list of likely candidates: age, sex, pregnancy, lactation, exercise, sunlight, disease, infection, occupational exposures, drugs, circadian and seasonal variations, diet, stress, fever, malnutrition, alcohol intake, tobacco or cannabis smoking and the functioning of the cardiovascular, gastrointestinal, hepatic, immunological and renal systems.[23]

Age

The neonate and infant[24]

Young human beings differ greatly from adults, not merely in size but also in the proportions and constituents of their bodies and the functioning of their physiological systems. These differences are reflected in the way the body handles and responds to drugs and are relevant to prescribing.

Absorption of drugs from the gastrointestinal tract is generally slower in neonates than in older children, although the proportion ultimately absorbed may be similar.

- Rectal absorption is efficient with an appropriate formulation and has been used for diazepam and theophyllines; this route may be preferred with an uncooperative infant.
- The intramuscular or subcutaneous routes tend to give unpredictable plasma concentrations, e.g. of digoxin or gentamicin, because of the relatively low proportion of skeletal muscle and fat. Intravenous administration is preferred in the seriously ill newborn.
- Drugs or chemicals that come in contact with the skin are readily absorbed as the skin is well hydrated and the stratum corneum is thin; overdose toxicity may result, e.g. with hexachlorophane used in

dusting powders and emulsions to prevent infection.

Distribution of drugs is influenced by the fact that total body water in the neonate amounts to 80% as compared to 65% in older children. Consequently:

- Weight-related priming doses of aminoglycosides, aminophylline, digoxin and frusemide are larger for neonates than for older children.
- Less extensive binding of drugs to plasma proteins is generally without clinical importance but there is a significant risk of elevation of plasma bilirubin following its displacement from protein binding sites by vitamin K, X-ray contrast media or indomethacin.
- The blood–brain barrier in the neonate is more readily penetrated by some drugs than in the adult.

Metabolism. Although the enzyme systems that inactivate drugs are present at birth, they are functionally immature, especially in the preterm baby, and especially for oxidation and for conjugation with glucuronic acid. Inability to conjugate and thus inactivate chloramphenicol causes the fatal grey syndrome in neonates. After the first weeks of life the drug metabolic capacity increases rapidly.

Elimination. Glomerular filtration, tubular secretion and reabsorption are low in the neonate (even lower in preterm babies) only reaching adult values in relation to body surface area at 2–5 months. Therefore drugs that are eliminated by the kidney (e.g. aminoglycosides, penicillins, diuretics) must be given in reduced dose; after about 6 months, body weight- or surface area-related daily doses are the same for all ages.

The elderly

The incidence of adverse drug reactions rises with age in the adult, especially after 65 years because of:

- the increasing number of drugs that they need to take because they tend to have multiple diseases

---

[23] Vessell E S 1982 Clin Pharm Therap 31: 1.
[24] A neonate is under 1 month and an infant is 1–12 months of age.

- poor compliance with dosing regimens
- bodily changes of ageing that require modification of dosage regimens.

Absorption of drugs may be slightly slower because gastrointestinal blood flow and motility are reduced but the effect is rarely important.

Distribution is influenced by the following changes:

- There is a significant decrease in lean body mass so that standard adult doses provide a greater amount of drug per kg.
- Total body water is less (and in general the distribution volume of water-soluble drugs is reduced) but body fat is increased, especially in males (and in general lipid-soluble drugs have larger distribution volume). Hence standard doses of drugs ought to be reduced, especially the priming doses of those that are water soluble.
- Plasma albumin concentration tends to be well maintained in the healthy elderly but may be reduced by chronic disease, giving scope for a greater proportion of unbound (free) drug; this may be important when priming doses are given.

Metabolism is reduced because liver mass and liver blood flow are decreased. Consequently:

- Metabolic inactivation of drugs is slower.
- Drugs that are normally extensively eliminated in first-pass through the liver appear in higher concentration in the systemic circulation and persist in it for longer. There is thus particular cause initially to use lower doses of most major tranquillisers, tricyclic antidepressants and cardiac antidysrhythmic agents.
- Capacity for hepatic enzyme induction appears to be lessened.

Elimination. Renal blood flow, glomerular filtration and tubular secretion decrease with age above 55 years, a decline that is not signalled by raised serum creatinine concentration because production of this metabolite is diminished by the age-associated diminution of muscle mass. Indeed, in the elderly, serum creatinine may be within the concentration range for normal young adults even when the creatinine clearance is 50 ml/min (127 ml/min in adult male). Particular risk of adverse effects arises with drugs that are eliminated mainly by the kidney and that have a small therapeutic ratio, e.g. aminoglycosides, chlorpropamide, digoxin, lithium.

Pharmacodynamic response may alter with age, to produce either a greater or lesser effect than is anticipated in younger adults.

- Drugs that act on the central nervous system appear to produce an exaggerated response in relation to that expected from the plasma concentration, and sedatives and hypnotics may have a pronounced hangover effect. These drugs are also more likely to depress respiration because vital capacity and maximum breathing capacity are lessened in the elderly.
- Response to β-adrenoceptor agonists and antagonists appears to be blunted in old age partly, it is believed, through reduction in the number of receptors.
- Baroreceptor sensitivity is reduced leading to the potential for orthostatic hypotension with drugs that reduce blood pressure.

Rules of prescribing for the elderly[25]

1. Think about the necessity for drugs. Is the diagnosis correct and complete? Is the drug really necessary? Is there a better alternative?

2. Do not prescribe drugs that are not useful. Think carefully before giving an old person a drug that may have major side-effects, and consider alternatives.

3. Think about the dose. Is it appropriate to possible alterations in the patient's physiological state? Is it appropriate to the patient's renal and hepatic function at the time?

4. Think about drug formulation. Is a tablet the most appropriate form of drug or would an injection, a suppository or a syrup be better? Is the drug suitably packaged for the elderly patient, bearing in mind any disabilities?

5. Assume any new symptoms may be due to

---

[25] By permission from Caird FI, ed. Drugs for the elderly. Copenhagen: WHO (Europe) 1985.

drug side-effects, or more rarely, to drug withdrawal. Rarely (if ever) treat a side-effect of one drug with another.

6. Take a careful drug history. Bear in mind the possibility of interaction with substances the patient may be taking without your knowledge, such as herbal or other non-prescribed remedies, old drugs taken from the medicine cabinet or drugs obtained from friends.

7. Use fixed-combinations of drugs only when they are logical and well studied and they either aid compliance or improve tolerance or efficacy. Few fixed-combinations meet this standard.

8. When adding a new drug to the therapeutic regimen, see whether another can be withdrawn.

9. Attempt to check whether the patient's compliance is adequate, e.g. by counting remaining tablets. Has the patient (or relatives) been properly instructed?

10. Remember that stopping a drug is as important as starting it.

Note. The *old* (80+ years) are particularly intolerant of neuroleptics (given for confusion) and of diuretics (given for ankle swelling that is postural and not due to heart failure) which cause adverse electrolyte changes. Both classes of drug may result in admission to hospital of semi-comatose 'senior citizens' who deserve better treatment from their juniors.

Pregnancy

As the pregnancy evolves, profound changes occur in physiology including fluid and tissue composition.

Absorption. Gastrointestinal motility is decreased but there appears to be no major defect in drug absorption except that reduced gastric emptying delays the appearance in the plasma of orally administered drugs, especially during labour. Absorption from an intramuscular site is likely to be efficient because tissue perfusion is increased due to vasodilatation.

Distribution. Total body water increases by up to 8 l creating a larger space within which water-soluble drugs may distribute. As a result of haemodilution, plasma albumin (normal 33–55 g/l) declines by some 10 g/l. Thus there is

scope for increased free concentration of drugs that bind to albumin, e.g. phenytoin. Unbound drug, however, is free to distribute and to be metabolised and excreted and the free (and pharmacologically active) concentration of phenytoin is unaltered, although the *total* plasma concentration is reduced. Therapeutic drug monitoring interpreted by concentrations appropriate for non-pregnant women thus may mislead. A useful general guide during pregnancy is to maintain concentrations at the lower end of the recommended range. Body fat increases by about 4 kg and provides a reservoir for lipid-soluble drugs.

Hepatic metabolism increases though not blood flow to the liver. Consequently, there is increased clearance of drugs such as phenytoin and theophylline, whose elimination rate depends on liver enzyme activity. Drugs that are so rapidly metabolised that their elimination rate depends on their delivery to the liver, i.e. on hepatic blood flow, have unaltered clearance, e.g. propranolol.

Elimination. Renal plasma flow almost doubles and there is more rapid loss of drugs that are excreted by the kidney, e.g. amoxicillin, whose dose should be doubled for systemic infections (but not for tract infections as penicillins are highly concentrated in the urine).

Placenta: see p. 88.

Disease

Diseases cause *pharmacokinetic changes* which include:

Absorption

● Surgery that involves resection and reconstruction of the gut may lead to malabsorption of iron, folic acid and fat soluble vitamins after partial gastrectomy, and of vitamin B_{12} after ileal resection.

● Delayed gastric emptying and intestinal stasis during an attack of migraine interferes with absorption of drugs.

● Severe low output cardiac failure or shock (with peripheral vasoconstriction) delays absorption from subcutaneous or intramuscular sites; reduced hepatic blood flow prolongs the presence in the plasma of drugs that are so rapidly extracted by the liver that removal depends on their rate of presentation to it, e.g. lignocaine.

Distribution. Hypoalbuminaemia, from any cause, e.g. burns, malnutrition, sepsis, allows a higher proportion of free (unbound) drug in plasma. Although free drug is available for metabolism and excretion, there remains a risk of enhanced or adverse responses especially with initial doses of those that are highly protein bound, e.g. phenytoin. Inflammation is associated with increase in the concentration of the acute-phase protein, α_1-acid glycoprotein, which binds a number of basic drugs, e.g. lignocaine, disopyramide, monitoring of which may thus give misleadingly high results.

Metabolism. Acute inflammatory disease of the liver (viral, alcoholic) and cirrhosis affect both the functioning of the hepatocytes and blood flow through the liver. Reduced extraction from the plasma of drugs that are normally highly cleared in first pass through the liver results in increased *systemic availability* of drugs such as propranolol, labetalol and chlormethiazole. Many other drugs exhibit prolonged $t_{\frac{1}{2}}$ and reduced clearance in patients with chronic liver disease, e.g. diazepam, tolbutamide, rifampicin (see Drugs and the liver, p. 541). Thyroid disease has the expected effects, i.e. drug metabolism is accelerated in hyperthyroidism and diminished in hypothyroidism.

Elimination. Disease of the kidney (p. 469) has profound effects on the pharmacokinetics and thence the actions of drugs that are eliminated by that organ.

Diseases cause *pharmacodynamic changes*, e.g.:

- *Asthmatic attacks* can be precipitated by beta-adrenoceptor blockers.
- *Malfunctioning of the respiratory centre* (raised intracranial pressure, severe pulmonary insufficiency) causes patients to be intolerant of opioids, and indeed any sedative may precipitate respiratory failure.
- *Myocardial infarction* predisposes to cardiac dysrhythmia with digitalis glycosides or sympathomimetics.
- *Myasthenia gravis* is made worse by quinine and quinidine and myasthenics are

intolerant of competitive neuromuscular blocking agents and aminoglycoside antibiotics.

Food

- The presence of food in the stomach, especially if it is fatty, delays gastric emptying. Plasma concentration of drugs including some antimicrobials, e.g. ampillin, rifampicin, may be much reduced if they are taken on a full stomach. More specifically, calcium, e.g. in milk, interferes with absorption of tetracyclines (by chelation).
- Substitution of protein for fat or carbohydrate in the diet is associated with an increase in drug oxidation rates. Some specific dietary factors induce drug metabolising enzymes, e.g. alcohol, methylxanthines (coffee, cola drinks, chocolate), charcoal grilled (broiled) beef, cabbage and Brussels sprouts.

Protein malnutrition causes changes that are likely to influence pharmacokinetics, e.g. loss of body weight, reduced hepatic metabolising capacity, hypoproteinaemia.

Alterations in drug action caused by diet may be termed drug:food interactions.

DRUG INTERACTIONS

When a drug is administered, a response is obtained; if a second drug is given and the response to the first drug is altered, a drug interaction is said to have occurred.[26] A drug interaction may be *desired* or *undesired*, i.e. *beneficial* or *harmful*. It is deliberately sought in treating tuberculosis and when naloxone is given to treat morphine overdose. It is an embarrassment when a woman taking a combined oestrogen/progestogen oral contraceptive for a desired interaction is prescribed a drug that is an enzyme inducer, with the result that she becomes pregnant.

Although dramatic unintended interactions attract most attention and are the principal subject of this section they should not distract attention

---

[26] The term drug:drug interaction is also used, to make the distinction from drug:food interactions.

from the many therapeutically useful interactions that are the basis of rational polypharmacy. These useful interactions are referred to throughout the book whenever it is relevant to do so.

Clinical importance of drug interactions

If doctors were to limit their prescribing to the list in Use of Essential Drugs (WHO) (p. 65) and were to prescribe four drugs for any patient at any one time, the number of possible combinations would be more than 64 million. There can be no doubt that the number of drug interactions that *might* occur in this imagined situation would be too large to commit to memory. But the observation that one drug can be shown measurably to alter the disposition or effect of another drug does not mean that the interaction is necessarily of clinical importance. In this section we highlight the circumstances in which clinically *important* interactions can occur, we describe their pharmacological basis, and provide a schematic framework to identify potential drug interactions during clinical practice.

Clinically important drug interactions become likely:

- with any drug for which precise control of plasma concentration is required and where *small* interference may alter it;
- with drugs that have a *steep dose response curve* and a *small therapeutic index* so that relatively small quantitative changes at the target site, e.g. receptor or enzyme, will lead to substantial changes in effect, as with digoxin or lithium;
- with drugs that are known enzyme inducers or inhibitors (p. 98).
- with drugs that exhibit saturable metabolism (zero-order kinetics), when small interference with kinetics may lead to large alteration of plasma concentration, e.g. phenytoin, theophylline;
- with drugs that are used long-term, where precise plasma concentrations are required, e.g. oral contraceptives, antiepilepsy drugs, cardiac antidysrhythmia drugs, lithium;

- when several drugs are used at the same time, for 'every time a physician adds to the number of drugs a patient is taking he may devise a novel combination that has a special risk;'[27]
- when multiple drugs are used to treat the same disease, for this increases the chance of their being given concurrently, e.g. theophylline and salbutamol given for asthma may cause cardiac dysrhythmia;
- in severely ill patients, for they may be receiving several drugs; signs of iatrogenic disease may be difficult to distinguish from those already present and their condition may be such that they cannot tolerate further adversity;
- in patients with significantly impaired liver or kidney function, for these are the principal organs that terminate drug action;
- in the elderly, for they tend to have multiple pathology, may receive several drugs concurrently, and are specially susceptible to adverse drug effects (p. 107).

Pharmacological basis of drug interactions

Some knowledge of the pharmacological basis of how one drug may change the action of another is useful in obtaining those interactions that are wanted, as well as in recognising and preventing those that are not.

Drug interactions are of two principal kinds:

1. *Pharmacodynamic interaction: both drugs act on the target site of clinical effect*, exerting synergism or antagonism. The drugs may act on the same or different receptors or processes, mediating similar biological consequences. Examples include: alcohol + benzodiazepine (to produce sedation), morphine + naloxone (to reverse opioid overdose), rifampicin + isoniazid (effective antituberculosis combination).

2. *Pharmacokinetic interaction: the drugs interact*

---

[27] Dollery CT Proceedings of the Royal Society of Medicine 1965; 58: 943.

remotely from the target site to alter plasma (and other tissue) concentrations so that the amount of the drug at the target site of clinical effect is altered, e.g. enzyme induction (rifampicin/warfarin), competition for plasma protein binding sites (sodium valproate/phenytoin).

Interaction may result in antagonism or synergism.

Antagonism occurs when the action of one drug opposes the action of another. Two drugs simply have opposite pharmacodynamic effects, e.g. histamine and adrenaline on the bronchi exhibit *physiological* or *functional antagonism*; or they compete reversibly for the same drug receptor, e.g. isoprenaline and β-adrenoceptor blockers exhibit *competitive antagonism*.

Synergism.[28] The probability that pharmacologists will, in the foreseeable future, agree on the terminology to describe drug synergism is remote. Therefore, the following will suffice. Synergism is of two sorts:

1. *Summation or addition* occurs when the effects of two drugs having the same action are additive, i.e. 2 + 2 = 4 (a β-adrenoceptor blocker plus a thiazide diuretic have an additive antihypertensive effect).

2. *Potentiation* (to make more powerful) occurs when one drug increases the action of another, i.e. 2 + 2 = 5. Sometimes the two drugs both have the action concerned (trimethoprim plus sulphonamide) and sometimes one drug lacks the action concerned (benserazide plus levodopa), i.e. 0 + 2 = 5.

Identifying potential drug interactions during clinical practice

Drugs can interact at any stage from when they are mixed with other drugs in a pharmaceutical formulation or by a clinician, e.g. in an i.v. infusion or syringe, to their final excretion either unchanged or as metabolites. When a drug is added to an existing regimen, a doctor can evaluate the possibility of an interaction logically by thinking through the usual sequence of processes to which a drug is subject and which are outlined earlier in this chapter, i.e. interactions may occur:

- outside the body
- at the site of absorption
- during distribution
- on receptors or body systems (pharmacodynamic interactions)
- during metabolism
- during excretion

INTERACTIONS OUTSIDE THE BODY

Intravenous fluids offer special scope for interactions (incompatibilities) when drugs are added to the reservoir, for a number of reasons. Drugs commonly are weak organic acids or bases. They are often insoluble and to make them soluble it is necessary to prepare salts. Plainly, the mixing of solutions of salts can result in instability which may or may not be evident from visible change in the solution, i.e. precipitation. Furthermore, the solutions have little buffering capacity and pH readily changes with added drugs. Dilution of a drug in the reservoir fluid may also lead to loss of stability.

Serious loss of potency can result from incompatibility between an infusion fluid and a drug that is added to it. Issues of compatibility are complex but specific sources of information are available in manufacturers' package inserts or from the hospital pharmacy. The general rule must be to consult these sources before ever adding a drug to an infusion fluid.

Mixing drugs prepared for i.v. injection may cause interaction, e.g. protamine zinc insulin contains excess of protamine which binds with some soluble insulin and reduces the immediate effect of the dose, if this is drawn up in the same syringe.

INTERACTIONS AT SITE OF ABSORPTION

In the complex environment of the gut there are opportunities for drugs to interfere with each other both directly and indirectly via alteration of

---

[28] Greek: *syn* together; *ergos* work.

gut physiology. Usually the result is to impair absorption.

Direct chemical interaction in the gut is a significant cause of reduced absorption. Antacids that contain aluminium and magnesium form insoluble complexes with tetracyclines, iron and prednisolone. Milk contains sufficient calcium to warrant its avoidance as a major article of diet when tetracyclines are taken. Cholestyramine interferes with absorption of thyroxine, digoxin and some acidic drugs, e.g. warfarin. Sucralfate reduces the absorption of phenytoin. Interactions of this type depend on both drugs being in the stomach at the same time, and can be prevented if the doses are separated by at least 2 hours.

Gut motility may be altered by drugs. Those having antimuscarinic effects, e.g. some antidepressants, and opioid analgesics, reduce gastric emptying and delay absorption of other drugs. Purgatives reduce the time spent in the small intestine and give less opportunity for the absorption of poorly soluble substances such as adrenal steroids and digoxin.

Alterations in gut flora by antimicrobials may potentiate oral anticoagulant by reducing bacterial synthesis of vitamin K in the large gut. There may also be an effect on enterohepatic recycling where bacteria release active drug from the conjugate.

Interactions other than in the gut are exemplified by the use of hyaluronidase to promote dissipation of a s.c. injection, and by the addition of vasoconstrictors, e.g. adrenaline, felypressin, to local anaesthetics to delay absorption and usefully prolong local anaesthesia.

INTERACTIONS DURING DISTRIBUTION

1. *Displacement from plasma protein binding sites* may contribute to adverse reaction. A drug that is extensively protein bound can be displaced from its binding site by a competing drug, so raising the free (and pharmacologically active) concentration of the first drug. Unbound drug, however, is available for distribution away from the plasma and for metabolism and excretion. Commonly, the result is that the free concen-

tration of the displaced drug soon returns close to its original value and any extra effect is transient.

For a displacement interaction to become clinically important, a second mechanism usually operates: thus sodium valproate can cause phenytoin toxicity because it *both* displaces phenytoin from its binding site on plasma albumin *and* inhibits its metabolism. Similarly aspirin and probenecid (and possibly other non-steroidal anti-inflammatory drugs) displace the folic acid antagonist methotrexate from its protein binding site *and* reduce its rate of active secretion by the renal tubules; the result is serious methotrexate toxicity. Bilirubin is displaced from its binding protein by sulphonamides, vitamin K, X-ray contrast media or indomethacin; in the neonate this may cause a significant risk of kernicterus, for its capacity to metabolise bilirubin is immature.

Direct interaction between drugs may also take place in the plasma, e.g. protamine with heparin; desferrioxamine with iron; dimercaprol with arsenic.

2. *Displacement from other tissue binding* may cause unwanted effects. When quinidine is given to patients who are receiving digoxin, the plasma concentration of free digoxin may double because quinidine displaces digoxin from binding sites in tissue (as well as plasma proteins). As with interaction due to displacement from plasma proteins, however, an additional mechanism contributes to the overall effect, for quinidine also impairs renal excretion of digoxin.

INTERACTIONS DIRECTLY ON RECEPTORS OR BODY SYSTEM (Pharmacodynamic interactions)

This category comprises specific interactions between drugs on the same receptor, to less precise interactions involving the same body organ or system; whatever the precise location, the result is altered drug action.

1. *Action on receptors* provides numerous examples. Beneficial interactions are sought in overdose, as with the use of naloxone for mor-

phine overdose (opioid receptor), of atropine for anticholinesterase, i.e. insecticide, poisoning (acetylcholine receptor), of isoprenaline for overdose with a β-adrenoceptor blocker (β-adrenoceptor), of phentolamine for the monoamine oxidase inhibitor-sympathomimetic interaction (α-adrenoceptor).

Unwanted interactions include the loss of antihypertensive effect of β-blockers when common cold remedies containing ephedrine, phenylpropanolamine or phenylephrine are taken, usually unknown to the doctor; their alpha-adrenoceptor agonist action is unrestrained in the β-blocked patient.

2. *Actions on body systems* provide scope for a variety of interactions. The following list shows something of the range of possibilities; others may be found under accounts of individual drugs:

Beta-adrenoceptor blockers lose some antihypertensive efficacy when *nonsteroidal anti-inflammatory drugs* (NSAIDs), especially indomethacin, are co-administered; the effect may involve inhibition of prostaglandin production by the kidney.

Diuretics, especially of the loop variety, lose efficacy if administered with NSAIDs; the mechanism may involve inhibition of prostaglandin synthesis, as above.

Potassium supplements, given with potassium-retaining diuretics, e.g. *amiloride, spironolactone*, or with ACE-inhibitors may cause dangerous hyperkalaemia.

Digoxin is more effective, but also more toxic in the presence of hypokalaemia, which may be caused by *thiazide* or *loop diuretics*.

Verapamil, given i.v. with a *β-blocker*, e.g. practolol, for supraventricular tachycardia may cause dangerous bradycardia since both drugs delay atrioventricular conduction.

Theophylline potentiates β-adrenergic effects, e.g. of *salbutamol*, and cardiac dysrhythmia may result during treatment of asthma.

Lithium toxicity may result if *thiazide* diuretic is co-administered; resorption of lithium by the proximal renal tubule is increased and plasma concentrations rise.

Central nervous system depressant drugs including *benzodiazepines, several H_1-receptor antihistamines, alcohol, phenothiazines, antiepilepsy drugs* interact to augment their sedative effects.

Loop diuretics and aminoglycoside antibiotics are both ototoxic in high dose; the chance of an adverse event is greater if they are administered together.

Aminoglycosides and *cephalosporins* may be nephrotoxic if given together, especially to elderly patients whose renal function is already impaired.

INTERACTIONS DURING METABOLISM

1. **Enzyme induction** by drugs and other substances (see p. 98) accelerates metabolism and is a cause of therapeutic failure; the following are examples:

Oral contraceptive steroids are metabolised more rapidly when an enzyme inducer is also taken, and unplanned pregnancy has occurred. In this circumstance an oral contraceptive of high oestrogen content may be substituted (or an alternative contraceptive method); if breakthrough bleeding occurs, the oestrogen content is not high enough. The metabolism of progestogens is also increased by enzyme induction.

Anticoagulant control with warfarin is dependent on a steady state of elimination by metabolism. Enzyme induction leads to accelerated metabolism of warfarin, loss of anticoagulant control and danger of thrombosis. Conversely, if a patient's anticoagulant control is stable on warfarin plus an inducing agent, there is a danger of haemorrhage if the inducing agent is discontinued because warfarin will be eliminated at a slower rate.

Chronic alcohol ingestion causing enzyme induction is a likely explanation of the tolerance shown by alcoholics to hydrocarbon anaesthetics and to tolbutamide.

Cyclosporin is at least 50% cleared by hepatic metabolism; its concentration in blood may be reduced due to enzyme induction by rifampicin, with danger of inadequate immunosuppression hazarding an organ or marrow transplant.

2. **_Enzyme inhibition_** by drugs (see p. 98) potentiates other drugs whose intensity and duration of action are limited by being metabolised. Adverse reactions may result. Enzyme inhibiting drugs may be classified thus:

● Some drugs appear to be non-specific metabolic inhibitors. Examples appear below; drugs with which they interact are also given but the list is not complete, and there should be a general awareness of the possibility of metabolic inhibition when the following drugs are used.

Cimetidine is an inhibitor of Phase 1 metabolism (p. 97) and so potentiates a large number of drugs, notably propranolol, theophylline, warfarin and phenytoin. Depending on the interacting drug, up to 50% inhibition of metabolism may occur when cimetidine 2000 mg/d is taken.

Erythromycin inhibits drug oxidising enzymes and impairs the metabolism of theophylline, warfarin, carbamazepine and methylprednisolone. The mean reduction in drug clearance is 20–25%.

Monoamine oxidase inhibitors (MAOI) are not completely selective for MAO and impair the metabolism of tricyclic antidepressants, of some sympathomimetics, e.g. phenylpropanolamine, amphetamine, of opioid analgesics, especially pethidine, and of mercaptopurine.

Quinolone antimicrobials interfere with the metabolism of several compounds, most notably theophylline, the clearance of which may be reduced by 50% by enoxacin; ciprofloxacin has a lesser inhibitory effect.

Sodium valproate inhibits the metabolism of phenytoin, phenobarbitone and primidone.

● Other drugs are more selective inhibitors, e.g.

DRUG	INHIBITS METABOLISM OF
allopurinol	azathioprine
dextropropoxyphene (in co-proxamol)	warfarin
metronidazole	ethanol
verapamil	carbamazepine

INTERACTIONS DURING EXCRETION

Clinically important interactions, both beneficial and potentially harmful, occur in the kidney.

Interference with passive diffusion. Reabsorption of a drug by the renal tubule can be reduced, and its excretion increased, by altering urine pH (see Drug overdose, p. 87, 140).

Interference with active transport. Organic acids are passed from the blood into the urine by active transport across the renal tubular epithelium. Penicillin is mostly excreted in this way. Probenecid, an organic acid that competes successfully with penicillin for this transport system, may be used to prolong the action of penicillin when repeated administration is impracticable, e.g. in sexually transmitted diseases, where compliance is notoriously poor. Interference with renal excretion of methotrexate by aspirin, zidovudine by probenecid and of digoxin by quinidine, contribute to the potentially harmful interactions with these combinations.

GUIDE TO FURTHER READING

Brodie M J, Feely J 1988 Adverse drug interactions. British Medical Journal 296: 845

Editorial 1987 Administration of drugs by the buccal route. Lancet 1: 666

Editorial 1988 Pharmacological adaptive responses to drugs. Lancet 1: 25

Editorial 1988 Intrathecal drugs. Lancet 1: 743

Feely J, Brodie M J 1988 Practical clinical pharmacology: drug handling and response. British Medical Journal 296: 1046

Montamat S C et al 1989 Management of drug therapy in the elderly. New England Journal of Medicine 321: 303

Rubin P C 1986 Prescribing in pregnancy: general principles. British Medical Journal 293: 1415

Rylance G W 1988 Prescribing for infants and children. British Medical Journal 296: 984

Unwanted effects of drugs: adverse reactions

BACKGROUND

Cur'd yesterday of my disease
I died last night of my physician.[1]

Nature is neutral, i.e. it has no 'intentions' towards humans, though it is often unfavourable to them. It is mankind, in its desire to avoid suffering and death, that decides that some of the biological effects of drugs are desirable (therapeutic) and others are undesirable (adverse). In addition to this arbitrary division, which has no fundamental biological basis, unwanted effects of drugs are promoted, or even caused, by numerous non-drug factors. Because of the variety of these factors, attempts to make a simple account of the unwanted effects of drugs must be imperfect.

There is general agreement that drugs prescribed for disease are themselves the cause of a serious amount of disease (adverse reactions), ranging from mere inconvenience to permanent disability and death.

Since drugs are intended to relieve suffering, patients find it peculiarly offensive that they can also cause disease. Therefore it is important to know how much disease they do cause and why they cause it, so that preventive measures can be taken.

It is not enough to measure the rate of adverse reactions to drugs, their nature and their severity,

---

[1] From, The remedy worse than the disease. Matthew Prior (1664–1721).

though accurate data on these are obviously useful. It is necessary to take, or to try to take, into account which effects are avoidable (by skilled choice and use) and which unavoidable (inherent in drug or patient). Also, different adverse effects can matter to a different degree to different people.

Since there can be no hope of eliminating all adverse effects of drugs it is necessary to evaluate patterns of adverse reaction against each other. One drug may frequently cause minor ill-effects but pose no threat to life, though patients do not like it and may take it irregularly, to their own detriment. Another drug may be pleasant to take, so that patients take it consistently, with benefit, but it may rarely kill someone. It is not obvious which drug is to be preferred.

Some patients, e.g. those with a history of allergy or previous reactions to drugs, are up to 4 times more likely to have another adverse reaction, so that the incidence does not fall evenly.

It is also useful to discover the causes of adverse reactions, where these are unknown, for such knowledge can be used to render avoidable what are at present unavoidable reactions.

Avoidable adverse effects will be reduced by more skilful prescribing and this means that doctors, amongst all the other claims on their time, must find time better to understand drugs, as well as to understand their patients and their diseases.

Estimates of the incidence and severity of adverse reactions to drugs are various, for reliable data are hard to get.

DEFINITION OF ADVERSE REACTION

Many unwanted effects of drugs are medically trivial, and in order to avoid inflating the figures of drug-induced disease, it is convenient to retain the term **side-effects** for minor effects of type A class (p. 121). The term **adverse reaction** should be confined to: harmful or seriously unpleasant effects occurring at doses intended for therapeutic (prophylactic or diagnostic) effect and which call for reduction of dose or withdrawal of the drug and/or forecast hazard from future administration; it is effects of this order that are of importance in evaluating drug-induced disease in the community.

Toxicity implies a direct action of the drug, often at high dose, damaging cells, e.g. liver damage from paracetamol overdose, eighth cranial nerve damage from gentamicin. All drugs, for practical purposes, are toxic in overdose and *overdose can be absolute or relative*; in the latter case an ordinary dose may be administered but may be toxic due to an underlying abnormality in the patient, e.g. disease of the liver or kidney. Mutagenicity, carcinogenicity and teratogenicity (see index) are special cases of toxicity.

Secondary effects are the indirect consequences of a primary drug action. Examples are: vitamin deficiency or opportunistic infection which may occur in patients whose normal bowel flora has been altered by antibiotics; diuretic-induced hypokalaemia causing digoxin intolerance; the Herxheimer reaction (probably due to products released by killed organisms, usually spirochaetes).

Intolerance means a low threshold to the normal pharmacological action of a drug. Individuals vary greatly in their susceptibility to drugs, those at one extreme of the normal distribution curve being intolerant of the drugs, those at the other, tolerant.

Idiosyncrasy (see Pharmacogenetics) implies an inherent qualitative abnormal reaction to a drug, usually due to genetic abnormality, e.g. porphyria.

CAUSATION: DEGREES OF CERTAINTY

Reliable attribution of a cause-effect relationship provides the biggest problem in this field. Karch and Lasagna[2] propose the following degrees of certainty for attributing adverse events to drugs:

Definite:
- time sequence from taking drug is reasonable
- event corresponds to what is known of drug

[2] JAMA 1975; 234: 1236.

	• event ceases on stopping drug
	• event returns on restarting drug (rarely advisable).
Probable:	• time sequence reasonable
	• corresponds to what is known of drug
	• ceases on stopping drug
	• not reasonably explained by patient's disease.
Possible:	• time sequence reasonable
	• corresponds to what is known of drug
	• could readily have been result of patient's disease or other therapy.
Conditional:	• time sequence reasonable
	• does not correspond to what is known of drug
	• could not reasonably be explained by the patient's disease.
Doubtful:	• event not meeting the above criteria.

Recognition of adverse drug reactions

When an unexpected event, for which there is no obvious cause, occurs in a patient already taking a drug, the possibility that it is drug-caused must always be considered.

PHARMACOVIGILANCE AND PHARMACOEPIDEMIOLOGY

The principal methods of collecting data on adverse reactions are:

• **Formal therapeutic trials**. These provide reliable data only on the commoner events as they involve small numbers of patients (hundreds); they detect an incidence of up to 1:200.

• **Epidemiological techniques** used for post marketing studies include:

The *observational cohort study*
The *case-control study*, described on p. 53.

These are extremely important in the detection and quantification of adverse reactions with incidence of 1:5000–1:10 000.

One form of observational cohort study is *prescription event monitoring*. Prescriptions for a drug (say, 20 000) are collected (in the UK this is made practicable by the existence of a National Health Service in which prescriptions are sent to regional offices for pricing and payment of the pharmacist). The prescriber is sent a questionnaire and asked to report all *events* that have occurred (not only suspected adverse reactions). By linking general practice and hospital records and death certificates, both prospective and retrospective studies can be done and unsuspected effects can be detected. Prescription event monitoring can be used routinely on newly licensed drugs and it can also be implemented quickly in response to a suspicion raised, e.g. by spontaneous reports.

• **Spontaneous reporting systems** depend on doctors' intuitions and willingness to respond. They are therefore erratic, but really have no upper limit of qualitative sensitivity and may detect the rarest events; they are plainly unreliable for quantification.

It is recommended[3] that for

Newer drugs: doctors should report all suspected reactions, i.e. any adverse or any unexpected event, however minor, which could conceivably be attributed to the drug.

Established drugs: doctors should report all serious suspected reactions even if the effect is well recognised.

• **Record linkage schemes**, see p. 54.
• **Population statistics** e.g. birth defect registers and cancer registers, are insensitive unless a drug-induced event is highly unusual or very frequent. If suspicions are aroused then case-control and observational cohort studies will be initiated.

Drug-induced illness

The discovery of drug-induced illness has been usefully analysed by Jick[3] thus:

---

[3] N Engl J Med 1977; 296: 481.

• Drug commonly induces an otherwise rare illness: this effect is likely to be discovered by clinical observation in the pre-registration (pre-marketing) formal therapeutic trials and the drug will almost always be abandoned; but some patients are normally excluded from such trials, e.g. pregnant women, and detection will then occur later, e.g. thalidomide.

• Drug rarely induces an otherwise common illness: this effect is likely to remain undiscovered.

• Drug rarely induces an otherwise rare illness: this effect is likely to remain undiscovered before the drug is released for general prescribing; the effect should be detected by informal clinical observation or during any special post-registration surveillance and confirmed by a case-control study (see above), e.g. chloramphenicol and aplastic anaemia, practolol and oculomucocutaneous syndrome.

• Drug commonly induces an otherwise common illness: this effect will not be discovered by informal clinical observation. If very common, it may be discovered in formal therapeutic trials and in case-control studies, but if only moderately common it may require observational cohort studies, e.g. sulphonylureas and cardiovascular mortality in diabetics.

• Both drug and illness rates in intermediate range: both case-control and cohort studies may be needed.

The practicalities of detecting rare adverse reactions

For reactions with no background incidence the number of patients required to give a good (95%) chance of detecting the effect is given in Table 8.1. Assuming that three events are required before any regulatory or other action should be taken, it shows the large number of patients that must be monitored to detect even a relatively high incidence adverse effect.

The problem can be many orders of magnitude worse if the adverse reactions closely resemble spontaneous disease with a background incidence in the population.

Table 8.1   Detecting rare adverse reactions[4]

Expected incidence of adverse reaction	Required number of patients for event		
	1 event	2 events	3 events
1 in 100	300	480	650
1 in 200	600	960	1 300
1 in 1 000	3 000	4 800	6 500
1 in 2 000	6 000	9 600	13 000
1 in 10 000	30 000	48 000	65 000

GENERAL DATA AND DISCUSSION

• Adverse reactions cause 2–3% of *consultations* in general practice.

• They cause up to 3% of *admissions* to acute care hospital wards (and 0.3% of general hospital admissions).

• *Overall incidence* in hospital in-patients is 10–20%, and possible prolongation of hospital stay in 2–10% of patients in acute medical wards.

• *Predisposing factors*: age over 60 years or under one month, female, previous history of adverse reaction, hepatic or renal disease.

• They *cause death* in up to 0.3% hospital in-patients (or 1% if intravenous fluids are included), largely in patients already seriously ill.

• They *most commonly occur early* in therapy (days 1–10).

• *Most common diseases of sufferers*: cardiovascular, diabetes mellitus, respiratory (infection, chronic obstructive lung disease).

• *Most common drugs*: digoxin, antimicrobials, diuretics, potassium, analgesics, tranquillisers, insulin, aspirin, adrenocortical steroids, antihypertensives, warfarin.

• *Mechanism*: type A 80%: type B 20% (p. 121)

• *They most commonly affect*: gastrointestinal tract, skin, mental alertness, plasma K concentration.

Caution. About 80% of well people not taking

[4] By permission from, Safety requirements for the first use of new drugs and diagnostic agents in man. Geneva: CIOMS (WHO) 1983.

any drugs admit on questioning to symptoms (often several) such as are commonly experienced as lesser adverse reactions to drugs. These symptoms are intensified (or diminished) by administration of a placebo. Thus, many symptoms may be wrongly attributed to drugs.

On the other hand people may take drugs without realising they are doing so. The quinine used as a flavour in 'tonic water' was responsible in the following example of intolerance:[5]

A man presented with a seven week history of tinnitus and hearing loss. He was diagnosed as having bilateral meningiomas. He escaped craniotomy when an alert doctor discovered the man's enormous intake of 'tonic water', stopped it and the patient recovered.[5]

It is important to avoid alarmist or defeatist extremes of attitude. Many treatments are dangerous, e.g. surgery, electroshock, drugs, and it is irrational to accept the risks of surgery for peptic ulcer or hernia and refuse to accept any risk at all from drugs for conditions of comparable seriousness.

Many patients whose death is deemed to be partly or wholly caused by drugs are dangerously ill already; justified risks may be taken in the hope of helping them; ill-informed criticism in such cases can act against the interest of the sick. On the other hand there is no doubt that some of these accidents are avoidable. Avoidability is often more obvious when reviewing the conduct of treatment after death, i.e. with hindsight, than it was at the time.

Sir Anthony Carlisle,[6] in the first half of the 19th century, said that *medicine is 'an art founded on conjecture and improved by murder'*. Although medicine has advanced so rapidly, there is still a ring of truth in that statement[7] to anyone who follows the introduction of new drugs and observes how, after the early enthusiasm, the reports of serious toxic effects appear.

---

[5] Yohalem S B. JAMA 1953; 153: 1304.

[6] Noted for his advocacy of the use of 'the simple carpenter's saw' in surgery.

[7] In the less candid language of our times the opinion has been repeated; 'The trend of greater risks for greater gain is likely to continue'. Royal Commission on Civil Liability and Compensation for Personal Injury. London: HMSO, Cmnd. 7045, 1978.

Another cryptic remark of this therapeutic nihilist was 'digitalis kills people' and this is true. William Withering in 1785 laid down rules for the use of digitalis that would serve today. Neglect of these rules resulted in needless suffering for patients with heart failure for more than a century until the therapeutic criteria were rediscovered. Any drug that is really worth using can do harm.

> It is an absolute obligation on doctors to use only drugs about which they have troubled to inform themselves.

Effective therapy depends not only on the *correct choice* of drugs but also on their *correct use*. This latter is sometimes forgotten and a drug is condemned as useless when it has been used in a dose or way which absolutely precluded a successful result; which can be regarded as a *negative adverse effect*.

CLASSIFICATION OF ADVERSE REACTIONS

Adverse reactions are of two principal kinds:

Type A (Augmented) reactions will occur in **everyone** if enough of the drug is given because they are due to excess of normal, predictable, dose-related, pharmacodynamic effects. They are common and skilled management reduces their incidence, e.g. postural hypotension, hypoglycaemia, hypokalaemia.

Type B (Bizarre) reactions will occur only in **some people**. They are not part of the normal pharmacology of the drug, are not dose-related and are due to unusual attributes of the patient interacting with the drug. These effects are predictable where the mechanism is known (though predictive tests may be expensive or impracticable), otherwise they are unpredictable for the individual, although the incidence may be known. The class includes unwanted effects due to inherited abnormalities (see Pharmacogenetics) and immunological processes (see Drug allergy). These account for most drug fatalities.

Three subordinate types may be recognised:

Type C (Continuous) reactions due to long-term use, e.g. analgesic nephropathy, tardive dyskinesia.

Type D (Delayed) reactions, e.g. teratogenesis, carcinogenesis.

Type E (Ending of use) reactions, e.g. rebound adrenocortical insufficiency.

CAUSES OF ADVERSE REACTIONS

When an unusual or unexpected event, for which there is no evident natural explanation, occurs in a patient already taking a drug, the possibility that the event is drug-caused must always be considered.

Adverse reactions to drugs are due to or promoted by:

Non-drug factors

- intrinsic to the patient: age, sex, genetics, tendency to allergy, disease, personality and habits.
- extrinsic to the patient: the prescriber, the environment.

Drug factors

- intrinsic to the drug:
  use of the drug
  interactions between drugs.

Note. Aspects of the two sections above, **Classification** and **Causes** appear throughout the book. Selected topics are discussed below.

Age

The very old and the very young are liable to be intolerant of many drugs, largely because the equipment for disposing of them in the body is less efficient. The young, it has been aptly said, are not simply 'small adults', and 'respect for their pharmacokinetic variability should be added to the list of our senior citizens' rights'.[8] The old are also frequently exposed to multiple drug therapy which predisposes to adverse effects (see also p. 108).

---

[8] Fogel B S New Engl J Med 1983; 308: 1600.

Genetics (see also Pharmacogenetics)

The **hepatic porphyrias** (acute intermittent p., variegate p., hereditary coproporphyria, p. cutanea tarda) are a rare group of genetically determined single enzyme defects. The greatest care in prescribing for these patients is required if serious illness is to be avoided. In healthy people forming haemoglobin for their erythrocytes the rate of haem synthesis is controlled by negative feedback according to the amount of haem present.

When more haem is needed there is increased production of the rate controlling enzyme delta-aminolaevulinic acid (ALA) synthase which provides the basis of the formation of porphyrin precursors of haem. But in people with porphyria one or other of the enzymes that convert the various porphyrins to haem is deficient and so porphyrins accumulate.

A vicious cycle occurs, less haem : more ALA synthase, more porphobilinogen (in the case of acute intermittent porphyria), the metabolism of which is blocked, and a clinical attack occurs. The exact precipitating mechanism of the clinical features of an acute attack of porphyria is uncertain, but it would be rational to use any safe means of depressing the formation of ALA synthase. Fructose (laevulose) will do this; up to 400 g have been given i.v. per day in acute attacks with apparent benefit within 24 hours; glucose may be substituted. Haematin infusion (haem arginate), by replenishing haem and so removing the stimulus to ALA synthase, has also been found effective if given early and may prevent chronic neuropathy.

Increase in the haem-containing hepatic oxidising enzymes of the cytochrome P_{450} group causes an increased demand for haem. Therefore drugs that induce these enzymes would be expected to precipitate acute attacks of porphyria and they do so; tobacco smoking may act by this mechanism.

It is of interest that those who inherited acute intermittent porphyria and variegate porphyria suffered no biological disadvantage from the natural environment and bred as well as the normal population until the introduction of barbiturates and sulphonamides. They are now

Table 8.2 Unsafe prescribing in acute porphyria

A. ALCURONIUM	* DIHYDROERGOTAMINE	LOPRAZOLAM	(PHENYLBUTAZONE)
ALPRAZOLAM	DILTIAZEM	LOXAPINE	* PHENYTOIN
ALUMINIUM PREPARATIONS	* DIMENHYDRINATE	LYSURIDE	PIROXICAM
AMINOGLUTETHIMIDE	DIPHENHYDRAMINE		* PIVAMPICILLIN
AMIDOPYRINE	DIPYRONE	M: MAPROTILINE	PRAZEPAM
AMIODARONE	(DOTHIEPIN)	MEBEVERINE	(PRILOCAINE)
(AMITRIPTYLINE)	DOXYCYCLINE	(MEFENAMIC ACID)	* PRIMIDONE
(AMPHETAMINES)	(DYDROGESTERONE)	MEGESTROL	(PROBENECID)
* AMYLOBARBITONE		MESTRANOL	* PROGESTERONE (/OGENS)
ANTIPYRINE	E: ECONAZOLE	MEPIVACAINE	PROMETHAZINE
ASTEMIZOLE	ENALAPRIL	* MEPROBAMATE	* PYRAZINAMIDE
AURANOFIN	ENFLURANE	MERCAPTOPURINE	
AZAPROPAZONE	* ERGOT COMPOUNDS	MERCURY COMPOUNDS	Q: QUINALBARBITONE
	ERYTHROMYCIN	MESTRANOL	
B. BACLOFEN	* ETHANOL	METHAMPHETAMINE	R: RIFAMPICIN
* BARBITURATES	ETHIONAMIDE	METHOHEXITONE	
BENDROFLUAZIDE	ETHOSUXIMIDE	METHOTREXATE	S: SIMVASTATIN
BROMOCRIPTINE	ETHOTOIN	METHOXYFLURANE	SODIUM AUROTHIOMALATE
BUSULPHAN	ETIDOCAINE	METHSUXIMIDE	(SODIUM VALPROATE)
	ETOMIDATE	* METHYLDOPA	SPIRONOLACTONE
C. CAPTOPRIL		* METHYPRYLONE	STANOZOLOL
* CARBAMAZEPINE	F: FENFLURAMINE	(METOCLOPRAMIDE)	SUCCINIMIDES
* CARISOPRODOL	(FLUCLOXACILLIN)	METYRAPONE	* SULPHADIMIDINE
(CEPHALOSPORINS)	* FLUFENAMIC ACID	MIANSERIN	* SULPHASALAZINE
(CHLORAMBUCIL)	FLUNARIZINE	MICONAZOLE	SULPHINPYRAZONE
* CHLORAMPHENICOL	FLUNITRAZEPAM	MINOXIDIL	SULPIRIDE
* CHLORDIAZEPOXIDE	FLUPENTHIXOL		SULTHIAME
CHLORMEZANONE	FLURAZEPAM	N: NALIDIXIC ACID	
* CHLORPROPAMIDE	(FRUSEMIDE)	NATAMYCIN	T: TAMOXIFEN
CIMETIDINE		(NANDROLONE)	TERFENADINE
CINNARIZINE	G:* GLUTETHIMIDE	(NICERGOLINE)	* THEOPHYLLINE
CLEMASTINE	GLYMIDINE	NIFEDIPINE	* THIOPENTONE
(CLOBAZAM)	GOLD	* NIKETHAMIDE	THIORIDAZINE
(CLOMIPRAMINE)	GRAMICIDIN	NITRAZEPAM	TILIDATE
(CLONAZEPAM) (has been used safely	* GRISEOFULVIN	(NITROFURANTOIN)	TINIDAZOLE
in seizure prophylaxis)	GUAIPHENESIN	NORETHYNODREL	TOLAZAMIDE
CLONIDINE		NORTRIPTYLINE	TOLBUTAMIDE
CLORAZEPATE	H:* HALOTHANE		TRANYLCYPROMINE
COCAINE	* HYDANTOINS	O:* ORAL CONTRACEPTIVES	TRAZODONE
(COLISTIN)	HYDRALAZINE	* ORPHENADRINE	TRIMETHOPRIM
	(HYDROCHLOROTHIAZIDE)	(OXAZEPAM)	TRIMIPRAMINE
D: DANAZOL	HYOSCINE BUTYLBROMIDE	OXPENTIFYLLINE	TROXIDONE
DAPSONE		OXYCODONE	
DEXFENFLURAMINE	I: * IMIPRAMINE	OXYMETAZOLINE	V: (VALPROATE SODIUM) (has been
DEXTROPROPOXYPHENE	ISOMETHEPTENE	OXYPHENBUTAZONE	used safely in seizure prophylaxis)
(DIAZEPAM) (has been used safely in	(ISONIAZID)	OXYTETRACYCLINE	VALPROMIDE
status epilepticus)	K: KETOCONAZOLE		VERAPAMIL
* DICHLORALPHENAZONE		P:* PENTAZOCINE	VILOXAZINE
DICLOFENAC	L: LIGNOCAINE	PHENELZINE	
DIETHYLPROPION	LOFEPRAMINE	* PHENOBARBITONE	Z: ZUCLOPENTHIXOL
		PHENOXYBENZAMINE	

We are grateful to Dr. M.R. Moore for permission to base these lists on the more comprehensive data supplied by the Porphyria Research Unit, Western Infirmary, Glasgow, UK.
* Drugs in bold type with asterisk have actually been associated with acute attacks.
(—) Bracketed drugs are those for which there is *conflicting* experimental evidence.
Absence of a drug from this list does *not* mean it is safe.

at serious disadvantage, for many other drugs can precipitate fatal acute attacks.

Apparently unexplained attacks of porphyria should be an indication for close enquiry into all possible chemical intake, e.g. surreptitious ingestion of mouthwash containing alcohol, eucalyptol, and menthol caused attacks in one patient. Studies showed that the mouthwash, in particular the eucalyptol, induced hepatic ALA-synthase activity.[9] Guaiphenesin is hazardous; it is included in a multitude of multi-ingredient cough medicines (often non-prescription). Patients must be educated to understand their condition and to protect themselves from themselves and from others, including prescribing doctors.

Patients (1 in 10 000 UK population) are so highly vulnerable that we provide a partial list of drugs known and believed to be hazardous (see Table 8.2).

Factors extrinsic to the patient

The prescriber. It is obvious that the choice of drug and the skill with which it is used will have an important bearing on the occurrence of adverse reactions. Obviously, unskilled administration of general anaesthetics or anticancer drugs, however well chosen, is more serious than unskilled administration of correctly chosen penicillin.

Drug regulatory authorities that collect and evaluate spontaneously reported adverse reactions seldom have information to allow them to determine whether an adverse reaction should be primarily attributed to the prescriber's choice or skill and so regarded as avoidable, rather than inherent to the drug and unavoidable.

The environment. Significant environmental factors causing adverse reactions to drugs include simple pollution by drugs, e.g. halothane in the air of surgical operating theatres causing abortions amongst female staff; penicillin in the air of hospitals or in milk (see below), causing allergy.

Drug metabolism may also be increased by hepatic enzyme induction from insecticide accumulation (DDT) and from alcohol and the tobacco habit, e.g. smokers require a higher dose of theophylline.

Antimicrobials used in feeds of animals for human consumption have given rise to concern in relation to the spread of resistant bacteria that may affect man.

---

[9] Bickers D R et al New Engl J Med 1975; 292: 1115.

Factors intrinsic to the drug or formulation: see Classification of adverse reactions, p. 121

Adverse reactions, usually type B, may occur to ingredients of a formulation other than the active drug, e.g. colouring, flavouring.

Interactions between drugs:
see p. 110

ALLERGY IN RESPONSE TO DRUGS

Allergic reactions to drugs are the resultant of the interaction of drug or metabolite (or a non-drug element in the formulation) with patient and disease, and subsequent re-exposure.

Lack of previous exposure is not the same as lack of history of previous exposure. Exposure is not necessarily medical, e.g. penicillins occur in dairy products following treatment of cattle (despite laws to prevent this), and penicillin antibodies are commonly present in those who deny ever having received the drug.

Immune responses to drugs may be harmful (allergy) or harmless; the fact that antibodies are produced does not mean a patient will necessarily respond to re-exposure with clinical manifestations; most of our population has antibodies to penicillins, but, fortunately, comparatively few are allergic to them.

Whilst macromolecules (proteins, peptides, dextran polysaccharides) can act as complete antigens, most drugs are simple chemicals (mol. wt. less than 1000) and act as *incomplete antigens* or *haptens*, which become complete antigens in combination with a body protein.

The chief *target organs* of *drug allergy* are the skin, respiratory tract, gastrointestinal tract, the blood and the blood vessels.

Drugs may elicit allergic reactions of all types:
Type I reactions. Immediate-type (anaphylactic). The drug causes formation of tissue-sensitising IgE antibodies that are fixed to mast cells or leucocytes; on subsequent administration the allergen (conjugate of drug or metabolite with tissue protein) reacts with these antibodies, activating but not damaging the cell to which they are fixed and causing release of

pharmacologically active substances, e.g. histamine, leukotrienes, prostaglandins, platelet-activating factor, and causing effects such as urticaria, anaphylactic shock and asthma. Allergy develops within minutes and lasts 1–2 hours.

Type II reactions. Autoallergy. The drug or metabolite combines with a protein in the body so that the body no longer recognises the protein as self, treats it as a foreign protein and forms antibodies which combine with the antigen and activate complement which damages cells, e.g. methyldopa or penicillin-induced haemolytic anaemia.

Type III reactions. Antigen and antibody form large complexes and activate complement. Small blood vessels are damaged or blocked. Leucocytes attracted to the site of reaction engulf the immune complexes and release pharmacologically active substances (including lysosomal enzymes), starting an inflammatory process. These reactions include serum sickness, glomerulonephritis, vasculitis and pulmonary disease.

Type IV reactions. Delayed (cell-mediated) allergy. Antigen-specific receptors develop on T-lymphocytes. Subsequent administration leads to a local or tissue allergic reaction, e.g. contact dermatitis.

Distinctive features of allergic reactions[10]

- No correlation with known pharmacological properties of the drug
- No linear relation with drug dose (very small doses may cause very severe effects)
- Often include rashes, angioedema, serum sickness syndrome, anaphylaxis and asthma; characteristics of classical protein allergy
- Require an induction period on primary exposure, but not on re-exposure
- Disappear on cessation of administration and reappear on re-exposure
- Occur in a minority of patients receiving the drug
- Condition may be temporary
- Desensitisation may be possible

Cross-allergy

Cross-allergy within a group of drugs is usual.

Why allergy is commoner with some drugs, e.g. penicillins, than with others and why the same drug produces different effects in different people is unknown; a genetic basis in the host is likely. In addition, the patients with allergic diseases, e.g. eczema, are more likely to develop allergy to the drugs.

Principal clinical manifestations and treatment

1. Urticarial rashes and angioneurotic oedema (types I, III). These are probably the commonest type of drug allergy. They are usually accompanied by itching. The eyelids, lips and face are usually most affected; oedema of the larynx is rare but may be fatal if tracheostomy is not done. Such reactions may be generalised, but frequently are worst in and around the area of administration of the drug. They respond to adrenaline (i.m. if urgent), ephedrine, H_1-receptor antihistamines and adrenal steroids.

2 a. Non-urticarial rashes (types I, II, IV). These occur in great variety; frequently they are weeping exudative lesions. It is often difficult to be sure when a rash is due to a drug. Apart from stopping the drug, treatment is non-specific; in severe cases an adrenal steroid should be tried. Skin sensitisation to antibiotics may be very troublesome, especially amongst those who handle them. See Drugs and the skin for more detail.

b. Diseases of the lymphoid system. Infectious mononucleosis (and lymphoma, leukaemia) is associated with an increased incidence (40%+) of characteristic maculopapular, sometimes purpuric, rash which is probably allergic, when an aminopenicillin (ampicillin, amoxycillin) is taken; patients may not be allergic to other penicillins.

3. Anaphylactic shock (type I) occurs with penicillin, anaesthetics (i.v.), iodine-containing radiocontrast media and a huge variety of other drugs. A severe fall in blood pressure occurs, with bronchoconstriction, angioedema (including

---

[10] Assem E-S K. In: Davies D M, ed Textbook of adverse drug reactions. London: Oxford University Press, 1991.

larynx) and sometimes death due to loss of fluid from the intravascular compartment. Anaphylactic shock usually occurs suddenly, in less than an hour after the drug, but within minutes if it has been given i.v. *Treatment is urgent*, as follows: first 0.5–1.0 ml of adrenaline injection (1 mg/ml: 1 in 1000) should be given i.m.[11] to raise the blood pressure and to dilate the bronchi; it may be repeated after 3 min according to the clinical condition. Noradrenaline lacks any useful bronchodilator action (β effect). The adrenaline should be accompanied by an H_1-receptor antihistamine (say, chlorpheniramine 10 mg i.v.) and hydrocortisone (100 mg i.m. or i.v.). The adrenal steroid may be of benefit by reducing vascular permeability and by suppressing further response to the antigen-antibody reaction. Benefit from an adrenal steroid is not immediate; it is unlikely to begin for 30 min and takes hours to reach its maximum. Any hospital ward or other place where anaphylaxis may be expected should have all the drugs and tools necessary to deal with it in one convenient kit, for when they are needed there is little time to think and none to run about from place to place. See Pseudo-allergic reactions (p. 128).

4 a. Pulmonary reactions: asthma (type I). Aspirin and other nonsteroidal anti-inflammatory drugs may cause an asthmatic attack which can be fatal; 0.25–1.0 ml of adrenaline injection (1 mg/ml s.c.) will usually cut short an attack; the other treatments for asthma are also effective. Whether this is an allergic or pseudo-allergic reaction or a mixture of the two is uncertain.

b. Other types of pulmonary reaction (type IV). These include syndromes resembling acute and chronic lung infections, pneumonitis, fibrosis and eosinophilia.

5. The serum-sickness syndrome (type III). This occurs about 1–3 weeks after administration.

Treatment is by an adrenal steroid, and as above if there is urticaria.

6. Blood disorders[12]
a. Thrombocytopenia (type II, but also pseudo-allergic). This has been reported occasionally after a large number of drugs, including: phenylbutazone, gold, sulphonamides, quinine, quinidine, phenazone (antipyrine), rifampicin, tetracycline, thiourea derivatives, thiazides, oestrogens. Adrenal steroids may help.

b. Granulocytopenia (type II, but also pseudo-allergic) sometimes leading to agranulocytosis, is a very serious allergy which may occur with many drugs, e.g. clozapine, carbamazepine, carbimazole, chloramphenicol, sulphonamides (including diuretic and hypoglycaemic derivatives), colchicine, gold. Amidopyrine and dipyrone are notorious in this respect and need never be used, as there are adequate substitutes. Precautionary leucocyte counts are often advised for drugs having special risk (sometimes more to protect the doctor than to protect the patient). If they are used they should be frequent, say 2–4-weekly, for onset can be sudden, around the period of maximum risk if this is known. Later, intervals may be longer or the precaution abandoned. The chief clinical manifestation of agranulocytosis is sore throat or mouth ulcers and patients should be warned to report such events immediately; but they should not be frightened into non-compliance with essential therapy. Treatment of agranulocytosis involves both stopping the drug responsible and giving a *bactericidal* drug, e.g. penicillin, to treat or prevent infection. If the blood picture does not rapidly improve following withdrawal of the drug an adrenal steroid plus an androgen, e.g. fluoxymesterone, should be given in severe granulocytopenia and in all cases of agranulocytosis, but proof of its beneficial effect is naturally hard to get.

c. Aplastic anaemia (type II, but not al-

---

[11] Not s.c., for intense local vasoconstriction added to the low blood pressure will result in low tissue perfusion and so in delayed absorption. In extreme urgency 0.5 ml diluted × 10 may be given slowly i.v. It can cause ventricular fibrillation, but this may be thought to be the lesser risk.

[12] Where cells are being destroyed in the periphery and production is normal, transfusion is useless or nearly so, as the transfused cells will be destroyed, though in an emergency even a short cell life (platelets, erythrocytes) may tip the balance usefully. Where the bone marrow is depressed, transfusion is useful and the transfused cells will survive normally.

ways allergic). About 50% of cases of aplastic anaemia may be drug-induced. Chloramphenicol is the most important cause but others include sulphonamides and derivatives (diuretics, antidiabetics), phenylbutazone, gold, perchlorate and some insecticides, e.g. dicophane (DDT). In the case of chloramphenicol, bone marrow depression is a normal pharmacological effect of the drug (type A reaction) although aplastic anaemia may also be due to idiosyncrasy or allergy (type B reaction).

Death occurs in about 50% of cases, and treatment is as for agranulocytosis, with, obviously, blood transfusion.

d. Haemolysis of all kinds is included here for convenience. There are three principal categories:

(i) Allergy (type II) occurs with methyldopa, levodopa, penicillin, quinine, quinidine, sulphasalazine and organic antimony. It may be that in some of these cases a drug-protein-antigen/antibody interaction involves erythrocytes casually, i.e. a true 'innocent bystander' phenomenon.

(ii) Dose-related pharmacological action on normal cells e.g. lead, benzene, phenylhydrazine, chlorates, methyl chloride (refrigerant), some snake venoms.

(iii) Idiosyncrasy (see Pharmacogenetics).

Precipitation of a haemolytic crisis may also occur with the above drugs in the rare chronic haemolytic states due to *unstable haemoglobins*. Treatment is to withdraw the drug, and an adrenal steroid is useful in severe cases if the mechanism is immunological. Blood transfusion may be needed.

7. Fever is common; a mechanism is the release of interleukin-1 by leucocytes into the circulation which acts on receptors in the hypothalamic thermoregulatory centre, releasing prostaglandin-E_1.

8. Collagen diseases (type II) and syndromes resembling them, e.g. systemic lupus erythematosus are sometimes caused by drugs, e.g. hydralazine, procainamide, isoniazid, sulphonamides. Adrenal steroids are useful.

9. Hepatitis and cholestatic jaundice are sometimes allergic (type II, see Drugs and the liver). Adrenal steroids may be useful.

10. Nephropathy of various kinds (types II, III) occurs as does damage to other organs, e.g. myocarditis. Adrenal steroid may be useful.

Diagnosis of drug allergy

This still depends largely on clinical criteria, history, type of reaction, response to withdrawal and systemic rechallenge (if thought safe to do so).

Simple patch skin testing is naturally most useful in diagnosing contact dermatitis, but it is unreliable for other allergies. Skin prick or intradermal injection tests (especially the latter) are more reliable in specialist hands, but they can cause anaphylactic shock. False negative and false positive results occur.

Detection of drug-specific circulating antibodies only proves that an immunological response has occurred; it does not prove clinical allergy. Development of reliable in vitro predictive tests, e.g. employing human tissue or leucocytes, is a matter of considerable importance, not merely to avoid hazard to patients but to avoid depriving them of a drug that may be useful; drug allergy, once it has occurred, is not necessarily permanent, e.g. less than 50% of patients giving a history of allergy to penicillin have a reaction if it is given again.

Hyposensitisation/desensitisation

Once patients become allergic to a drug, it is better that they should never again come into contact with it. However, this can be inconvenient, for instance in allergy to antituberculosis drugs in both patients and in nurses. Such people can be hyposensitised by giving very small amounts of allergen, which are than gradually increased (usually every few hours) until a normal dose is tolerated. This may have been done under cover of a corticosteriod and a β-adrenoceptor agonist (both of which inhibit mediator synthesis and release). An antihistamine (H_1-receptor) may be added if an adverse reaction occurs. A full kit for treating anaphylactic shock should be handy.

The ease and safety of hyposensitisation varies with different drugs; penicillin is troublesome (see p. 161) and antituberculosis drugs generally less so. Hyposensitisation may only be temporary.

The mechanism underlying hyposensitisation is not understood but may involve the production by the patient of blocking antibodies that complete successfully for the allergen but whose combination with it is innocuous; or the threshold of cells to the triggering antibodies may be raised. Sometimes allergy is to an ingredient of the preparation other than the essential drug and merely changing the preparation is sufficient. Impurities are sometimes responsible and purified penicillins and insulins reduce the incidence of reactions.

Prevention of allergic reactions

Prevention is important since these reactions are unpleasant and may be fatal; it provides good reason for taking a drug history. Patients should always be told when they are thought to be allergic to a drug. It is essential that if a patient says he is allergic to some drug then that drug should not be given without careful enquiry that may include testing. But if the drug must be given there are precautions, e.g. rapid (rush) hyposensitisation with use of prophylactic drugs, as above.

The assumption that patients are all either ignorant or stupid has caused deaths: a young man was admitted to hospital for an interval appendicectomy, but had a sore throat and a slight fever. The house surgeon said this would soon clear up with penicillin, but the patient at once protested, saying that he was seriously allergic to penicillin. The doctor said that in that case he would use another drug, but in fact he gave penicillin and the patient died from anaphylactic shock.[13,14]

A doctor has also been known, when choosing an alternative drug to avoid a reaction, to prescribe inadvertently another drug from the same group, because the proprietary name gave no indication of the nature of the drug; another good reason for adopting the commonsense system of one drug, one sensible non-proprietary name.

Repeated blood counts in patients taking drugs known to cause allergic blood disorders, especially agranulocytosis, appear at first sight to be desirable, but as the onset is ordinarily abrupt they commonly fail to give protection and may give a false sense of security.[15] In addition, spontaneous fluctuations in the number of granulocytes make the interpretation of such counts difficult, especially in children. Routine blood counts are probably not worth doing except with drugs having a particularly high incidence, e.g. clozapine. The best protection normally is to tell the patients to report at once any fever, enlarged lymph nodes or sore throat (evidence of infection)[16] and to stop taking the drug until they have obtained advice (see granulocytopenia, p. 126).

The only way completely to prevent allergic reaction to drugs is to cease to use drugs; but at least the unnecessary use of drugs for trivial complaints should be avoided.

Pseudo-allergic reactions

These are effects that mimic allergic reactions but have no immunological basis. They are largely genetically determined and are due to release of endogenous biologically active substances (e.g. histamine and leukotrienes) by the drug, probably through a variety of mechanisms, direct and indirect, including complement activation leading to formation of polypeptides that affect mast cells as in true immunological reactions. Some drugs may cause both allergic and pseudo-allergic reactions.

Pseudo-allergic effects mimicking type I reac-

---

[13] Quoted in: Rosenheim M L et al eds. Sensitivity reactions to drugs. Oxford: Blackwell Scientific Publications, 1958.

[14] Failure to ask a patient about previous adverse reaction to penicillin before starting treatment has been judged negligent in the courts.

[15] Though, where a drug that causes bone marrow depression as a pharmacological dose-related effect, blood counts are part of the essential routine monitoring of therapy, e.g. anticancer drugs.

[16] Though one patient's agranulocytosis was first manifested clinically by an acute infection of pre-existing haemorrhoids.

tions (above) are called *anaphylactoid*, and they occur with aspirin and other nonsteroidal anti-inflammatory drugs (indirect action as above) (see also pulmonary reactions, above); corticotrophin (direct histamine release): i.v. anaesthetics and a variety of other drugs i.v. (morphine, tubocurarine, dextran, radiographic contrast media) and inhaled (cromoglycate). Severe cases are treated as for true allergic anaphylactic shock (above) from which, at the time, they are not distinguishable.

Type II reactions are mimicked by the haemolysis induced by drugs (antimalarials, sulphonamides and oxidising agents) and fava beans in subjects with inherited abnormalities of erythrocyte enzymes or haemoglobin.

Type III reactions are mimicked by nitrofurantoin (pneumonitis) and penicillamine (nephropathy). Lupus erythematosus due to drugs (procainamide, isoniazid, phenytoin) may be pseudo-allergic.

Miscellaneous adverse reactions

Reactions to *intravenous injections* are fairly common — hypotension, renal pain, rigors and fever, especially if the injection is very rapid. Some are due to foreign substances in the solutions and some just due to excessive delivery of the drug to the brain.

EFFECTS OF PROLONGED ADMINISTRATION: CHRONIC ORGAN TOXICITY

Eye. Toxic cataract can be due to chloroquine (retina also affected) and related drugs, adrenal steroids (topical and systemic), phenothiazines, naphthalene, carbromal, ergot, dinitrophenol, galactose, lactose, paradichlorobenzene and alkylating agents. Corneal opacities occur with amiodarone, phenothiazines and chloroquine. Retinal injury with thioridazine (particularly, of the neuroleptics), chloroquine and indomethacin.

Kidney: see Analgesic nephropathy.

Liver: see Alcohol.

Uterus: Prolonged postmenopausal oestrogen replacement therapy causes endometrial cancer (see below). See also, Chronic pharmacology, p. 14.

Carcinogenesis: see also p. 38. Mechanisms of carcinogenesis are complex; prediction from animal tests is uncertain and causal attribution in man has to be based on epidemiological studies. The principal mechanisms are:

- **Alteration of DNA (genotoxicity, mutagenicity).** Many chemicals or their metabolites act by causing mutations, activating oncogenes; those substances that are used as medicines include griseofulvin and alkylating cytotoxic drugs used in the treatment of cancer. Leukaemias and lymphomas are the most common malignancies.
- **Immunosuppression**. The immune system has a role in suppressing cancers (immune surveillance). A wide range of cancers develops in immunosuppressed patients, e.g after organ transplantation.
- **Hormonal.** Long-term use of oestrogen replacement in postmenopausal women induces endometrial cancer.

Combined oestrogen/progestrogen oral contraceptives may both suppress and enhance cancers (see p. 604).

Stilboestrol caused vaginal adenosis and cancer in the offspring of mothers who took it during pregnancy in the hope of preventing miscarriage. It was used for this purpose for decades after its introduction in the 1940s, on purely theoretical grounds. Controlled therapeutic trials were not done and there is no valid evidence of therapeutic efficacy. Male fetuses developed non-malignant genital abnormalities.

Carcinogenesis due to medicines requires drug exposure to be prolonged,[17] i.e. months or years; the cancers develop most commonly over 3–5 years and often years after treatment has ceased.

Incidence of second cancers in patients treated for primary cancer can be as high as 15 times the normal rate. The use of immunosuppression in, e.g. rheumatoid arthritis and organ transplants, also increases the incidence of cancers.

---

[17] Carcinogens that are effective after a single dose in animals are known, e.g. nitrosamines.

ADVERSE EFFECTS ON REPRODUCTION (see also p. 38)

The embryo/fetus. Drugs may act on the embryo and fetus:

Directly (thalidomide, cytotoxic, drugs, antithyroid drugs): any drug affecting cell division enzymes, protein synthesis, or DNA synthesis, is a potential teratogen, e.g. many antibiotics.

Indirectly
- on the placenta (vitamin A, isotretinoin)
- on the uterus (vasoconstrictors reduce blood supply and cause fetal anoxia);
- on the mother's hormone balance and biochemistry;
- on the father's sperm (uncertain).

Tests in animals are poor predictors for man. Proposals to test drugs on pregnant women who await abortion have met with both practical and ethical problems. Drugs can cross the placenta, see p. 88.

Early pregnancy. Drugs can affect the embryo before the placenta is formed, causing abortion or interfering with organogenesis. The most vulnerable period for major anatomical abnormality, i.e. *teratogenesis* (*teratos*: monster), is weeks 3–10 of intrauterine life, which corresponds to about 5–12 weeks after the first day of the last menstruation. Before that time drugs are likely to cause abortion, and after it the organs are formed and abnormalities are less anatomically dramatic; thus the activity of a teratogen is most devastating soon after implantation, at a time when the woman may not know she is pregnant.

Selective interference can produce characteristic anatomical abnormalities, and this was one factor that caused thalidomide to be so readily recognised; the others were the previous rarity of phocomelia and the widespread use of the drug.

Teratogenic effects can occur at doses that do not harm the mother and they are associated with increased intrauterine mortality, i.e. if the abnormality is gross enough, abortion occurs.

Drugs known to be teratogenic include anticancer drugs, warfarin, alcohol, adrenocortical steroids and isotretinoin. For an account of thalidomide see p. 65.

Drugs which are probably teratogenic include antiepileptics and sex hormones in general. Tobacco smoking retards fetal growth; it does not cause anatomical abnormalities in man as far as is known.

Innumerable drugs including aspirin, gastric antacids, co-trimoxazole, iron, neuroleptics, benzodiazepines and diuretics have come under suspicion.

Naturally the subject is a highly emotional one for prospective parents. Much depends on dose and stage of pregnancy. A definitive list of drugs is not practicable; the topic must be followed in the current literature.

Late pregnancy. Because the important organs are already formed, drugs will not cause the gross anatomical defects that can occur when they are given in early pregnancy. Administration of hormones, androgens or progestogens, can cause fetal masculinisation; iodide and antithyroid drugs in high dose can cause fetal goitre, as can lithium; tetracyclines can interfere with tooth and bone development.

Inhibitors of prostaglandin synthase (aspirin, indomethacin) may delay onset of labour and, in the fetus, it is possible they may interfere with cardiovascular function (maintenance of a patent ductus arteriosus is dependent on prostaglandins, which relax the ductus muscle).

It is probable that drug allergy in the mother can also occur in the fetus and it is possible that the fetus may be sensitised where the mother shows no effect, e.g. neonatal thrombocytopenia from thiazide diuretics.

The suggestion that congenital cataract (due to denaturation of lens protein) might be due to drugs has some support in man. Chloroquine and chlorpromazine are concentrated in the fetal eye. Since both can cause retinopathy it would seem wise to avoid them in pregnancy if possible.

Anticoagulants in pregnancy: see p. 478.

Drugs given to the mother just **prior to labour** can cause postnatal effects: CNS depressants may persist in and affect the baby for days after birth; chloramphenicol can cause collapse due to failure to conjugate it; vasoconstrictors can cause fetal distress by reducing uterine blood supply; β-adrenoceptor blockers may impair fetal response to hypoxia; sulphonamides displace bilirubin from plasma protein (risk of kernicterus); anticoagulants can cause haemorrhage.

Babies born to mothers dependent on opioids may show a physical withdrawal syndrome.

Drugs given during labour. Any drug that depresses respiration in the mother can cause respiratory depression in the newborn; opioid analgesics are notorious in this respect, but there can also be difficulty with any sedatives and general anaesthetics; they may also cause fetal distress by reducing uterine blood flow, and prolong labour by depressing uterine muscle.

Drugs used to relax the uterus in premature labour, e.g. β-adrenoceptor agonists (isoxsuprine) may affect the fetal circulation at birth. Diazepam (and other depressants) in high doses may cause hypotonia in the baby and possibly interfere with suckling. There remains the possibility of later behavioural effects due to impaired development of the central nervous system due to psychotropic drugs used during pregnancy; such effects have been shown in animals, including impaired ability to learn their way around mazes.

The possibility has been raised by case-control studies that childhood cancer may be promoted by drugs, e.g. pethidine, given to the mother during labour; studies continue.

Detection of teratogens. Anatomical abnormalities are the easiest to detect. Non-anatomical (functional) effects can also occur, though it is not appropriate to use the term teratogenesis (see definition above). They include effects on brain biochemistry which may have late behavioural consequences. No doubt these are usually adverse, though it is possible that prenatal exposure to drugs may enhance learning or memory (nootropism).

There is a substantial spontaneous background incidence in the community (up to 2%) so that the detection of a low-grade teratogen that increases the incidence of one of the commoner abnormalities presents an intimidating task. Also, most teratogenic effects are probably multifactorial.

Detection of teratogens will be accomplished by combinations of the techniques previously described.

In this emotionally charged area it is indeed hard for the public and especially for parents of an affected child to grasp that:

The concept of absolute safety of drugs needs to be demolished. It has been suggested that a particular antinauseant used in pregnancy (Debendox, Bendectin)[18] should have been taken off the market until it could be proved to be safe. In real life it can never be shown that a drug (or anything else) has no teratogenic activity at all, in the sense of never being a contributory factor in anybody under any circumstances. This concept can neither be tested nor proved.

Let us suppose for example, that some agent doubles the incidence of a condition that has natural incidence of 1 in 10 000 births. If the hypothesis is true, then studying 20 000 pregnant women who have taken the drug and 20 000 who have not may yield respectively two cases and one case of the abnormality. It does not take a statistician to realise that this signifies nothing, and it may need ten times as many pregnant women (almost half a million) to produce a statistically significant result. This would involve such an extensive multicentre study that hundreds of doctors and hospitals have to participate. The participants then each tend to bend the protocol to fit in with their clinical customs and in the end it is difficult to assess the validity of the data. Alternatively, a limited geographical basis may be used, with the trial going on for many years. During this time other things in the environment change, so again the results would not command our confidence. If it were to be suggested that there was something slightly teratogenic in milk, the hypothesis would be virtually untestable.

In practice we have to make up our minds which drugs may reasonably be given to pregnant women. Do we start from a position of presumed guilt or from one of presumed innocence? If the former course is chosen then we cannot give any drugs to pregnant women because we can never prove that they are completely free of teratogenic influence. It therefore seems that we must start from a position of presumed innocence and then take all possible steps to find out if the presumption is correct.

Finally, we must put the matter in perspective by considering the benefit/risk ratio. The problem of prescription in pregnancy cannot be considered from the point of view of only one side of the

---

[18] A combination of antimuscarinic (dicyclomine, later omitted), antihistamine (doxylamine) and vitamin (pyridoxine).

equation. Drugs are primarily designed to do good, and if a pregnant woman is ill it is in the best interests of her baby and herself that she gets better as quickly as possible. This often means giving her drugs. We can argue about the necessity of giving drugs to prevent vomiting, but there is no argument about the need for treatment of women with meningitis, septicaemia or venereal disease.

What we must try to avoid is medication by the media or prescription by politicians. A public scare about a well-tried drug will lead to wider use of less-tried alternatives. We do not want to be forced to practice the kind of defensive medicine that is primarily designed to avoid litigation. The best decisions for patients are made by well-informed doctors.[19]

General discussion

Whilst everyone will wish to avoid giving to women drugs that have been shown to cause fetal abnormalities in animals, they will also properly be reluctant at present to accept the corollary that failure to induce such abnormalities in animals means that a drug is safe.

Human toxic effects not predicted from animal experiments are often reversible, but even the most optimistic enthusiasts for drugs must shrink from the thought that their hands wrote prescriptions resulting in deformed, surviving babies.

Clinical data are, at present, inevitably open to doubt, and any list of suspected drugs must, so slight is our knowledge, become obsolete and misleading very quickly. This topic must, therefore, be followed in the periodical press and manufacturers' up-to-date Data Sheets.

It is possible that some drugs in common use may be undetected low-grade teratogens. In one retrospective (case-control) study of the drug consumption of mothers of infants with congenital abnormalities it was found that more of these took aspirin, antacids, amphetamine, barbiturates, iron, cough medicines and sulphonamides in early pregnancy than did those in the control group (mothers of infants without congenital abnormalities). The authors acknow-

ledge that such studies do not give proof of cause, e.g. a drug may be taken to control symptoms of a disease that causes the abnormality. But they conclude that it would be wise to avoid these drugs (prescribed or self medication) on which suspicion falls unless there is a specific indication for them, not only during known pregnancy but also in any women of childbearing age in whom conception is likely; a counsel of perfection, perhaps.

The medical profession clearly has a grave duty to refrain from all inessential prescribing of drugs with, say, less than 10–15 years' widespread use behind them, for all women of childbearing potential. It is not sufficient safeguard merely to ask a woman if she is or may be pregnant (the natural reluctance to broach this subject to unmarried women may, even in our permissive society, act as a salutary check to casual prescribing), but it will also be necessary to consider the possibility of a woman who evidently is not pregnant at the time of prescribing, becoming so whilst taking the drug.

Since morning sickness of pregnancy occurs during the time when the fetus is vulnerable, it is specially important to restrict drug therapy of this symptom to a minimum; but severe vomiting with its accompanying biochemical changes may itself harm the fetus.

Thus, before a drug is condemned as a cause of fetal damage, it is necessary to consider whether the disease for which it was given, or other intercurrent disease, might perhaps be responsible. Since the only way to be certain whether a drug causes fetal damage in man is to test it in man, it is necessary that doctors should (a) suspect a drug-induced abnormality when it occurs and (b) report it to a central organisation (UK Committee on Safety of Medicines) or to a national register of all birth defects (such a register ideally should be kept plus a full drug history of the mother from prior to conception). Unfortunately, none of these requirements is easily satisfied. Minor congenital abnormalities are common in the absence of drug therapy and some may be virtually undetectable, e.g. reduced intelligence or learning ability. Human frailty also causes any reporting system based on voluntary

---

[19] By permission from Smithells R W. In: Hawkins D F, ed. Drugs and pregnancy. Edinburgh: Churchill-Livingstone, 1983.

cooperation to be less than perfect. For example, the UK Committee on Safety of Medicines has found that when a letter exhorting doctors to report drug reactions is sent out, there is a large, but very short-lived increase in reports.

In addition, the more cautiously a new drug is introduced, the more difficult it is going to be to detect, by epidemiological methods, a capacity to cause fetal abnormality. This is especially so if the abnormality produced is already fairly common.

The possibility of fetal abnormalities resulting from drugs taken by the father exists but has only begun to be explored in animals.

Male reproductive function

Impotence may occur with drugs affecting autonomic sympathetic function, e.g. antihypertensives.

Spermatogenesis is reduced by sulphasalazine and mesalazine (reversible) and by cytotoxic anticancer drugs (reversible and irreversible).

Causation of birth defects due to abnormal sperm remain uncertain.

GUIDE TO FURTHER READING

Black S 1963 Inhibition of immediate-type hypersensitivity response by direct suggestion under hypnosis. British Medical Journal 1: 952

Bochner B S et al 1991 Anaphylaxis. New England Journal of Medicine 324: 1785

Brennan T A et al 1991 Incidence of adverse events and negligence in hospitalized patients. New England Journal of Medicine 324: 370
(also Leape L L et al Nature of adverse events: 377)

Herbst A L 1984 Diethylstilboestrol exposure — 1984 [effects of exposure during pregnancy on mother and daughters]. New England Journal of Medicine 311: 1433

Hurwitz N 1969 Predisposing factors in adverse reactions to drugs. British Medical Journal 1:536, admission to hospital due to drugs, 539

Inman W H W 1981 Postmarketing surveillance of adverse drug reactions in general practice. British Medical Journal 282: 1131,1216

Jick H 1974 Drugs–remarkably non-toxic. New England Journal of Medicine 291: 824

Kramer M S et al 1979 An algorithm for the operational assessment of adverse reactions. Journal of the American Medical Association 242: 623

Park B K et al 1988 The immunological basis of adverse drug reactions. British Journal of Clinical Pharmacology 26: 491

Rawlins M D 1984 Postmarketing surveillance of adverse reaction to drugs. British Medical Journal 288: 879

Rawlins M D 1988 Spontaneous reporting of adverse drug reactions. British Journal of Clinical Pharmacology 26: 1,7

Scott J L et al 1965 A controlled double-blind study of the hematologic toxicity of chloramphenicol. New England Journal of Medicine 272: 1137

Poisoning, drug overdose, antidotes

SELF POISONING

Deliberate self-poisoning. A curious by-product of the modern 'drug and prescribing explosion' is the rise in the incidence of non-fatal deliberate self-harm. The majority of people who do this lack serious suicidal intent and are termed *parasuicide.* In over 90% of instances, poisoning is the means chosen, usually by medicines taken in overdose. Two or more drugs are taken in over 30% of episodes, not including alcohol which is also taken in over 50% of the instances. Repeated episodes are not rare.[1] Prescribed drugs are used in over 75% of episodes but teenagers tend to favour non-prescribed analgesics available by direct sale, e.g. paracetamol and aspirin, which is important bearing in mind their potentially serious toxicity. The mortality rate of self-poisoning is very low (less than 1% of acute hospital admissions), but 'completed' suicides by poisoning still number 3500 per annum in England and Wales.

Accidental self-poisoning causing admission to hospital occurs predominantly amongst children under 5 years, usually with medicines left within reach or with domestic chemicals, e.g. bleach, detergents.

---

[1] An extreme example is that of a young man who, over a period of 6 years, was admitted to hospital following 82 episodes of self-poisoning, 31 employing paracetamol; he had had a disturbed, unhappy upbringing and had been expelled from both the Danish Navy and the British Army. Prescott L F et al Br Med J 1978; 2: 1399.

PRINCIPLES OF TREATMENT

Successful treatment of acute poisoning depends on a combination of speed and common sense as well as on the nature of the poison, the amount taken and the time which has since elapsed. Some 80% of those admitted to hospital require only observation and general supportive measures while they metabolise and eliminate the poison. About 15% require a specific antidote or some measure to increase elimination, when appropriate. Intensive care facilities are needed by only 5%. In the UK the centres of the National Poisons Information Service provide information and advice over the telephone throughout the day and night.[2]

Poison-specific measures

Identification
Prevention of further absorption
Specific antidotes
Acceleration of elimination

General measures
Initial assessment and resuscitation

Supportive measures
Psychiatric and social assessment

POISON-SPECIFIC MEASURES

Identification of the poison(s)

The key pieces of information are: the identity of the substance(s) taken, the dose(s) and the time that has since elapsed. Adults may be sufficiently conscious to give some indication of the poison or refer to it in a suicide note, or there may be other circumstantial evidence. Rapid (1–2 h) drug 'screens' of plasma or urine are available but are best reserved for seriously ill or unconscious patients in whom the cause of coma is unknown. Analysis of plasma for specific substances is essential in suspected cases of paracetamol or iron poisoning, to indicate which patients should receive antidotes; it is also re-

quired for salicylate, lithium and some sedative drugs, e.g. trichloroethanol derivatives, phenobarbitone, when a decision is needed about using urine alkalinisation, haemodialysis or haemoperfusion. Response to a specific antidote may provide a diagnosis, e.g. dilatation of constricted pupils and increased respiratory rate after i.v. naloxone (opioid poisoning) or arousal from unconsciousness in response to i.v. flumazenil (benzodiazepine poisoning).

Prevention of further absorption of the poison

From the environment

When a poison has been inhaled or absorbed through the skin, the patient should be taken from the toxic environment, contaminated clothing removed and the skin cleansed.

From the gut

Gastric lavage is best confined to the adult who is believed to have taken a significant amount of a toxic substance within 4–6 h, or longer in the case of drugs that delay gastric emptying, e.g. aspirin, tricyclic antidepressants, sympathomimetics, theophylline, opioids. Lavage is probably worth undertaking in any *unconscious* patient, who is believed to have ingested poison, regardless of the interval after ingestion, and provided the airways are protected by a cuffed endotracheal tube. Paradoxically, lavage may wash an ingested substance *into* the small intestine, enhancing its absorption; thus patients who have ingested tricyclic antidepressants or centrally depressant drugs must be monitored closely after the procedure.

The passing of a gastric tube, naturally, takes second place to emergency resuscitative measures, institution of controlled respiration or suppression of convulsions. Nothing is gained by aspirating the stomach of a corpse.

Emesis, in conscious patients only, is preferred for children and may also be used for adults who refuse gastric lavage; it has the advantage of being applicable on first seeing the

---

[2] For telephone numbers see the British National Formulary (BNF).

patient, whereas gastric lavage should be done in hospital. Emesis is induced by Ipecacuanha Emetic Mixture, Pediatric (BNF), 10 ml for a child 6–18 months, 15 ml for an older child and 30 ml for an adult, i.e. all ages may receive the same preparation but in a different dose, which is followed by a tumblerful of water and may be repeated after 20 minutes. The active constituent of ipecacuanha is emetine which itself can cause prolonged vomiting, diarrhoea and drowsiness that may be confused with effects of the ingested poison. Even / fully conscious patients may develop aspiration pneumonia after ipecacuanha.

Both emesis and lavage are *contraindicated* for corrosive poisons when there is a risk of perforation of the gut, and for petroleum distillates as the danger of causing inhalational chemical pneumonia outweighs that of leaving the substance in the stomach.

Cathartics or whole-bowel irrigation[3] are appropriate for the removal of sustained-release formulations. These formulations are now common, e.g. aspirin, theophylline, iron. Patients have died from failure to recognise the danger of continued release of drug from such products, after apparently successful gastric lavage.

Oral adsorbents. Activated charcoal (Carbomix, Medicoal) consists of a very fine black powder prepared from vegetable matter, e.g. wood pulp, coconut shell, which is 'activated' by an oxidising gas flow at high temperature to create a network of fine (10–20 nm) pores to give it an enormous surface area in relation to weight ($1000 \text{ m}^2/\text{g}$). This binds to, and thus inactivates, a wide variety of compounds in the gut; exceptions are listed below. Indeed, activated charcoal comes nearest to fulfilling the long-sought notion of a 'universal antidote'.[4] It should be given as soon as possible after a poison has been ingested, when a significant amount remains unabsorbed and, to be most effective, about 10 times as much charcoal as poison, weight for weight, is needed; in the adult an initial dose of 50–100 g is usual. If the patient is vomiting, the charcoal should be given through a naso-gastric tube.

Activated charcoal appears to be relatively safe but constipation or mechanical bowel obstruction may accompany repeated use. Aspiration of charcoal into the lungs can cause hypoxia through obstruction and arteriovenous shunting. Charcoal binds to and so inactivates ipecacuanha but may be used after *successful* emesis with that substance; methionine, used for paracetamol poisoning, is also adsorbed. *Iron, lithium* and *organic solvents* and *corrosive agents* are *not* absorbed by charcoal.

Other oral adsorbents have specific uses. Fuller's earth and bentonite (both natural forms of aluminium silicate) bind and inactivate the herbicides, paraquat (activated charcoal is superior) and diquat; cholestyramine and colestipol adsorb warfarin.

Specific antidotes[5]

Specific antidotes reduce or abolish the effects of poisons through a variety of mechanisms, which may be categorised as follows:

- on *receptors*, which may be stimulated, blocked or bypassed
- on *enzymes*, which may be inhibited or reactivated
- by *displacement* from tissue binding sites
- by *exchanging* with the poison

---

[3] Magnesium sulphate may be used; alternatively, irrigation with large volumes of a polyethylene glycol-electrolyte solution, e.g. Provide, by mouth causes minimal fluid and electrolyte disturbance (it was developed for preparation for colonoscopy).

[4] For centuries it was supposed not only that there could be, but that there actually was, a single antidote to all poisons. This was Theriaca Andromachi, a formulation of 72 (a magical number) ingredients amongst which particular importance was attached to the flesh of a snake (viper). The antidote was devised by Andromachus whose son was physician to the Roman Emperor, Nero (AD 54–68).

[5] Mithridates the Great (?132–63 BC) king of Pontus (in Asia Minor) was noted for 'ambition, cruelty and artifice'. 'He murdered his own mother . . . . and fortified his constitution by drinking antidotes' to the poisons with which his domestic enemies sought to kill him (Lemprière). When his son also sought to kill him, Mithridates was so disappointed that he compelled his wife to poison herself. *He* then tried to poison himself, but in vain; the frequent antidotes which he had taken in the early part of his life had so strengthened his constitution that he was immune. He was obliged to stab himself, but had to seek the help of a slave to complete his task. Modern physicians have to be content with less comprehensively effectively antidotes, some of which are listed in Table 9.1.

Table 9.1 Antidotes, indications and modes of action

Antidote	Indication	Mode of action
acetylcysteine	paracetamol, chloroform, carbon tetrachloride	replenishes depleted glutathione stores
atropine	cholinesterase inhibitors e.g. organophosphorus insecticides	blocks muscarinic cholinoceptors
benztropine	drug-induced movement disorders	blocks muscarinic cholinoceptors
benzylpenicillin	amatoxin (*Amanita phalloides*)	displaces toxin from plasma albumin and enhances urinary excretion
calciumedetate	lead	chelates lead ions
calcium gluconate	hydrofluoric acid, fluorides	binds or precipitates fluoride ions
desferrioxamine	iron	chelates ferrous ions
dicobalt edetate	cyanide and derivatives e.g. acrylonitrile	chelates to form non-toxic cobalti- and cobalto-cyanides
digoxin-specific antibody fragments (FAB)	digitalis glycosides	binds free glycoside in plasma, complex excreted in urine
dimercaprol (BAL)	arsenic, copper, gold, lead, inorganic mercury	chelates metal ions
ethanol	ethylene glycol, methanol	competitively inhibits alcohol and acetaldehyde dehydrogenases, preventing formation of toxic metabolites
flumazenil	benzodiazepines	competes for benzodiazepine receptors
glucagon	β-adrenoceptor antagonists	bypasses blockade of the beta-adrenoceptor; stimulates cyclic AMP formation with positive cardiac inotropic effect
isoprenaline	β-adrenoceptor antagonists	competes for β-adrenoceptors
methionine	paracetamol	replenishes depleted glutathione stores
naloxone	opioids	competes for opioid receptors
neostigmine	antimuscarinic drugs	inhibits acetylcholinesterase, causing acetylcholine to accumulate at cholinergic receptor sites
oxygen	carbon monoxide	competitively displaces carbon monoxide from binding sites on haemoglobin
penicillamine	copper, gold, lead, elemental mercury (vapour), zinc	chelates metal ions
phenoxybenzamine	hypertension due to α-adrenoceptor agonists, e.g. with MAOI, clonidine, ergotamine	competes for α-adrenoceptors (long-acting)
phentolamine	as above	competes for α-adrenoceptors (short-acting)
phytomenadione (vitamin K_1)	coumarin (warfarin) and indandione anticoagulants	replenishes vitamin K

Table 9.1 (cont'd)

Antidote	Indication	Mode of action
pralidoxime	cholinesterase inhibitors, e.g. organophosphorus insecticides	competitively reactivates cholinesterase
propranolol	β-adrenoceptor agonist drugs, ephedrine, theophylline, thyroxine	competes for β-adrenoceptors
protamine	heparin	binds ionically to neutralise
Prussian blue (ferric ferrocyanide)	thallium (in rodentocides)	exchanges for thallium
Unithiol	lead, elemental and organic mercury	chelates metal ions

- by *replenishment* of an essential substance
- by *binding* to the poison (including *chelation*).

Table 9.1 illustrates these mechanisms with antidotes that are of therapeutic value.

Chelating agents

Chelating agents are used for poisoning with heavy metals. They incorporate the metal ions into an inner ring structure in the molecule (Greek, *chele* = claw) by means of chemical groups called ligands (Latin, *ligare* = to bind); effective agents form stable, biologically inert complexes that are excreted in the urine.

Dimercaprol (BAL, British Anti-Lewisite) was synthesised during a systematic study of possible antagonists to arsenical vesicant war gases such as Lewisite. Arsenic and other metal ions are toxic in relatively low concentration because they combine with the –SH groups of essential enzymes, thus inactivating them. Dimercaprol provides –SH groups which combine with the metal ions to form relatively harmless ring compounds which are excreted, mainly in the urine. As dimercaprol, itself, is oxidised in the body and renally excreted, repeated administration is necessary to ensure that an excess is available until all the metal has been eliminated. Adverse effects are common, particularly with larger doses and include nausea and vomiting, lachrymation and salivation, paraesthesiae, muscular aches and pains, urticarial rashes, tachycardia and a raised blood pressure. Gross overdosage may cause overbreathing, muscular tremors, convulsions and coma.

Unithiol (dimercaptopropanesulphonate, DMPS) is a new agent which effectively chelates lead and mercury; it appears to be well tolerated.

Sodium calciumedetate is the calcium chelate of the disodium salt of ethylenediamine-tetra-acetic acid (calcium EDTA). Its effectiveness is due to its capacity to exchange, in lead poisoning, calcium for lead: the lead chelate is excreted in the urine, leaving behind a harmless amount of calcium. Dimercaprol may usefully be combined with sodium calciumedetate when lead poisoning is severe, e.g. with encephalopathy. Adverse effects are fairly common, and include hypotension, lachrymation, nasal stuffiness, sneezing, muscle pains and chills. Renal damage can occur.

Dicobalt edetate. Cobalt forms stable, non-toxic complexes with cyanide. It is toxic (especially if the wrong diagnosis is made and no cyanide is present), causing hypertension, tachycardia and chest pain; cobalt poisoning is treated by giving sodium calciumedetate and i.v. glucose.

Penicillamine (dimethylcysteine) is a metabolite of penicillin that contains –SH groups; it may be used to chelate lead and also copper (see Hepatolenticular degeneration). Its principal use is for rheumatoid arthritis (see Index).

Desferrioxamine (see iron).

Acceleration of elimination of the poison

Techniques for eliminating poisons have a role that is limited, but important when applicable.[6] Each method depends, directly or indirectly, on removing drug from the circulation and successful use requires that:

- the poison should be present in high concentration in the plasma relative to that in the rest of the body, i.e. it should have a small distribution volume;
- the poison should dissociate readily from any plasma protein binding sites;
- the effects of the poison should relate to its plasma concentration.

Methods used are:

Alteration of urine pH and diuresis

By manipulation of the pH of the glomerular filtrate, a drug can be made to ionise, become less lipid soluble and thus remain in the renal tubular fluid, then to be eliminated in the urine (see p. 87). Maintenance of a good urine flow helps this process but 'it is the alteration of tubular fluid pH that is important'.[7] The practice of forcing diuresis with frusemide and large volumes of i.v. fluid does not add significantly to drug clearance but may cause fluid overload.

Alkalinisation may be used for *salicylate* (> 500 mg/l + metabolic acidosis, or in any case > 750 mg/l), *phenobarbitone* (75–150 mg/l) or *chlorophenoxy herbicides*, e.g. 2,4-D, MCPA. The objective is to maintain a urine pH of 7.5–8.5 by an i.v. infusion of sodium bicarbonate. Available preparations of sodium bicarbonate vary between 1.2 and 8.4% (1 ml of the 8.4% preparation contains 1 mmol of sodium bicarbonate) and the concentration given will depend on the patient's fluid needs. Supplementation with infusion of dextrose 5% may be necessary; hypokalaemia should be corrected (by adding potassium 10–20

mmol) preferably before commencing alkalinisation, which will itself lower plasma potassium.

Acidification may be used for severe, acute *amphetamine, dexfenfluramine, quinine* or *phencyclidine* poisoning. The objective is to maintain a urine pH of 5.5–6.5 by giving i.v. infusion of arginine hydrochloride (10 g) or lysine hydrochloride (10 g) over 30 min, followed by ammonium chloride (4 g) 2-hourly by mouth. It is rarely necessary.

Peritoneal dialysis

Peritoneal dialysis involves instilling appropriate fluid into the peritoneal cavity. Poison in the blood enters the dialysis fluid down the concentration gradient. The fluid is then drained and replaced. The technique requires little equipment; it is effective for lithium and methanol poisoning. Adequate peritoneal blood flow is essential; it becomes inefficient if the patient is hypotensive.

Haemodialysis and haemoperfusion

Both haemodialysis and haemoperfusion are substantially more effective than peritoneal dialysis. They involve establishing a temporary extracorporeal circulation, usually from an artery to a vein in the arm. In haemodialysis a semipermeable membrane separates blood from dialysis fluid and the poison passes passively from the blood, where it is present in high concentration, into the fluid. The principle of haemoperfusion is that blood flows over activated charcoal or an appropriate ion-exchange resin which adsorbs the poison. Loss of blood cells and activation of the clotting mechanism are largely overcome by coating the charcoal with an acrylic hydrogel which does not reduce adsorbing capacity, though the patient must be anticoagulated with heparin.

Such artificial methods of removing poison from the body are invasive, demand skill and experience on the part of the operator and are expensive in manpower. Their use should therefore be confined to cases of severe, prolonged or progressive clinical intoxication, when high plasma concentration indicates a dangerous degree of poisoning, and when removal by

---

[6] Vale J A 1990 Methods to increase poison elimination. In: Catto G R D, ed. Drugs and the kidney. Dordrecht: Kluwer, p. 65.
[7] Prescott L F et al. Br Med J 1982; 285: 1383.

haemoperfusion or dialysis constitutes a significant addition to natural methods of elimination.

- Haemodialysis is effective for:
  salicylate (> 750 mg/l + renal failure, or in any case > 900 mg/l), isopropanol (present in aftershave lotions and window-cleaning solutions), lithium and methanol.
- Haemoperfusion is effective for:
  phenobarbitone (> 100–150 mg/l, but repeat-dose activated charcoal by mouth appears to be as effective, see below) and other barbiturates, ethchlorvynol, glutethimide, meprobamate, methaqualone, theophylline, trichloroethanol derivatives.

Repeated doses of activated charcoal

Activated charcoal by mouth not only prevents absorption of ingested drug in the gut (see above), it also adsorbs drug that is secreted in the bile or that diffuses from the blood into the gut lumen if the concentration there is lower. Given in repeated doses, e.g. 50 g × 6/d, charcoal thus *accelerates elimination* and has been found effective for poisoning with phenobarbitone and carbamazepine. Accumulating evidence suggests that charcoal thus administered may achieve a place in the management of several forms of poisoning.

GENERAL MEASURES
Initial assessment and resuscitation

The initial clinical review should include a search for known consequences of poisoning, which include: impaired consciousness with flaccidity (benzodiazepines, alcohol, trichloroethanol) or with hypertonia (tricyclic antidepressants, antimuscarinic agents), hypotension, shock, cardiac dysrhythmia, evidence of convulsions, behavioural disturbances (psychotropic drugs), hypothermia, aspiration pneumonia and cutaneous blisters, burns in the mouth (corrosives).

Maintenance of an adequate oxygen supply to the body is the first priority. A systolic blood pressure of 80 mm Hg can be tolerated in a young person but a level below 90 mm Hg will imperil the brain or kidney of the elderly. Expansion of the venous capacitance bed is the usual cause of shock in acute poisoning and blood pressure may be restored by placing the patient in the head-down position to encourage venous return, or by the use of a colloid plasma expander such as gelatin or hetastarch. External cardiac compression may be necessary and should be continued till the cardiac output is self-sustaining, which may be a long time when the patient is hypothermic or poisoned with cardiodepressant drugs, e.g. tricyclic antidepressants, β-adrenoceptor blockers. The airway must be sucked clear of oropharyngeal secretions or regurgitated matter.

Supportive treatment

The salient fact is that patients recover from most poisonings provided they are adequately ventilated, hydrated and perfused, for, in the majority of cases, the most efficient mechanisms of elimination are the patients' own and, given time, they will eliminate all the poison. Patients require the standard care of the unconscious, with special attention to the problems introduced by poisoning which are outlined below.

Airway maintenance is essential, with efficient bronchial toilet to remove secretions. Some patients require a cuffed endotracheal tube but seldom for more than 24 h. Inspired air should be humidified to avoid drying and crusting of the airways.

Ventilation needs should be assessed, if necessary supported by blood gas analysis. A mixed respiratory and metabolic acidosis is common. Hypoxia may be corrected by supplementing the inspired air with oxygen but mechanical ventilation is necessary if there is significant hypercapnia i.e. if the Pa CO_2 exceeds 6.5 kPa. *Aspiration pneumonia* should be treated with appropriate antimicrobials, e.g. cefuroxime and metronidazole.

Plasma biochemistry should be monitored and appropriate measures taken, e.g. for acid-base disturbance, hypokalaemia or hypoglycaemia.

Hypotension is common and in addition to the resuscitative measures indicated above, infusion of a combination of dopamine and dobutamine in low dose may be required to maintain renal perfusion.

Convulsions should be treated if they are persistent or protracted. Diazepam i.v. is the first choice.

Cardiac dysrhythmia frequently accompanies poisoning, e.g. with tricyclic antidepressants, theophylline, β-adrenoceptor blockers. Acidosis, hypoxia and electrolyte disturbance are often important contributory factors; the emphasis of therapy should be to correct these and to resist the temptation to resort to an antidysrhythmic drug. If dysrhythmia leads to persistent peripheral circulatory failure, then an appropriate drug ought to be used, e.g. a β-blocker for poisoning with a sympathomimetic drug.

Hypothermia may occur if temperature regulation is impaired by CNS depression. Core temperature must be monitored by a low-reading rectal thermometer, while the patient is nursed in a heat retaining 'space blanket'.

Immobility may lead to pressure lesions of peripheral nerves, cutaneous blisters and necrosis over bony prominences, and rhabdomyolysis, the latter being a cause of acute renal failure. These are avoided by good nursing care.

The urinary bladder can be emptied reflexly by gentle suprapubic pressure, catheterisation being reserved for the minority of patients who remain unconscious for more than 12 h.

Psychiatric and social assessment

Most cases of self-poisoning are precipitated by interpersonal or social problems, which should be addressed. Genuine psychiatric illness ought to be identified and treated.

SOME POISONINGS (for medicines: see individual drugs)

Poisonings by chemicals and metals

Cyanide causes tissue anoxia by chelating the ferric part of the intracellular respiratory enzyme, cytochrome oxidase. Poisoning may occur as a result of self-administration of hydrocyanic (prussic) acid, by accidental exposure in industry, through inhaling smoke from burning polyurethane foams in furniture, through ingesting amygdalin which is present in the kernels of several fruits including apricots, almonds and peaches (constituents of the unlicensed anticancer agent, Laetrile), or from excessive use of sodium nitroprusside for severe hypertension.[8] The symptoms of acute poisoning reflect tissue anoxia, with dizziness, palpitations, a feeling of chest constriction and anxiety; characteristically the breath smells of bitter almonds. In more severe cases there is acidosis and coma. Inhaled hydrogen cyanide may lead to death within minutes but when it is ingested as the salt several hours may elapse before the patient is seriously ill. Chronic exposure damages the nervous system causing peripheral neuropathy, optic atrophy and nerve deafness.

The principles of specific therapy are:

- Dicobalt edetate (Kelocyanor) to chelate the cyanide is the treatment of choice when the diagnosis is certain. The dose is 300–600 mg given i.v. over one minute, followed by a further 300 ml if recovery is not evident within one minute.
- Alternatively, a two-stage procedure may be followed by i.v. administration of:
  (1) sodium nitrite, which rapidly converts haemoglobin to methaemoglobin, the ferric ion of which takes up cyanide as cyanmethaemoglobin (up to 40% methaemoglobin can be tolerated);
  (2) sodium thiosulphate, which more slowly detoxifies the cyanide by permitting the formation of thiocyanate. When the

---

[8] Or in other more bizarre ways. 'A 23-year-old medical student saw his dog (a puppy) suddenly collapse. He started external cardiac message and a mouth-to-nose ventilation effort. Moments later the dog died, and the student felt nauseated, vomited and lost consciousness. On the victim's arrival at hospital, an alert medical officer detected a bitter almonds odour on his breath and administered the accepted treatment for cyanide poisoning after which he recovered. It turned out that the dog had accidentally swallowed cyanide, and the poison eliminated through the lungs had been inhaled by the master during the mouth-to-nose artificial respiration.' J Amer Med Ass 1983: 249, 353.

diagnosis is uncertain, administration of thiosulphate plus oxygen is a safe course.

There is evidence that oxygen, especially if at high pressure (hyperbaric), overcomes the cellular anoxia in cyanide poisoning; the mechanism is uncertain, but oxygen should be administered.

Methanol is widely available as a solvent and in paints and antifreezes. It may be consumed as a substitute for ethanol; the acute effect is less than that of ethanol, i.e. the subject is less 'drunk', but it is the toxic metabolites that make methanol intoxication so serious; as little as 10 ml may cause permanent blindness and 30 ml may kill. Methanol, like ethanol, is metabolised by zero-order processes that involve the hepatic alcohol and aldehyde dehydrogenases, but whereas ethanol forms acetaldehyde and acetic acid which are partly responsible for the unpleasant effects of 'hangover', methanol forms formaldehyde and formic acid. Blindness may be due to retinal aldehyde dehydrogenase (for the interconversion of retinol and retinene) allowing the local formation of formaldehyde. Acidosis is due to the formic acid, which itself enhances pH-dependent hepatic lactate production, so that lactic acidosis is added.

The clinical features are severe malaise, vomiting, abdominal pain and tachypnoea (due to the acidosis). Loss of visual acuity and scotomata indicate ocular damage and, if the pupils are dilated and non-reactive, permanent loss of sight is probable. Coma and circulatory collapse may follow.

Therapy is directed at:

- *Correcting the acidosis.* The outcome largely depends on achieving this, and sodium bicarbonate is given i.v. in doses up to 2 mol in a few hours, carrying an excess of sodium which must be managed. Methanol is metabolised slowly and the patient may relapse if bicarbonate administration is discontinued too soon.
- *Inhibiting methanol metabolism.* The dehydrogenase enzymes have a greater affinity for ethanol than for methanol and administering ethanol to occupy the enzymes is an effective means of preventing metabolism of methanol to its toxic products. A single oral dose of ethanol 1 ml/kg (as a 50% solution or as the equivalent in gin or whisky) is followed by 0.25 ml/kg/h orally or i.v., aiming to maintain the blood ethanol at about 100 mg/100 ml until no methanol is detectable in the blood.
- *Eliminating methanol* and its metabolites by dialysis. Haemodialysis is 2–3 times more effective than is peritoneal dialysis. Folinic acid 30 mg i.v. six-hourly may protect against retinal damage by enhancing formate metabolism.

Ethylene glycol is readily accessible as a constituent of antifreezes for car radiators. It has been used criminally to give 'body' and sweetness to white table wines. The substance itself is not toxic but metabolism to glycolate and oxalate causes acidosis and renal damage, and usually the situation is further complicated by lactic acidosis. In the first 12 hours after ingestion the patient appears as though intoxicated with alcohol but does not smell of that; subsequently there is increasing acidosis, pulmonary oedema and cardiac failure, and in 2–3 days renal pain and tubular necrosis develop because calcium oxalate crystals form in the urine.

In addition to general supportive measures against shock and respiratory distress, acidosis is corrected with i.v. sodium bicarbonate and hypocalcaemia with calcium gluconate. As with methanol (above), ethanol is given competitively to inhibit the metabolism of ethylene glycol and haemodialysis is used to eliminate the poison.

Hydrocarbons, e.g. paraffin oil (kerosene), petrol (gasoline), benzene, chiefly cause CNS depression and pulmonary damage from inhalation. It is vital to avoid aspiration into the lungs during attempts to remove the poison or in spontaneous vomiting. Gastric aspiration should be performed only if a cuffed endotracheal tube is efficiently in place, if necessary after anaesthetising the subject.

Volatile solvent abuse or 'glue sniffing', is common among teenagers, especially males. The success of the modern chemical industry provides easy access to these substances as adhesives, dry cleaners, air fresheners, deodorants, aerosols and other products. Various techniques of administration are employed: viscous products may be inhaled from a plastic bag, liquids from a handkerchief or plastic bottle. The immediate euphoriant and excitatory effects are replaced by confusion, hallucinations and delusions as the dose is increased. Chronic abusers, notably of toluene, develop peripheral neuropathy, cerebellar disease and dementia; damage to the kidney, liver heart and lungs also occurs with solvents. Over 50% of deaths from the practice follow cardiac dysrhythmia, probably caused by sensitisation of the myocardium to catecholamines and by vagal inhibition from laryngeal stimulation when aerosol propellants are sprayed into the throat.

Standard cardiorespiratory resuscitation and antidysrhythmia treatment are used for acute solvent poisoning. Toxicity from carbon tetrachloride and chloroform involves the generation of phosgene which is inactivated by cysteine, and by glutathione which is formed from cysteine; treatment with N-acetylcysteine, as for poisoning with paracetamol, is therefore recommended. The lead content of some petrols may cause additional specific toxicity in petrol 'sniffers', and appropriate therapy is needed (see below).

> **Heavy metal poisonings.** Specific chelating agents are listed in Table 9.1. Treatments of choice are for:
> *lead*: sodium calciumedetate, or penicillamine in less severe cases
> *mercury* (inorganic, e.g. $HgCl_2$): dimercaprol
> *mercury* (elemental, i.e. vapour, and organic, i.e. alkylmercury): unithiol or penicillamine
> *copper*: penicillamine

Poisoning by herbicides and pesticides

Organophosphorus pesticides are anticholinesterases; poisoning and its management are described on p. 385. Organic *carbamates* are similar.

Dinitro-compounds. Dinitrophenol, abandoned as an explosive, had a short career in the therapy of obesity, but it was so toxic that it shortened life more than obesity does. The rationale for its use was that it increases the metabolic rate by uncoupling oxidative phosphorylation, so that the surplus fat would be used up. Related compounds, dinitro-orthocresol (DNOC) and dinitrobutylphenol (DNBP) are used as selective weed killers and insecticides, and cases of poisoning occur accidentally, e.g. when safety precautions are ignored. These substances can be absorbed through the skin and the hands: face or hair are usually stained yellow. Symptoms and signs indicate the very high metabolic rate; copious sweating and thirst are early warning signs and may proceed to dehydration and vomiting, weakness, restlessness, tachycardia and deep, rapid breathing, convulsions and coma. Treatment is urgent and consists of cooling the patient and attention to fluid and electrolyte balance. It is essential to differentiate this type of poisoning from that due to anticholinesterases (p. 385) because atropine given to patients poisoned with dinitro-compound will stop sweating and may cause death from hyperthermia.

Organochlorine pesticides, e.g. DDT, may cause convulsions in acute overdose. Treat as for status epilepticus.

Rodenticides include warfarin and thallium (see Table 9.1); for strychnine, which causes convulsions, give diazepam.

Paraquat is a widely used herbicide which is extremely toxic if it is ingested; a mouthful of commercial solution taken and spat out may be enough to kill. Ulceration and sloughing of the oral and oesophageal mucosa are prominent. Some days later renal tubular necrosis develops and later there is pulmonary oedema followed by pulmonary fibrosis; whether the patient lives or dies depends largely on the condition of the lung. Treatment is *urgent* and includes gastric lavage, activated charcoal or aluminium silicate (Fuller's earth) by mouth as adsorbents, and osmotic purgation (magnesium sulphate). Haemodialysis or haemoperfusion may have a role in the first 24 h, the rationale being that reducing the plasma concentration by these methods protects the kidney, failure of which allows the slow but relentless accumulation of paraquat in the lung.

Diquat is similar but the late pulmonary changes may not occur.

Poisoning by biological substances

Many plants form substances that are important for their survival either by enticing animals which disperse their spores, or by repelling potential predators. Poisoning occurs when children eat berries or chew flowers, attracted by their colour; adults may mistake non-edible for edible varieties of salad plants and fungi (mushrooms) for they may resemble each other closely and are greatly prized by epicures.

The range of toxic substances which these plants produce is reflected in a diversity of symptoms which, however, may be grouped broadly thus:

- *Atropinic*, e.g. from deadly nightshade and thorn apple, causing blurred vision, dry mouth, flushed skin, dilated pupils, confusion and delirium.
- *Nicotinic*, e.g. from hemlock and laburnum, causing salivation, dilated pupils, vomiting, convulsions and respiratory paralysis.
- *Muscarinic*, e.g. from *Inocybe* and *Clitocybe* mushrooms, causing salivation, lachrymation, perspiration, bradycardia and bronchoconstriction, also hallucinations.
- *Hallucinogenic*, e.g. from psilocybin-containing mushrooms (liberty cap), which may be taken specifically for this effect ('magic mushrooms').
- *Cardiovascular*, e.g. from foxglove, mistletoe and lilly-of-the-valley which contain cardiac glycosides that cause vomiting, diarrhoea and cardiac dysrhythmia.
- *Hepatotoxic*, e.g. from *Amanita phalloides* (death cap mushroom), from *Senecio* (ragwort) and *Crotalaria* and from 'bush teas' prepared from these plants in the Caribbean. Aflatoxin, from *Aspergillus flavus*, a fungus which contaminates foods, is probably a cause of primary liver cancer.
- *Convulsant*, e.g. from hemlock, water dropwort and cowbane, which contain the related and very dangerous substances, oenanthotoxin and cicutoxin.
- *Cutaneous irritation*, e.g. directly with nettle, or dermatitis following sensitisation with primula.
- *Gastrointestinal symptoms*, nausea, vomiting, diarrhoea and abdominal pain occur with numerous plants.

Treatment of plant poisonings consists mainly of activated charcoal to adsorb toxin in the gastrointestinal tract. Inducing emesis with ipecacuanha may make the diagnosis more difficult for vomiting is often the earliest sign of poisoning. Convulsions should be controlled with diazepam. In 'death cap' mushroom poisoning, penicillin may be used to displace toxin from plasma albumin, provided haemodialysis is being used, which latter may also benefit the renal failure.

INCAPACITATING AGENTS
(harassing, disabling, anti-riot agents)

Harassing agents may be defined as chemical agents that are capable when used in field conditions, of rapidly causing a temporary disablement that lasts for little longer than the period of exposure.[9]

The pharmacological requirements for a safe and effective harassing agent must be stringent (it is hardly appropriate to refer to benefit versus risk). As well as potency and rapid onset and offset of effect in open areas under any atmospheric condition, it must be safe in confined spaces where concentration may be very high and may affect an innocent, bedridden invalid should a projectile enter a window.

CS (chlorobenzylidene malononitrile, a tear gas) is a favoured substance at present. This is a solid that is disseminated as a solid or particulate aerosol by including it in a pyrotechnic mixture. The spectacle of its dissemination has been rendered familiar by television. It is not a gas, it is an aerosol or smoke. The particles aggregate and settle to the ground in minutes so that the risk of prolonged exposure out of doors is not great.

---

[9] Health aspects of chemical and biological weapons. Geneva: WHO 1970.

According to the concentration of CS to which a person is exposed, the effects vary from a slight pricking or peppery sensation in the eyes and nasal passages up to the maximum symptoms of streaming from the eyes and nose, spasm of the eyelids, profuse lachrymation and salivation, retching and sometimes vomiting, burning of the mouth and throat, cough and gripping pain in the chest.[10]

The onset of symptoms occurs immediately on exposure (an important factor from the point of view of the user) and they disappear dramatically;

At one moment the exposed person is in their grip. Then he either stumbles away, or the smoke plume veers or the discharge from the grenade stops, and, immediately, the symptoms begin to roll away. Within a minute or two, the pain in the chest has gone and his eyes, although still streaming, are open. Five or so minutes later, the excessive salivation and pouring tears stop and a quarter of an hour after exposure, the subject is essentially back to normal.[10]

Exposed subjects absorb small amounts only, and the plasma $t_{\frac{1}{2}}$ is about 5 s.

Investigations of the effects of CS are difficult in 'field use', but some have been done and at present there is no evidence that even the most persistent rioter will suffer any permanent effect. The hazard to the infirm or sick seems to be low, but plainly it would be prudent to assume that asthmatics or bronchitics could suffer an exacerbation from high concentrations, though bronchospasm does not occur in normal people. Whether or not CS can cause unconsciousness is uncertain and is difficult to investigate for, 'in the highly charged circumstance of a riot, unconsciousness can occur for a variety of reasons', and deliberate use of CS in training operations has induced panic and fainting at first contact. Vomiting seems to be due to swallowing contaminated saliva. Transient looseness of the bowels may follow exposure. Hazard from CS is probably confined to situations where the missiles are projected into enclosed spaces.

CN (chloroacetophenone, a tear gas) is generally used as a solid aerosol or smoke; solutions (Mace) are used at close quarters.

CR (dibenzoxazepine) was put into production in 1973 after testing on 150 army volunteers. In addition to the usual properties (above) it may induce a transient rise in intraocular pressure which is dismissed by the investigators as unimportant on the grounds 'of the likely youth of those against whom CR will be used'.[11] Its solubility allows use in water 'cannons'.

'Authority' is reticent about the properties of all these substances and no further important information is readily available.

This brief account has been included, because, in addition to helping victims, even the most well-conducted and tractable students and doctors may find themselves exposed to CS smoke in our troubled world; and some may even feel it their duty to incur exposure. The following points are made:

- Wear disposable plastic gloves, for the object of treating the sufferer is frustrated if the physician becomes affected.
- Contaminated clothing should be put in plastic bags and skin should be washed with soap and water. Showering or bathing may cause symptoms to return by releasing the agent from contaminated hair. Cutaneous erythema is usual and blistering may occur with high concentrations of CS and CN in warm, moist conditions.
- The eyes should be left to irrigate themselves; raised intraocular pressure may cause acute glaucoma in those over 40 years.

Drugs used for torture, interrogation and judicial execution

Regrettably, drugs have been and are being used for torture, sometimes disguised as 'interrogation' or 'aversion therapy'. Facts are, not surprisingly, hard to obtain, but it seems that suxamethonium, hallucinogens, thiopentone, neuroleptics, amphetamines, apomorphine and cyclophosphamide have been employed to hurt, frighten, confuse or debilitate in such ways as callous ingenuity can devise. When the definition of criminal activity

---

[10] Home Office Report of the enquiry into the medical and toxicological aspects of CS. pt II. London: HMSO, Cmnd 4775, 1971.

[11] Editorial 1973 Lancet 2: 1184.

becomes perverted to include activities in defence of human liberty, the employment of drugs offers inducement to inhuman behaviour. Such use, and any doctors or others who engage in it, or who misguidedly allow themselves to believe that it can be in the interest of victims to monitor the activity by others, must surely be outlawed.

It might be urged that it is justifiable to use drugs to protect society by discovering serious crimes such as murder. There is no such thing as a 'truth drug' in the sense that it guarantees the truth of what the subject says. There always must be uncertainty of the truth of evidence, obtained with drugs, e.g. thiopentone, that cannot be independently confirmed. But accused people, convinced of their own innocence, sometimes volunteer to undergo such tests. The problem of discerning truth from falsehood remains.

In some countries drugs are used for judicial execution, e.g. combinations of thiopentone, potassium, curare.

GUIDE TO FURTHER READING

Amnesty International 1973 Report on torture. Duckworth, London

Ashton C H 1990 Solvent abuse. Little progress after twenty years. British Medical Journal 300: 135

Davies J E 1987 Changing profile of pesticide poisoning. New England Journal of Medicine 316: 807

Editorial 1984 Chemical and bacteriological warfare in the 1980s. Lancet 2: 141

Editorial 1988 Complications of chronic volatile substance abuse. Lancet 2: 431

Ferner R E, Rawlins M D 1989 Chemical weapons. Easy to make, hard to destroy. British Medical Journal 298: 767

Meredith T J, Vale J A 1988 Carbon monoxide poisoning. British Medical Journal 296: 77

Proudfoot A T 1986 A star treatment for digoxin overdose? British Medical Journal 293: 643

Ridker P M, McDermott W V 1989 Comfrey herb tea and hepatic veno-occlusive disease. Lancet 1: 657

Volans G N 1987 Monitoring the safety of over the counter drugs. British Medical Journal 295: 797

World Health Organization 1970 Health aspects of chemical and biological weapons. Geneva

10

Infection I: chemotherapy

SYNOPSIS

Infection is a major category of human disease and skilled management of antimicrobial drugs is of the first importance. The term chemotherapy is used for the drug treatment of parasitic infections in which the parasites (viruses, bacteria, protozoa, fungi, worms) are destroyed or removed without injuring the host. The use of the term to cover all drug or synthetic drug therapy needlessly removes a distinction which is convenient to the clinician and has the sanction of long usage. By convention the term is used to include therapy of cancer.

- Classification of antimicrobial drugs
- How antimicrobials act
- General principles of antimicrobial therapy
- Use of antimicrobial drugs: choice of antimicrobials; combinations of drugs; chemoprophylaxis and suppressive therapy
- Problems with antimicrobial drugs: resistance to drugs; opportunistic infection; masking of infections; treatment failure
- Antimicrobial drugs of choice (reference table)

History

Many substances that we now know to possess therapeutic efficacy have been used in the past. The Ancient Greeks used male fern, and the Aztecs chenopodium, as intestinal anthelminthics. The Ancient Hindus treated leprosy with chaulmoogra. For hundreds of years moulds have been applied to wounds, but, despite the introduction of mercury as a treatment for syphilis (16th century), and the use of cinchona bark against malaria (17th century), the history of modern rational chemotherapy did not begin until the late 19th century.

The differential staining of tissues and bacteria was an obvious instance of chemicals distinguishing between the parasite and host, and gave hope of usefully selective toxicity. Aniline dyes were used for staining, and when it was shown that these dyes could also kill bacteria, Ehrlich[1] successfully tried their effect on infected experimental animals. Ehrlich thus developed the idea of chemotherapy and he invented the word. In 1906 he wrote:

In order to use chemotherapy successfully, we must search for substances which have an affinity for the cells of the parasites and a power of killing them greater than the damage such substances cause to the organism itself . . . . This means . . . *we must learn to aim, learn to aim with chemical substances.*

---

[1] Paul Ehrlich (1854–1915), the German scientist who was the pioneer of chemotherapy and discovered the first cure for syphilis.

His efforts resulted in the introduction of arsphenamine (Salvarsan) for the treatment of syphilis, later superseded by penicillin.

The antimalarials pamaquin and mepacrine were developed from dyes and in 1935 the first sulphonamide, linked with a dye (Prontosil), was introduced as a result of systematic studies by Domagk.[2] The results obtained with sulphonamides in puerperal sepsis, pneumonia and meningitis were dramatic and caused a revolution in scientific and medical thinking.

In 1928, Fleming[3] accidentally rediscovered the long-known ability of penicillium fungi to suppress the growth of bacterial cultures. Attempts to isolate the active principle (penicillin) from the crude preparations were made, but lack of appreciation of its potentialities as well as the difficulty of preparing enough for experiments caused it to be put aside as a curiosity.

In 1939, principally as an academic exercise, Florey[4] and Chain[5] undertook an investigation of antibiotics, i.e. substances produced by micro-organisms that are antagonistic to the growth or life of other micro-organisms.[6] They prepared penicillin, discovered its *systemic* in addition to its local chemotherapeutic power against experimental infections in mice, and confirmed its remarkable lack of toxicity.[7] When the preparation was administered to a man with combined staphylococcal and streptococcal septicaemia there was dramatic improvement; unfortunately the manufacture of penicillin (in the Pathology Laboratory) could not keep pace with the requirements (it was also extracted from the patient's urine and re-injected); it ran out and the patient later succumbed to infection. Subsequent development, however, amply demonstrated the remarkable therapeutic efficacy of penicillin.

Since 1939 large programmes of screening fungi and bacteria for antibiotic production have been conducted. That nothing is beneath the notice of some investigators is illustrated by the discovery of antibacterial substances in the anal gland secretion of the Argentine ant and in the faeces of blow-fly larvae.

CLASSIFICATION OF ANTIMICROBIAL DRUGS

Antimicrobial agents may be classified according to the type of organism against which they are active and in this book follow the sequence:

Antibacterial drugs
Antiviral drugs
Antifungal drugs
Antiprotozoal drugs
Anthelminthic drugs

Antimicrobial drugs may also be classified broadly into those that are:

- *bacteriostatic*, i.e. act primarily by arresting bacterial growth, such as sulphonamides, tetracyclines and chloramphenicol, and those that are
- *bactericidal*, i.e. which act primarily by killing bacteria, such as penicillins, cephalosporins, aminoglycosides, isoniazid and rifampicin.

The classification is somewhat arbitrary because most bacteriostatic drugs can be shown to be bac-

---

[2] Gerhard Domagk (1895–1964), bacteriologist and pathologist who made his discovery while working in Germany. Awarded the 1939 Nobel prize for Physiology or Medicine, he had to wait until 1947 to receive the gold medal because of Nazi policy at the time.
[3] Alexander Fleming (1881–1955). He researched for years on antibacterial substances that would not be harmful to humans. His findings on penicillin were made at St. Mary's Hospital, London.
[4] Howard Walter Florey (1898–1969), Professor of Pathology at Oxford University.
[5] Ernest Boris Chain (1906–79). Biochemist. Fleming, Florey and Chain shared the 1945 Nobel prize for Physiology or Medicine.
[6] Strictly, the definition should refer to substances that are antagonistic *in dilute solution* for it is necessary to exclude various metabolic products such as alcohol and hydrogen peroxide.

[7] The importance of this discovery for a nation at war was obvious to these workers, but the time, July 1940, was unpropitious, for invasion was feared. The mood of the time is shown by the decision that by the time the invaders reached Oxford, the essential records and apparatus for making penicillin would have been deliberately destroyed; but the productive strain of *Penicillium* mould was to be secretly preserved by several of the principal workers smearing the spores of the mould into the linings of their ordinary clothes where it could remain dormant but alive for years; any member of the team who escaped (wearing the right clothes) could use it to start the work again. Macfarlane G. Howard Florey. Oxford: 1979.

tericidal at high concentrations. It does retain a certain usefulness in that when a bacteriostatic drug is used, the defence mechanisms of the body are relied on to destroy the organisms whose multiplication has been stopped by the drug. These mechanisms are inadequate for the purpose, e.g. for infective endocarditis and for infections in those whose immune systems are compromised by disease or drugs. In these cases, bactericidal drugs should be used.

Bactericidal drugs act most effectively on rapidly dividing organisms. Thus a bacteriostatic drug, by reducing multiplication, may protect the organism from a bactericidal drug. Such mutual *antagonism* of antimicrobials may be clinically important, but the matter is complex for drugs are not purely bactericidal or bacteriostatic at all concentrations.

HOW ANTIMICROBIALS ACT

It should always be remembered that drugs are seldom the sole instruments of cure. The natural defences of the body perform the final elimination of infection. Where these are seriously inadequate the choice of a drug that will actually *kill* the organism and its management gain prime importance.

Antimicrobials act at different sites in the target organism as follows:

- *The cell wall.* This gives the bacterium its characteristic shape and provides protection against the much lower osmotic pressure of the environment. Bacterial growth involves breakdown and extension of the wall; interference with its function allows the cell to absorb water so that it bursts. As the cells of higher, e.g. human, organisms do not possess this type of wall, drugs that act here are especially selective; obviously, the drugs are effective only against growing cells. They include: penicillins, cephalosporins, vancomycin, bacitracin, cycloserine.
- *The cytoplasmic membrane* inside the cell wall is the site of most of the microbial cell's biochemical activity. Drugs that interfere with its function include: polyenes (nystatin, amphotericin), polymyxins (colistin, polymyxin B).

- *Protein synthesis.* Drugs that interfere at various points with the build-up of peptide chains on the ribosomes of the organism include: chloramphenicol, erythromycin, fusidic acid, tetracyclines, aminoglycosides.
- *Nucleic acid metabolism.* Drugs may interfere
1. directly with microbial DNA, e.g. quinolones, or with RNA, e.g. rifampicin;
2. indirectly, e.g. sulphonamides, trimethoprim.

GENERAL PRINCIPLES OF ANTIMICROBIAL CHEMOTHERAPY

The following principles, many of which apply to drug therapy in general, are a guide to good practice with antimicrobial agents.

- *Make a diagnosis* as precisely as is possible, defining the site of infection, the organism(s) responsible and their sensitivity to drugs. This objective will be more readily achieved if all relevant biological samples for the laboratory are taken before treatment is begun.
- *Remove barriers to cure*, e.g. lack of free drainage of abscesses, obstruction in the urinary or respiratory tracts.
- *Decide whether chemotherapy is really necessary.* As a general rule, acute infections require chemotherapy whilst chronic infections may not. Chronic abscess, empyema or osteomyelitis respond poorly, although chemotherapeutic cover is essential if surgery is undertaken in order to avoid a flare-up of infection or its dissemination due to the breaking down of tissue barriers. Even some acute infections such as gastroenteritis are better managed symptomatically than by antimicrobials.
- *Select the best drug.* This involves consideration of:

1. *specificity*; for ideally the antimicrobial activity of the drug should match that of the infecting organisms. Indiscriminate use of broad-spectrum drugs encourages opportunistic infections. There are however times when 'best guess' chemotherapy of reasonably broad spectrum must be given because of the absence of precise identification of the responsible microbe.

2. *pharmacokinetic factors*; to ensure that the chosen drug is capable of reaching the site of infection in adequate amounts, e.g. by crossing the blood–brain barrier.
3. *the patient*; who may previously have exhibited allergy to antimicrobials or whose routes of elimination may be impaired, e.g. by renal disease.

• *Administer the drug* in optimum *dose* and *frequency* and by the most appropriate *route(s)*. Inadequate dose may lead to the development of microbial resistance. In general, intermittent dosing is preferred to continuous infusion. Plasma concentration monitoring is often a guide to the adequacy of therapy.

• *Continue therapy* until apparent cure has been achieved. If an infection deserves treatment, it probably deserves at least 5 days. There are many exceptions to this, such as typhoid fever, tuberculosis and infective endocarditis, in which relapse is possible long after apparent clinical cure and so the drugs are continued for a longer time, determined by experience.

• *Test for cure.* In some infections, microbiological proof of cure is desirable because disappearance of symptoms and signs occurs before the organisms are eradicated, e.g. urinary infections. Microbiological examination must be done, of course, after withdrawal of chemotherapy.

• *Prophylactic chemotherapy* for surgical and dental procedures should be of very limited duration. It should start *at the time of surgery* to reduce the risk of producing resistant organisms prior to surgery and continue for, say 48 h.

• *Carriers of pathogenic organisms*, in general, should not be treated to remove the organisms for it is better to allow natural re-establishment of a normal flora.

USE OF ANTIMICROBIAL DRUGS
Choice of antimicrobials

The general rule is that selection of antimicrobials should be based on identification of the microbe and sensitivity tests. All appropriate specimens (blood, pus, urine, sputum, cerebro-

spinal fluid) *must* therefore be taken for examination before administering any antimicrobial.

This process inevitably takes time and therapy must usually be started on the basis of the 'best guess', from which point of view infections may be categorised as those in which:

• choice of antimicrobial follows automatically from the clinical diagnosis because the causative organism is always the same, and is virtually always sensitive to the same drug, e.g. segmental pneumonia in a young person which is almost always caused by *Streptococcus pneumoniae* (penicillin), some haemolytic streptococcal infections, e.g. scarlet fever, erysipelas (penicillin), typhus (tetracycline), leprosy (dapsone with rifampicin);
• the infecting organism is identified by the clinical diagnosis, but no assumption can be made as to its sensitivity to any one antimicrobial, e.g. tuberculosis;
• the infecting organism is not identified by the clinical diagnosis, e.g. in urinary tract infection or meningitis.

In the second and third categories particularly, choice of an antimicrobial may be guided by:

1. knowledge of the likely pathogens in the clinical situation. Trimethoprim is a reasonable first choice for lower urinary tract infection (coliform organisms), and benzylpenicillin for meningitis in the adult (meningococcal or pneumococcal);
2. simple staining tests. The antimicrobial may be selected in the knowledge that the organism is a Gram-positive or Gram-negative coccus or bacillus. It is necessary to know the approximate range of antimicrobial drugs for organisms so classified; a penicillin may be indicated when Gram-positive cocci are found or an aminoglycoside if Gram-negative bacilli are present.

Modification of treatment can be made later if necessary, after identification and sensitivity tests. Treatment otherwise should be changed only after adequate trial, usually 3 days, for over-hasty alterations cause confusion and tend to produce resistant organisms. Lack of bacteriological assistance is not an excuse for indiscriminate polypharmacy.

Combinations of antimicrobials

A critical attitude is essential towards the use of two or more antimicrobials, prescribed separately to suit the patient and the infection. The indications for use of two or more antimicrobials are:

- *To obtain potentiation*, i.e. an effect unobtainable with either drug alone, e.g. co-trimoxazole for gonorrhoea; penicillin plus gentamicin for enterococcal endocarditis.
- *To delay development of drug resistance*, especially in chronic infections, e.g. tuberculosis.
- *To broaden the spectrum of antibacterial activity* in a known mixed infection or where treatment is essential before a diagnosis has been reached; full doses of each drug are needed.

Selection. A bacteriostatic drug, by reducing multiplication, may protect the organism from a bactericidal drug (see above, antagonism). When a combination must be used blind, it is preferable to use two bacteriostatic or two bactericidal drugs.

Chemoprophylaxis and pre-emptive suppressive therapy

It is sometimes assumed that what a drug can cure it will also prevent, but this is not necessarily so.

The basis of effective, true, chemoprophylaxis is the use of a drug to prevent infection by one organism of virtually uniform susceptibility, e.g. benzylpenicillin against a group A streptococcus. But the term chemoprophylaxis is commonly extended to include suppression of *disease* as well as prevention of *infection*. The main categories of chemoprophylaxis may be summarised as follows:

- *True prevention of infection*: rheumatic fever,[8] urinary tract infection.
- *Prevention of opportunistic infections*, e.g. due to commensals getting into the wrong place (bacterial endocarditis after dentistry and peritonitis

after bowel surgery). Note that these are both high risk situations of short duration; prolonged administration of drugs before surgery would result in the areas concerned (mouth and bowel) being colonised by drug-resistant organisms with potentially disastrous results (see below). Immunocompromised patients, e.g. with treated leukaemia, benefit from chemoprophylaxis.

- *Suppression* of existing infection before it causes overt disease, e.g. tuberculosis, malaria, animal bites.
- *Prevention of exacerbations* of a chronic infection, e.g. bronchitis, in cystic fibrosis.
- *Prevention of spread amongst contacts* (in epidemics and/or sporadic cases). Spread of influenza A can be partially prevented by amantadine; in an epidemic of meningitis, or when there is a case in the family, rifampicin may be used; very young and fragile non-immune child contacts of pertussis *might* benefit from erythromycin.

Prophylaxis of bacterial infection can be achieved often by doses that are inadequate for therapy. Details of the practice of chemoprophylaxis are given in the appropriate sections.

Attempts to use drugs routinely in groups specially at risk to prevent infection by a range of organisms, e.g. pneumonia in the unconscious or in patients with heart failure and in the newborn after prolonged labour, have not only failed but have sometimes permitted infections with less susceptible organisms. Attempts routinely to prevent bacterial infection secondary to virus infections (e.g. in respiratory tract infections, measles) have not been sufficiently successful to outweigh the disadvantages of drug allergy and infection with drug-resistant bacteria. It is probably generally better to be alert for complications and then to treat them vigorously, than to try to prevent them.

---

[8] Rheumatic fever is caused by a large number of types of Group A streptococci and immunity is type specific. Recurrent attacks are commonly due to infection with different strains of these, all of which are sensitive to penicillin and so chemoprophylaxis is used. Acute glomerulonephritis is also due to group A streptococci. But only a few types cause it, so that natural immunity is more likely to protect and, in fact, second attacks are rare. Therefore, chemoprophylaxis is not used.

Chemoprophylaxis in surgery

The principles governing use of antimicrobials in this context are as follows.

- Chemoprophylaxis is justified:

1. when the risk of infection is high because of bacteria in the viscus which is being operated on, e.g. the large bowel;
2. when the patient has a susceptible organ, e.g. diseased heart valves;
3. when the patient is generally susceptible to infection, e.g. patients who are neutropenic due to treatment of leukaemia.

- Antimicrobials should be selected with a knowledge of the likely pathogens at different sites.
- Antimicrobials should be given i.v., i.m. or occasionally rectally at the beginning of anaesthesia and for no more than 48 h. Specific instances are:

1. *colorectal surgery*, because there is a high risk of infection with *Escherichia coli*, clostridia and bacteroides which inhabit the gut (a cephalosporin plus metronidazole is satisfactory);
2. *gastric surgery*, for colonisation of the stomach with gut organisms (above) occurs especially when acid secretion is low, e.g. in gastric malignancy, following use of a histamine H_2-receptor antagonist or following previous gastric surgery to reduce acid (usually a cephalosporin alone provides adequate chemoprophylaxis);
3. *gynaecological surgery*, because the vagina contains bacteroides, streptococci, coliforms and anaerobes (metronidazole and a cephalosporin are used). Chemoprophylaxis is indicated for hysterectomy, by the vaginal and by the abdominal route, and for perineal floor repair but probably not for other elective procedures;
4. *leg amputation*, because there is a risk of gas gangrene in an ischaemic limb (see p. 193), and the mortality is high (penicillin should be given, or metronidazole for the patient with allergy to penicillin),
5. *insertion of prostheses*; chemoprophylaxis may be justified because infection almost invariably means that the artificial joint, valve or vessel must be replaced.

PROBLEMS WITH ANTIMICROBIAL DRUGS

Resistance to drugs

Microbial resistance to antimicrobials is a matter of great importance; if sensitive strains are supplanted by resistant ones, then a valuable drug may become useless. The availability of effective antimicrobials in the future requires that drug development keep pace with drug resistance. For several years β-lactamase-producing staphylococci were a grave clinical problem and killed many people.

Origins of resistance in clinical practice are:

- *Selection* of primary or naturally resistant strains. In the course of therapy, the naturally sensitive strains are eliminated and those naturally resistant proliferate and occupy the biological space created by the drug.
- *Spontaneous mutation* with selective multiplication of the resistant strain so that it eventually dominates as above.
- *By transmission of genes from other organisms*, the commonest and most important mechanism. Genetic material may be transferred, e.g. in the form of *plasmids* which are strands of DNA that lie outwith the chromosomes and contain genes capable of controlling various metabolic processes including formation of β-lactamases (that destroy penicillins and cephalosporins), and enzymes that inactivate aminoglycosides. Alternatively genetic transfer may occur through a bacteriophage (a virus which infects bacteria), particularly in the case of staphylococci.

Limitation of resistance to antimicrobials may be achieved by:

- avoidance of indiscriminate use by ensuring that the indication for, dose of and duration of treatment are appropriate;
- using antimicrobial combinations in selected circumstances, e.g. tuberculosis;
- constant monitoring of resistance patterns in a hospital or community;
- restricting drug use, which involves agreement between clinicians and microbiologists, e.g. by limiting the use of the newest member of a group of

antimicrobials so long as the currently-used drugs are effective.

Opportunistic infection

When any antimicrobial drug is used, there is usually suppression of part of the normal bacterial flora of the patient, which varies according to the drug. Often, this causes no ill effects, but sometimes a drug-resistant organism, freed from competition, proliferates to an extent which can even be fatal. The principal responsible organisms are *Candida albicans* and pseudomonads. The mere presence of such organisms in diagnostic specimens does not mean they are causing disease.

Antibiotic-associated colitis is an example of an opportunistic infection. Almost any antimicrobial that can alter bowel flora may initiate this condition but the drugs most commonly associated are lincomycin, clindamycin, amoxycillin, ampicillin and cephalosporins. It takes the form of an acute, non-specific colitis (*pseudomembranous colitis*) with diarrhoeal stools containing blood, or mucus, abdominal pain, leucocytosis and dehydration. A history of antibiotic use in the previous 3 weeks, even if the drug therapy has been stopped, should alert the physician to the diagnosis which is confirmed by proctosigmoidoscopy and the isolation of *Clostridium difficile* or its toxin from the stools; it is this toxin that causes the colitis, which responds to vancomycin 125 mg by mouth, 6-hourly for 5 days.

A special problem of opportunistic infection arises in patients whose *immune systems are compromised* by disease or drugs. Bacterial infection causes about two-thirds of deaths in such patients, the remainder being mainly due to fungi. Treatment should be prompt, initiated before the results of bacteriological tests are known and usually involves combinations of bactericidal drugs administered parenterally.

Masking of infections

Masking of infections by chemotherapy is an im-portant possibility. The risk cannot be entirely avoided but it can be minimised by intelligent use of antimicrobials. For example, a course of penicillin adequate to cure gonorrhoea may prevent simultaneously contracted syphilis from showing primary and secondary stages and a serological test for syphilis should be done 3 months after treatment for gonorrhoea.

Treatment failure

Treatment failure may be due to:

- Drug resistance, natural or acquired.
- The organism isolated not being the cause of the disease.
- Treatment begun too late to save patient.
- Suboptimal use of drug (inadequate dose, interval between doses too long, duration of course too short, unsuitable route).
- Barriers to adequate access of drug to organism, which may be natural (e.g. poor entry into eye, cerebrospinal fluid) or pathological (e.g. abscess, fibrosis).
- Reduced host defences due to disease (e.g. AIDS, hypogammaglobulinaemia, leukaemia, diabetes, cystic fibrosis) or immuno-suppression (e.g. anticancer drugs or adrenal steroids).

ANTIMICROBIAL DRUGS OF CHOICE

Table 10.1 is provided for reference. It is a summary of the choice of antimicrobial drugs and owes its form and much of its contents to *Medical Letter on Drugs and Therapeutics* (USA) (1990). We are very grateful to the Chairman of the Editorial Board for permission to use this material.

The Table should be read in conjunction with the text. There is some repetition between text and table, but presenting the data in different ways can be helpful. Note also some differences for there is no single correct procedure for each infection. Tables on drugs for viruses, fungi, protozoa and helminths are provided in Chapter 13.

Table 10.1 Reference data on antimicrobial drugs of choice

Infecting organism	Drug(s) of first choice	Alternative drugs[1]
Gram-positive cocci		
Enterococcus		
endocarditis or other severe infection	benzylpenicillin or amoxycillin with gentamicin	vancomycin with gentamycin
uncomplicated urinary tract infection	amoxycillin	trimethoprim or nitrofurantoin
*Staphylococcus aureus or *epidermidis*		
non-penicillinase-producing	benzylpenicillin or phenoxymethylpenicillin	a cephalosporin or vancomycin or erythromycin or clindamyein
penicillinase-producing	cloxacillin or flucloxacillin	a cephalosporin or vancomycin or erythromycin or clindamycin
methicillin-resistant	vancomycin or teicoplanin	trimethoprim or ciprofloxacin or sodium fusidate or rifampicin
Streptococcus pyogenes (Group A) and Groups C and G } *Streptococcus, Group B* }	benzylpenicillin or phenoxymethylpenicillin or amoxycillin	erythromycin or a cephalosporin or vancomycin
Streptococcus, viridans group (endocarditis)	benzylpenicillin with or without gentamicin	vancomycin or a cephalosporin
Streptococcus, anaerobic	benzylpenicillin	metronidazole
*Streptococcus pneumoniae (pneumococcus)	benzylpenicillin or phenoxymethylpenicillin or amoxycillin	erythromycin or a cephalosporin or vancomycin (or chloramphenicol for meningitis)
Gram-negative cocci		
Moraxella (Branhamella) *catarrhalis*	co-amoxiclav	erythromycin or a tetracycline
*Neisseria gonorrhoeae (gonorrhoea)	amoxycillin (+ probenecid) or ciprofloxacin	spectinomycin
Neisseria meningitidis (meningitis)	benzylpenicillin	chloramphenicol
Gram-positive bacilli		
Bacillus anthracis (anthrax)	benzylpenicillin	erythromycin or a tetracycline
Clostridium perfringens (gas gangrene)	benzylpenicillin	metronidazole or clindamycin
Clostridium tetani (tetanus)	benzylpenicillin	a tetracycline
Clostridium difficile (pseudomembranous colitis)	vancomycin (oral)	metronidazole
Corynebacterium diphtheriae (diphtheria)	erythromycin	benzylpenicillin
Listeria monocytogenes (listeriosis)	amoxycillin with or without gentamicin	erythromycin with gentamicin
Enteric Gram-negative bacilli		
*Bacteroides		
oropharyngeal strains	benzylpenicillin	metronidazole or clindamycin
gastrointestinal strains	metronidazole	co-amoxiclav or clindamycin or imipenem
*Campylobacter jejuni	ciprofloxacin or erythromycin	tetracycline

Table 10.1 (Cont'd)

Infecting organism	Drug(s) of first choice	Alternative drugs[1]
Enterobacteriaceae e.g Enterobacter aerogenes Escherichia coli Klebsiella pneumoniae Proteus spp.		
lower urinary tract	trimethoprim or an oral cephalosporin	ciprofloxacin
septicaemia	gentamicin or cefuroxime or cefotaxime	ciprofloxacin or imipenem
Salmonella typhi (typhoid fever)	ciprofloxacin	co-trimoxazole or choramphenicol
other Salmonella	ciprofloxacin	trimethoprim or mecillinam
Shigella	ciprofloxacin	trimethoprim or ampicillin
Yersinia enterocolitica	co-trimoxaxole	ciprofloxacin
Other Gram-negative bacilli		
Bordetella pertussis (whooping cough)	erythromycin	ampicillin
Brucella (brucellosis)	a tetracycline with streptomycin	co-trimoxazole or rifampicin with a tetracycline
Calymmatobacterium granulomatis (granuloma inguinale)	a tetracycline	amoxycillin or co-trimoxazole
Gardnerella (Haemophilus) *vaginalis* (anaerobic vaginosis)	metronidazole	amoxycillin
Haemophilus ducreyi (chancroid)	erythromycin	co-trimoxaxole or ciprofloxacin
Haemophilus influenzae		
meningitis, epiglottitis, arthritis or other serious infections	cefotaxime or chloramphenicol	amoxycillin
upper respiratory infections and bronchitis	amoxycillin	co-amoxiclav or cefuroxime
Legionella pneumophila (legionnaires' disease)	erythromycin with or without rifampicin	
Pasteurella multocida (from animal bites)	benzylpenicillin	a cephalosporin or erythromycin
Pseudomonas aeruginosa		
urinary tract infection	ciprofloxacin (or another quinolone) or carfecillin	gentamicin
other infections	ciprofloxacin or piperacillin or azlocillin with gentamicin	ceftazidime or imipenem
Vibrio cholerae (cholera)	tetracycline	ciprofloxacin
Acid fast bacilli		
Mycobacterium tuberculosis	isoniazid with rifampicin with pyrazinamide	ethambutol or capreomycin or cycloserine or streptomycin or kanamycin
Mycobacterium leprae (leprosy)	dapsone with rifampicin with or without clofazimine	

Table 10.1 (Cont'd)

Infecting organism	Drug(s) of first choice	Alternative drugs[1]
Actinomycetes		
Actinomyces israelii (actinomycosis)	benzylpenicillin	a tetracycline
Nocardia	a sulphonamide	co-trimoxazole or amikacin or minocycline
Chlamydiae		
Chlamydia psittaci (psittacosis)	tetracycline	chloramphenicol
Chlamydia trachomatis		
trachoma	tetracycline (topical plus oral)	a sulphonamide (topical plus oral)
inclusion conjunctivitis	tetracycline (topical plus oral)	a sulphonamide (topical plus oral)
urethritis	tetracycline or erythromycin	
lymphogranuloma venereum	tetracycline	
Chlamydia pneumoniae (TWAR strain)	tetracycline	
Mycoplasma		
Mycoplasma pneumoniae	erythromycin or tetracycline	
Ureaplasma urealyticum	erythromycin	tetracycline
Rickettsia		
Q fever, typhus	tetracycline	chloramphenicol or co-trimoxazole
Spirochaetes		
Borrelia burgdorferi (Lyme disease)	tetracycline	benzylpenicillin
Borrelia recurrentis (relapsing fever)	tetracycline	benzylpenicillin or erythromycin
Leptospira (leptospirosis)	benzylpenicillin	tetracycline
Treponema pallidum (syphilis)	benzylpenicillin	tetracycline
Treponema pertenue (yaws)	benzylpenicillin	tetracycline

* Resistance may be a problem; sensitivity tests should be performed.
[1] Suggested alternatives do not necessarily comprise all options.

GUIDE TO FURTHER READING

Colebrook L, Kenny M 1939 Treatment with prontosil of puerperal infections. Lancet 2: 1319

Geddes A M 1988 Antibiotic therapy — a resume. Lancet 2: 286

Mackowiak P A 1982 The normal microbiological flora. New England Journal of Medicine 307: 83

Pollock A V 1988 Surgical prophylaxis — the emerging picture. Lancet 1: 225

Styrt B, Gorbach S L 1989 Recent developments in the understanding of the pathogenesis and treatment of anaerobic infections. New England Journal of Medicine 321: 240 (part 1), 298 (part 2)

Wise R 1987 Prescribing in pregnancy: antibiotics. British Medical Journal 294: 42

Wise R 1987 Antimicrobial agents: a widening choice. Lancet 2: 1251

Wolfson J S, Swartz S W 1985 Serum bacterial activity as a monitor of antibiotic therapy. New England Journal of Medicine 312: 968

11

Infection II: antibacterial drugs

SYNOPSIS

The range of antibacterial drugs is wide and affords the clinician scope to select with a knowledge of the likely or proved pathogen(s) and of factors relevant to the patient, e.g. allergy, renal disease.

Antibacterial drugs are here discussed in groups according to their molecular structure, for members of each group have the same mechanism of action, are usually handled by the body in a similar way and have the same range of adverse effects.

Table 10.1 is a general reference for this chapter.

Classification

- **Beta-lactams**, structure of which contains a β-lactam ring. The major subdivisions are the *penicillins* whose official names include or end in 'cillin' and the *cephalosporins* and *cephamycins* which are recognised by the inclusion of 'cef' or 'ceph' in their official names. Lesser categories of β-lactams include the *carbapenems* and *monobactams*.
- **Aminoglycosides**. Those that are derived from streptomyces end in 'mycin', e.g. tobramycin. Others include gentamicin (from *Micromonospora purpurea* which is not a fungus, hence the spelling as 'micin') and semisynthetic drugs, e.g. amikacin.
- **Sulphonamides**. Usually their names contain 'sulpha' or 'sulfa'.
- **Tetracyclines**, as the name suggests, are four-ringed structures and their names end in '-cycline'.
- **Azoles** all contain an azole ring and the names end in '-azole', e.g. metronidazole.
- **Quinolones** are structurally related to nalidixic acid; the names of the most recently introduced members of the group end in '-oxacin', e.g. ciprofloxacin.
- **Macrolides**: erythromycin.
- **Others**. A number of important antibacterial agents do not bear a close structural relationship to any of the above groups and these are described individually.

BETA-LACTAMS

PENICILLINS

Penicillin is produced by growing one of the penicillium moulds in deep tanks. According to the variety of fungus and the composition of the medium either benzylpenicillin (penicillin G) or phenoxymethylpenicillin (penicillin V) results.

In 1957 the penicillin nucleus (6-amino-penicillanic acid) was made by fermentation and it became possible to add various side-chains and so to make semisynthetic penicillins with different properties.

It is important to recognise that not all penicillins have the same antibacterial spectrum and that it is necessary to choose between a number of penicillins just as between antimicrobials of different structural groups, as is shown below.

PENICILLINS

Narrow spectrum
(natural penicillins)

benzylpenicillin
phenoxymethylpenicillin
phenethicillin

Antistaphylococcal penicillins
(β-lactamase resistant)

cloxacillin flucloxacillin
methicillin

Broad spectrum

ampicillin amoxycillin
bacampicillin
pivampicillin
talampicillin mezlocillin

Mecillinams
(active against
Gram-negative
bacteria excluding
P. aeruginosa)

mecillinam
pivmecillinam

Antipseudomonal

Carboxypenicillins

carbenicillin
carfecillin ticarcillin
temociillin

Ureidopenicillins

azlocillin
piperacillin

A general account of the penicillins follows and then of the individual drugs in so far as they differ.

Mode of action is by interference with synthesis of the peptidoglycan layer of the cell wall which normally protects the bacterium from its environment. The cell becomes incapable of withstanding the osmotic gradient between its interior and its environment so that it swells and explodes. Penicillins are thus bactericidal and are only effective against multiplying organisms, as resting organisms are not making new cell wall. The main defence of bacteria against penicillins is to produce enzymes, *β-lactamases*, which open the β-lactam ring and terminate their activity. The remarkable safety of the penicillins is due to the fact that human cell walls have a different structure that is unaffected by penicillin.

Pharmacokinetics. Benzylpenicillin is destroyed by gastric acid and is unsuitable for oral use. Others, e.g. phenoxymethylpenicillin, resist acid and are absorbed in upper small bowel. The plasma $t_\frac{1}{2}$ of penicillins is usually <2 h; they are distributed mainly in the body water and enter well into the CSF if the meninges are inflamed. Penicillins are organic acids and their rapid clearance from plasma is due to secretion into renal tubular fluid by the anion transport mechanism in the kidney. Renal clearance therefore greatly exceeds the glomerular filtration rate (127 ml/min). The excretion rate of penicillin can be usefully delayed by concurrently giving probenecid which competes successfully for the transport mechanism. Dosage of penicillins may need to be reduced for patients with severely impaired renal function.

Adverse effects. The main hazard with the penicillins is *allergic reactions*. These occur in up to 10% of patients and include itching, rashes (eczematous or urticarial), drug fever and angioneurotic oedema. Rarely, there is anaphylactic shock which can be fatal. Allergies are least likely when penicillins are given orally and most likely with local application or with procaine penicillin i.m. Metabolic opening of the β-lactam ring creates a highly reactive penicilloyl group which binds with tissue proteins to form the major antigenic determinant. The anaphylactic reaction involves specific IgE antibodies which can be detected in the plasma of susceptible persons.

There is *cross-allergy* between all the various forms of penicillin probably due in part to their common structure, and in part to the degradation products common to them all. *Partial cross-allergy* exists between penicillins and cephalosporins (10%) which is of particular concern when the reaction to either group of anti-microbials has been angioneurotic oedema or anaphylactic shock.

When attempting to *predict* whether a patient will have an allergic reaction, a reliable history of a previous adverse response to penicillin is valuable. Immediate-type reactions such as urticaria, angio-oedema and anaphylactic shock can probably be taken to indicate allergy, but interpretation of maculopapular rashes is more difficult. Since an alternative drug can usually be found, a penicillin is best avoided if there is suspicion of allergy, although the condition is undoubtedly overdiagnosed and may be transient (see below).

When the history of allergy is not clear-cut and it is necessary to prescribe a penicillin, an *intradermal test* for allergy may be performed using standard amounts of a mixture of a major determinant (benzylpenicilloyl polylysine) and minor determinants, e.g. benzylpenicillin itself, of the allergic reaction; appearance of a flare and weal reaction greater than 3 mm or more in diameter after 10–15 min indicates a positive response. In fact, only about 10% of patients with a history of 'penicillin allergy' respond, which suggests that many who are so labelled are not, or are no longer, allergic to penicillin. Patients in whom there is reliable evidence of susceptibility to penicillin anaphylaxis, and who need penicillin for overwhelming bacterial infection may be desensitised by giving increasing doses of penicillin orally and i.v. over 4 h.[1] The procedure should be undertaken in an intensive care unit.

Other adverse effects include diarrhoea due to alteration in normal intestine flora which may lead to opportunist infection with pseudomonads or *Candida albicans*, although this is uncommon. Neutropenia is a risk if penicillins (or other β-lactam antibiotics) are used in high dose and usually for a period of longer than 10 days. Rarely the penicillins cause anaemia, sometimes haemolytic. Penicillins are presented as their sodium or potassium salts which are inevitably taken in significant amounts if high dose of antimicrobial is used. Physicians should be aware of this unexpected source of sodium or potassium especially in patients with renal or cardiac disease. Extremely high plasma penicillin concentrations cause convulsions.

Narrow spectrum penicillins

Benzylpenicillin (penicillin G)

Benzylpenicillin is used when high plasma concentration is required. The short $t_{\frac{1}{2}}$ (0.5 h) means that reasonably spaced doses have to be large to maintain a therapeutic concentration. Only the extraordinary lack of dose-related toxicity of penicillin allows the resulting fluctuations to be acceptable. Benzylpenicillin is eliminated by the kidney, about 80% being actively secreted by the renal tubule and this can be blocked usefully by probenecid, e.g. to treat bacterial endocarditis, where very large doses may be needed, to reduce frequency of injection for small children or for single dose therapy as in gonorrhoea.

Uses (see Table 10.1). Benzylpenicillin is highly active against *Streptococcus pneumoniae* and the Lancefield group A, β-haemolytic streptococci. Viridans streptococci are usually sensitive unless the patient has recently received penicillin. *Streptococcus faecalis* is less susceptible and especially for endocarditis; penicillin should be combined with an aminoglycoside, usually gentamicin. Benzylpenicillin is the drug of choice for infections due to *Neisseria meningitidis* (meningococcal meningitis), *Bacillus anthracis* (anthrax), *Clostridium perfringens* (gas gangrene) and *Clostridium tetani* (tetanus), *Treponema pallidum* (syphilis), *Leptospira* spp. (leptospirosis) and *Actinomyces israelii* (actinomycosis). The sensitivity of *Neisseria gonorrhoeae* varies in different parts of the world, and in some resistance is rife. *Staphy-*

[1] Sullivan T J et al. J Allergy Clin Immunol 1982; 69: 275, Stark B J et al. J Allergy Clin Immunol 1987; 79: 523.

lococcus aureus is sensitive except for strains that produce β-lactamase, and these are the majority.

Adverse effects are in general uncommon, apart from allergy (above). It is salutary to reflect that the first clinically useful true antibiotic (1942) is also amongst the least toxic.

Preparations and dosage for injection. Benzylpenicillin may be given i.m. or i.v. (by bolus injection or by continuous infusion). For a sensitive infection, benzylpenicillin 300 to 600 mg $\times$ 6 h^2 is enough. This is obviously inconvenient in domiciliary practice and 600 mg $\times$ 12 h can be used, but because renal excretion is rapid, the minimum blood concentration will fall below that of the same total dose given at shorter intervals. Thus, the maximum blood concentration rises hugely with a big dose, but the *duration* of effect increases only little. If infrequent dosage is unavoidable, a mixture of benzylpenicillin and one of its long-acting variants it used (see below).

For relatively insensitive infections and where sensitive organisms are in avascular tissue (infective endocarditis) 7.2–14.4 g are given daily i.v. in divided doses. For such cases it is useful, especially with children (who receive lower doses), to block active renal tubular excretion with probenecid, to get higher blood concentrations for a longer time with smaller volumes of injection. When an infection is subdued, a change may be made to the oral route (phenoxymethyl-penicillin, or amoxycillin which is better absorbed).

Procaine penicillin, given i.m. only, is a stable salt and liberates benzylpenicillin over 12–24 h, according to the dose administered, on average 360 mg $\times$ 12–24 h. There is no general agreement on its place in therapy. It is probably best to use benzylpenicillin in the most severe infections, especially at the outset, as procaine penicillin will not give therapeutic blood concentrations for some hours after injection.

Benethamine penicillin is a poorly soluble salt of benzylpenicillin which provides sustained low plasma concentrations; it is combined with

sodium benzylpenicillin and procaine penicillin (Triplopen) in a single i.m. injection which gives prompt and subsequently prolonged plasma concentrations of benzylpenicillin over 2 days.

Preparations and dosage for oral use. Phenoxymethylpenicillin (penicillin V), is resistant to gastric acid and so reaches the small intestine intact where it is moderately well absorbed. It is less active than benzylpenicillin against *N. gonorrhoeae* and *N. meningitidis*, and so is unsuitable for use in gonorrhoea and meningococcal meningitis. It is a satisfactory substitute for benzylpenicillin against *Strep. pneumoniae*, *Strep. pyogenes* and *Staph. aureus*, especially after the acute infection has been brought under control. The dose is 250–500 mg $\times$ 6 h.

Alternative oral, semisynthetic, acid-resistant penicillins, each with its slightly varying relative potency against particular organisms include benzathine penicillin and phenethicillin.

All oral penicillins are best given on an empty stomach to avoid the absorption delay caused by food.

Antistaphylococcal penicillins

Certain bacteria produce β-lactamases which open the β-lactam ring that is common to all penicillins, and thus terminate the antibacterial activity. Drugs that resist the action of staphylococcal β-lactamase do so by their possession of an acyl side-chain which protects the β-lactam bond by preventing the enzyme getting access to it. The drugs do have activity against other bacteria for which penicillin is indicated, but benzylpenicillin is *substantially* more active against these organisms — up to 20 times more so in the cases of pneumococci, β-haemolytic streptococci and Neisseria. Hence, when infection is mixed, it may be necessary to give benzylpenicillin as well as a β-lactamase-resistant drug. These include:

Cloxacillin (t$_{\frac{1}{2}}$ 0.5 h) resists degradation by gastric acid and is absorbed from the gut, but food interferes with absorption.

Flucloxacillin (t$_{\frac{1}{2}}$ 1 h) is more fully absorbed and so gives higher blood concentration than does cloxacillin.

---

^{2} 600 mg = 1000 000 units, 1 mega-unit.

Methicillin is destroyed by gastric acid and so must be injected i.m. or i.v.: its use is now virtually confined to laboratory tests of bacterial sensitivity.

Broad spectrum penicillins

The activity of these semisynthetic penicillins extends beyond the Gram-positive and Gram-negative cocci which are susceptible to benzylpenicillin, and includes many Gram-negative bacilli. They do not resist β-lactamases and are therefore ineffective against organisms that produce these enzymes.

As a general rule these agents are rather less active than benzylpenicillin against Gram-positive cocci, but more active than the β-lactamase-resistant penicillins (above). They have very useful activity against *Strep. faecalis* and many strains of *Haemophilus influenzae*. *Enterobacteriaceae* are variably sensitive and laboratory testing for sensitivity is important in infections with these organisms. The differences between the members of this group are pharmacological rather than bacteriological.

Ampicillin (t_2^1 1 h) is acid-stable and is moderately well absorbed when swallowed. The oral dose is 0.25–1 g × 6–8 h; or i.m. or i.v. 250–500 mg × 4–6 h. Approximately one-third of a dose appears unchanged in the urine. The drug is concentrated in the bile.

Talampicillin is an ester of ampicillin which itself is microbiologically inactive; it is de-esterified in the gut mucosa or liver to release ampicillin to the systemic circulation, i.e. it is a prodrug. The ester is better absorbed than ampicillin itself, which results in higher blood concentrations for equivalent doses.

Pivampicillin and *bacampicillin* are other prodrugs which release ampicillin in vivo.

Amoxycillin (t_2^1 1 h) is a structural analogue of ampicillin which is better absorbed from the gut (especially after food), and for the same dose achieves approximately double the plasma concentration. Diarrhoea appears to be less frequent with amoxycillin than with ampicillin. The oral dose is 250 mg × 8 h; a parenteral form is available.

Co-amoxiclav (Augmentin). *Clavulanic acid* is a β-lactam compound which has little intrinsic antibacterial activity but which is important because it binds to β-lactamases and thereby competitively protects the penicillin, so potentiating it against bacteria which owe their resistance to production of β-lactamases, i.e. clavulanic acid acts as a 'suicide' inhibitor. It is formulated in tablets as its potassium salt (equivalent to 125 mg of clavulanic acid) in combination with amoxycillin (250 mg), as co-amoxiclav, and is a satisfactory oral treatment for infections due to β-lactamase-producing organisms, notably in the respiratory or urinary tracts. It should be used when β-lactamase-producing amoxycillin resistant organisms are either suspected or proven by culture. The dose is one tablet × 8 h.

Adverse effects. Diarrhoea may be troublesome with ampicillin but the incidence (12%) is less with prodrugs of ampicillin and with amoxycillin. Ampicillin and its analogues have a peculiar capacity to cause a macular rash resembling measles or rubella, and usually unaccompanied by other signs of allergy. These rashes are very common in patients with disease of the lymphoid system, notably infectious mononucleosis (and may sometimes declare this diagnosis when used for sore throat), and in lymphoid leukaemia. A macular rash should not be taken to imply allergy to other penicillins which tend to cause a true urticarial reaction. Patients with renal failure and those taking allopurinol for hyperuricaemia also seem more prone to ampicillin rashes.

Mezlocillin (t_2^1 1 h) is a ureidopenicillin (see below) whose antibacterial activity better allows its classification with the broad spectrum drugs. It is active against some ampicillin-resistant organisms, more active than azlocillin against the common Gram-negative organisms, but less active than the other ureidopenicillins against *Pseudomonas aeruginosa*.

Mecillinams (closely related to the broad spectrum penicillins)

Mecillinam (t_2^1 1 h) is active principally against

Gram-negative bacteria including *Escherichia coli*, salmonellae and shigellae but excluding *P. aeruginosa*. It has reliably low susceptibility to some common β-lactamases and therefore is active against some ampicillin-resistant *Enterobacteriaceae*. Mecillinam is not absorbed from the gastrointestinal tract. It may be used parenterally in severe infection due to Gram-negative bowel.

Pivmecillinam is an inactive ester which is hydrolysed to mecillinam in the intestinal wall and is suitable for oral therapy. Its main use is in urinary tract infection caused by organisms resistant to other oral antimicrobials.

Antipseudomonal penicillins

Carboxypenicillins

These in general have the same antibacterial spectrum as ampicillin (and are susceptible to β-lactamases), but have the additional capacity to destroy *P. aeruginosa* and indole-positive *Proteus spp.*

Carbenicillin ($t_\frac{1}{2}$ 1 h) is given parenterally; ticarcillin (below) or a ureidopenicillin is now preferred for severe infection.

Carfecillin, an inert ester of carbenicillin, is absorbed from the gut and is suitable for infection of the urinary tract because the released carbenicillin is concentrated and eliminated by the kidney; the plasma concentrations attained, however, are too low to treat systemic infections.

Ticarcillin ($t_\frac{1}{2}$ 1 h) is similar to carbenicillin but is 4 times more active against *P. aeruginosa*. It is given by i.m. or slow i.v. injection or by rapid i.v. infusion. Combination with clavulanic acid (Timentin) provides greater activity against β-lactamase-producing organisms.

Temocillin ($t_\frac{1}{2}$ 5 h) is a derivative of ticarillin active solely against Gram-negative organisms; these include the respiratory pathogens *H. influenza* and *Branhamella catarrhalis*, and the *Enterobacteriaceae* but excludes *P. aeruginosa* and *Bacteroides fragilis*. Temocillin has been used to treat urinary infection and septicaemia. Diarrhoea, rash and pain at the site of i.m. injection may occur.

Notes. 1. Both carbenicillin and ticarcillin are presented as disodium salts and each 1 g delivers about 5.4 mmol of sodium; this source of sodium should be borne in mind when treating patients with impaired cardiac or renal function.

2. Carboxypenicillins inactivate aminoglycosides if both drugs are administered in the same syringe or intravenous infusion bottle.

Ureidopenicillins

These are adapted from the ampicillin molecule, with a side-chain derived from urea. Their major advantage is efficacy against *P. aeruginosa*; e.g. *azlocillin* is 8 times more active than carbenicillin against this organism. They are degraded by β-lactamases. Ureidopenicillins must be administered parenterally and are eliminated is the urine. Accumulation in patients with poor renal function however, is less than with other penicillins because 25% is excreted in the bile. An unusual feature about their kinetics is that, as dose is increased, plasma concentration rises disproportionately, i.e they exhibit *saturation (zero-order) kinetics*.

Ureidopenicillins, as monosodium salts, on average deliver about 2 mmol of sodium per gram of antimicrobial. For pseudomonas septicaemia, a ureidopenicillin plus an aminoglycoside provides a synergistic effect *but* the co-administration in the same fluid results in inactivation of the aminoglycoside (as with carboxypenicillins, above).

Azlocillin ($t_\frac{1}{2}$ 1 h), highly effective against *P. aeruginosa* infections, is less so than the other ureidopenicillins against other common Gram-negative organisms.

Piperacillin ($t_\frac{1}{2}$ 1 h) has the same or slightly greater activity as azlocillin against *P. aeruginosa* but is more effective against the common Gram-negative organisms.

Mezlocillin: see p. 163.

CEPHALOSPORINS

Cephalosporins were first obtained from a fungus *Cephalosporium* cultured from the sea near a Sardinian sewage outfall in 1945; their molecular structure is closely related to that of penicillin, and many semisynthetic forms have been introduced. They now comprise a group of antibiotics having a wide range of activity and low toxicity. The term cephalosporins will be used here in a general sense although some are strictly cephamycins (cefoxitin) or oxacephems (latamoxef).

Mode of action is similar to the penicillins, i.e. the cephalosporins impair bacterial cell wall synthesis and hence are bactericidal.

Addition of various side-chains on the cephalosporin molecule confers variety in pharmacokinetic and antibacterial activities. The β-lactam ring can be protected by such structural manoeuvering, which results in compounds with improved activity against Gram-negative organisms. Cephalosporins resist attack by β-lactamases but bacteria develop resistance to them by other means.

Pharmacokinetics. Usually, cephalosporins are excreted unchanged in the urine, but some, including cefotaxime, form a desacetyl metabolite. Many are actively secreted by the renal tubule, a process which can be blocked usefully with probenecid; ceftazidime and latamoxef are eliminated solely by glomerular filtration and so are not affected by probenecid. In general, the dose of cephalosporins should be reduced in patients with poor renal function. Cephalosporins in general have a $t_\frac{1}{2}$ of 1–4 h (see Table 11.1). Wide distribution in the body allows treatment of infection at most sites, including bone, soft tissue and muscle.

Data on cephalosporins, including their antibacterial activity, appear in Table 11.1.

Uses of cephalosporins. *Oral cephalosporins* are used to treat urinary tract infections, especially those due to enterobacteria resistant to other agents. Exacerbations of chronic bronchitis also respond when these are caused by *Strep. pneumoniae*.

Parenteral cephalosporins, especially those of the third generation, are effective against many Gram-negative organisms and may be used as follows:

- A cephalosporin combined with metronidazole is a reasonable best guess initial treatment for severe abdominal

---

Classification of cephalosporins

By convention the injectable cephalosporins have been categorised into *generations* having broadly similar antibacterial and pharmacokinetic properties; newer agents have rendered this classification less precise but it retains sufficient usefulness to be presented below.

First generation injectables have useful antistaphylococcal activity and comprise *cephazolin* and *cephradine*, together with *cephalothin* (which is now little used).

Orally-active cephalosporins can be considered microbiologically equivalent to the first generation injectables and comprise *cephalexin, cephradine, cefaclor* and *cefadroxil*.

Second generation injectables have antistaphylococcal activity but also cover certain Gram-negative organisms, e.g. *H. influenzae* and *Enterobacteriaceae*. They comprise *cefuroxime, cephamandole* and *cefoxitin*.

Third generation injectables are mainly effective against Gram-negative organisms and less against staphylococci. They comprise *cefotaxime, cefsulodin, ceftazidime, ceftizoxime* and *latamoxef*.

---

infection, when the likely organisms are enterobacteria, staphylococci and *Bacteroides fragilis*.

- Many biliary infections are due to enterobacteria and parenteral cephalosporins are useful both for prophylaxis in surgery and for treatment of established biliary sepsis.
- Patients with urinary tract infection due to multiply-resistant bacteria may develop bacteraemia after urinary tract instrumentation; prior administration of a parenteral cephalosporin reduces the bacterial load in the urine and avoids this complication.
- Gonorrhoea due to penicillin-resistant gonococci may be treated with a single intramuscular dose of a cephalosporin, e.g. cefotaxime.

Adverse effects. Cephalosporins have a low incidence of adverse effects. The most usual are *allergic* reactions of the penicillin type. *There is cross-allergy between penicillins and cephalosporins* involving about 10% of patients; if a patient has

Table 11.1 The cephalosporins

Drug	$t_{\frac{1}{2}}$ (h)	Excretion in urine (%)	Dose (g/d)	Staph. aureus	H. influenzae	Activity against Entero-bacter-iaceae*	P. aeruginosa	B. fragilis
Oral drugs								
Cefaclor	1	86	0.75–4.0	++	+	++	0	0
Cefadroxil	2	88	1.0–2.0	++	+	++	0	0
Cephalexin	1	88	1.0–6.0	++	0/+	++	0	0
Cefixime	4	20	0.2–0.4	+	++	++	0	0
Parenteral drugs *First generation*								
Cephalothin	1	50	6.0–12.0	+++	+++	++	0	+
Cephazolin	2	90	1.0–4.0	+++	++	++	0	+
Cephradine (also oral)	1	86	2.0–8.0 (1.0–2.0)	++	0/+	++	0	0
Second generation								
Cefoxitin	1	90	3.0–12.0	++	++	+++	0	+++
Cefuroxime (also oral)	1	80	2.25–6.0 (0.5–1.0)	+++	+++	+++	0	0
Cephamandole	1	75	1.5–12.0	+++	+++	+++	0	0
Third generation								
Cefotaxime	1	50	3.0–12.0	++	+++	+++	+/++	0/+
Cefsoludin sodium	2	90	1.0–4.0	++	++	0	+++	0/+
Ceftazidime	2	88	3.0–6.0	++	+++	+++	+++	0/+
Ceftizoxime	1	90	2.0–8.0	++	+++	+++	+/++	0/+
Latamoxef disodium	3	88	2.0–12.0	++	+++	+++	+/++	+

Note: The data in this table are drawn from various sources but substantially from Wise R Lancet 1982; 2: 140 with permission which is gratefully acknowledged (DRL, PNB).
+++ = 10% of the peak serum concentration attained with this drug exceeds the mean MIC (minimum inhibitory concentration)
++ = 50% of the peak serum concentration exceeds the mean MIC
+ = 100% of the peak serum concentration exceeds the mean MIC
0 = no useful activity
* This family contains the common Gram-negative, fermentative, intestinal flora except *P. aeruginosa*; certain strains may be considered more resistant.

had a severe or immediate allergic reaction or if skin testing for penicillin allergy is positive (see p. 161), then a cephalosporin should not be used. If cephalosporins are continued for more than 2 weeks, thrombocytopenia, neutropenia, interstitial nephritis or abnormal liver function tests may occur; these reverse on stopping the drug. Some cephalosporins, especially latamoxef, interfere with blood coagulation factors and cause haemorrhage. Latamoxef and other cephalosporins may cause a disulfiram type of response after ingestion of alcohol.

OTHER BETA-LACTAM ANTIBIOTICS
Carbapenem

Imipenem ($t_{\frac{1}{2}}$ 1 h) is a derivative of an antibiotic derived from the fungus *Streptomyces cattleya*; it has the widest spectrum of all currently available antibiotics, being bactericidal against most Gram-positive and Gram-negative aerobic and anaerobic pathogenic bacteria. It is inactivated by metabolism in the kidney and is potentially toxic to renal tubules; combining imipenem with *cilastatin* (as Primaxin), a specific inhibitor of dihydropeptidase, prevents both renal inactivation and toxicity. In terms of imipenem, 1–2 g/d is given by i.v. infusion in 3–4 doses; reduced doses are recommended when renal function is impaired. It may cause gastrointestinal upset, blood disorders, allergic reactions, confusion and convulsions.

Monobactam

Aztreonam is active against Gram-negative bacteria including *P. aeruginosa, H. influenzae* and *N. meningitidis* and *gonorrhoea*. Its different molecular structure may be an advantage in penicillin-allergic patients. Adverse effects include gastrointestinal upset, hepatitis, thrombocytopenia and neutropenia.

AMINOGLYCOSIDES

In the purposeful search that followed the demonstration of the clinical efficacy of penicillin, streptomycin was obtained from *Streptomyces griseus* in 1944, cultured from a heavily manured field, and also from a chicken's throat. Aminoglycosides resemble each other in their mode of action, therapeutic and toxic, and their pharmacokinetic properties; the main differences in usage reflect variation in their range of antibacterial activity; cross-resistance is variable.

Mode of action. The aminoglycosides are bactericidal. They act inside the cell by binding to the ribosomes in such a way that incorrect amino acid sequences are entered into peptide chains. The abnormal proteins which result are fatal to the microbe.

Pharmacokinetics. Aminoglycosides are water-soluble and do not readily cross cell membranes. Poor absorption from the intestine necessitates their administration i.v. or i.m. and they distribute mainly to the extracellular fluid; transfer into the cerebrospinal fluid is poor even when the meninges are inflamed.

Their $t_{\frac{1}{2}}$ is 2–5 h and they are eliminated unchanged mainly by glomerular filtration and attain high concentrations in the urine. Significant accumulation occurs in the renal cortex unless there is severe renal parenchymal disease.

Dose reduction is necessary to compensate for varying degrees of renal impairment, including that of normal ageing, and schemes have been developed to assist in prescribing for these patients.[3] Plasma concentration should be measured regularly and frequently in such patients, and indeed it is good practice to monitor it, even if renal function is normal.

Antibacterial activity. Aminoglycosides are in general active against aerobic Gram-negative organisms; individual differences in activity are given below. *Bacterial resistance* to aminoglycosides is an increasing problem, notably by acquisition of *plasmids* (see p. 154) which mediate the formation of drug destroying enzymes.

Uses include:

- *Gram-negative bacillary infection*, particularly septicaemia, pelvic and abdominal sepsis. Gentamicin remains the drug of choice but tobramycin should be preferred for infections caused by *P. aeruginosa*. Amikacin has the widest antibacterial spectrum of the aminoglycosides but is best reserved for infection caused by gentamicin-resistant organisms. An aminoglycoside may be included in the initial best guess regimen for treatment of serious septicaemia before the causative organism(s) is identified.

- *Bacterial endocarditis*. An aminoglycoside, usually gentamicin, should comprise part of the antimicrobial combination for enterococcal, streptococcal or staphylococcal infection of the heart valves, and for the therapy of clinical endocarditis which fails to yield a positive blood culture.

- *Other infections*: tuberculosis, tularaemia, plague, brucellosis.

- *Topical uses*. Neomycin and framycetin, whilst too toxic for systemic use, are effective for topical treatment of infections of the conjunctiva or external ear. They are used in antimicrobial combinations to sterilise the bowel of patients who are to receive intense immunosuppressive therapy.

---

[3] Mawer G E et al Br J Clin Pharmacol 1974;1:45, Dettli L. Clin Pharmacokinet 1976;1: 126.

Adverse reactions. Aminoglycosides may cause toxicity of the following types:

- *8th nerve toxicity. Auditory* impairment appears to be more common with amikacin, neomycin and kanamycin and *vestibular* toxicity with streptomycin, gentamicin and tobramycin but these differences between drugs are not always clearcut. The drugs are toxic to sensory hair cells in the cochlea and the vestibular organ. Tinnitus may give warning of auditory nerve damage. Early signs of vestibular toxicity include motion-related headache, dizziness or nausea and are indications to stop or to readjust the dosing schedule, for ototoxicity is irreversible. Serious ototoxicity can occur with topical application, including ear drops.

- *Nephrotoxicity.* Dose-related changes, which are usually reversible, occur in renal tubular cells, where aminoglycosides accumulate. Low blood pressure, loop diuretics, and advanced age are recognised as added risk factors. Neomycin, gentamicin and amikacin are more nephrotoxic than tobramycin and netilmicin.

- *Neurotoxicity.* Large amounts of streptomycin instilled into the pleural or peritoneal cavities may cause respiratory paralysis due to competitive neuromuscular block (curare-like), particularly in patients who have received muscle relaxants or who have myasthenia gravis.

- Other reactions include rashes, drug fever with eosinophilia and haematological abnormalities, including marrow depression, haemolytic anaemia and bleeding due to antagonism of factor V.

Individual aminoglycosides

Gentamicin is active against aerobic Gram-negative bacilli including *Esch. coli, Enterobacter, Klebsiella pneumoniae, Proteus* (indole positive) and *P. aeruginosa*. In the best guess treatment of septicaemia, gentamicin should be combined with a β-lactam antibiotic or an anti-anaerobic agent, e.g. metronidazole, or with both. Gentamicin is a drug of choice for serious Gram-negative septicaemia and it is effective for abdominal and pelvic sepsis, when combined with an agent effective against *B. fragilis*, e.g. metronidazole. In streptococcal and enterococcal endocarditis gentamicin is combined with benzylpenicillin, in staphylococcal endocarditis with an antistaphylococcal penicillin, and in enterococcal endocarditis with ampicillin.

Dose is 2–5 mg/kg body weight per day (the highest dose for more serious infections) in 3 equally divided doses and should achieve a peak serum concentration of 5 mg/l 1 h after i.m. or i.v. injection (>10 mg/l is dangerous), and a trough concentration of less than 2 mg/l just before the next injection on an 8-hourly regimen. Therapy should rarely exceed 7 days. Gentamicin applied to the eye gives effective corneal and aqueous humour concentrations.

Tobramycin is similar to gentamicin; in particular, it is more active against most strains of *P. aeruginosa*.

Amikacin is mainly of value against gentamicin-resistant organisms. It is 3 times less potent than gentamicin but can be given safely in higher doses. Peak plasma concentrations should be kept between 20–30 mg/l and trough concentrations below 10 mg/l.

Netilmicin is a semisynthetic aminoglycoside which is active against some strains of bacteria that resist gentamicin and tobramycin; evidence suggests that it may be less ototoxic and nephrotoxic.

Neomycin is principally used topically for skin, eye and ear infections and, by some, to reduce the bacterial load in the colon in preparation for bowel surgery, or in hepatic failure. Enough absorption can occur from both oral and topical use to cause eighth cranial nerve damage, especially if there is renal impairment.

Framycetin is similar to neomycin in use and in toxicity.

Streptomycin has been superseded by rifampicin, isoniazid and ethambutol in the first-choice treatment of tuberculosis.

Kanamycin can be used as a reserve drug in tuberculosis.

SULPHONAMIDES AND SULPHONAMIDE COMBINATIONS

Sulphonamides, amongst the first successful chemotherapeutic agents, now have their place in medicine mainly as combinations with trimethoprim. Their mode of action illustrates well the important pharmacological principle of *competi-* *tive inhibition* (see Fig. 11.1). Sulphonamides are bacteriostatic. Humans do not synthesise folic acid inside the body but use preformed folate from leafy vegetables; their cells are thus unharmed by the metabolic effect of sulphonamides.

A sulphonamide forms an effective *combination* with trimethoprim because trimethoprim interferes with the next metabolic step, the conversion

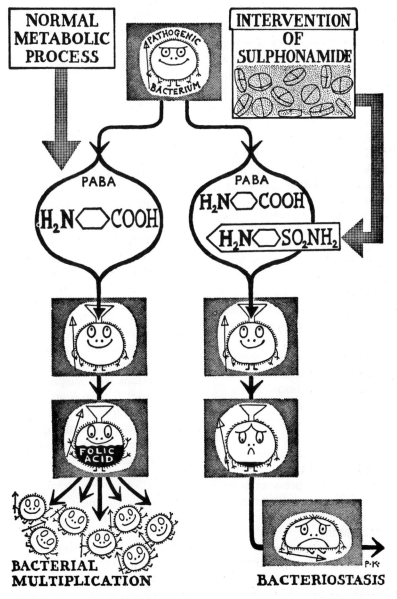

Fig. 11.1 The mode of action of sulphonamides, illustrating the principle of competition

of folic acid to folinic (tetrahydrofolic) acid. The inhibition of successive steps in the synthesis of DNA and RNA potentiates the effect of both drugs. Although humans also convert folic to folinic acid, the sensitivity of the enzyme that is inhibited (dihydrofolate reductase) is much greater in bacteria, so that trimethoprim is relatively safe.

Pharmacokinetics. Sulphonamides for systemic use are absorbed rapidly from the gut. Sulphadiazine enters CSF more readily than others. The principal metabolic path is acetylation and the capacity to acetylate is genetically determined in a bimodal form, i.e. there are slow and fast acetylators (see Pharmacogenetics) but the differences are of limited practical importance in therapy. Both the parent drug and its microbiologically inactive acetylated form enter the glomerular filtrate and the urine is the principal mode of excretion.

Sulphonamides may be classified according to pharmacokinetic properties as follows:

- *Well absorbed by mouth with intermediate* $t_{\frac{1}{2}}$, e.g. sulphadiazine ($t_{\frac{1}{2}}$ 10 h) and sulphadimidine (sulphamethazine) ($t_{\frac{1}{2}}$ approx. 6 h, dose dependent); they are given 4–8 hourly.
- *Well absorbed by mouth with long* $t_{\frac{1}{2}}$, e.g. sulfametopyrazine ($t_{\frac{1}{2}}$ 40 h); it is given once weekly. The incidence of adverse reactions is relatively high, especially of the serious Stevens–Johnson syndrome (a severe form of erythema multiforme); it is rarely used.
- *Poorly absorbed*: calcium sulphaloxate has been used for preoperative bowel preparation and for gut infections, but is now rarely used.
- *Topical application*: silver sulphadiazine is used for prophylaxis and treatment of infected burns, leg ulcers and pressure sores because of its wide antibacterial spectrum (which includes pseudomonads).
- *Miscellaneous*: sulphasalazine (salicylazosulphapyridine) is used in inflammatory bowel disease (see p. 538); in effect the sulphapyridine component acts as a carrier to release the active 5-aminosalicylic acid in the colon.

- *Sulphonamide-trimethoprim combination*. Co-trimoxazole (sulphamethoxazole plus trimethoprim); the optimum synergistic effect against most susceptible bacteria is achieved with trimethoprim 80 mg plus sulphamethoxazole 400 mg. Each drug is well absorbed from the gut, has a $t_{\frac{1}{2}}$ of 10 h and is 80% excreted by the kidney; consequently, the dose of co-trimoxazole should be reduced when renal function is impaired.

Uses. Co-trimoxazole very largely replaced the use of a sulphonamide alone. In turn, trimethoprim on its own has been found to be as effective in many conditions for which the combination was used, and causes fewer adverse reactions. The following is an assessment of the current position:

- Co-trimoxazole is the treatment of choice for pneumonia due to *Pneumocystis carinii*, a life-threatening infection in immunosuppressed patients. Co-trimoxazole is also indicated for infections with *Nocardia asteroides*.
- Co-trimoxazole may be used to treat typhoid and paratyphoid infections (but ciprofloxacin is preferred); and bacillary dysentery due to strains of Shigella resistant to amoxycillin.
- Co-trimoxazole has largely been replaced by trimethoprim alone for (a) urinary tract infections with susceptible organisms which include: *Esch. coli* and proteus species but not pseudomonads and (b) respiratory tract infections, especially due to the common pathogens *Strep. pneumoniae* and *H. influenzae*.

Dose of co-trimoxazole is 2 tabs by mouth twice daily for most infections.

Adverse effects of sulphonamides include malaise, diarrhoea, mental depression and rarely cyanosis, which latter is due to methaemoglobinaemia. These may all be transient and are not necessarily indications for stopping the drug. Crystalluria may occur particularly with rapidly excreted sulphonamides. *Allergic reactions* include: rash, fever, hepatitis, agranulocytosis, purpura, aplastic anaemia, peripheral neuritis, a serum-sickness-like syndrome and polyarteritis nodosa. Rarely, severe skin reactions including erythema multiforme bullosa (Stevens–Johnson syndrome) and toxic epidermal necrolysis (Lyell's syndrome) occur. Haemolysis may occur in glucose-6-phosphate dehydrogenase-deficient subjects. Co-trimoxazole in high dose may cause macrocytic anaemia due to interference with conversion of folic to folinic acid. Co-trimoxazole should not be used in pregnancy because of the possible teratogenic effects of inducing folate deficiency.

Trimethoprim

Subsequent to its extensive use in combination with sulphonamides, trimethoprim has emerged as a broad spectrum antimicrobial of considerable efficacy on its own. It is active against many Gram-positive and Gram-negative aerobic organisms excepting *P. aeruginosa*; the emergence of resistant organisms is becoming a problem. Trimethoprim is effective as sole therapy in treating urinary and respiratory tract infections due to susceptible organisms and for prophylaxis of urinary tract infections. The dose is 200 mg twice daily by mouth for acute urinary tract or respiratory tract infections. Adverse effects are fewer than with co-trimoxazole and include: skin rash, anorexia, nausea, vomiting, abdominal pain and diarrhoea.

TETRACYCLINES

Tetracyclines have a broad range of antimicrobial activity and differences between individual members are small.

Mode of action. Tetracyclines interfere with protein synthesis by binding to bacterial ribosomes. They are bacteriostatic.

Pharmacokinetics. Most tetracyclines are only partially absorbed from the alimentary tract, enough remaining in the intestine to alter the flora and give rise to troublesome and sometimes dangerous complications such as pseudomembranous colitis. Dairy products reduce absorption to a degree but antacids and iron preparations do so much more, by chelation to calcium, aluminium and iron. Tetracyclines are distributed throughout the body; they cross the placenta. Tetracyclines are excreted mainly unchanged in the urine and should be avoided when renal function is severely impaired. Exceptionally among the tetracyclines, doxycycline and minocycline are eliminated by non-renal routes and may be used in patients with impaired renal function because of this property.

Uses. Tetracyclines are active against nearly all Gram-positive and Gram-negative pathogenic bacteria. As drugs of *first* choice, however, they are used for infection with Chlamydiae (e.g. psittacosis, trachoma, pelvic inflammatory disease, lymphogranuloma venereum), Mycoplasma (pneumonia), Rickettsia (e.g. Q fever, typhus), *Vibrio cholerae* (cholera) and Borrelia (Lyme disease, relapsing fever). (For use in acne, see p. 645.)

An unexpected use for a tetracycline occurs in the treatment of chronic hyponatraemia due to the syndrome of inappropriate antidiuretic hormone secretion (SIADH) for which demeclocycline is effective when water restriction has failed. Demeclocycline produces a state of unresponsiveness to ADH probably by inhibiting the formation and action of cyclic-AMP in the renal tubule. It is convenient to use in SIADH because this action is both dose-dependent and reversible.

Adverse reactions. Heartburn, nausea and vomiting due to gastric irritation, are common. Attempts to reduce this with milk or antacids impair absorption of tetracyclines. Loose bowel movements occur, due to alteration of the bowel flora, and this sometimes develops into diarrhoea and *opportunistic infection* may supervene. Disorders of epithelial surfaces, perhaps due partly to vitamin B complex deficiency and partly due to mild opportunistic infection with yeasts and moulds, lead to sore mouth and throat, black hairy tongue, dysphagia and perianal soreness. Vitamin B preparations may prevent or arrest alimentary tract symptoms.

Tetracyclines are selectively taken up in the teeth and growing bones of the fetus and of children, due to their chelating properties with calcium phosphate. This causes dental enamel hypoplasia with pitting, cusp malformation, yellow or brown pigmentation and increased susceptibility to caries. After the fourteenth week of pregnancy and in the first few months of life, even short courses can be damaging. Prevention of discolouration of the permanent front teeth requires that tetracyclines be avoided from the last 2 months of pregnancy to 4 years, and of other teeth until 8 years of age (or 12 years if the third molars are valued). Prolonged tetracycline therapy can also stain the fingernails at all ages.

The effects on the bones after they are formed in the fetus are of less clinical importance because pigmentation has no cosmetic disadvantage and a short spell of delayed growth may not matter. Whether serious anatomical deformity can result from administration in early pregnancy is not known. No serious growth disorders have yet been reported amongst children with chronic respiratory disease taking tetracycline continuously.

Tetracyclines act by inhibiting bacterial protein synthesis but the same effect occurring in man causes blood urea to rise (the *antianabolic* effect). The increased nitrogen load can be clinically important in renal failure, in surgical or injured patients, in those with poor general nutrition and in the elderly.

Tetracyclines also induce photosensitisation and other rashes. Liver and pancreatic damage can occur, especially in pregnancy and with renal disease, when the drugs have been given i.v. Rarely tetracyclines cause benign intracranial hypertension.

Individual tetracyclines

Tetracycline ($t_\frac{1}{2}$ 6 h) may be taken as representative of most tetracyclines. Because of incomplete absorption from the gut the i.m. and i.v. doses need be less than half of the oral dose to be similarly effective. Tetracycline is eliminated by the kidney and in the bile. The dose is 250–500 mg 6-hourly by mouth, 100 mg 6–8 hourly i.m. or 500 mg twice daily by i.v. infusion (maximum 2 g/d).

Doxycycline ($t_\frac{1}{2}$ 16 h) is well absorbed from the gut, even after food. It is excreted in the bile, in the faeces which it re-enters by diffusing across the small intestinal wall and, to some extent, in the urine. These non-renal mechanisms compensate effectively when renal function is impaired and no reduction of dose is necessary: 200 mg is given on the first day, then 100 mg/d.

Minocycline ($t_\frac{1}{2}$ 15 h) is also well absorbed from the gut, even after a meal. It is partly metabolised in the liver and partly excreted in the bile and urine. Dose reduction is not necessary when renal function is impaired; 200 mg initially is followed by 100 mg twice daily. Minocycline but not other tetracyclines may cause a reversible vestibular disturbance with dizziness, tinnitus and impaired balance, especially in females.

Other tetracyclines include chlortetracycline, clomocycline, demeclocycline (see above) and oxytetracycline.

AZOLES

This group includes:

- Metronidazole and tinidazole (antibacterial and antiprotozoal) which are described here.
- Fluconazole, itraconazole, clotrimazole, econazole, ketoconazole, isoconazole and miconazole which are described under Antifungal drugs.
- Nimorazole which is used for trichomoniasis.
- Mebendazole and thiabendazole which are described under Anthelminthic drugs.

Metronidazole

In anaerobic microorganisms (but not in aerobic microorganisms which it also enters) metronidazole is converted into an active form by reduction of its nitro group: this binds to DNA and prevents nucleic acid formation; it is bacteristatic.

Pharmacokinetics. Metronidazole is well absorbed after either oral or rectal administration and distributes to achieve sufficient concentration to eradicate infection in liver, gut wall and pelvic tissues. It is eliminated in the urine, partly unchanged and partly as metabolites. The $t_{\frac{1}{2}}$ is 8 h.

Uses. Metronidazole is active against a wide range of anaerobic bacteria and also protozoa. Its clinical indications are:

- Treatment of sepsis to which anaerobic organisms, e.g. *Bacteroides* spp., anaerobic cocci, are contributing, notably postsurgical infection, intra-abdominal infection, and septicaemia but also wound and pelvic infection, osteomyelitis and abscesses of brain or lung.
- Prevention of postoperative infection in which anaerobic bacteria may be expected to play a part, especially after bowel surgery.
- Pseudomembraneous colitis.
- Trichomoniasis of the urogenital tract in both sexes.
- Amoebiasis (*Entamoeba histolytica*), whether symptomless carriers of cysts or intestinal and extra-intestinal infection.
- Giardiasis (*Giardia lamblia*).
- Acute ulcerative gingivitis and dental infections (*Fusobacterium spp.*).
- Anaerobic vaginosis (*Gardnerella vaginalis*).

Dose. Established anaerobic infection is treated with metronidazole by mouth 400 mg × 8 h; by rectum 1 g × 8 h for 3 days followed by 1 g × 12 h; or by i.v. injection 0.5 g × 8 h; treatment should continue for up to 7 days. Prophylaxis of anaerobic infection after surgery requires the same doses for 2 days, starting just before the operation.

Adverse effects include nausea, vomiting, diarrhoea, furred tongue and an unpleasant metallic taste in the mouth; also headache, dizziness and ataxia. Rashes, urticaria and angioedema occur. Peripheral neuropathy occurs if treatment is prolonged and epileptiform seizures if the dose is high. Large doses of metronidazole are carcinogenic in rodents and the drug is mutagenic in bacteria; however, long-term studies have failed to discover oncogenic effects in humans.

A disulfiram-like effect occurs with alcohol because metronidazole inhibits alcohol and aldehyde dehydrogenase; patients should be warned appropriately.

Tinidazole is similar to metronidazole but has a longer $t_{\frac{1}{2}}$ (13 h). It is excreted mainly unchanged in the urine. The indications for use and adverse effects are essentially those of metronidazole. The longer duration of action of tinidazole may be an advantage; e.g. in giardiasis, trichomoniasis and acute ulcerative gingivitis, tinidazole 2 g by mouth in a single dose is as effective as a course of metronidazole.

QUINOLONES

The first widely used quinolone was nalidixic acid which, though effective for urinary tract infections, has little systemic activity. It was subsequently found that fluorination of the quinolone structure produced compounds that were up to 60 times more active than nalidixic acid and killed a wider range of organisms. Their mode of action is complex but includes inhibiting DNA gyrase, the enzyme that maintains the helical twists in DNA; they are bactericidal. In general quinolones are particularly active against Gram-negative organisms, are usefully active against Gram-positive organisms but are not effective against anaerobes.

Pharmacokinetics. Quinolones are well absorbed from the gut, are widely distributed in body tissues and are eliminated by renal excretion, hepatic metabolism and biliary secretion.

Uses vary between individual members (see below).

Adverse effects include gastrointestinal upset, CNS effects (dizziness, headache, confusion, convulsions) and allergic reactions (rash, pruritus, arthralgia and photosensitivity). Some quinolones are potent enzyme inhibitors and impair the metabolic inactivation of other drugs, increasing their effect (see below). Quinolones cause arthropathy in immature animals and should be avoided in children and growing adolescents.

Individual members of the group include:

Ciprofloxacin ($t_{\frac{1}{2}}$ 3 h) is effective against a range of bacteria but particularly the Gram-negative including salmonella, shigella, campylobacter, neisseria and pseudomonads; it has less activity against Gram-positive bacteria such as *Strep. pneumoniae* and *Strep. faecalis*. Chlamydia are sensitive but most anaerobes are not. Ciprofloxacin is indicated for infections of the urinary, gastrointestinal and respiratory tracts, tissue infections, gonorrhoea and septicaemia caused by sensitive organisms. The dose is 250–750 mg × 2/d by mouth, 200 mg × 2/d i.v. but should be halved when the glomerular filtration rate is <20 ml/min. To discourage the emergence of resistant strains, it is a good policy to reserve ciprofloxacin for infections caused by organisms that are resistant to other drugs. Ciprofloxacin impairs the metabolism of *theophylline* and of warfarin, both of which should be monitored carefully when there is co-administration.

Acrosoxacin ($t_\frac{1}{2}$ 7 h) is effective as a single 300 mg oral dose for gonorrhoea; it is usually reserved for patients who are allergic to penicillin or for organisms that are resistant to that drug.

Cinoxacin ($t_\frac{1}{2}$ 2 h) is used for urinary tract infections, but not when renal function is impaired.

Enoxacin ($t_\frac{1}{2}$ 5 h) may be used for urinary tract and (systemically) for cutaneous infections, and gonorrhoea. It enhances the effect of theophylline and warfarin by inhibiting their metabolism.

Ofloxacin ($t_\frac{1}{2}$ 4 h) is indicated for urinary and respiratory tract infections and gonorrhoea.

Nalidixic acid ($t_\frac{1}{2}$ 6 h) is now used principally for the prevention of urinary tract infection. It may cause haemolysis in glucose-6-phosphate dehydrogenase deficient subjects.

MACROLIDES

Erythromycin

Erythromycin acts by binding to ribosomes and interfering with protein synthesis; it is bacteriostatic.

Absorption after oral administration is best with erythromycin estolate, even if there is food in the stomach. Hydrolysis of the estolate in the body releases the active erythromycin which diffuses readily into most tissues; the $t_\frac{1}{2}$ is approx. 2 h (dose dependent) and elimination is almost exclusively via the bile and faeces.

Uses

- Erythromycin is the drug of choice for *Mycoplasma pneumoniae* in children, although

in adults a tetracycline may be preferred.
- First choice treatment for infection with *Legionella* spp. (Legionnaires' disease) is erythromycin with or without rifampicin.
- Erythromycin is a first choice treatment for diphtheria (including carriers), pertussis and for some chlamydial infections.
- In gastroenteritis caused by *Campylobacter jejuni*, erythromycin is effective in eliminating the organism from the faeces, although it does not necessarily reduce the duration of the symptoms.
- Erythromycin is an effective alternative choice for penicillin-allergic patients infected with *Staph. pyogenes*, *Strep. pneumoniae* or *Treponema pallidum*.
- Acne, see p. 645.

Dose is 250 mg × 6 h or twice this in serious infection. The ethylsuccinate and stearate esters of erythromycin produce lower plasma concentrations of the active drug than does the same dose of the estolate.

Adverse reactions. Erythromycin is remarkably non-toxic, but the estolate can cause cholestatic hepatitis with abdominal pain and fever which may be confused with viral hepatitis, acute cholecystitis or acute pancreatitis. This is probably an allergy, and recovery is usual but the estolate should not be given to a patient with liver disease. Other allergies are rare. Gastrointestinal disturbances, particularly diarrhoea, occur but, the antibacterial spectrum being narrower than with tetracycline, opportunistic infection is less troublesome.

Erythromycin is an enzyme inhibitor and interferes with the metabolic inactivation of some drugs, e.g. warfarin, carbamazepine and theophylline, increasing their effects.

Azithromycin has been introduced for adult streptococcal pharyngitis and chlamydial infections of the cervix and urethra.

OTHER ANTIMICROBIALS

Chloramphenicol

Chloramphenicol was obtained in 1947 from a streptomyces found in a soil sample from a mulched field in Venezuela, and from a compost heap in Illinois. It was soon made synthetically. Chloramphenicol interferes with bacterial protein synthesis by ribosomes. It is primarily bacteriostatic but also may be bactericidal against *H. influenzae*, *N. meningitidis* and *Bacteroides* spp.

Pharmacokinetics. Chloramphenicol tastes bitter; it is available as the base for oral use in capsules and as two esters: the palmitate which is tasteless and is used as a suspension and the succinate which is soluble and is given i.m. or i.v. Absorption of the base from the alimentary tract is efficient but the palmitate ester must be hydrolysed by pancreatic lipase in the small intestine before the active chloramphenicol is released and absorbed. Chloramphenicol succinate is hydrolysed to the active chloramphenicol and there is much individual variation in the capacity to perform this reaction. Chloramphenicol is inactivated by conjugation with glucuronic acid in the liver: In the *neonate*, the processes of hydroxylation and glucuronidation are slow, and plasma concentrations are extremely variable (see below). Monitoring of plasma concentration is therefore essential in the neonate and infant, and in the adult with serious infection. Chloramphenicol penetrates well into all tissues including the CSF and brain. The $t_{\frac{1}{2}}$ is 4 h in adults.

Uses. The decision to use chloramphenicol is influenced by its rare but serious toxic effects (see below):

- There is a case for initiating treatment of bacterial *meningitis* with chloramphenicol plus benzylpenicillin, until the causal organism is identified. When the organism is *H. influenzae*, type B, chloramphenicol should be continued and the benzylpenicillin stopped. Similarly, in the initial treatment of *brain abscess*, chloramphenicol is given with penicillin.
- Chloramphenicol may be used for salmonella infections (typhoid fever, salmonella septicaemia) but ciprofloxacin is preferred.
- Chloramphenicol penetrates well into the ocular aqueous and vitreous humours after either topical or systemic administration and is effective treatment for ocular infections.

The dose is, by mouth 500 mg 6-hourly, and by i.m. or i.v. injection or i.v. infusion 50 mg/kg daily in divided doses 6-hourly. For *topical* use ear-drops (5 and 10%), eye-drops (0.5%) and an ophthalmic ointment (1%) are available.

Adverse reactions include gastrointestinal upset which tends to be mild. Optic and peripheral neuritis occur with prolonged use (which should be avoided) but are uncommon. The systemic use of chloramphenicol is dominated by the fact that it can cause rare though serious reactions. *Bone marrow damage* is of two types: 1. a dose-dependent, reversible depression of erythrocyte, platelet and leucocyte formation that occurs early in treatment (type A adverse drug reaction); 2. an idiosyncratic, non-dose-related, and usually *fatal aplastic anaemia* which tends to develop during, or even weeks after, prolonged treatment, and sometimes on re-exposure to the drug (type B reaction); it has also occurred with eye drops. The danger is remote enough for a physician habitually to prescribe chloramphenicol for such diseases and yet not to see a case of aplastic anaemia during an entire career. This has led some to discount the risk (about 1:18 000–50 000 courses), but to many it is intolerable that trivial disease should be treated with chloramphenicol. It may be detected at an early and recoverable stage by frequent examination of the blood. The *'grey' syndrome* occurs in neonates as circulatory collapse in which the skin develops a cyanotic grey colour. It is caused by high chloramphenicol plasma concentration due to failure of the liver to conjugate, and of the kidney to excrete the drug.

Clindamycin

Clindamycin binds to bacterial ribosomes to inhibit protein synthesis. Its antibacterial spectrum is similar to that of erythromycin (with which there is partial cross-resistance) and benzylpenicillin, but it has the useful additional property of efficacy against *B. fragilis*, an anaerobe that is involved in gut-associated sepsis. Clindamycin is well absorbed from the gut and distributes to most body tissues including bone, but only small quantities reach the eye and cerebrospinal fluid. The drug is metabolised by the liver and enterohepatic cycling occurs with bile concentrations 2–5 times those of plasma. Significant excretion occurs by the gut.

Uses

- Bone or joint infections, because the drug penetrates these tissues well and is active against *Staph. aureus*.
- Intra-abdominal sepsis and non-sexually transmitted infection of the genital tract in the female, both of which usually involve anaerobes resistant to penicillins: in these circumstances, clindamycin is usually combined with an aminoglycoside.
- Anaerobic infection caused by penicillin-resistant organisms outwith the nervous system: anaerobic organisms often cause orodental sepsis, aspiration pneumonia and lung abscess and here clindamycin may prove efficacious should penicillin fail or be contraindicated.

The dose is 150–300 mg × 6 h by mouth; 0.6–2.7 g/d by slow i.v. infusion or i.m. in 2–4 divided doses.

The most serious *adverse effect* is antibiotic-associated (pseudomembranous) colitis (see p. 155) due to opportunistic infection of the bowel with *Clostridium difficile* which produces an enterotoxin; clindamycin should be stopped if any diarrhoea occurs.

Lincomycin has largely been replaced by clindamycin.

Sodium fusidate

Sodium fusidate is a steroid antimicrobial which is used almost exclusively against β-lactamase-producing staphylococci. These bacteria fairly rapidly become resistant and the drug should be combined with another antistaphylococcal drug, e.g. flucloxacillin. Sodium fusidate is readily absorbed from the gut and distributes widely in body tissues including bone. It is metabolised and very little is excreted unchanged in the urine; the $t_{\frac{1}{2}}$ is 5 h.

Sodium fusidate is a valuable drug for treating severe staphylococcal infections, including osteomyelitis. The dose is 500 mg × 8 h; an intravenous preparation is available. In an ointment or gel, sodium fusidate is used topically for staphylococcal skin infection and as a cream is applied to eradicate the staphylococcal nasal carrier state. It is well tolerated but mild gastrointestinal upset occurs. Jaundice occurs, particularly with i.v. administration.

Spectinomycin

Spectinomycin is active against Gram-negative organisms but its clinical use is confined to gonorrhoea in patients allergic to penicillin, or to infection with gonococci that are β-lactamase resistant. The steady growth of resistant gonococci, particularly the penicillinase-producing type, suggests that spectinomycin will continue to have a significant role in this disease, although resistance to it is reported.

Vancomycin

Vancomycin acts on multiplying organisms by inhibiting cell wall formation. It is bactericidal against several species of Gram-positive and Gram-negative cocci.

Vancomycin is poorly absorbed from the gut and, there being no satisfactory intramuscular preparation, is given i.v. for systemic infections. It distributes effectively into body tissues and the $t_{\frac{1}{2}}$ is 6 h; it is eliminated by the kidney.

Vancomycin is the drug of choice for antibiotic-associated pseudomembranous colitis (due to *C. difficile* or less commonly to staphylococci) in a dose of 125 mg × 6 h by mouth. Combined with an aminoglycoside, it may be given i.v. for streptococcal endocarditis in patients who are allergic to benzylpenicillin. It may also be used for serious infection with multiply resistant staphylococci. It is advisable to monitor plasma concentration.

The main disadvantage to vancomycin is auditory damage. Tinnitus and deafness may improve if the drug is stopped. Nephrotoxicity and allergic reactions also occur. Rapid i.v. infusion may cause a maculopapular rash possibly due to histamine release (the 'red man' syndrome).

Teicoplanin is structurally related to vancomycin and is active against Gram-positive bacteria. The $t_{\frac{1}{2}}$ of 50 h allows once daily administration. It is used for serious infection with Gram-positive bacteria including endocarditis, and peritonitis in patients undergoing chronic ambulatory peritoneal dialysis.

Minor antimicrobials

These are included because they are effective topically without serious risk of allergy, although toxicity limits or precludes their systemic use.

Mupirocin is active against both Gram-positive and Gram-negative organisms including those commonly associated with skin infections. It is available as an ointment for use, e.g. in folliculitis and impetigo, and to eradicate nasal staphylococci, e.g. in carriers of resistant organisms.

Polypeptide antibiotics. *Colistin* is effective against Gram-negative organisms particularly *P. aeruginosa*. It is used for bowel sterilisation in neutropenic patients, is included in bladder irrigation fluids and topically is applied to skin, including external ear infections. *Polymyxin B* is also active against Gram-negative organisms, particularly *P. aeruginosa*. Its principal use now is in bladder irrigation fluids and topically for skin, eye and external ear infections. *Gramicidin* is used in various topical applications as eye- and ear-drops, combined with neomycin and framycetin.

GUIDE TO FURTHER READING

Brumfitt W, Hamilton-Miller J 1989 Methicillin-resistant *Staphylococcus aureus*. New England Journal of Medicine 320: 1188

Donowitz G R, Mandell G L 1988 Beta-lactam antibiotics. New England Journal of Medicine 318: 419, 490

Finch R 1990 The penicillins today. British Medical Journal 300: 1289

Holgate S 1988 Penicillin allergy: how to diagnose and when to treat. British Medical Journal 296: 1213

Neu H C 1987 Clinical use of the quinolones. Lancet 2: 1319

12

Infection III: chemotherapy of bacterial infections

SYNOPSIS

We live in a world heavily populated by microorganisms of astonishing diversity. Most of these exist in our external environment but certain classes are normally harboured within our bodies. Depending on the circumstances, infectious disease can arise from organisms living exogenously or endogenously, and a knowledge of common pathogens at specific sites often provides a good basis for rational initial therapy.

This chapter considers the bacteria that cause disease in particular body systems, the drugs that are used to combat them, and how they are best used. It considers organisms that infect:

- Blood
- Paranasal sinuses and ears
- Throat
- Bronchi, lungs and pleura
- Endocardium
- Meninges
- Intestines
- Urinary tract
- Genital tract
- Eye
- Also mycobacteria, that infect many sites

Table 10.1 is a general reference for this chapter.

INFECTION OF THE BLOOD

Septicaemia is a medical emergency. Accurate microbiological diagnosis is of the first importance and blood cultures should be taken *before* starting antimicrobial therapy. Usually, the infecting organism(s) is not known and treatment must be instituted on the basis of a 'best guess'. The clinical circumstances may provide some clues:

- When septicaemia follows gastrointestinal or genital tract surgery, *Escherichia coli* (or other Gram-negative bacteria), anaerobic bacteria, *e.g. Bacteroides*, or streptococci are likely pathogens; the following combinations are effective: gentamicin plus amoxycillin plus metronidazole or cefuroxime plus metronidazole.

- Septicaemia related to urinary tract infection usually involves *Esch. coli* (or other Gram-negative bacteria), enterococci or, less commonly, *P. aeruginosa*: gentamicin plus amoxycillin or cefotaxime alone are indicated.

- Neonatal septicaemia is usually due to streptococci or coliforms, occasionally to *P. aeruginosa* and cefotaxime alone, or with netilmicin, is used.

- Staphylococcal septicaemia may be suspected where there is an abscess, e.g. of bone or lung, and flucloxacillin is indicated. Toxic shock syndrome occurs in circumstances that include: healthy women using vaginal tampons, abortion or childbirth, cutaneous or subcutaneous infection. The clinical problem is due to toxins produced by staphylococci and, while not strictly an infection of the blood, flucloxacillin is used to eliminate the source.

Antimicrobials should be given parenterally in septicaemia.

HA-1A (human antibody-1A, Centoxin) (t$\frac{1}{2}$ 16 h). The pathophysiology of circulatory collapse in septicaemia is complex (see p. 403). It is commonly due to the endotoxin of Gram-negative organisms, a component of the bacterial cell wall which induces the release of mediators of shock and tissue damage. It is now possible to neutralise the endotoxin directly with human IgM monoclonal antibody and forestall its adverse systemic reactions. Evidence indicates that following a single 100 mg i.v. injection the beneficial effect is rapid and mortality is reduced substantially. Adverse effects of HA-1A are infrequent and comprise mild allergic reactions. HA-1A thus appears to be a valuable addition to antimicrobial therapy for gram-negative septicaemia.

INFECTION OF PARANASAL SINUSES AND EARS

Sinusitis

Infection of the paranasal sinuses causes significant morbidity. Since oedema of the mucous membrane hinders the removal of pus, a logical first step is to restore normal drainage with a sympathetomimetic vasoconstrictor, e.g. ephedrine nasal drops. The common infecting organisms (*Streptococcus pneumoniae, Haemophilus influenzae, Streptococcus pyogenes, Moraxella (Branhamella) catarrhalis*) usually respond to amoxycillin (with or without clavulanic acid) or to doxycycline.

In chronic sinusitis, correction of the anatomical abnormalities (polypi, nasal septum deviation) is often important. Very diverse organisms, many of them normal inhabitants of the upper respiratory tract, may be cultured, e.g. anaerobic streptococci, *Bacteroides* spp., and a judgement is required as to whether any particular organism is acting as a pathogen. Choice of antibiotic should be guided by culture and sensitivity testing; therapy may need to be prolonged.

Otitis media

Mild cases, characterised by pinkness or infection

of the eardrum, often resolve spontaneously and need only analgesia and observation. They are normally viral. A bulging, inflamed eardrum indicates bacterial otitis media usually due to *Strep. pneumoniae, H. influenzae, Moraxella* (Branhamella) *catarrhalis, Strep. pyogenes (Group A)* or *Staphylococcus aureus*. Amoxycillin is satisfactory. Chemotherapy has not removed the need for myringotomy when pain is very severe, and also for later cases, as sterilised pus may not be completely absorbed and may leave adhesions that impair hearing. Chronic infection presents a similar problem to that of chronic sinus infection, above.

INFECTION OF THE THROAT

Pharyngitis is normally viral but the more serious cases may be caused by *Strep. pyogenes* (Group B) which is always sensitive to benzylpenicillin. *Strep. pneumoniae* and *H. influenzae* may be secondary invaders. Unfortunately, streptococcal sore throats cannot be clinically differentiated from the non-streptococcal with any certainty. Prevention of complications is more important than relief of the symptoms which seldom last long.

There is no general agreement whether chemotherapy should be employed in mild endemic sore throat; the disease usually subsides in a few days, septic complications are uncommon and rheumatic fever rarely follows. It is reasonable to withhold penicillin unless streptococci are cultured or the patient develops a high fever. Severe or epidemic sore throat is likely to be streptococcal and benzylpenicillin should be given to prevent these complications. Ideally, it should be continued for 10 days but compliance is bad once the symptoms have subsided and 5 days should be the minimum objective. For patients in general practice phenoxymethylpenicillin, or amoxycillin, which are more reliably absorbed, may be used. In a closed community, chemoprophylaxis of unaffected people to stop an epidemic may be considered, for instance with phenoxymethylpenicillin 125 mg × 2/d orally, for a period depending on the course of the epidemic, or a single intramuscular injection of benzathine penicillin 900 mg.

In *scarlet fever* and *erysipelas*, the infection is invariably streptococcal (Group B) and benzylpenicillin should be used even in mild cases, to prevent rheumatic fever and nephritis.

Chemoprophylaxis

Chemoprophylaxis of streptococcal (Group B) infection should be undertaken in patients who have had one attack of rheumatic fever. It is continued for at least 5 years, or until aged 20, whichever is the longer period, although some hold that it should continue for life, for histological study of atrial biopsies shows that the cardiac lesions may progress despite absence of clinical activity. Chemoprophylaxis should be continued for life after a second attack of rheumatic fever. A single attack of acute nephritis is not an indication for chemoprophylaxis but in the rare cases of nephritis in which recurrent haematuria occurs after sore throats, chemoprophylaxis should be used. Ideally, chemoprophylaxis should continue throughout the year, but if the patient is unwilling to submit to this, at least the colder months should be covered. The choice between daily phenoxymethylpenicillin by mouth or 3-weekly benzathine penicillin injections will depend on an assessment of patient preference and likely compliance.

Adverse effects are uncommon. Patients taking penicillin prophylaxis are liable to have penicillin resistant Group A streptococci (viridans type) in the mouth, so that during even minor dentistry, e.g. scaling, there is a risk of bacteraemia and thus of infective endocarditis with a penicillin-resistant organism in those with any residual rheumatic heart lesion. The same risk applies to urinary, abdominal and chest surgery, and patients need special chemoprophylaxis (see Endocarditis). Patients taking penicillins are also liable to carry resistant staphylococci.

Other causes of pharyngitis

Vincent's infection (microbiologically complex, includes anaerobes, spirochaetes) responds readily to benzylpenicillin; a single i.m. dose of 600 mg is often enough except in a mouth needing dental treatment, when relapse may follow. Metronidazole 200 mg × 8 h by mouth for 3 days is also effective.

Diphtheria (Corynebacterium diphtheriae). Antitoxin 10 000–30 000 units i.m. or 40 000–100 000 units i.v. in 2 divided doses 0.5–2 h apart is given to neutralise toxin already formed according to the severity of the disease. Erythromycin or benzylpenicillin is also used, to prevent the production of more toxin by destroying the bacteria.

Whooping-cough (Bordetella pertussis). Chemotherapy is needed in children who are weak, have damaged lungs or are under 3 years old. Erythromycin is usually recommended at the catarrhal stage and should be continued for 14 days. It may curtail an attack if given early enough but is not dramatically effective; it also reduces infectivity. A corticosteroid, salbutamol, and physiotherapy may be helpful for relief of symptoms, but reliable evidence of efficacy is lacking.

INFECTION OF THE BRONCHI, LUNGS AND PLEURA

Bronchitis

Most cases of acute bronchitis are viral; where bacteria are responsible the usual organisms are *Strep. pneumoniae* or *H. influenzae* and these respond well to amoxycillin or trimethoprim. In *chronic bronchitis*, suppressive chemotherapy, generally needed only during the colder months, should be considered for patients with symptoms of pulmonary insufficiency, recurrent acute exacerbations or permanently purulent sputum. It is reasonable first to try intermittent therapy, and only to use continuous therapy if it fails. Suitable regimens are amoxycillin 250 mg × 8 h by mouth or trimethoprim 200 mg × 12 h by mouth. For *intermittent therapy*, the patient is given a supply of the drug and is told to take it in full dose at the first sign of a 'chest' cold, e.g. purulent sputum, and to stop it after 3 days if there is rapid improvement. Otherwise, the patient should continue the drug until recovery takes place. If the exacerbation lasts for more than 10 days, there is a need for clinical reassessment. The main effect of *continuous therapy* is to reduce the duration of acute exacerbations rather than their number, perhaps because the exacerbations are initiated by virus infection which promotes secondary bacterial invasion.

Pneumonias

The clinical setting is a useful guide to the causal organism and hence to the best guess early choice of antimicrobial.

Pneumonia in previously healthy people (community acquired)

- Disease that is *segmental or lobar* in distribution is almost certainly caused by *Strep. pneumoniae* (pneumococcus). *H. influenzae* is also a cause, although it more often leads to exacerbations of chronic bronchitis. Benzylpenicillin is the treatment of choice if pneumococcal pneumonia can be diagnosed with certainty; alternatively, amoxycillin is used, and erythromycin in a penicillin-allergic patient.
- Pneumonia following *influenza* is often caused by *Staph. aureus*, and sodium fusidate and flucloxacillin are used in combination.
- *Atypical* cases of pneumonia may be caused by *Mycoplasma pneumoniae* which may be epidemic, or more rarely *Chlamydia psittaci* (psittacosis) or *Coxiella burnetii* (Q fever) and a tetracycline should be given. Treatment of psittacosis should continue for 10 days after the fever has settled and in mycoplasma pneumonia and Q fever a total· of 3 weeks' treatment may be needed to prevent relapse.

Pneumonia in people with chronic lung disease

- Normal commensals of the upper respiratory tract proliferate in damaged lungs especially following viral infections, pulmonary congestion or pulmonary infarction. Mixed infection is therefore common, and since *H. influenzae* and *Strep. pneumoniae* are often the pathogens, amoxycillin or trimethoprim are reasonable choices.

- *Klebsiella pneumoniae* tends to cause lung infection in the debilitated elderly and abscesses form, particularly in the upper lobes: cefotaxime plus an aminoglycoside is recommended.
- In hospitalised patients, *Staph. aureus* should be considered as the cause of a pneumonia.
- *Moraxella* (Branhamella) *catarrhalis*, a commensal of the oropharynx, may be a pathogen in lower respiratory tract infections, especially in patients with chronic lung disease, lung cancer, or those taking a corticosteroid; amoxycillin may fail because many strains produce β-lactamase but the organism is sensitive to co-amoxiclav or erythromycin.

Pneumonia in immunocompromised patients

Pneumonia is a common infection, e.g. in acquired immunodeficiency syndrome (AIDS) or in those who are receiving immunosuppressive drugs.

- Common pathogenic bacteria may be responsible *(Staph. aureus, Strep. pneumoniae)* but often organisms of lower natural virulence (viruses, fungi) are causal and strenuous efforts should be made to identify the microbe including, if feasible, bronchial washings or lung biopsy. Until the pathogen is known the patient should receive broad-spectrum antimicrobial treatment, such as an aminoglycoside plus amoxycillin.
- Aerobic Gram-negative bacilli, e.g. *Enterobacteriaceae*, *Klebsiella* spp., are pathogens in half of the cases and respond to cefotaxime or ·ceftazidime.
- An important respiratory pathogen in this group is the protozoon *Pneumocystis carinii*, which should be treated with co-trimoxazole 120 mg/kg/d by mouth or i.v. in 4 divided doses for 14 days, or with pentamidine (see p. 208).
- *P. aeruginosa* may cause pneumonia in these patients; for treatment, see Reference data on antimicrobial drugs of choice p. 156.

Legionnaires' disease

Legionella pneumophila responds to erythromycin 2–4 g/d i.v. in divided doses but rifampicin may be added in more severe infections.

Pneumonia due to anaerobic microorganisms

Pneumonia is often caused by aspiration of material from the oropharynx, or due to the presence of other lung pathology such as pulmonary infarction or bronchogenic carcinoma. The pathogens include anaerobic streptococci, *Bacteroides* spp. and *Fusibacterium*, and the diagnosis may be missed unless anaerobic cultures of fresh material are taken. Treatment for several weeks with cefuroxime plus metronidazole may be needed to prevent relapse.

Pulmonary abscess is treated according to the organism identified and with surgery if necessary.

Empyema is treated according to the organism isolated and with aspiration and drainage.

ENDOCARDITIS

When suspicion is high enough, three blood cultures should be taken over a few hours and antimicrobial treatment commenced. Delay in treating only exposes the patient to the risk of grave cardiac damage or systemic embolism.

Streptococci and staphylococci are causal in 80% of cases with viridans group streptococci, the most common pathogen. In narcotic addicts, *Staph. aureus* is the most likely organism. Culture-negative endocarditis (up to 20% of cases) is usually due to prior antimicrobial therapy or to special culture requirements of the microbe; it is best regarded as being due to streptococci and treated accordingly.

Elements of the treatment of infective endocarditis

- High doses of *bactericidal* drugs are needed because the organisms are relatively inaccessible in avascular vegetations on valves and the host reaction is negligible.
- Drugs should be given parenterally *at least initially* and preferably by intravenous bolus injection which achieves the necessary high peak concentration to penetrate the relatively avascular vegetations. The antimicrobial

should never be added to the infusion reservoir whose only purpose is to keep open the route into the vein.

- The infusion site should be changed every 2–3 days to prevent opportunistic infection, which is usually with staphylococci or fungi. Alternatively, use may be made of a central subclavian venous line sited with careful attention to aseptic technique.
- Prolonged therapy is needed, usually 4 weeks, and in the case of infected prosthetic valves at least 6 weeks. The patient should be reviewed one month after completing the antimicrobial treatment.
- Dosage must be adjusted according to the sensitivity of the infecting organism and therapy may be regarded as adequate if a 1:8 dilution of the patient's plasma kills it (serum bactericidal titration test).

The following regimens will serve:

1. Initial treatment[1] should comprise benzylpenicillin 1.2–2.4 g, 4-hourly plus gentamicin 80 mg, 8 or 12-hourly by i.v. injection (synergy allows this low dose of gentamicin and minimises risk of adverse effects); if *Staph. aureus* is suspected, sodium fusidate 500 mg, 8-hourly by mouth should be added. Patients allergic to penicillin should be treated with vancomycin 1 g i.v. over 60 min 12-hourly.

2. When an organism has been identified and its sensitivity to drugs determined:

Viridans group streptococci: benzylpenicillin plus gentamicin i.v. for at least 4 weeks or, if the organism is very sensitive, for 2 weeks followed by amoxycillin 1 g, 8-hourly by mouth for 2 weeks.

Streptococcus faecalis (Group D): benzylpenicillin plus gentamicin i.v. (as above) for at least 4 weeks.

Staph. aureus: flucloxacillin 2 g, 4-hourly by i.v. injection plus either gentamicin 80–120 mg, 8-hourly i.v. or sodium fusidate 500 mg, 8-hourly by mouth.

---

[1] Further details appear in Report of a Working Party of the British Society for Antimicrobial Chemotherapy. Lancet 1985; 2: 815.

Staphylococcus epidermidis has a predilection for prosthetic valves and should be managed as for *Staphylococcus aureus* if the organism is sensitive; but even if this is so, valve replacement may be needed.

Coxiella or *Chlamydia* : tetracycline 750 mg, 8-hourly by mouth reducing after 4–6 weeks to 250 mg, 12-hourly. Valve replacement is advised in most cases but some may continue indefinitely on tetracycline.

Fungal endocarditis: amphotericin plus flucytosine are used.

Culture-negative endocarditis: benzylpenicillin plus gentamicin are given for 6 weeks.

Prophylaxis of infective endocarditis

Transient bacteraemia is provoked by dental procedures, surgical incision of the skin, instrumentation of the urinary tract, parturition and even seemingly innocent activities such as brushing the teeth or chewing toffee. Bacteraemia does not always lead to endocarditis in people with *acquired* or *congenital* heart defects but experience shows that such individuals are at risk from bacteraemia and are protected by antimicrobials given prophylactically. The drugs are given as a *short* course in *high* dose at the *time* of the procedure to avoid emergence of resistant organisms. The recommendations that follow are taken from a Report of a Working Party of the British Society for Antimicrobial Chemotherapy.[2] Not every contingency is covered, because antimicrobial prophylaxis may be needed for patients *with cardiac defects* whenever surgery or instrumentation is undertaken on tissue that is heavily colonised or infected. The physician should exercise a clinical judgement that relates to individual circumstances. Doses quoted are for adults; those for children are given in the Report. All oral drugs should be taken under supervision.

Dental procedures

Under local or no anaesthesia

1. Adults who are *not allergic* to penicillins and who have not taken penicillin more than once in the previous month should receive amoxycillin 3 g by mouth 1 h before the procedure.

2. Patients *allergic* to penicillins should receive erythromycin stearate 1.5 g by mouth, 1–2 h before the procedure, followed by 0.5 g 6 h later. *Alternatively*, clindamycin 600 mg by mouth may be taken 1 h before the procedure.

Under general anaesthesia

1. Patients who are *not allergic* to penicillins and who have not taken penicillin more than once in the previous month should receive amoxycillin 1 g in 2.5 ml 1% lignocaine i.m. just before induction plus 0.5 g by mouth 6 h later. *Alternatively* amoxycillin 3 g may be taken by mouth, followed by 3 g by mouth as soon as possible after operation; or amoxycillin 3 g plus probenecid 1 g may be taken by mouth 4 h before operation.

2. *Special risk* patients, i.e. with prosthetic valves, or with penicillin allergy, with previous endocarditis are subject to separate recommendations (see Report).

Other procedures

The Report[2] should be consulted for recommendations on:
Surgery or instrumentation of the upper respiratory tract,
Genitourinary surgery or instrumentation,
Obstetric and gynaecological procedures,
Gastrointestinal procedures.

MENINGITIS

Accurate bacteriological diagnosis and speed of initiating treatment are the major factors determining the fate of the patient.

Drugs must be given i.v.; the regimens below provide the recommended therapy, with alternatives for patients allergic to first choices. Intrathecal therapy is now considered unnecessary, and can be dangerous, e.g. encephalopathy with penicillin.

---

[2] Report. Lancet 1990; 1: 88. Permission to quote from the Report is gratefully acknowledged.

Initial therapy should be sufficient to kill all pathogens, which are likely to be:

- All ages over 5 years. *N. meningitidis* and *Strep. pneumoniae*: benzylpenicillin should be given. *H. influenzae* is much less common but if it is suspected, e.g. in a patient with head injury, chloramphenicol or cefotaxime should be used instead of benzylpenicillin.
- Children under 5 years[3] *H. influenzae* and *N. meningitidis* are commonest, and *Strep. pneumoniae* less so: give a cephalosporin, e.g. cefuroxime or cefotaxime; alternatively benzylpenicillin plus chloramphenicol are used.
- Neonates.[3] *Esch. coli* or Group B streptococci: give cefotaxime or ceftazidime. Ampicillin must be added if *Listeria monocytogenes* is suspected.

Subsequent therapy. When the infecting organism has been identified, specific therapy is given below. Intravenous administration should continue until the patient is capable of taking drugs by mouth. Antimicrobials (except aminoglycosides) enter well into the CSF when the meninges are inflamed; relapse may be due to restoration of the blood : CSF barrier as inflammation is reduced.

N. meningitidis: benzylpenicillin 7.2 g/d. Alternatively *cefotaxime* 6–12 g/d or chloramphenicol 2–4 g/d is given. Hydrocortisone should be added if there is evidence of adrenocortical insufficiency (Waterhouse-Friderichsen syndrome). Treatment should continue for 5 days after the patient has become afebrile.

Strep. pneumoniae: benzylpenicillin 9.6 g/d. Alternatively chloramphenicol 2–4 g/d or cefuroxime 9–g/d or cefotaxime 6–12 g/d is given. Treatment should continue for 10 days after the patient has become afebrile and the physician should be aware of the risk of subsequent relapse.

H. influenzae: chloramphenicol 2–4 g/d or cefotaxime 6–12 g/d or cefuroxime 9 g/d is given. Treatment should continue for 10 days after the temperature has settled.

---

[3] Dexamethasone i.v., given early, improves outcome, probably by reducing meningeal cytokine production (Odio C M et al N Engl J Med 1991; 324: 1525).

Chemoprophylaxis

The three common pathogens (below) are spread by respiratory secretions. Asymptomatic nasopharyngeal carriers seldom develop meningitis but they may transmit the pathogens to close personal contacts. Rifampicin by mouth is effective at reducing carriage rates.

Meningococcal disease often occurs in epidemics, in closed communities but also in isolated cases. Close personal contacts should receive rifampicin 600 mg × 12 h for 2 days.

Haemophilus meningitis has an infectivity similar to that of meningococcal meningitis. Rifampicin 600 mg/day may be given for 4 days.

Pneumococcal meningitis tends to occur in isolated cases and chemoprophylaxis is not at present recommended.

INFECTIONS OF THE INTESTINES

Antimicrobial therapy should be reserved for specific conditions with identified pathogens which have shown to be shortened by drug therapy. Not all acute diarrhoea is infective for it can be caused for example by bacterial toxins, dietary indiscretions, anxiety and by drugs. Even if diarrhoea is infective, it may be due to viruses or if it is bacterial, antimicrobial agents may not reduce the duration of symptoms and may aggravate the condition by causing opportunistic infection. Maintenance of water and electrolyte balance, either by i.v. infusion or orally with a glucose-electrolyte solution together with an antimotility drug (except in small children) are the mainstays of therapy in such cases (see Oral rehydration therapy, p. 536).

Some specific intestinal infections do benefit from chemotherapy:

Campylobacter jejuni. Erythromycin will eliminate the organism from the stools; whether the drug alters the clinical course of the disease is less certain but a 5-day course is worth giving if the illness is severe or turns out to be protracted.

Shigella. Mild disease requires no specific antimicrobial therapy but toxic shigellosis with high fever should be treated with amoxycillin or trimethoprim or ciprofloxacin.

Salmonella. An antimicrobial should be used for *severe salmonella gastroenteritis*, or for *bacteraemia or salmonella enteritis* in an immunocompromised patient. The choice lies between ciprofloxacin amoxycillin or co-trimoxazole, according to the sensitivity of the pathogen.

Typhoid fever is a generalised infection and requires treatment with chloramphenicol, ciprofloxacin, amoxycillin or co-trimoxazole; the i.v. route should be used if administration by mouth is unsuitable. A longer period of treatment may be required for those who develop complications such as osteomyelitis or abscess.

A carrier state develops in a few individuals who have no symptoms of disease but who can infect others. Organisms reside in the biliary or urinary tracts. Chloramphenicol is bacteriostatic to Salmonellae and should *not* be used to treat the carrier state for there is no local defence reaction to eradicate the immobilised organisms. Amoxycillin in high dose for 3 months may be successful for what can be a very difficult problem.[4] Cholecystectomy may be needed.

Esch. coli is a normal inhabitant of the bowel but some *enterotoxigenic* strains are pathogenic and are a frequent cause of travellers' diarrhoea. Co-trimoxazole, or trimethoprim, or doxycycline may be given for a moderate or severe attack: they reduce symptoms and shorten its duration (see Travellers' diarrhoea, p. 537).

Staph. aureus. Staphylococcal enteritis, although rare may complicate abdominal surgery, shock or antimicrobial therapy. Dehydration, shock and electrolyte imbalance should be treated vigorously. Vancomycin by mouth or flucloxacillin by mouth and i.v. is effective.

Vibrio cholerae. The cause of death in cholera is electrolyte and fluid loss in the stools which may exceed one 1/hr. The most important aim of treatment is replacement and maintenance of water and electrolytes with oral or intravenous electrolyte solutions. Tetracycline, given early,

significantly reduces the amount and duration of diarrhoea and eliminates the organism from the faeces (thus lessening the contamination of the environment). Carriers may be treated by tetracycline by mouth in high dose for 3 days.

Suppression of bowel flora is useful in *hepatic insufficiency*. Here, absorption of products of bacterial breakdown of protein (ammonium, amines) in the intestine lead to cerebral symptoms and even to coma. In acute coma, neomycin 6 g/d should be given by gastric tube; as prophylactic, 1–4 g/d may be given to patients with protein intolerance who fail to respond to dietary protein restriction.

Sterilisation of bowel may be necessary in preparation for certain forms of intensive antineoplastic therapy which seriously impair natural defences, to prevent opportunistic infection. Combinations of drugs are used, e.g. framycetin, colistin, nystatin and amphotericin.

Chemoprophylaxis in surgery: see p. 154.

Antibiotic-associated colitis: see p. 155.

Peritonitis is usually a mixed infection and antimicrobial choice must take account of coliforms, anaerobes and streptococci; a combination of gentamicin, amoxycillin plus metronidazole or of cefuroxime plus metronidazole is usually effective.

INFECTIONS OF THE URINARY TRACT (excluding sexually transmitted infections)

Common pathogens include *Esch. coli*, *Proteus spp.*, *Klebsiella pneumoniae*, *P. aeruginosa*, *Enterococci* and *Staphylococcus saprophyticus*. Identification of the causative organism and of its sensitivity to drugs are important because of the range of organisms and the prevalence of resistant strains.

For infection of the lower urinary tract a low dose may be effective, as many antimicrobials are concentrated in the urine. *Infections of the substance of the kidney require the doses needed for any systemic infection.* Elimination of infection is hastened by a large urine volume (over 1.5 1/day) and by frequent micturition.

---

[4] The most famous carrier was Mary Mallon ('Typhoid Mary') who worked as a cook in New York City, USA, using various assumed names and moving through several different households. She caused at least 10 outbreaks with 51 cases of typhoid fever and 3 deaths. To protect the public, she was kept in detention for 23 years.

Drug treatment of urinary tract infection falls into several categories:

Lower urinary tract infection

Initial treatment with trimethoprim, ampicillin, or an oral cephalosporin is usually satisfactory. Therapy should normally last 5 days and may need to be altered once the results of bacterial sensitivity are known. Single dose therapy with *amoxycillin* 3 g by mouth may be sufficient to cure uncomplicated lower urinary tract infection.

Upper urinary tract infection

Acute pyelonephritis may be accompanied by septicaemia and it is advisable to start with gentamicin plus amoxycillin or alternatively cefotaxime alone. This is an infection of the kidney substance and needs adequate *blood* as well as *urine* concentrations.

Recurrent urinary tract infection

Attacks following rapidly with the same organism may be *relapses* and indicate a failure to eliminate the original infection. Attacks with a longer interval between them and produced by differing bacterial types may be regarded as due to *reinfection*, presumably from a source outside the urinary tract. In treating a relapse it is wise to use a drug capable of achieving high tissue concentrations, e.g. trimethoprim. Repeated short courses of antimicrobials should overcome most recurrent infections but, if this fails, 7–14 days of high dose treatment may be given, following which continuous low-dose prophylaxis may be needed.

Asymptomatic infection

This may be found by routine urine testing of pregnant women or patients with known structural abnormality of the urinary tract. Such infection may explain micturition frequency or incontinence in the elderly. Appropriate antimicrobial therapy should be given. Amoxycillin or a cephalosporin is preferred in pregnancy.

Prostatitis

The commonest pathogens are Gram-negative aerobic bacilli. Trimethoprim or ciprofloxacin or erythromycin are effective and, being lipid-soluble, penetrate the prostate in adequate concentration; they may usefully be combined. Response to a single, short course is often good, but recurrence is common and a patient can be regarded as cured only if he has been symptom-free and off antimicrobials for a year.

Chemoprophylaxis of urinary infections

Chemoprophylaxis is sometimes undertaken in patients liable to recurrent attacks or acute exacerbations of ineradicable infection. It may prevent subclinical renal damage in schoolgirls who are found to have asymptomatic bacteriuria on routine screening. Nitrofurantoin (0.5–1.0 g/d), nalidixic acid (0.5–1.0 g/d) or trimethoprim (100 mg/d) are satisfactory. The drugs are best given as a single dose at night time.

Tuberculosis of the genitourinary tract is treated on the principles described for pulmonary infection (p. 189).

Special drugs for urinary tract infections

General antimicrobials are used for urinary tract infections and described elsewhere. A few agents are used solely for infection of the urinary tract:

Nitrofurantoin ($t_{\frac{1}{2}}$ 30 min), a synthetic antimicrobial, is active against the majority of urinary pathogens except pseudomonads. It is well absorbed from the gastrointestinal tract and is concentrated in the urine; but plasma concentrations are too low to treat infection of kidney tissue. Excretion is reduced when there is renal insufficiency, rendering the drug both more toxic and less effective. The main use of nitrofurantoin is now for prophylaxis. Adverse effects include nausea and vomiting and diarrhoea. Polyneuritis occurs especially in patients with significant renal impairment, in whom the drug is contraindicated. Allergic reactions include rashes, generalised urticaria and pulmonary infiltration with lung consolidation or pleural effusion.

Nalidixic acid: see p. 174.

Hexamine is an obsolete urinary antiseptic.

GENITAL TRACT INFECTIONS

A general account of orthodox literature is given below, but treatment is increasingly the prerogative of specialists, who, as is so often the case, get the best results.

Gonorrhoea

The problem of resistant *Neisseria gonorrhoeae* is increasing, and selection of a particular drug will depend on sensitivity testing and a knowledge of resistance patterns in different geographical locations. Effective treatment requires exposure of the organism briefly to a high concentration of the drug. Single dose regimens are practicable as well as being obviously desirable for social reasons, including compliance. The following schedules are effective:

Uncomplicated anogenital infections: amoxycillin with probenecid; spectinomycin or ciprofloxacin may be used for penicillin-allergic patients.

Pharyngeal gonorrhoea responds less well to the single dose regimen, and tetracycline in high dose is needed for 7 days.

Co-existent infection. Chlamydia trachomatis is frequently present with *N. gonorrhoeae* and tetracycline for 7 days will limit the incidence of chlamydial urethritis if it is suspected.

Non-gonococcal urethritis

The vast majority of cases of urethritis with pus in which gonococci cannot be identified, are due to sexually-transmitted organisms, usually *C. trachomatis* and sometimes *Ureaplasma urealyticum*. Tetracycline or erythromycin is effective.

Pelvic inflammatory disease

Pathogens include *C. trachomatis*, *N. gonorrhoeae* and *Mycoplasma hominis*. A combination of antimicrobials may be required, e.g. metronidazole plus doxycycline.

Syphilis

Treponema pallidum is always sensitive to penicillin.

Primary and *secondary* syphilis are effectively treated by procaine penicillin i.m. daily for 10–21 days. If it is suspected that the patient may not comply with this course, a single i.m. injection of benzathine penicillin may be given. Tetracycline or erythromycin may be used for penicillin-allergic patients.

Tertiary syphilis should have the same treatment, ensuring that it continues for 3 weeks.

Congenital syphilis in the newborn should be treated with benzylpenicillin for 10 days at least.

A *pregnant* woman with syphilis should be treated as for primary syphilis, in each pregnancy, some advocate, in order to avoid all danger to children. Therapy is best given between the third and sixth month, as there may be a risk of abortion if it is given earlier.

Results of treatment of syphilis with penicillin are excellent; virtually 100% cure is achieved in seronegative cases, but the cure rate is lower in seropositive cases. Follow-up of all cases is essential, for 5 years if possible.

The *Herxheimer* (or Jarisch-Herxheimer) reaction may be due to the massive slaughter of spirochaetes resulting in the release of toxic substances. As pyrexia, it is common during the few hours after the first penicillin injection; other features include tachycardia, headache, myalgia and malaise which last up to a day. It cannot be prevented by giving graduated doses of penicillin. An adrenal steroid may stop it and should probably be given if a reaction is specially to be feared, e.g. in a patient with syphilitis aortic valve disease; prednisolone 30 mg/d by mouth for 2 days before and for 1 day after the antimicrobial, will serve.

Chancroid

The causal agent, *Haemophilus ducreyi*, normally responds to erythromycin.

Granuloma inguinale

Calymmatobacterium granulomatis infection is

treated with ampicillin or co-trimoxazole or a tetracycline.

Non-specific vaginitis (anaerobic vaginosis)

This is a common form of vaginal inflammation in which neither *Trichomonas vaginalis* nor *Candida albicans* can be isolated. There is evidence to associate the condition with *Gardnerella vaginalis*, and anaerobic organisms, especially of the *Bacteroides* species, the latter being responsible for the characteristic odour of the vaginal discharge. The condition responds well to a single 2 g dose of metronidazole.

Specific vaginitis

Candida vaginitis: see p. 198.
Trichomonas vaginitis: see p. 173, 208.

EYE INFECTIONS

Superficial infections, caused by a variety of organisms, are treated by chloramphenicol, framycetin or neomycin in drops (or ointments where drops are inconvenient), e.g. at night. Gentamicin or tobramycin are used for *P. aeruginosa*, and fusidic acid for *Staph. aureus*. Preparations often contain hydrocortisone or prednisolone, but the steroid may mask the progress of the infection, and should it be applied with an antimicrobial to which the organism is resistant (bacterium or virus), may make the disease worse by suppressing protective inflammation. Local chemoprophylaxis without corticosteroid is used to prevent secondary bacterial infection in virus conjunctivitis.

Chlamydial conjunctivitis. In the developed world, the genital (D-K) serotypes of the organism are responsible and the reservoir and transmission is maintained by sexual contact. Endemic trachoma in developing countries is usually caused by serotypes A, B and C. In either case, tetracycline is effective. Alternatively, pregnant or lactating women may receive erythromycin.

Herpes keratitis: see p. 196. It is *essential* that a corticosteroid should never be put on the eye; the disease is exacerbated and permanent blindness can result.

MYCOBACTERIAL INFECTIONS
Pulmonary tuberculosis

Drug therapy has transformed tuberculosis from a disabling and often fatal disease into one in which almost 100% cure is obtainable. Chemotherapy was formerly protracted, but a better understanding of the mode of action of anti-tuberculosis drugs has allowed the development of effective short-course regimens. Success requires that:

- a large number of actively multiplying bacilli be killed: isoniazid achieves this.
- persisters, i.e. semi-dormant bacilli that metabolise slowly or intermittently be killed: rifampicin and pyrazinamide are the most efficacious.
- the emergence of drug resistance be prevented by multiple therapy to suppress drug-resistant mutants that exist in all large bacterial populations: isoniazid and rifampicin are best.

All short-course regimens therefore include isoniazid, pyrazinamide and rifampicin.

After extensive clinical trials, the following daily regimens have been found satisfactory:

1. Isoniazid and rifampicin for 6 months, with pyrazinamide for the first 2 months.
2. isoniazid and rifampicin for 6 months plus streptomycin (or ethambutol) and pyrazinamide for the first 2 months.
3. isoniazid and rifampicin for 9 months plus ethambutol for the first 2 months.

Ethambutol or streptomycin should be used if there is a high prevalence of drug-resistant organisms, or if the patient is severely ill with extensive active lesions.

When compliance seems likely to be poor, the 6-monthly regimen (1 above) can be altered to *fully supervised intermittent* chemotherapy, i.e. less than daily, given thrice weekly, without loss of therapeutic efficacy. The dose of each drug, except for rifampicin, must be increased.

All the regimens are highly effective, with relapse rates of 1–2% in those who continue for 6 months; even if patients default after say, 4 months, tuberculosis can be expected to recur in only 10–15%. Drug resistance seldom develops with of these any regimens.

In some countries the cost of rifampicin and pyrazinamide may preclude or restrict their use. Longer duration, i.e. 8–12 month, regimens are then used, with these drugs given for shorter periods and with greater reliance on streptomycin and thioacetazone, which are less expensive.

Special problems

Resistant organisms. Initial resistance occurs in about 4% of patients, usually to isoniazid, but very rarely to rifampicin or ethambutol. By contrast, atypical mycobacteria are usually resistant to most standard drugs; their virulence is low but they can produce serious infection in immunocompromised patients which may respond, e.g. to erythromycin or a quinolone or a tetracycline, often in combination.

Chemoprophylaxis may be either *primary*, i.e. the giving of antituberculosis drugs to uninfected individuals, which is seldom justified, or *secondary*, which is the treatment of infected but symptom-free individuals, e.g. those known to be in contact with the disease and who develop a positive tuberculin reaction. Secondary chemoprophylaxis may be justified in children under the age of 3 because they have a high risk of disseminated disease; isoniazid alone for 6 months may be used since there is little risk of resistant organisms emerging.

Pregnancy. Drug treatment should never be interrupted or postponed during pregnancy. On the general principle of limiting exposure of the fetus, the standard 3-drug, 6-month course (1 above) is best. Streptomycin should be excluded from any regime (danger of fetal eighth cranial nerve damage).

Non-respiratory tuberculosis. The principles of treatment — multiple therapy and prolonged follow-up — are the same as for respiratory tuberculosis. In only a few cases is surgery now necessary. It should always be preceded and followed by chemotherapy. Many chronic tuberculous lesions may be relatively inaccessible to drugs as a result of avascularity of surrounding tissues and treatment frequently has to be prolonged, and dosage high, especially if damaged tissue cannot be removed by surgery, e.g. tuberculosis of bones.

Meningeal tuberculosis. It is essential to use isoniazid and pyrazinamide which penetrate well into the CSF. Rifampicin enters inflamed meninges well but non-inflamed meninges less so. An effective regimen is isoniazid, rifampicin, pyrazinamide and streptomycin. Treatment may need to continue for much longer than modern short course chemotherapy for pulmonary tuberculosis.

Tuberculosis of the skin, particularly lupus vulgaris, usually responds well. Some physicians have given isoniazid alone but it is preferable to give two drugs.

Adrenal steroid and tuberculosis. In pulmonary tuberculosis a corticosteroid may be given to severely ill patients. It reduces the reaction of the body to tuberculoprotein and buys time for the chemotherapy to take effect. It also causes the patient to feel better much more quickly.

In the absence of effective chemotherapy, an adrenal steroid will cause tuberculosis to extend and it should never be used alone, e.g. for another disease, if tuberculosis is suspected.

Antituberculosis drugs

Isoniazid (INH, INAH, isonicotinic acid hydrazide)

Isoniazid is selectively effective against *Mycobacterium tuberculosis* and has little or no activity against other bacteria: it is bactericidal (mechanism uncertain) against actively multiplying bacilli whether within macrophages or at extracellular sites. Isoniazid is well absorbed from the alimentary tract and is distributed throughout the body water, readily crossing tissue barriers and entering cells and cerebrospinal fluid. It should always be given in cases where there is special risk of meningitis (miliary tuberculosis and primary infection). Isoniazid is inactivated by conjugation with an acetyl group and the rate of the reaction is bimodally distributed. The $t_{\frac{1}{2}}$ is 1 h in fast and 3 h in slow acetylators; steady-state plasma concentration in fast acetylators is less than half that in slow acetylators but standard oral doses (5 mg/kg/d) on daily regimens give adequate tuberculocidal concentrations in both groups.

Isoniazid is in general well tolerated. The most severe adverse effect is liver damage which may range from moderate elevation of hepatic enzymes to severe hepatitis and death. It is probably caused by a chemically reactive metabolite(s), e.g. acetylhydrazine. Most cases develop within the first 8 weeks of therapy and liver function tests should be monitored monthly during this period at least.

Isoniazid is a structural analogue of pyridoxine and accelerates its excretion, the principal result of which is peripheral neuropathy with numbness and tingling of the feet, motor involvement being less common. Neuropathy is more frequent in slow acetylators, malnourished people, the elderly and those with liver disease and alcoholism. Such patients should receive pyridoxine 10 mg/d by mouth, which prevents neuropathy and does not interfere with the therapeutic effect; some prefer simply to give pyridoxine to all patients. Other adverse effects include mental disturbances, incoordination, optic neuritis and convulsions.

Isoniazid inhibits the metabolism of phenytoin, carbamazepine and ethosuximide, increasing their effect.

Rifampicin (rifampin)

Rifampicin has bactericidal activity against the tubercle bacillus, comparable to that of isoniazid.

It acts by inhibiting RNA synthesis and is particularly effective against mycobacteria that lie semidormant within cells. Rifampicin has a wide range of antimicrobial activity and *other uses* include leprosy, severe Legionnaires' disease (with erythromycin), and the chemoprophylaxis of meningococcal meningitis.

Rifampicin is well absorbed from the gastro-intestinal tract. It penetrates well into most tissues. Entry into the CSF when meninges are inflamed is sufficient to maintain therapeutic concentrations at normal oral doses but transfer is reduced as inflammation subsides in about 1 or 2 months. Enterohepatic recycling takes place, and eventually about 60% of a single dose is eliminated in the faeces; urinary excretion of unchanged drug also occurs. The $t_{\frac{1}{2}}$ is 4 h after initial doses, but shortens on repeated dosing because rifampicin is a very effective enzyme inducer and increases its own metabolism (as well as that of several other drugs, see below).

The oral dose is 450–600 mg/d (as a single dose); combined rifampicin and isoniazid tablets are available (Rimactazid).

Rifampicin rarely causes serious toxicity. Adverse reactions include flushing and itching with or without a rash, and thrombocytopenia. Rises in plasma bilirubin and hepatic enzymes may occur when treatment starts but are often transient and are not necessarily an indication for stopping the drug; fatal hepatitis has however occurred. *Intermittent* dosing, i.e. less than twice weekly, either as part of a regimen or through poor compliance promotes certain effects that probably have an immunological basis, namely, an influenza-like syndrome (malaise, headache and fever, shortness of breath and wheezing), acute haemolytic anaemia and acute renal failure sometimes with haemolysis, sometimes without. Red discolouration of urine, tears and sputum occurs which is harmless, and is a useful check that the patient is taking the drug. Rifampicin also causes an orange discolouration of soft contact lenses.

Rifampicin is a powerful *enzyme inducer* and speeds the inactivation of numerous drugs, including warfarin, oral contraceptives, narcotic analgesics, oral antidiabetic agents, phenytoin and dapsone. Appropriate increase in dosage is required to compensate for increased drug metabolism.

Pyrazinamide

Pyrazinamide is a derivative of nicotinamide and is included in first-choice combination regimens because of its particular ability to kill persisters, i.e. mycobacteria that are semidormant, often within cells. It is well absorbed from the gastrointestinal tract and metabolised in the liver, very little unchanged drug appearing in the urine; the $t_{\frac{1}{2}}$ is 9 h. The dose is 20–30 mg/kg by mouth to a maximum of 3 g daily in 3–4 doses.

Adverse effects include hyperuricaemia and arthralgia, which is relatively frequent with daily but less so with intermittent dosing and, unlike gout, affects both large and small joints. Pyrazinoic acid, the principal metabolite of pyrazinamide, inhibits renal tubular secretion of urate. Symptomatic treatment is usually sufficient and it is rarely necessary to discontinue pyrazinamide because of arthralgia. Hepatitis, which was particularly associated with high doses, is not a problem with modern short-course schedules. Sideroblastic anaemia and urticaria also occur.

Ethambutol

Ethambutol, being bacteristatic, is used in conjunction with other antituberculosis drugs to delay or prevent the emergence of resistant bacilli. It is well absorbed from the gastrointestinal tract and enters most body tissues including the lung; in tuberculous meningitis, sufficient may reach the CSF to inhibit mycobacterial growth but insignificant amounts cross into the CSF if the meninges are not inflamed. The $t_{\frac{1}{2}}$ is 4 h. Excretion is mainly by the kidney, by tubular secretion as well as by glomerular filtration; the dose should be reduced when renal function is impaired.

In recommended oral doses (15 mg/kg per day) (taking account of reduced renal function), ethambutol is relatively non-toxic. The main problem is *optic neuritis* (unilateral or bilateral) causing loss of visual acuity, central scotomata, occasionally also peripheral vision loss and red-green colour blindness. The changes reverse if treatment is stopped promptly; if not, the patient may go blind. It is prudent to note any history of eye disease and to get baseline tests of vision before starting treatment with ethambutol. The drug should not be given to a patient whose vision is much reduced and who may not notice

further minor deterioration. Patients should be told to make a point of reading small print in newspapers (with each eye separately) and if there is any deterioration to stop the drug immediately and seek advice. Patients who cannot understand and comply should be given alternative therapy, if possible. The need for repeated specialist ophthalmological monitoring is controversial. Peripheral neuritis occurs but is rare.

Streptomycin: see page 168.

Thiacetazone

Thiacetazone ($t_{\frac{1}{2}}$ 13 h) is tuberculostatic and is used with isoniazid to inhibit the emergence of resistance to the latter drug. It is absorbed from the gastrointestinal tract, partly metabolised and partly excreted in the urine. Adverse reactions include gastrointestinal symptoms, conjunctivitis and vertigo. More serious effects are erythema multiforme, haemolytic anaemia, agranulocytosis, cerebral oedema and hepatitis.

Alternative or *reserve* drugs are used where there are problems of drug intolerance and bacterial resistance. They are in this class because of either greater toxicity or of lesser efficacy and include: ethionamide (gastrointestinal irritation, allergic reactions), capreomycin (nephrotoxic), cycloserine (CNS toxicity), and kanamycin (see Aminoglycosides). Sodium aminosalicylate (para-aminosalicylic acid, PAS) is now obsolete.

Leprosy

Effective treatment of leprosy is complex and requires much experience to obtain the best results. Problems of *resistant* leprosy now requires that multiple drug therapy be used and involve:

- for *paucibacillary* disease: dapsone and rifampicin for 6 months;
- for *multibacillary* disease: dapsone, rifampicin and clofazimine for 2 years. Follow-up for 4–8 years may be necessary.

Dapsone ($t_{\frac{1}{2}}$ 24 h), a bacteriostatic sulphone (related to sulphonamides), has for many years been the standard drug for the treatment of all forms of leprosy but irregular and inadequate duration of treatment with a single drug have allowed the emergence of resistance, both primary and secondary, now a major problem in control of the disease. Adverse effects are gastrointestinal symptoms and allergic reactions including erythema nodosum leprosum.

Rifampicin (see above) is bactericidal, and is safe and effective when given once monthly: contact between patients and health workers at these intervals is feasible in most countries and boosts compliance, for the swallowing of medicines by the patient can be witnessed.

Clofazimine (t_2^1 70 days) has a leprostatic action and an anti-inflammatory effect that prevents erythema nodosum leprosum. It causes gastro-intestinal symptoms. Reddish discolouration of the skin and other cutaneous lesions also occur, and may persist for months after the drug has been stopped.

Other antileprotics include ethionamide and prothionamide. Thalidomide (see index) despite its notorious past still finds a use in the control of allergic lepromatous reactions.

Other bacterial infections

Burns. Infection may be substantially reduced by application of silver sulphadiazine cream. Substantial absorption can occur from any raw surface and use of an aminoglycoside, e.g. neomycin, preparations can cause ototoxicity.

Gas gangrene. The skin between the waist and the knees is normally contaminated with anaerobic faecal organisms. However assiduous the skin preparation for orthopaedic operations or thigh amputations, it will not kill the spores. Surgery done for vascular insufficiency where tissue oxygenation may be poor is likely to be followed by infection. *Clostridium perfringens (welchii)* is sensitive to benzlypenicillin which should be used for prophylaxis in such operations.

Wounds. Systemic chemoprophylaxis is necessary for several days at least in dirty wounds where sutures have to be left below the skin, and in penetrating wounds of body cavities. Benzyl-penicillin is probably best, but in the case of penetrating abdominal wounds, metronidazole should be added, intravenously (see also tetanus). Weak iodine solution is an effective skin antiseptic where the patient is not allergic. It is, however, inactivated by serum so that its painful application to wounds is punishment, not therapy; povidone iodine is preferred.

Abscesses and infections in bone and serous cavities are treated according to the antimicrobial sensitivity of the organism concerned but require high doses because of poor penetration. Local instillation of the drug may be needed.

In *osteomyelitis,* early treatment is urgent to prevent bone necrosis. Bacteriological identification is of great importance and blood for culture (50% of cases are positive) should be taken before therapy begins; indeed, aspiration of the bone to get the organism has been advocated. As the organism is commonly *Staph. aureus,* flucloxacillin and sodium fusidate should be used. Treatment is required for weeks. Surgery is often needed in late cases.

Actinomycosis. Actinomyces israelii is sensitive to several drugs but access is poor because of granulomatous fibrosis. High doses of benzyl-penicillin are given for several weeks. Surgery is likely to be needed.

Leptospirosis. To be most effective, chemotherapy should be started within 4 days of the onset of symptoms. Benzylpenicillin is recommended; a Herxheimer reaction may be induced (see syphilis). General supportive management is important, including attention to fluid balance and observation for signs of hepatic, renal or cardiac failure.

GUIDE TO FURTHER READING

Editorial 1988 Chemotherapy of leprosy. Lancet 2: 487

Eykyn S J 1988 Staphylococcal sepsis. The changing pattern of disease and therapy. Lancet 1: 100

Finch R 1988 Skin and soft tissue infections. Lancet 1: 164

Geddes A M 1988 Antibiotic therapy — a resumé. Lancet 1: 286

Gorbach S 1987 Bacterial diarrhoea and its treatment. Lancet 2: 1378

Hughes W T 1987 *Pneumocystis carinii* pneumonitis. New England Journal of Medicine 317: 1021

Jones D M 1989 Control of meningococcal disease. British Medical Journal 298: 542

Macfarlane J T 1987 The treatment of lower respiratory infections. Lancet 2: 1446

Macintyre I M C, Munro A 1990 Pelvic inflammatory disease. British Medical Journal 300: 1090

Mackowiak P A 1982 The normal microbial flora. New England Journal of Medicine 307: 83

Welsby P D, Golledge C L 1990 Meningococcal meningitis. A diagnosis not to be missed. British Medical Journal 300: 1150

Williams G 1990 The toxic shock syndrome. British Medical Journal 300: 960

Wolff S M 1991 Monoclonal antibodies and the treatment of Gram-negative bacteraemia and shock. New England Journal of Medicine 324: 486

Ziegler E J et al 1991 Treatment of Gram-negative bacteraemia and septic shock with HA-1A human monoclonal antibody against endotoxin. New England Journal of Medicine 324: 429

13

Infection IV: chemotherapy of viral, fungal, protozoal and helminthic infections

SYNOPSIS

- **Viruses** present a more difficult problem of chemotherapy than do higher organisms, e.g. bacteria, for they are intracellular parasites that participate in the metabolism of host cells. Identification of differences between viral and human metabolism however have led to the development of effective antiviral agents, whose roles are increasingly well defined.
- **Fungus** infections range from inconvenient skin conditions to life-threatening systemic diseases; the latter have become more frequent as opportunistic infections in patients immunocompromised by drugs or AIDS.
- **Protozoal** infections. Malaria is the major transmissible parasitic disease. The life cycle of the plasmodium that is relevant to prophylaxis and therapy is described. Drug resistance is a real problem and differs with geographical location, time and type of plasmodium.
- **Helminthic** infestations cause considerable morbidity. The drugs that are effective against these organisms are summarised.

CHEMOTHERAPY OF VIRAL INFECTIONS

Antiviral agents are most active when viruses are replicating. The earlier that treatment is given therefore, the better the results. An important difficulty is that a substantial amount of viral multiplication has often taken place before symptoms occur. Apart from primary infection, viral illness is often the consequence of reactivation of latent virus in the body. In both cases, patients whose immune systems are compromised, suffer particularly severe illness.

CLASSIFICATION OF ANTIVIRUS DRUGS

Drugs that directly impair virus replication

For herpes simplex and varicella-zoster virus infections: acyclovir, idoxuridine, vidarabine
For human immunodeficiency virus (HIV) infection: zidovudine
For cytomegalovirus (CMV) infection: ganciclovir, foscarnet
For respiratory syncytial virus (RSV) infection: tribavirin
For influenza A: amantadine

Drugs that modulate the host immune system

alpha interferons, inosine pranobex
An overview of the place of these agents in therapy is given in Table 13.1.

Viruses are capable of developing resistance to antimicrobial drugs, just as are bacteria, with similar implications for the individual patient, for the community and for drug development.

Table 13.1 Drugs of choice for virus infections

Organism	Drug of choice	Alternative
Cytomegalovirus (CMV)	ganciclovir	foscarnet (for CMV retinitis in HIV patients)
Hepatitis B or C	interferon alfa-2a	
Herpes simplex		
keratitis	acyclovir (topical)	idoxuridine or vidarabine (topical)
labial	acyclovir (topical and/or systemic)	
genital	acyclovir (topical and/or systemic)	
encephalitis	acyclovir	vidarabine
disseminated	acyclovir	vidarabine
Human immuno-deficiency virus (HIV)	zidovudine	
Influenza A	amantadine	
Respiratory syncytial virus	tribavirin	
Varicella-zoster	acyclovir	vidarabine

INDIVIDUAL DRUGS

Drugs that directly impair virus replication

Acyclovir

Acyclovir (Zovirax) is a prodrug; it inhibits viral DNA synthesis only after phosphorylation by virus-specific thymidine kinase, which accounts for its high therapeutic index. Only 20% is absorbed from the gut, but this is sufficient for the systemic treatment of some infections. It distributes widely in the body; the concentration in CSF is approximately half that of plasma, and the brain concentration may be even less. These differences are taken into account in dosing for viral encephalitis. The drug is excreted in the urine. The $t_{\frac{1}{2}}$ is 3 h.

Indications for acyclovir are expanding and include:

- *Herpes simplex.*
  1. skin infections, including initial and recurrent labial and genital herpes (as a cream), most effectively when new lesions are forming; skin and mucous membrane infections (as tablets or oral suspension);
  2. ocular keratitis (as an ointment);
  3. prophylaxis in the immunocompromised (oral, as tablets or suspension);
  4. encephalitis, disseminated disease (i.v.). Acyclovir-resistant herpes simplex virus has been reported in patients with AIDS.
- *Varicella-zoster.* Shingles or generalised, in immunocompetent persons (as tablets or suspension, and best within 48 h of the appearance of the rash), and in immunocompromised persons (i.v.).

Adverse reactions are remarkably few. The ophthalmic ointment causes a mild transient stinging sensation and a diffuse superficial punctate keratopathy which clears when the drug is stopped. Oral or i.v. use is associated with gastrointestinal symptoms, headache and neuropsychiatric reactions. Extravasation with i.v. use causes severe local inflammation.

Idoxuridine

Idoxuridine was the first widely used antivirus drug. It replaces its analogue thymidine in the DNA of viruses, preventing their multiplication, but it is also incorporated into the DNA of host cells, notably of bone marrow, liver and kidney, causing toxicity which precludes systemic use; but it is effective *topically* for ocular and cutaneous herpes simplex with few adverse reactions. It is superseded by acyclovir.

Vidarabine

Vidarabine ($t_{\frac{1}{2}}$ 4 h) is an analogue of adenine deoxyriboside, a natural nucleoside, and acts by inhibiting viral DNA-polymerase. It is poorly soluble and is given by slow i.v. infusion in large fluid volume, or used topically.

Vidarabine may be used for varicella, herpes zoster and herpes simplex infections, but acyclovir is preferred.

Gastrointestinal symptoms occur but lessen as the drug is continued. High doses induce pancytopenia and megaloblastosis. Neurological effects include parkinsonian tremor, ataxia, myoclonus, hallucinations, confusion and coma.

Amantadine

Amantadine is effective against influenza A; it acts by interfering with the uncoating and release of viral genome into the host cell. It is well absorbed from the gastrointestinal tract and is eliminated in the urine ($t_{\frac{1}{2}}$ 12 h). Amantadine may be used orally for the *prevention and treatment of infection with influenza A* (but not B) virus. Those most likely to benefit include the debilitated, persons with respiratory disability and people living in crowded conditions, especially during an influenza epidemic.

Adverse reactions include dizziness, nervousness, lightheadedness and insomnia. Drowsiness, hallucinations, delirium and coma may occur in patients with impaired renal function. Convulsions may be induced, and amantadine should be avoided in epileptic patients.

Amantadine for Parkinson's disease: see p. 312.

Zidovudine (Retrovir)

Human immunodeficiency virus replicates by converting its single stranded RNA into double stranded DNA which is incorporated into host DNA; this crucial conversion, the *reverse* of the normal cellular transcription of nucleic acids, is accomplished by the enzyme *reverse transcriptase*. Zidovudine, as the active triphosphate, has a high affinity for reverse transcriptase and is integrated by it into the viral DNA chain whose further elongation is thereby prevented. The drug must be present continuously to prevent viral alteration of the host DNA, which is permanent once it occurs.

Zidovudine is well absorbed from the gastrointestinal tract (it is available only as capsules) and is rapidly cleared from the plasma ($t_{\frac{1}{2}}$ 1 h); concentrations in CSF are approximately half those in plasma. The drug is inactivated mainly by metabolism but 25% is excreted unchanged by the kidney.

Zidovudine is indicated for serious manifestations of human immunodeficiency virus infection in patients with acquired immunodeficiency syndrome (AIDS) or AIDS-related complex., i.e. those with opportunistic infection, constitutional or neurological symptoms; treatment reduces the frequency of opportunistic infections and may prolong survival.

Adverse reactions early in treatment may include anorexia, nausea, vomiting, headache, dizziness, malaise and myalgia, but tolerance develops to these and usually the dose need not be altered. More serious are anaemia and neutropenia which develop when the dose is high, and with advanced disease. A toxic myopathy may develop with long-term use.

Ganciclovir

Ganciclovir is similar to acyclovir in its mode of action. It is given i.v. and is eliminated in the urine, mainly unchanged; the $t_{\frac{1}{2}}$ is 4 h. Ganciclovir is active against several types of virus but because of toxicity, its use is limited to *life-* or *sight-threatening* cytomegalovirus infection in immunocompromised patients. Ganciclovir resistant cytomegalovirus has been reported.

Adverse reactions include neutropenia and thrombocytopenia which are usually but not always reversible after withdrawal. Concomitant use of potential marrow-depressant drugs, e.g. co-trimoxazole, amphotericin B, zidovudine, should be avoided. Other reactions are fever, rash, gastrointestinal symptoms, confusion and seizure (the last especially if imipenem is co-administered).

Foscarnet is used for *retinitis* due to cytomegalovirus in patients with human immunodeficiency virus infection when ganciclovir is contraindicated. It causes numerous adverse effects, including renal toxicity.

Tribavirin is a synthetic nucleoside which is administered by inhalation as an aerosol or nebulised solution for severe respiratory syncytial virus bronchiolitis in infants and children. Systemic absorption by this route is negligible and no serious adverse effects are reported.

Drugs that modulate the host immune system

Interferons

Virus infection stimulates the production of protective glycoproteins (*interferons*) which act: 1. directly on uninfected cells to induce enzymes that degrade viral RNA; 2. indirectly by stimulating the immune system. Interferons also modify cell regulatory mechanisms and inhibit neoplastic growth. They are classified alpha, beta or gamma according to their antigenic and physical properties. Alfa interferons (subclassified -2a, -2b, and -N1) are effective against conditions that include hairy cell leukaemia, chronic myelogenous leukaemia, recurrent or metastatic renal cell carcinoma, Kaposi's sarcoma in AIDS patients (an effect that may be partly due to its activity against HIV) and *condylomata accuminata* (genital warts). Evidence also shows that interferon alpha-2a improves the manifestations of hepatitis B and C infection.

Adverse reactions are common and include an influenza-like syndrome (naturally-produced interferon may cause the symptoms of influenza), fatigue and depression which respond to lowering of the dose. Other effects are anorexia (sufficient to induce weight loss), convulsions, hypotension, hypertension, cardiac dysrhythmias and marrow depression. Interferons inhibit the metabolism of theophylline, increasing its effect.

Inosine pranobex

This drug is reported to stimulate the host immune response to virus infection and has been used for mucocutaneous herpes simplex and genital warts (but acyclovir is superior). It is administered by mouth and metabolised to uric acid, so should be used with caution in patients with hyperuricaemia or gout.

CHEMOTHERAPY OF FUNGAL INFECTIONS

Widespread use of immunosuppressive chemotherapy and the emergence of AIDS have contributed to a rise in the incidence of opportunistic infection ranging from comparatively trivial cutaneous infections to systemic disease that demand prolonged treatment with potentially toxic agents.

TREATMENT

Superficial mycoses

Dermatophyte infections (ringworm, tinea)

Longstanding remedies such as Compound Benzoic Acid Ointment (Whitfield's ointment) is still acceptable for mild infections but a topical imidazole (clotrimazole, econazole, miconazole, sulconazole), which is also effective against candida, is now usually preferred. Tioconazole is the only imidazole that is effective topically for nail infections. Griseofulvin orally should be used for extensive nail or scalp tinea infection.

Candida infections

Cutaneous infection is generally treated with topical amphotericin, clotrimazole, econazole, miconazole or nystatin. Local hygiene is also important. An underlying explanation should be sought if a patient fails to respond to these measures, e.g. diabetes, the use of a broad-spectrum antibiotic or of immunosuppressive drugs.

Candidiasis of alimentary tract mucosa responds to amphotericin, fluconazole, ketoconazole, miconazole or nystatin as lozenges (to suck, for oral infection), gel (held in the mouth before swallowing), suspension or tablets.

Vaginal candidiasis is treated by clotrimazole, econazole, isoconazole, ketoconazole, miconazole or nystatin as pessaries or vaginal tablets or cream inserted once or twice a day with cream or ointment on surrounding skin. Failure may be due to a concurrent intestinal infection causing reinfection and nystatin tablets may be given by mouth 8-hourly with the local treatment. The male sexual partner may use a similar antifungal ointment for his benefit and for hers (reinfection).

Systemic mycoses

The principal features are summarised in Table 13.2.

ANTIFUNGAL AGENTS

Polyene antibiotics

These act by binding tightly to sterols present in cell membranes. The resulting deformity of the

Table 13.2 Drugs of choice for systemic fungal infections

Infection	Drug of first choice	Alternative
Aspergillosis	amphotericin	no dependable alternative
Blastomycosis	amphotericin or ketoconazole[1]	see footnote[2]
Candidiasis oesophageal	fluconazole or ketoconazole	low doses of amphotericin
deep	amphotericin with or without flucytosine	no dependable alternative
Chromoblasto-mycosis	flucytosine	no dependable alternative
Coccidiomycosis	amphotericin or ketoconazole[1]	see footnote[2]
Cryptococcosis	amphotericin with or without flucytosine	fluconazole
Histoplasmosis	amphotericin or ketoconazole[1]	see footnote[2]
Mucormycosis	amphotericin	no dependable alternative
Paracoccidioido-mycosis	amphotericin or ketoconazole[1]	a sulphonamide[2]
Sporotrichosis cutaneous	iodide, heat	see footnote[2]
deep	amphotericin	see footnote[2]

[1] Patients with severe illness, meningitis, AIDS or some other causes of immunosuppression should receive amphotericin.
[2] Itraconazole may prove effective.
(This Table is drawn substantially from the Medical Letter on Drugs and Therapeutics (USA; 1990). We are grateful to the Chairman of the Editorial Board for permission to publish the material. DRL, PNB)

membrane allows leakage of intracellular ions and enzymes, causing cell death. Those polyenes that have useful antifungal activity bind selectively to ergosterol, the most important sterol in fungal (but not mammalian) cell walls.

Amphotericin

Amphotericin is negligibly absorbed from the gut and must be given by i.v. infusion for systemic infection; its activity is terminated by metabolism. The $t_\frac{1}{2}$ is 15 days, i.e. after stopping treatment, drug persists in the body for several weeks.

Amphotericin is at present *the drug of choice for most systemic fungal infections* (see Table 13.2). The diagnosis of systemic infection must be firmly established because toxicity to amphotericin is significant. The presence of fungus in the blood may be due to a contaminated intravenous needle, or in the urine due to an indwelling catheter, without causing disease; tissue biopsy and culture may be necessary. A conventional course of treatment lasts 6–12 weeks during which at least 2 g of amphotericin is given. Oral use for intestinal candidiasis requires higher dose.

Adverse reactions. Although gradual escalation of the dose limits toxic effects, they may have to be tolerated in life-threatening infection. Renal impairment is invariable, although amphotericin need not be stopped until serum creatinine has risen to 200 micromol/l; the same dose may then be resumed after 3–5 days. Hypokalaemia (due to distal renal tubular acidosis) may necessitate replacement therapy. Other adverse effects include: anorexia, nausea, vomiting, malaise, abdominal, muscle and joint pains, loss of weight, anaemia, hypomagnesaemia and fever. Symptoms may be alleviated by aspirin, an antihistamine (H_1) or an antiemetic. Severe febrile reactions are mitigated by hydrocortisone 25–50 mg before each infusion.

Nystatin

Nystatin is too toxic for systemic use. It is not absorbed from the alimentary canal and is used to prevent or treat superficial *candidiasis* of the mouth, oesophagus or intestinal tract (as suspension, tablets or pastilles), for vaginal candidiasis (pessaries) and cutaneous infection (cream, ointment or powder).

Azoles

The antibacterial, antiprotozoal and anthelminthic members of this group are described in the appropriate sections.

Antifungal azoles comprise:

- *Imidazoles* (ketoconazole, miconazole, clotrimazole, isoconazole, tioconazole) interfere with fungal oxidative enzymes to cause lethal accumulation of hydrogen peroxide, and also reduce the formation of ergosterol, an important constituent of the fungal cell wall which thus becomes permeable to intracellular constituents. Lack of selectivity in these actions results in important adverse effects.
- *Triazoles* (fluconazole, itraconazole) damage the fungal cell membrane by inhibiting a demethylase enzyme; they have greater selectivity against fungi, better penetration of the CNS, resistance to degradation, and cause less endocrine disturbance than do the imidazoles.

Ketoconazole

Ketoconazole is well absorbed from the gut (poorly where there is gastric hypoacidity, see below), is widely distributed in tissues but concentrations in CSF and urine are low; its action is terminated by metabolism ($t_{\frac{1}{2}}$ 8 h). Ketoconazole is effective by mouth for systemic mycoses (see Table 13.2). It is less toxic but less effective than amphotericin, which may be preferred where the illness is severe, e.g. meningitis or AIDS. Impairment of steroid synthesis by ketoconazole confers other uses: 1. inhibition of testosterone formation causes striking clinical benefit in patients with advanced prostatic cancer, notably for bone pain; 2. patients with hyperadrenalcorticism may be improved by its inhibition of cortisol synthesis.

Adverse reactions include nausea, giddiness, headache, pruritus and photophobia. Impairment

of testosterone synthesis may cause gynaecomastia and decreased libido in men. Of particular concern is impairment of liver function, ranging from transient elevation of hepatic transaminases and alkaline phosphatase to severe injury and death. Liver damage may progress despite discontinuing ketoconazole.

Drugs that lower gastric acidity, e.g. antacids, histamine H_2-receptor antagonists, impair the absorption of ketoconazole from the gastrointestinal tract. Inhibition of drug metabolism by ketoconazole leads to increased effects of oral anticoagulants, phenytoin and cyclosporin, and a disulfiram-like reaction with alcohol. Concurrent use of rifampicin, by enzyme induction, markedly reduces the plasma concentration of ketoconazole.

Miconazole is an alternative. Clotrimazole is an effective topical agent for dermatophyte, yeast, and other fungal infections (intertrigo, athletes' foot, ringworm, pityriasis versicolor, fungal nappy rash). Econazole and sulconazole are similar. Tioconazole is used for fungal nail infections and isoconazole for vaginal candidiasis.

Fluconazole

Fluconazole is absorbed from the gastrointestinal tract and is excreted largely unchanged by the kidney ($t_{\frac{1}{2}}$ 24 h). It is effective by mouth for oropharyngeal and oesophageal candidiasis, and i.v. for systemic candidiasis and cryptococcosis (including cryptococcal meningitis). It may cause gastrointestinal discomfort, headaches, elevation of liver enzymes and allergic rash. Animal studies demonstrate embryotoxicity and fluconazole ought not to be given to pregnant women. High doses increase the effects of phenytoin, cyclosporin and warfarin.

Itraconazole is an alternative (see Table 13.2).

Other antifungal drugs

Griseofulvin

Griseofulvin was the first drug to be effective, taken by mouth, against superficial fungus infections in man. Its precise mode of action is complex but efficacy depends on its capacity to bind to keratin as it is being formed in the cells of the nail-bed, hair follicles and skin, for dermatophytes specifically infect keratinous tissues. Griseofulvin does not kill fungus already established, it merely prevents infection of new keratin so that the duration of treatment is governed by the time that it takes for infected keratin to be shed; on average, hair and skin infection should be treated for 4–6 weeks while toenails may need a year or more. Relapse will occur if treatment is stopped while infected keratin is still in the body. Local hygiene therefore remains important. Treatment must continue for a time after both visual and microscopic evidence have disappeared.

Fat in a meal enhances absorption of griseofulvin; it is metabolised in the liver and induces hepatic enzymes ($t_{\frac{1}{2}}$ 22 h).

Griseofulvin is effective against all superficial ringworm (dermatophyte) infections but is ineffective against pityriasis versicolor, superficial candidiasis and all systemic mycoses.

Adverse reactions include gastrointestinal upset, rashes, photosensitivity, headache, and various central nervous system disturbances (see porphyria).

Flucytosine

Flucytosine (5-fluorocytosine) interferes with fungal nucleic acid synthesis. It is well absorbed from the gut, penetrates effectively into tissues and almost all is excreted unchanged in the urine ($t_{\frac{1}{2}}$ 4 h). The dose should be reduced for patients with impaired renal function, and the plasma concentration should be monitored. The drug is well tolerated when renal function is normal. *Candida albicans* rapidly becomes resistant to flucytosine which ought not to be used alone; it may be combined with amphotericin (see Table 13.2) but this increases the risk of adverse effects (leucopenia, thrombocytopenia, enterocolitis).

Potassium iodide is given by mouth to treat cutaneous sporotrichosis.

CHEMOTHERAPY OF PROTOZOAL INFECTIONS[1]

MALARIA

Over 90 million cases of malaria occur each year; in socioeconomic impact, it is the most important of the transmissible parasitic diseases.

History

Quinine as cinchona bark was introduced into Europe from South America in 1633. It was used for all fevers, amongst them malaria. Further advance in the chemotherapy of malaria was delayed until 1880, when Laveran[2] finally identified the parasites in the blood.

Mepacrine (quinacrine) was introduced in 1930 but did not displace quinine until in 1942 the Japanese armies captured South East Asia and the Pacific Islands, which had supplanted South America as the source of quinine. The withdrawal of quinine supplies from the Allied forces precipitated a military crisis and mepacrine was hastily manufactured to meet it.

It was vital that the dose of mepacrine necessary to enable troops to fight in hyperendemic areas without serious casualties from malaria should be quickly found. Physical stress is believed to promote malarial relapses and so, at a base in North Australia, trials of mepacrine were carried out under conditions simulating those of jungle warfare. Volunteers were first exposed to the bites of infected mosquitoes. They were then injected with adrenaline or insulin, put half-naked into, and kept immobile in, a refrigerator at −9°C for one hour or 'worked or exercised in tropical climate at the hottest time of the year to a point verging on physical exhaustion'. Some were 'taken over hills for 6–10

[1] Material for this section is drawn substantially from WHO Model Prescribing Information. Drugs used in parasitic diseases. World Health Organization, Geneva 1990. We are very grateful to the World Health Organization for their permission to use this source. DRL, PNB.
[2] Charles Louis Alphonse Laveran (1845–1922), Professor of Medicine, Paris (France); Nobel prize winner.

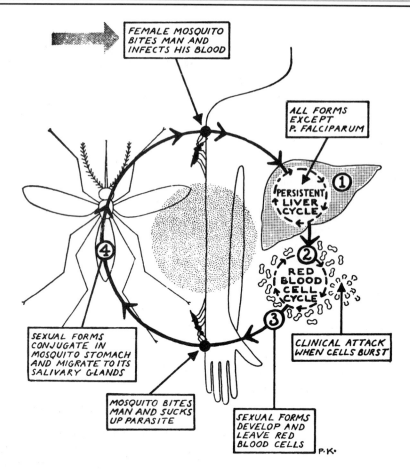

Fig. 13.1 Life cycle of the malaria parasite. The numbers are referred to in the text

miles, induced to swim against a stream until they were tired out, and were then walked back over the hills at as fast a pace as possible by a specially trained sergeant major'. Others marched 80–85 miles over mountains in 3 days or were put into a decompression chamber. Mepacrine was an effective prophylactic under all these conditions.[3]

Since this time, numerous antimalarial drugs have been made, and there is a choice of remedies.

Life cycle of malaria parasite and sites of drug action (Fig. 13.1)

The principal features of the life cycle of the malaria parasite must be known in order to understand its therapy. Female anopheles mosquitoes require a blood meal for egg production and in the process of feeding they inject salivary fluid containing sporozoites into humans. Since no drugs are effective against sporozoites, *infection* with the malaria parasite cannot be prevented.

Hepatic cycle (site 1 in Fig. 13.1)

Sporozoites enter liver cells where they develop into schizonts which form large numbers of merozoites which, usually after 5–16 days but sometimes after months or years, are released into the circulation. *Plasmodium falciparum* is an exception in that it has no persistent hepatic cycle. Primaquine, proguanil and tetracyclines (*tissue schizontocides*) act at this site and are used for:

---

[3] Fairley N H. Trans Roy Soc Trop Med Hyg 1945; 38: 311.

- *Radical cure*, i.e. an attack on persisting hepatic forms (hypnozoites, i.e. sleeping) once the parasite has been cleared from the blood; this is most effectively accomplished with primaquine; proguanil is only weakly effective.
- *Preventing* the hepatic cycle from becoming established. This is also called causal prophylaxis. Primaquine is too toxic for prolonged use; proguanil is weakly effective. Doxycycline may be used short-term.

Erythrocyte cycle (site 2 in Fig. 13.1)

Merozoites enter red cells where they develop into schizonts which form more merozoites which are released when the cells burst giving rise to the features of the clinical attack. The merozoites re-enter red cells and the cycle is repeated. Chloroquine, quinine, mefloquine, proguanil, pyrimethamine, and tetracyclines (*blood schizontocides*) kill the asexual forms. Drugs which act on this stage in the cycle of the parasite may be used for:

- *Treatment* of acute attacks of malaria.
- *Prevention* of attacks by early destruction of the erythrocytic forms. This is called suppressive prophylaxis.

Sexual forms (site 3 in Fig. 13.1)

Some merozoites differentiate into male and female gametocytes in the erythrocytes and can only develop further if they are ingested by a mosquito where they form sporozoites (site 4 in Fig. 13.1) and complete the transmission cycle.

Quinine, mefloquine, chloroquine and primaquine (gametocytocides) act on sexual forms and prevent *transmission* of the infection because the patient becomes non-infective and the parasite fails to develop in the mosquito (site 4 in the diagram).

In summary, drugs may be selected for:

- Treatment of clinical attacks
- Prevention of clinical attacks
- Radical cure.

Drugs used to treat malaria, and their principal actions are classified in Table 13.3.

Table 13.3 Antimalarial drugs and their locus of action

Drug	Biological activity	
	Blood schizontocide	Tissue schizontocide
4-Aminoquinolone		
chloroquine	++	0
Arylaminoalcohols		
quinine	++	0
mefloquine	++	0
Antimetabolites		
proguanil	+	+
pyrimethamine	+	0
sulfadoxine	+	0
dapsone	+	0
Antibiotics		
tetracycline	+	+
doxycycline	+	+
minocycline	+	+
8-Aminoquinolone		
primaquine	0	+

Drug-resistant malaria

Drug-resistant parasites constitute a persistent problem. *Plasmodium falciparum* is now resistant to chloroquine in many parts of the world. Areas of *high risk* for resistant parasites include Sub-Saharan Africa, Latin America, Oceania (Papua New Guinea, Solomon Islands, Vanuatu) and some parts of South-East Asia. The physician who is not familiar with the resistance pattern in the locality from which patients have come or to which they are going, is well advised to check the current position.

Chemotherapy of an acute attack of malaria[4]

Successful management demands attention to the following points of principle:

- Whenever possible, the diagnosis should be confirmed before treatment by examination of blood smears.

---

[4] Treatment regimens vary in detail; those quoted here for benign and falciparum malaria accord with the recommendations in the British National Formulary 1991.

- Drugs used to treat *Plasmodium falciparum* malaria must always be selected with regard to the prevalence of local patterns of drug resistance.
- Patients should be supervised to ensure they swallow the prescribed tablets. If they are vomited, the same dose must immediately be readministered.
- Patients not at risk of reinfection should be re-examined several weeks after treatment for signs of recrudescence which may result from inadequate chemotherapy or survival of persistent hepatic forms.

Benign malaria

This is usually due to *Plasmodium vivax* or, less commonly, *Plasmodium ovale* or *Plasmodium malariae*; the drug of choice is *chloroquine*, which should be given by mouth as follows:

- initial dose: 600 mg (base)[5], then 300 mg as a single dose 6–8 h later
- second day, 300 mg as a single dose
- third day, 300 mg as a single dose.

The total dose of chloroquine base over 3 days should be 25–30 mg/kg. This is sufficient for *P. malariae* infection but, for *P. vivax* and *P. ovale*, eradication of the hepatic parasites is necessary to prevent relapse, by:

- primaquine, 15 mg/d for 14–21 days started after the chloroquine course has been completed.

Falciparum malaria

P. falciparum is now resistant to chloroquine in most parts of the world and it should not be used.

The regimen depends on the condition of the patient.

1. *If the patient can swallow* and there are no serious complications such as impairment of consciousness, treatment may be either with *quinine* or *mefloquine* as follows:

   a. A *quinine salt*[6] 600 mg × 8 h by mouth for 7 days is followed by *pyrimethamine* plus *sulfadoxine* (Fansidar) 3 tablets as a single dose. Where there is Fansidar resistance, *tetracycline* 250 mg × 6 h, should be given *concurrently* with the quinine for 7 days.

This additional therapy is necessary as quinine alone tends to be associated with a higher rate of relapse.

   b. Mefloquine 20 mg/kg (base) by mouth may be given as 2 divided doses 6–8 h apart; it is not necessary to add Fansidar or tetracycline.

2. *Seriously ill* patients should be treated with a quinine salt 20 mg/kg as a loading dose[7] (maximum 1.4 g) infused i.v. over 4 h, followed 8 h later by a maintenance infusion of 10 mg/kg (maximum 700 mg) infused over 4 h, every 8 h,[8] until the patient can swallow tablets to complete the 7-day course. Fansidar should be given subsequently, or tetracycline concurrently, as above.

Chemoprophylaxis of malaria

Because of drug resistance, no single widely available regimen offers assured protection to everybody, but the following approaches apply:

- Prophylaxis requires that there be aqeduate concentration of drug in the blood when the first infected mosquito bites. This can be achieved within hours using a priming dose as in acute malaria if necessary, but prudence counsels that subjects become accustomed to the idea of prophylaxis by commencing a week or at least 1 or 2 days before entering a risk area. That a week

---

[5] The active component of many drugs, whether acid or base, is relatively insoluble and may present a problem in formulation. This is overcome by adding an acid to a base or vice versa and the weight of the salt differs according to the acid or base component, i.e. chloroquine base 150 mg ≡ chloroquine sulphate 200 mg ≡ chloroquine phosphate 250 mg (approximately). Where there may be variation, therefore, the amount of drug prescribed is expressed as the weight of the *active* component, in the case of chloroquine, the base.

[6] Acceptable as quinine hydrochloride, dihydrochloride or sulphate, but not quinine bisulphate which contains less quinine.
[7] The loading dose should *not* be given if the patient has received quinine, quinidine, mefloquine or possibly chloroquine in the previous 12–24 h.
[8] Reduced to 5–7 mg/kg if the infusion lasts for >72 h.

is necessary 'to get the blood concentration up' is a pharmacokinetic misconception. Prophylaxis should continue for 6 weeks after leaving an endemic area to kill parasites that are acquired about the time of departure, are still incubating in the liver and will develop into the erythrocyte phase.

• Where the risk of exposure to malaria is low the following are satisfactory:

chloroquine 300 mg (as base) once weekly,
or
proguanil hydrochloride 200 mg once daily.

• Where the risk of exposure to malaria is variable or high give:

chloroquine 300 mg (base) once weekly
and
proguanil hydrochloride 200 mg once daily.

• Where multiple-drug resistance is reported, mefloquine and doxycycline have been used but more information is required about the clinical performance of both drugs.

• Many travellers at risk of exposure to *P. falciparum*, resistant to both chloroquine and proguanil, need to rely primarily on protection against mosquito bites and prompt treatment should fever occur.

• Approaches to prophylaxis are maintained under constant review by the World Health Organization which publishes an annually-revised booklet 'Vaccination Certificate Requirements and Health Advice for International Travel'; the British National Formulary, issued 6-monthly, contains recommendations that apply particularly to UK residents. These or other appropriate sources ought to be consulted before specific advice is given.

• *Naturally acquired immunity* offers the most reliable protection for people living permanently in endemic areas (below). Repeated attacks of malaria confer partial immunity and the disease often becomes no more than an occasional inconvenience. Vaccines to confer active immunity are under development.

The *partially immune* should as a rule not take a prophylactic. The reasoning is that they will slowly lose their immunity because of the resulting absence of the red cell cycle which is needed to sustain immunity; should they then cease to use the prophylactic they are left highly vulnerable to the disease. There are however **exceptions** to this general advice and the partially immune may *or* should use a prophylactic:

1. if it is virtually certain that they will never abandon its use;
2. if they go to another malarial area where the strains of parasite may differ;
3. during the last few months of pregnancy in areas where *P. falciparum* is prevalent, to avert the risk of miscarriage.

Antimalarial drugs and pregnancy

Women living in endemic areas in which *P. falciparum* remains sensitive to chloroquine should take chloroquine prophylactically throughout pregnancy. It may also be used in full dose to treat chloroquine-sensitive infections. Proguanil can also be safely taken during pregnancy. Quinine is the only widely available drug that is acceptable as suitable for treating chloroquine-resistant infections during pregnancy. Mefloquine is teratogenic in animals and should not be used during pregnancy and for 3 months after.

Notes on individual antimalarial drugs

Chloroquine

Chloroquine is concentrated within parasitised red cells and complexes with plasmodial DNA. It is active against the blood forms and also the gametocytes (formed in the mosquito) of *P. vivax*, *P. ovale* and *P. malariae*; it is effective against the blood parasites of some strains of *P. falciparum* and also its immature gametocytes. Chloroquine is readily absorbed from the gut and is concentrated several-fold in various tissues, e.g. liver, spleen, heart, kidney, cornea and retina; the $t_\frac{1}{2}$ of 50 days reflects slow release from these sites. A priming dose is used in order to achieve adequate free plasma concentration (see acute malaria, above). Chloroquine is mainly inactivated by metabolism but about one-quarter is excreted unchanged in the urine.

Adverse effects are infrequent at doses normally used for malaria treatment and prophylaxis, but are more common with the higher or prolonged doses given for resistant malaria or for rheumatoid arthritis or lupus erythematosus (see index).

Corneal deposits of chloroquine may be asymptomatic or may cause halos around lights or photophobia. These are not a threat to vision and reverse when the drug is stopped. But retinal toxicity is more serious and may be irreversible. Hyperpigmentation of the retina may be seen and the functional defect can take the form of scotomas, photophobia, defective colour vision and decreased visual acuity resulting, in the extreme case, in blindness.

Other reactions include pruritus, which may be intolerable and is common in Africans, headaches, gastrointestinal disturbance, precipitation of acute intermittent porphyria in susceptible individuals, mental disturbances and interference with cardiac rhythm, the latter especially if the drug is given intravenously in high dose (it has a quinidine-like action). Overdose causes pulmonary oedema, convulsions, cardiac dysrhythmias and coma; as little as 50 mg/kg can be fatal. Supportive therapy including early mechanical ventilation, diazepam for convulsions, and other symptomatic treatment are required.

Quinine

Quinine can bind to plasmodial DNA to prevent protein synthesis but its exact mode of action remains uncertain. It is used to treat *P. falciparum* malaria in areas of multiple-drug-resistant *P. falciparum*. Apart from its antiplasmodial effect, quinine is used for myotonia and muscle cramps because it prolongs the muscle refractory period. Dilute solutions of quinine are included in tonics and aperitifs because of its bitter taste.

Quinine is well absorbed from the alimentary tract and is almost completely metabolised in the liver ($t_\frac{1}{2}$ 14 h).

Adverse effects include tinnitus, diminished auditory acuity, headache, blurred vision, nausea and diarrhoea (common to quinine, quinidine, salicylates and called cinchonism). Idiosyncratic reactions are uncommon but pruritus, urticaria and rashes occur. Hypoglycaemia may be significant when quinine is given by i.v. infusion and supplementary glucose may be required.

When large amounts are taken, e.g. to induce abortion or in attempted suicide, ocular disturbances, notably constriction of the visual fields may occur, and even complete blindness, the onset of which may be very sudden. Vomiting, abdominal pain and diarrhoea result from local irritation of the gastrointestinal tract. Quinidine-like effects include hypotension, disturbance of atrioventricular conduction and cardiac arrest. Emesis or gastric lavage should be undertaken and activated charcoal given. Supportive measures are employed thereafter as no specific therapy has proven benefit.

Quinidine, the D-isomer of quinine, has antimalarial activity, but is used mainly as a cardiac antidysrhythmic.

Mefloquine

Mefloquine is similar in several respects to quinine although it does not intercalate with plasmodial DNA. It is used to treat acute attacks of malaria due to multiple-drug-resistant strains of *P. falciparum*, and for prophylaxis of travellers to areas where multiple-drug-resistant strains of *P. falciparum* are prevalent. Mefloquine is rapidly absorbed from the gastrointestinal tract and its action is terminated by metabolism ($t_\frac{1}{2}$ 22 days). Avoid in hepatic or renal impairment.

Adverse effects include nausea, dizziness, disturbance of balance, vomiting, abdominal pain, diarrhoea and loss of appetite. More rarely, hallucinations, seizures and psychoses occur. Mefloquine should be avoided in patients taking β-adrenoceptor and calcium channel antagonists for it causes sinus bradycardia; quinine can potentiate these and other dose-related effects of mefloquine. Use of mefloquine is contraindicated in those whose activities require fine coordination or spatial performance, e.g. airline crews.

Proguanil (chloroguanide)

Proguanil inhibits dihydrofolate reductase which converts folic to folinic acid, deficiency of which results in inhibition of plasmodial cell division. Plasmodia, like some bacteria and unlike humans, cannot make use of preformed folic acid. Pyrimethamine and trimethoprim, which share this mode of action, are collectively known as the 'antifols'. Their plasmodicidal action is markedly enhanced by combination with sulphonamides or sulphones because there is inhibition of sequential steps in folate synthesis (see also co-trimoxazole, p. 169).

Proguanil (t_2^1 14 h) is moderately well absorbed from the gut and is excreted in the urine either unchanged or as an active metabolite. Being little stored in the tissues, proguanil must be used daily when given for prophylaxis, its main use, particularly in pregnant women and non-immune individuals. In prophylactic doses, it is well tolerated.

Pyrimethamine/sulfadoxine (Fansidar)

Pyrimethamine (t_2^1 4 days) is seldom used alone; it is combined with sulfadoxine (t_2^1 8 days) to act synergistically to inhibit folic acid metabolism (see 'antifols', above); both drugs are excreted in the urine, pyrimethamine partly as metabolites. The combination is used to treat acute attacks of malaria caused by susceptible strains of *P. falciparum*; a single dose of pyrimethamine 75 mg plus sulfadoxine 1.5 g (3 tablets) usually suffices.

Adverse effects to pyrimethamine include anorexia, abdominal cramps, vomiting, ataxia, tremor, seizures and megaloblastic anaemia. Suphonamide-induced allergic reactions can be severe, e.g. erythema multiforme, Stevens–Johnson syndrome and toxic epidermal necrolysis. Because of its 'antifol' action the combination should not be used by pregnant women.

Primaquine

Primaquine interferes with plasmodial mitochondrial function. It is used to eliminate the hepatic forms of *P. vivax* and *P. ovale* after standard chloroquine therapy when the risk of subsequent re-exposure is absent or slight. Primaquine is well absorbed from the gastrointestinal tract, is only moderately concentrated in the tissues and is rapidly metabolised (t_2^1 6 h).

Adverse effects include anorexia, nausea, abdominal cramps, methaemoglobinaemia and haemolytic anaemia especially in patients with genetic deficiency of erythrocyte glucose-6-phosphate dehydrogenase. In such persons, the risk of haemolytic anaemia is greatly reduced by giving primaquine at weekly intervals for 8 weeks.

AMOEBIASIS

Infection occurs when mature cysts are ingested and pass into the colon where they divide into trophozoites; these forms either enter the tissues or re-form cysts. Amoebiasis occurs in two forms, both of which need treatment.

- *Bowel lumen amoebiasis* is asymptomatic and trophozoites (non-infective) and cysts (infective) are passed into the faeces. Treatment is directed at eradicating cysts with a luminal amoebicide; diloxanide is the most widely used.
- *Tissue-invading amoebiasis* gives rise to dysentery, hepatic amoebiasis and liver abscess. A systemically-active drug (tissue amoebicide) effective against trophozoites must be used, e.g. metronidazole, tinidazole. Parenteral forms of these are available for patients too ill to take drugs by mouth. In severe cases of amoebic dysentery, tetracycline lessens the risk of opportunistic infection, perforation and peritonitis when it is given in addition to the systemic amoebicide.

Treatment with tissue amoebicides should always be followed by a course of a luminal amoebicide to eradicate the source of the infection.

Dehydroemetine (from ipecacuanha) is less toxic than the parent emetine; it is claimed by some authorities to be the most effective tissue amoebicide. It is reserved for dangerously-ill patients, but these are more likely to be vulnerable to its cardiotoxic effects. When dehydroemetine is used to treat amoebic liver abscess, chloroquine should also be given.

The drug treatment of other protozoal infections is summarised in Table 13.4.

Notes on some drugs for protozoal infections

Benznidazole is rapidly absorbed from the alimentary tract. Adverse effects include rashes which, if severe and accompanied by fever and purpura, are reason to stop the drug. Peripheral neuritis, leucopenia and agranulocytosis also occur.

Table 13.4 Drugs for some protozoal infections

Infection	Comment
Giardiasis	*Metronidazole, tinidazole* or *mepacrine*; family and institutional contacts should also be treated.
Leishmaniasis	
visceral	*Sodium stibogluconate* or *meglumine antimoniate*; resistant cases may benefit from combining antimonials with *allopurinol, pentamidine* or *amphotericin.*
cutaneous	Mild lesions heal spontaneously; *antimonials* may be injected intralesionally.
Pneumocystosis (*Pneumocystis carinii*)	*Sulphamethoxazole/trimethoprim* in high dose; intolerant or resistant cases may benefit from *pentamidine.*
Toxoplasmosis	*Pyrimethamine/sulphadiazine* for chorioretinitis, and active toxoplasmosis in immunodeficient patients; *folinic acid* is used to counteract the inevitable megaloblastic anaemia. *Spiramycin* for primary toxoplasmosis in pregnant women.
Trichomoniasis	*Metronidazole, tinidazole* or *nimorazole* are effective.
Trypanosomiasis	
African	*Pentamidine* and *suramin* are effective during the early stages but are ineffective for the later neurological manifestations for which *melarsoprol* should be used, or *eflornithine,* or *nifurtimox.*
American	*Benznidazole* or *nifurtimox* are effective in the early stages.

Diloxanide may cause troublesome flatulence, and pruritus and urticaria may occur.

Dehydroemetine is less toxic than the parent emetine but adverse effects include pain at the site of injection, weakness and muscular pain, hypotension, praecordial pain and cardiac dysrhythmias.

Sodium stibogluconate is an organic pentavalent antimony compound; it may cause anorexia, vomiting, coughing and substernal pain.

Meglumine antimoniate is similar.

Pentamidine must be administered parenterally as it is unreliably absorbed from the gastrointestinal tract; it does not enter the CSF. It frequently causes nephrotoxicity, which is reversible; acute hypotension and syncope are common after rapid i.v. injection. Pancreatic damage may cause hypoglycaemia due to insulin release.

Melarsoprol is an organic arsenical compound. Adverse effects include encephalopathy, myocardial damage, proteinuria and hypertension.

Mepacrine was formerly used as an antimalarial; it may cause gastrointestinal upset, occasional acute toxic psychosis, hepatitis and aplastic anaemia.

Suramin does not cross the blood–brain barrier; it forms stable complexes with plasma protein and is detectable in urine for up to 3 months after the last injection. It may cause tiredness, anorexia, malaise, polyuria, thirst and tenderness of the palms and soles.

Nifurtimox. Adverse effects include: anorexia, nausea, vomiting, gastric pain, insomnia, headache, vertigo, excitability, myalgia, arthralgia and convulsions. Peripheral neuropathy may necessitate stopping treatment.

CHEMOTHERAPY OF HELMINTHIC INFECTIONS

Helminths have complex life-cycles, special knowledge of which is required by those who treat infections. Table 13.5 will suffice here. Drug resistance has not so far proved to be a clinical problem, though it has occurred in animals on continuous chemoprophylaxis.

Table 13.5 Drugs for helminthic infections

Infection	Drug	Comment
Cestodes (tapeworms)		
Beef tapeworm *Taenia saginata*	niclosamide or praziquantel	Praziquantel cures with single dose
Pork tapeworm *Taenia solium*	niclosamide or praziquantel	
Cysticercosis *Taenia solium*	praziquantel	Treat in hospital as dying and disintegrating cysts may cause cerebral oedema
Fish tapeworm *Diphyllobothrium latum*	niclosamide or praziquantel	
Hydatid disease *Echinococcus granulosus*	mebendazole or albendazole	Surgery for operable cyst disease
Nematodes (intestinal)		
Ascariasis *Ascaris lumbricoides*	pyrantel or levamisole	Piperazine is effective but less well tolerated. Broad spectrum anthelminthics (mebendazole may be used where nematode infection is endemic)
Hookworm *Ancylostoma duodenale* *Necator americanus*	mebendazole, albendazole, bephenium or pyrantel	Anaemic patients require iron. Pyrantel cures with single dose
Stronglyoidiasis *Strongyloides stercoralis*	albendazole	Thiabendazole is effective but causes nausea
Threadworm (pinworm) *Enterobius vermicularis*	mebendazole, albendazole piperazine or pyrantel	
Whipworm *Trichuris trichiuria*	thiabendazole	
Nematodes (tissue)		
Cutaneous larva migrans *Ancylostoma braziliense* *Ancylostoma caninum*	thiabendazole	Calamine lotion for symptomatic relief
Guinea worm *Dracunculus medinensis*	metronidazole	Rapid symptom relief
Trichinellosis *Trichinella spiralis*	mebendazole, albendazole or pyrantel	Prednisolone may be needed to suppress allergic and inflammatory symptoms
Visceral larva migrans *Toxocara canis* *Toxocara cati*	diethylcarbamazine	Progressive escalation of dose lessens allergic reactions to dying larvae; prednisolone suppresses inflammatory response in ophthalmic disease
Lymphatic filariasis *Wuchereria bancrofti* *Brugia malayi* *Brugia timori*	diethylcarbamazine	Destruction of microfilaria may cause an immunological reaction (see below)
Onchocerciasis (river blindness) *Onchocerca volvulus*	ivermectin	Cures with single dose. Suppressive treatment; a single annual dose prevents significant complications
Schistosomiasis		
Intestinal *Schistosoma mansoni* *Schistosoma japonicum*	praziquantel	Oxamniquine only for Schistosoma mansoni. Metriphonate only for Schistosoma haematobium

Table 13.5 (Cont'd)

Infection	Drug	Comment
Urinary *Schistosoma haematobium*	praziquantel	
Flukes		
Intestinal) Lung) Liver)	praziquantel	

Notes on drugs for helminth infections

Diethylcarbamazine kills both microfilaria and adult worms. Fever, headache, anorexia, malaise, urticaria, vomiting and asthmatic attacks following the first dose are due to products of destruction of the parasite.

Ivermectin may cause immediate reactions due to the death of the microfilaria (see diethylcarbamazine). It can be effective in a single dose.

Levamisole paralyses the musculature of sensitive nematodes which, unable to maintain their anchorage, are expelled by normal peristalsis. It may cause abdominal pain, nausea, vomiting, headache and dizziness.

Mebendazole blocks glucose uptake by nematodes. Mild gastrointestinal discomfort may be caused. Albendazole is similar.

Metriphonate is an organophosphorus anticholinesterase compound that was originally used as an insecticide. Adverse effects include abdominal pain, nausea, vomiting, diarrhoea, headache and vertigo.

Niclosamide blocks glucose uptake by intestinal tapeworms. It may cause mild gastrointestinal symptoms.

Oxamniquine may cause headache, vomiting, diarrhoea, hallucinations and excitation.

Piperazine may cause hypersensitivity reactions, neurological symptoms and may precipitate epilepsy.

Praziquantel kills both adult worms and larvae. It is extensively metabolised. It may cause nausea, headache, dizziness and drowsiness; it cures with a single dose (or divided doses in one day).

Pyrantel depolarises neuromuscular junctions of susceptible nematodes which are expelled in the faeces. It cures with a single dose. It may induce gastrointestinal disturbance, headache, dizziness, drowsiness and insomnia.

Thiabendazole inhibits cellular enzymes of susceptible helminths. Gastrointestinal, neurological and hypersensitivity reactions, and crystalluria may be induced.

GUIDE TO FURTHER READING

Breckenridge A 1989 Risks and benefits of prophylactic antimalarial drugs. British Medical Journal 299: 1057

Bruce-Chwatt L J 1988 Three hundred and fifty years of the Peruvian fever bark. British Medical Journal 296: 1486

Crumpacker C S 1989 Molecular targets of antiviral therapy. New England Journal of Medicine 321: 163

Davey P G 1990 New antiviral and antifungal drugs. British Medical Journal 300: 793

Douglas R G Jr 1990 Prophylaxis and treatment of influenza. New England Journal of Medicine 322: 443

Editorial 1988 Urinary tract candidosis. Lancet 2: 1000

Editorial 1989 Ascariasis. Lancet 1: 997

Hirsch M S, Schooley R T 1989 Resistance to antiviral drugs: the end of innocence. New England Journal of Medicine 320: 313

Sonino N 1987 The use of ketoconazole as an inhibitor of steroid production. New England Journal of Medicine 317: 812

14

Arthritis and anti-inflammatory drugs

SYNOPSIS

Everyone has personal experience of inflammation and pain and there are many long-term sufferers from rheumatoid arthritis and osteoarthritis. The processes that underlie the phenomenon of inflammation are now better understood, and so are the modes of action of drugs that are used to treat it.

- Inflammation
- NSAIDs and their effects
- Classification of NSAIDs
- Drug treatment of rheumatoid disease
- Drugs and gout

INFLAMMATION

The classic signs of inflammation have long been recognised; the tissues become *red, swollen, tender* or *painful*, there is local heat and the patient may be febrile. At a microscopic level the capillaries become more permeable and fluid and other elements from the blood leak into the tissue spaces, leucocytes and other phagocytic cells migrate into the area, and rupture of cell lysosomes releases lytic enzymes into the tissues.

The inflammatory response in rheumatoid arthritis is manifested by an acute inflammatory exudate of neutrophil leucocytes into the synovial space and chronic inflammation of the synovial tissues. The former appears to involve an antigen–antibody interaction with complement; leucocytes are attracted into the synovial space to phagocytose the antigen-antibody-complement complexes and in doing so they liberate lysosomal enzymes that damage tissues including cartilage. Macrophages in the hypertrophied synovial tissue are stimulated to produce proteases and collagenases which contribute further to the destruction of collagen and bone.

Pharmacological interest in inflammation was stimulated by the discovery that the process is accompanied by the local liberation of chemical mediators that include histamine, 5-hydroxytryptamine, bradykinin and *eicosanoids*. The latter comprise a group of unsaturated fatty acids all with a 20-carbon structure[1] which are short-lived,

---

[1] The Greek word for 20 is *eicosa*, hence the term eicosanoid.

extremely potent and formed in almost every tissue in the body. Individual mediators differ in their importance to various types of inflammation; e.g. histamine, is necessary for the type of response seen in urticaria but not that of rheumatoid arthritis and H_1-receptor antihistamines are effective in the former but not in the latter.

Eicosanoids however, are involved in most types of inflammation and it is on manipulation of their biosynthesis that most present anti-inflammatory therapy is based. Their biosynthetic paths are shown in Figure 14.1.

The following points about Figure 14.1 are relevant:

● Arachidonic acid is mainly stored in phospholipids of cell walls, from which it is mobilised largely by the action of phospholipase A. Corticosteroids prevent the formation of arachidonic acid by inducing the synthesis of an inhibitory polypeptide called lipocortin; thus by inhibiting the subsequent formation of both prostaglandins and leukotrienes they exert a powerful anti-inflammatory effect.

● Arachidonic acid is further metabolised:

1. by cyclo-oxygenase, which changes the linear fatty acids into the cyclical structures of the *prostaglandins.* Evidence that various prostaglandins are components of inflammation includes the following: minute quantities of prostaglandin E_2 (PG E_2) and prostacyclin (PG I_2) cause erythema and increase local blood flow; PG E_2 and PG $F_{2\alpha}$ cause intense local pain when given i.m. or s.c. to induce abortion; PG E_1 infused subdermally with histamine causes itching; PG E_2 is associated with the production of fever. *Nonsteroidal anti-inflammatory drugs (NSAIDs) exert their anti-inflammatory effects by inhibiting cyclo-oxygenase* (prostaglandin synthase). The same inhibition permits their effects on platelets (see p. 487).

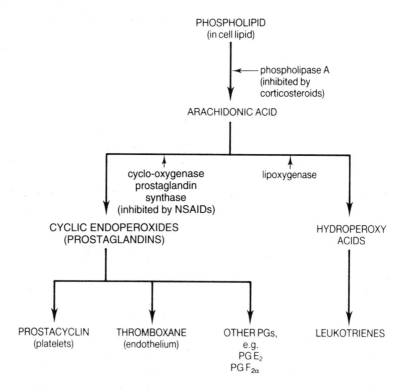

Fig. 14.1 Biosynthetic paths of eicosanoids (see text for description)

Synthetic analogues of prostaglandins have found, or are finding, uses in medicine.

PG I_2: *epoprostenol* (inhibits platelet aggregation, used for extracorporeal circulation), *iloprost, ciprostene* (peripheral vascular disease, Raynaud's disease).

PG E_1: *alprostadil* (used to maintain the patency of the ductus arteriosus in neonates with congenital heart defects), *misoprostol* (prophylaxis of peptic ulcer associated with NSAIDs), *gemeprost* (used as pessaries to soften the uterine cervix and dilate the cervical canal prior to vacuum aspiration for termination of pregnancy).

PG E_2: *dinoprostone* (used as pessaries to induce labour).

PG $F_{2\alpha}$: *dinoprost* (for induction of labour and termination of pregnancy).

2. by *lipoxygenase* to straight-chain hydroperoxy acids and then to *leukotrienes* which cause increased vascular permeability, vasoconstriction, bronchoconstriction, as well as chemotactic activity for leucocytes (whence their name). Inhibitors of lipoxygenase are being evaluated and are likely to find uses in inflammatory and allergic conditions.

NONSTEROIDAL ANTI-INFLAMMATORY DRUGS (NSAIDs) AND THEIR EFFECTS

Several types of drug influence the inflammatory process or its manifestations and they do so by a variety of actions. They include the adrenal glucocorticoid steroids, immunosuppressive agents, colchicine, chloroquine, penicillamine and gold salts; these drugs are described elsewhere in the chapter. The class of drug described here, of which aspirin is the prototype (nonsteroidal anti-inflammatory drugs), is worthy of separate consideration for its members, although structurally heterogeneous, possess a single common mode of action which is *to block prostaglandin biosynthesis* by cyclo-oxygenase (above). This action is reflected in the range of effects both beneficial and adverse which the individual members share, as follows:

Effects

Analgesia: NSAIDs are effective against pain of mild to moderate intensity. Their maximum efficacy is much lower than that of the opioids but they do not cause dependence (but see analgesic nephropathy).

Anti-inflammatory action: this is useful in several conditions including rheumatoid arthritis, osteoarthritis, musculoskeletal disorders and pericarditis.

Antipyretic action: cytokines, e.g. interleukin-I, produced at sites of inflammation stimulate prostaglandin synthesis in the hypothalamus, and this is blocked by NSAIDs.

Platelet function is reduced because formation of thromboxane is prevented; this action is used to protect against vascular occlusion (see p. 487).

Prolongation of gestation and labour: prostaglandin synthesis by the uterus increases substantially in the hours before parturition. Inhibition of prostaglandin synthesis, e.g. by indomethacin, has been used to prevent premature labour, but it causes transient constriction of the ductus arteriosus in some fetuses. A β_2-adrenoceptor agonist, e.g. salbutamol, is preferred.

Patency of the ductus arteriosus is maintained by prostaglandins and, when the ductus remains patent after birth, an attempt may be made to close it by giving indomethacin, to escape the alternative of surgical ligation.

Primary dysmenorrhoea is associated with the production of large quantities of prostaglandins in the uterus and with uterine hypercontractility; this is the rationale for its treatment with an NSAID, e.g. mefenamic acid.

Gastric or intestinal mucosal damage is the commonest adverse effect of the NSAIDs. Mucosal prostaglandins inhibit acid secretion and further appear to exert a cytoprotective effect by promoting the secretion of mucus and by strengthening resistance of the mucosal barrier to back-diffusion of acid from the gastric lumen to the submucosal tissues where it causes damage. Inhibition of prostaglandin biosynthesis is believed to account for the erosions, ulceration and bleeding caused by NSAIDs; toxicity relates to anti-inflammatory potency, i.e. it is least with paracetamol and greatest with drugs such as indomethacin. Prophylactic use of a prostaglandin analogue, misoprostol, may be justified in some patients with NSAID-induced peptic ulcer. Ulceration and stricture of the small bowel may also be caused by NSAIDs, and in some patients there is occult blood loss, diarrhoea and malabsorption, i.e. a clinical syndrome indistinguishable from Crohn's disease.

Urticaria, severe rhinitis and asthma occur in susceptible individuals, e.g. with nasal polyposis, who are exposed to NSAIDs, notably aspirin; the mechanism may involve inhibition of synthesis of bronchodilator prostaglandins (see index: Pseudo-allergic reactions).

Fluid and electrolyte balance may be disturbed through inhibition of synthesis of the renal prostaglandins which have an important influence in salt and water homeostasis.

Analgesic nephropathy. Mixtures of NSAIDs (rather than single agents) taken repeatedly cause grave and often irreversible renal damage, notably chronic interstitial nephritis, renal papillary necrosis and acute renal failure; these effects appear to be due at least in part to ischaemia through inhibition of formation of locally-produced vasodilator prostaglandins. The condition is most common in people who take high doses over years, e.g. for severe chronic rheumatism and patients with personality disorder. Whilst analgesic nephropathy appears to be associated with long-term abuse of NSAID mixtures, strong evidence that phenacetin was

particularly responsible has rendered this drug obsolete.[2]

Abuse of phenacetin and possibly of paracetamol may also lead to the development of cancer of the renal pelvis and ureters.

Interactions. NSAIDs are involved in certain significant drug interactions. Antihypertensive drugs and diuretics may be rendered less effective because of sodium retention due to NSAIDs. There is increased risk of renal impairment with NSAIDs, e.g. indomethacin, administered with diuretics, e.g. triamterene, and with ACE inhibitors. Renal tubular excretion of the cytotoxic drug methotrexate is impaired by NSAIDs and co-administration may cause toxicity. NSAIDs also delay the excretion of lithium by the kidney and may cause lithium toxicity. All NSAIDs are extensively protein-bound and may transiently increase the anticoagulant effect of warfarin by displacing it from its binding protein, notably azapropazone which also inhibits warfarin metabolism. The risk of bleeding may also be increased by the antiplatelet action, e.g. of aspirin, as well as by gut mucosal damage.

---

[2] Phenacetin abuse and toxicity. Although phenacetin was introduced in 1887, it was not until 1953 that suspicion was aroused that this NSAID might cause renal damage. During the influenza pandemic of 1918 a physician to a big factory in a Swedish town prescribed an antipyretic powder containing phenacetin, phenazone (an NSAID) and caffeine. There was substantial mortality from the epidemic, but survivors thought they felt fitter and reinvigorated during convalescence if they took the powder and they continued to take it after recovery. Consumption increased and many families 'could not think of beginning the day without a powder. Attractively wrapped packages of powder were often given as birthday presents.' The phenacetin consumption of the town was about 10 times as great as in a similar Swedish town. Deaths from renal insufficiency rose in the phenacetin town, but not in the control town, and in the decade of 1952–61 they were more than 3 times as many. An investigation was resisted by the factory workers and there was even an instance of organised burning of a questionnaire on powder-taking. It was eventually discovered that most of those who used the powders did so, not for pain, but to maintain a high working pace, from 'habit', or to counter fatigue (an effect probably due to the caffeine).

Eventually the rising death rate brought home to the consumers the gravity of the affair, something that has yet to be achieved for cigarette smoking or alcohol drinking. Grimlund K. Acta Med Scand 1964; 174: suppl. 405.

CLASSIFICATION OF NSAIDs

Despite the general similarity of actions of the NSAIDs, there are important differences between individual members of the group. These are most readily reflected in their anti-inflammatory effect which provides a basis for their clinical classification into those with:

1. Weak anti-inflammatory effect
   - Paracetamol.
2. Mild to moderate anti-inflammatory effect
   - Propionic acid derivatives: fenbufen, fenoprofen, flurbiprofen, ibuprofen, indoprofen, ketoprofen, naproxen.
   - Fenamic acid derivative: mefenamic acid.
   - Non-acidic drug: nabumetone.
3. Strong anti-inflammatory effect
   - Salicylic acid derivatives: aspirin, benorylate, choline magnesium trisalicylate, diflunisal, salsalate.
   - Pyrazolone derivatives: azapropazone, oxyphenbutazone, phenylbutazone.
   - Acetic acid derivatives: diclofenac, etodolac, indomethacin (indometacin), sulindac, tiaprofenic acid, tolmetin.
   - Oxicam derivatives: piroxicam, tenoxicam.

There is some overlap of the groups since effect also depends on dose but the classification broadly holds true. In the interests of simplification, licence has on occasion been taken in fitting drugs to the above chemical groupings, e.g. azapropazone, etodolac. Some detail on individual drugs follows.

Drug with weak anti-inflammatory effect

Paracetamol (acetaminophen)

This is a popular domestic analgesic and antipyretic for adults and children. Its analgesic therapeutic efficacy is equal to that of aspirin but in therapeutic doses it has no useful antiinflammatory effects, i.e. it inhibits prostaglandin synthesis in the brain but hardly at all in the periphery. Paracetamol (Panadol) is effective in mild to moderate pain such as that of headache or dysmenorrhoea and it is also useful in patients who should avoid aspirin because of gut intolerance, a bleeding tendency or allergy, or because they are aged <12 years.

Pharmakocinetics. Paracetamol ($t_\frac{1}{2}$ 2 h) is well absorbed from the alimentary tract and is inactivated in the liver principally by conjugation as glucuronide and sulphate. Minor metabolites of paracetamol are also formed of which one oxidation product, N-acetyl-p-benzoquinone-imine, is highly reactive chemically. This substance is normally rendered harmless by conjugation with glutathione. But the supply of hepatic glutathione is limited and if the amount of the paracetamol metabolite formed is greater than the glutathione available, then the metabolite is able to oxidise thiol (SH-) groups of key enzymes, which causes cell death. This explains why paracetamol, normally a safe drug, can give rise to hepatic necrosis in overdose. Indeed, severe hepatic damage can result from 10 g (20 tablets), taken in one dose, which is only 2.5 times the recommended maximum daily clinical dose (4.0 g). Patients whose hepatic enzymes are induced as a result of taking drugs or alcohol may be especially at risk in minor overdose as their livers may form more of the toxic metabolite.

The oral dose is 0.5–1 g × 4–6 h to a maximum of 4 g in a day.

Adverse effects with occasional use are few. The drug may rarely cause skin rash and allergy. It is well tolerated by the stomach because the peripheral cyclo-oxygenase inhibitory effect is weak. Long-term daily use may however predispose to chronic renal disease.[3]

Acute paracetamol overdose. The liver is most at risk but acute renal tubular necrosis also occurs, partly in association with fulminant hepatic failure and partly because the kidney also contains the oxidising enzymes that form the toxic metabolite (above). Plasma bilirubin, hepatic enzymes, e.g. aspartate aminotransferase, and prothrombin time, are useful to assess liver

---

[3] Sandler DP, et al. New Engl J Med 1989: 320; 1238.

damage. The clinical signs (jaundice, abdominal pain, hepatic tenderness) do not become apparent for 24–48 h and liver failure, when it occurs, does so between 2 and 7 days of the overdose. It is vital that this delay be remembered for lives can be saved only by effective anticipatory action (see below). The plasma concentration of paracetamol is of predictive value; if it is below 200 mg/l (1.32 mmol/l) at 4 h after ingestion, or below 50 mg/l (0.33 mmol/l) at 12 h, then serious hepatic damage is unlikely.

The general principles for treating drug overdose apply (Ch. 9). If the patient is seen early, activated charcoal by mouth can reduce absorption, but the decision to use it must take into account its capacity to bind an oral antidote (methionine). Hepatic failure should be managed along conventional lines with lactulose, vitamin K, i.v. fluids including glucose. *Specific therapy* is directed at replenishing the store of liver glutathione which combines with and so diminishes the amount of toxic metabolite available to do harm (see above). Glutathione itself cannot be used as it penetrates cells poorly but N-acetylcysteine (NAC) (Parvolex) and methionine are effective as they are precursors for the synthesis of glutathione. NAC is more effective because its conversion into glutathione requires fewer enzymes; also, it is administered by i.v. infusion which is an advantage if the patient is vomiting. Clearly the earlier such therapy is instituted the better. It is most effective if administered within 10 h of the overdose but evidence suggests that treatment after up to 36 h yet provides benefit. Once the liver, and the kidney, are seriously damaged NAC or methionine is ineffective. Therefore:

- in cases in which plasma concentration in relation to time after the overdose indicates likelihood of significant liver damage give NAC i.v. 150 mg/kg in dextrose 5% (200 ml) over 15 min; then 50 mg/kg in dextrose 5% (500 ml) over 4 h; then 100 mg/kg in dextrose 5% (1000 ml) over 16 h, to a total of about 300 mg/kg in 20 h;
- in cases in which significant liver damage appears unlikely give methionine by mouth 2.5 g × 4 h, up to 10 g in total.

A paracetamol-methionine combination (Pameton) has been produced, the methionine content ensuring that hepatic glutathione concentrations are maintained when the drug is used in therapeutic (and over-) dose.

Drugs with mild to moderate anti-inflammatory effect

Propionic acid derivatives

Ibuprofen (Brufen) is typical of the group. It is well absorbed after an oral dose and is inactivated by metabolism; $t_{\frac{1}{2}}$ is 2 h.

Others include fenbufen ($t_{\frac{1}{2}}$ 10 h), fenoprofen ($t_{\frac{1}{2}}$ 3 h), flurbiprofen ($t_{\frac{1}{2}}$ 4 h), ketoprofen ($t_{\frac{1}{2}}$ 1 h) and naproxen ($t_{\frac{1}{2}}$ 14 h). They all have similar properties and are most useful in painful conditions such as mild rheumatoid disease and musculoskeletal disorders. Patients often prefer one or another. Naproxen and fenbufen are suitable for twice-daily dosing.

The main advantage over aspirin is a lower incidence of adverse effects particularly in the gastrointestinal tract, and especially with ibuprofen at low dose. Nevertheless epigastric discomfort, activation of peptic ulcer and bleeding may occur. Other effects include headaches, dizziness, fever and rashes.

Fenamic acid derivative

Mefenamic acid (Ponstan) ($t_{\frac{1}{2}}$ 4 h) is slowly absorbed from the small intestine and is eliminated partly unchanged and partly as metabolites in the urine and faeces. It is used for mild to moderate pain where inflammation is not marked, e.g. muscular, dental and traumatic pain and headache, and also for dysmenorrhoea and menorrhagia due to uterine dysfunction. The principal adverse effects are haemolytic anaemia, upper abdominal discomfort, peptic ulcer and diarrhoea. Elderly patients who take mefenamic acid may develop non-oliguric renal failure especially if they become dehydrated, e.g. by diarrhoea; the drug should be avoided or used with close supervision in the elderly.

Non-acidic drug

Nabumetone is unlike most other NSAIDs in that it is non-acidic, but its major active metabolite is an acid and a potent inhibitor of prostaglandin synthesis. Nabumetone is extensively metabolised in first pass through the liver and the $t_{\frac{1}{2}}$ of the major metabolite is 24 h. In rheumatoid arthritis and osteoarthritis, nabumetone 1000 mg once daily is as effective as aspirin 3600 mg in divided doses, and it is used for these conditions. The commonest adverse effects experienced with it are dyspepsia with or without epigastric pain, diarrhoea and rash.

Drugs with marked anti-inflammatory effect

Aspirin

Aspirin (acetylsalicylic acid) was introduced in 1899 and remains the prototype NSAID; it is by far the commonest form in which salicylate is taken. The bark of the willow (Salix) contains salicin from which salicylic acid may be derived; it was used for fevers in the 18th century as a cheap substitute for imported cinchona (quinine) bark.

Mode of action. Aspirin is rapidly hydrolysed to salicylic acid in the plasma. Both substances are therapeutically active, by inhibiting prostaglandin synthesis, although by different mechanisms. Salicylic acid is highly irritant to the stomach and aspirin or salicylic acid derivatives are used instead; they have similar anti-inflammatory, antipyretic and analgesic effects. This account refers generally to aspirin.

The principal effects of aspirin are:

Anti-inflammatory
Analgesic
Antiplatelet
Antipyretic
On urate excretion
Respiratory stimulant
Metabolic
Hypoprothrombinaemic

- *Anti-inflammatory effect* is marked (see mode of action, above).

- *Analgesic effect* is mild, being less than that of codeine. It seems to be due to both central and peripheral action. Aspirin is most effective against mild pain of somatic as opposed to visceral origin.
- *Antiplatelet effect* follows irreversible inhibition (by acylation) of platelet cyclo-oxygenase and reduced production of thromboxane (see p. 487); the result is prolongation of the bleeding time. This action of aspirin is valuable in occlusive arterial disease.
- *Antipyresis*. Aspirin acts in the hypothalamus to place at a lower level the set point of temperature regulation which is controlled by prostaglandin synthesis (see above). It does not affect temperature raised by exercise or heat and does not lower normal temperature.
- *Urate excretion*. Renal tubular reabsorption of urate is reduced by aspirin (both substances are transported by the same mechanism), but in doses that are too high to be of value in gout. Aspirin antagonises the action of uricosuric drugs which all act by decreasing tubular reabsorption of urate. *Low* doses of aspirin (less than 2 g/day) inhibit urate secretion, causing urate *retention*.
- *Respiratory stimulation* is a characteristic of aspirin intoxication and occurs both directly by stimulation of the respiratory centre and indirectly through increased CO_2 production (see below).
- *Metabolic effects* including increased O_2 consumption and CO_2 production are important and understanding them aids the management of poisoning (see below).
- *Hypoprothrombinaemia* occurs with large doses (>5 g/d) of aspirin. The effect may be due to competition between salicylate and vitamin K, for it is preventable and reversible by vitamin K_1. Severe haemorrhage is rare.

Pharmacokinetics. Aspirin (acetylsalicylic acid) is well absorbed from the stomach and upper intestinal tract; hydrolysis removes the acetyl group, a process that has a $t_{\frac{1}{2}}$ of 15 min, and the resulting salicylate ion is, in turn, inactivated largely by conjugation with glycine. At low therapeutic doses this reaction proceeds by first-order kinetics with a $t_\frac{1}{2}$ of about 4 h but at higher therapeutic doses and in overdose the process becomes progressively saturated, i.e. kinetics become zero-order, the $t_\frac{1}{2}$ can be as much as 20 h, and most of the drug in the body is present as the salicylate. The problem in overdose therefore is the removal of salicylate which is achieved by alkalinising the urine (see below).

A reasonably steady plasma concentration can be maintained if salicylate is given 6-hourly by mouth but if a high dose is given repeatedly there is risk of accumulation to toxic amounts; tinnitus is a useful warning sign.

Uses. Aspirin relieves mild to moderate pain of non-visceral origin, e.g. headache, dysmenorrhoea, osteoarthritis, myalgia. The anti-inflammatory action is valuable for conditions in which an inflammatory reaction is prominent, e.g. rheumatoid disease, Still's disease and acute rheumatic fever. For cardiovascular uses, see p. 488.

Preparations and dosages. There is a plethora of commercial preparations, plain, buffered, soluble, effervescent, enteric-coated, sustained-release. A properly compounded Aspirin Tablet, Dispersible (single dose 300–900 mg) and a reliable enteric-coated preparation will suffice for most patients. Forms made for the purpose, e.g. dispersible, effervescent, should be dissolved in water and drunk.

Salicylic acid derivatives

Benorylate (Benoral) is an ester of aspirin and paracetamol which, being non-ionic and lipid soluble, is well absorbed from the gut; it is also less irritant to the stomach and causes less blood loss from it than does aspirin. When benorylate is hydrolysed in the liver and plasma, paracetamol and aspirin are released.

Diflunisal (Dolobid) is a fluorophenyl derivative of salicylic acid. Its elimination is saturable and the $t_\frac{1}{2}$ may be 5–20 h. Diflunisal compares favourably with aspirin in the treatment of osteoarthritis and it may cause fewer gastric adverse effects, although diarrhoea is more common; it is also uricosuric. There may be cross allergy with aspirin.

Aloxiprin (Palaprin Forte) is a condensation product of aspirin and aluminium hydroxide: it is an alternative to soluble aspirin.

Salsalate (Disalcid) is an ester that is hydrolysed to salicylic acid in the blood.

Methyl salicylate (oil of wintergreen) is too irritant to be used internally. It is used in counter-irritant liniments. Its smell sometimes attracts children; if they drink it, treatment is urgent.

Adverse reactions to aspirin and salicylic acid derivatives

These are in general those described earlier for NSAIDs, but some aspects merit further comment.

- *Gastrointestinal effects.* About 1 in 15 of the population cannot take aspirin without symptoms (heartburn, epigastric distress, vomiting). The characteristic lesion is a superficial gastric erosion and bleeding from this is enhanced by the antiplatelet effect (see above). *Occult blood loss* (usually 5 ml/d above control value of 0.7 ml) occurs in most people taking aspirin long term, sometimes sufficient to cause iron-deficiency anaemia. The site of bleeding is predominantly the stomach and anything that reduces the concentration of aspirin applied to the mucous membrane or increases ionisation, e.g. sodium bicarbonate, (so that it is less lipid-soluble and less will penetrate gastric mucosal cells) decreases the liability to erosion and blood loss. A rapidly dispersing tablet, or one that makes a buffered solution and is then swallowed with much fluid, e.g. Alka-Seltzer, is least likely to cause trouble. Enteric-coated aspirin causes less blood loss, for the small intestine is less affected than the stomach, but absorption is delayed for 6 or more hours, so that this preparation is unsuitable for occasional analgesia, though well suited for long-term medication, as in rheumatoid arthritis.

A history of taking aspirin recently is more common in patients with *overt gastroduodenal haemorrhage*, particularly those with acute erosions. The risk seems to be greatest in those who take aspirin frequently or in large dose but some patients suffer profuse gastric haemorrhage as a result of taking a single dose of aspirin. The latter appears to be an idiosyncratic response, possibly in individuals who have a minor haemostatic abnormality. Any patient with evidence of a mild defect in haemostatis, e.g. prolonged bleeding after teeth extraction, should be advised to treat aspirin with particular caution.

Aspirin is plainly best avoided in patients with disease of the upper gastrointestinal tract, particularly with a history of peptic ulcer, but any proposal that it should be abandoned in favour of newer analgesics ignores the fact that it has been used successfully for decades by the public and the medical profession, despite these effects. Considering that thousands of tons are eaten annually, serious adverse effects from aspirin are uncommon.

- *Salicylism* (the symptoms of too high dose) is expressed as tinnitus and hearing difficulty, dizziness, headache and confusion.
- *Allergy.* Aspirin is a common cause of allergic or pseudo-allergic symptoms and signs. Patients exhibit severe rhinitis, urticaria, angioedema, asthma or shock. Those who already suffer from recurrent urticaria, nasal polyps or asthma are more susceptible.
- *Reye's syndrome.* There is moderately strong evidence that aspirin is a cause of the rare Reye's syndrome (encephalopathy, liver injury) in children and teenagers recovering from febrile viral infections (respiratory, varicella). Paracetamol should be preferred for such febrile illnesses in children under 12 years. Parents should be educated not to use aspirin as most such administration is on their own initiative, not prescribed.

Overdose

The typical clinical picture of moderate overdose (plasma salicylate 500–750 mg/l) consists of nausea, vomiting, epigastric discomfort, tinnitus, deafness, hyperpnoea, headache, sweating, pyrexia, hypokalaemia and restlessness. With a large overdose (plasma salicylate >750 mg/l) these symptoms may be followed by pulmonary oedema, convulsions and coma with severe dehydration and ketosis. Despite the fact that aspirin reduces platelet activity and salicylates cause hypoprothrombinaemia and adverse effects on the stomach, gastric erosions and bleeding are uncommon after salicylate overdose.

Metabolic changes are important and understanding them aids the management of poisoning. As the plasma salicylate concentration rises the following occur:

- *Respiratory alkalosis* develops, directly due to stimulation of the respiratory centre, and indirectly by increased CO_2 production (from increased peripheral O_2 consumption due to uncoupling of oxidative phosphorylation).
- *Blood pH* thus rises, and is compensated by renal loss of bicarbonate which is necessarily accompanied by sodium and potassium ions as well as water; dehydration and hypokalaemia result. The reduction of plasma bicarbonate deprives the body of one of its buffering systems so that it becomes particularly vulnerable to metabolic acidosis.
- *Metabolic acidosis* is the result of several factors including accumulation of lactic and pyruvic acids due to toxic interference with Kreb's cycle enzymes, and stimulation of lipid metabolism causing increased production of ketone bodies. Late toxic respiratory depression may also cause CO_2 retention.

Adults who have taken a single large quantity usually develop a *respiratory alkalosis* but when poisoning is severe a *metabolic acidosis* follows; commonly a mixed acid-base disturbance is found.

Children under 4 years tend not to exhibit the respiratory alkalosis but readily develop severe *metabolic acidosis*, perhaps because poisoning more often occurs during prolonged therapy and the initial phase of alkalosis may not be apparent.

Serial measurements of plasma salicylate are necessary to monitor the course of the overdose, for the concentration may rise during the initial phases.

The general measures described in Chapter 9 apply to management but the following are relevant specifically for salicylate overdose.

- Gastric lavage (or therapeutic emesis with syrup of ipecacuanha in children) is worth undertaking up to 24 h after overdose for tablets may lie as an insoluble mass in the stomach. Activated charcoal is worth giving as it adsorbs both salicylate that has not been absorbed from the gut and also drug that diffuses from the blood into the gut.
- Hypoprothrombinaemia may be treated by giving vitamin K_1 i.v.
- Fluid and electrolyte repair. Correction of dehydration, which can be severe due to sweating, vomiting and overbreathing, is of the first importance. The i.v. route should be used for moderate or severe poisoning. As hypokalaemia is usual and hypoglycaemia is common, dextrose 5% with added potassium will often be indicated.
- Acid-base disturbance. Patients showing alkalosis or mixed alkalosis/acidosis with normal blood pH need no therapy directed to changing the blood acid-base balance but, if hyperventilation and alkalosis cause tetany, calcium gluconate should be given i.v. Sodium bicarbonate is used to correct metabolic acidosis (blood pH < 7.2) and to alkalinise the urine to remove salicylate (below).
- Removal of salicylate from the body by alkalinising the urine is rational (see p. 140). The practical importance of pH is shown by the fact that the amount of salicylate in urine at pH 8 is 4 times that at pH 7. A high plasma salicylate concentration may be halved in about 8 h by this procedure. Maintenance of a high urine flow rate by infusing fluid i.v. assists this process but forcing a diuresis, e.g. with a loop diuretic in high dose, does not improve salicylate clearance; the high pH of the urine is of much greater importance than its volume.

- Haemodialysis or haemoperfusion can be undertaken in specially equipped centres and are indicated when the plasma salicylate exceeds 900 mg/l. Exchange transfusion can be used for children. The decision to use these techniques should not be left until a person is moribund; patients, particularly children, poisoned by aspirin, can die in a few hours.

Pyrazolone derivatives

Azapropazone (Rheumox) has anti-inflammatory, analgesic, antipyretic and uricosuric effects. It is well absorbed from the gut, is mainly excreted unchanged in urine and has a $t_{\frac{1}{2}}$ of 20 h. Azapropazone is used to treat pain and inflammation in rheumatoid disease and other musculoskeletal disorders. Adverse effects are those to be expected of NSAIDs. Azapropazone interferes with the metabolism of phenytoin and enhances the effects of that drug.

Phenylbutazone, because of its toxicity (gastrointestinal, hepatic, renal, bone marrow), is now rarely indicated except to treat ankylosing spondylitis under specialist supervision.

Oxyphenbutazone, which is similar, remains available as an ointment for ocular inflammation, e.g. iridocyclitis.

Acetic acid derivatives

Indomethacin (indometacin) (Indocid) is a highly effective anti-inflammatory, analgesic and antipyretic agent. Absorption from the gut is rapid and almost complete, it is inactivated by metabolism and the $t_{\frac{1}{2}}$ is 6 h. Indomethacin is used to relieve moderate to severe pain and inflammation due to rheumatoid disease, acute musculoskeletal disorders and gout; it is also effective for pain due to pericardial inflammation after myocardial infarction. The oral dose is 25–50 mg × 2–3/d to a maximum of 200 mg/d; a suppository of 100 mg at night is effective for relief of morning stiffness. Adverse effects of indomethacin relate to its strong anti-inflammatory effect and include masking of symptoms and signs of infection. Gastric irritation with ulcer formation, bleeding and perforation occur. Headache is common, often similar to migraine, and is attributed to cerebral oedema; it can be limited by starting at a low dose and increasing only gradually. Vomiting, dizziness and ataxia occur. Indomethacin may aggravate pre-existing renal disease. Thus the drug is best avoided where there is gastroduodenal, renal or central nervous system disease or in the presence of infection; it is not recommended for children. Allergic reactions occur and there is cross-reactivity with aspirin. Indomethacin may cause salt and fluid retention; it reduces the effectiveness of diuretic drugs (and may cause renal failure with triamterene) and counteracts the antihypertensive action of β-adrenoceptor antagonists, possibly by inhibiting renal prostaglandin synthesis.

Sulindac (Clinoril) (t_2^1 7 h) is structurally related to indomethacin. It is a prodrug, i.e. the substance itself is relatively inactive but it is converted into an active sulphide metabolite (t_2^1 18 h) in the body and by the gut flora. Sulindac is used for pain and inflammation in rheumatoid disease, musculoskeletal disorders and in gout. Its anti-inflammatory action is less than that of indomethacin, but so is its gastric and central nervous system toxicity. Adverse effects on the kidney may be less likely as, unusually among the NSAIDs, the active (sulphide) metabolite of sulindac does not inhibit *renal* prostaglandin synthesis.

Diclofenac (Voltarol) (t_2^1 2 h) is used for moderate pain and inflammation due to rheumatoid disease and musculoskeletal disorders. Gastrointestinal and central nervous system and other adverse effects occur in common with other members of this group.

Tolmetin (Tolectin) (t_2^1 1 h) has an anti-inflammatory action that is greater than aspirin but less than indomethacin. It is used to relieve pain and inflammation in rheumatoid disease and musculoskeletal disorders. Allergic (anaphylactic) reactions appear to be more common with tolmetin and may occur in those who are not allergic to aspirin or other NSAIDs.

Etodolac (Lodine) (t_2^1 7 h) for rheumatoid and osteoarthritis appears to be well tolerated.

Ketorolac (t_2^1 5 h) may be given by i.m. injection.

Oxicam derivatives

Piroxicam (Feldene) has an anti-inflammatory action that is approximately equal to that of indomethacin. It is completely absorbed from the gastrointestinal tract and the long t_2^1 (45 h) is partly due to enterohepatic cycling which helps to maintain the plasma concentration. Steady state plasma concentrations appear not to alter significantly with age. Piroxicam is used for rheumatoid disease, musculoskeletal disorders and gout in a dose of 10–30 mg/d in single or divided amounts. Adverse effects are those to be expected with NSAIDs, gastrointestinal and central nervous system complaints being the commonest.

Tenoxicam is similar, except that its t_2^1 of 72 h indicates that steady state will only be reached after at least 2 weeks.

Topical use of NSAIDs

Felbinac (Traxam), a metabolite of fenbufen, and piroxicam (Feldene) are available as gels, and ibuprofen (Proflex) as a cream for topical use on the skin for relief of symptoms caused by soft tissue trauma. The objective is to produce therapeutic local concentrations without (undesirable) systemic effects.

Oxyphenbutazone is used as an ointment for ocular inflammation.

DRUG TREATMENT OF RHEUMATOID DISEASE

Rheumatoid disease affects 1–3% of the population of Europe and North America. Best results are obtained with early treatment, physiotherapy, and drugs.

Drug therapy is used:

● To relieve pain, inflammation and muscle
stiffness with NSAIDs.
● To modify the course of the disease or
induce remission when these measures fail
and there is radiological evidence of
progressive joint destruction.

CHOICE OF DRUGS IN RHEUMATOID ARTHRITIS

● **NSAIDs** should be used first, usually a
propionic acid derivative. The choice of drug
will depend on the amount of pain or
inflammation present and on patient tolerance.
When inflammation is prominent, a NSAID
with potent anti-inflammatory action (and more
risk of adverse effects), e.g. indomethacin or
piroxicam, is appropriate. Local injections of
corticosteroid are valuable for individual joints
that are more severely affected.
● **Second line drugs** should be used when
inflammatory symptoms persist and when
radiological evidence indicates progression of
joint damage. Evidence suggests that these
drugs *slow* the progress of the disease
although they may not reduce the *ultimate*
degree of deformity and disability. There is
now a tendency to employ them earlier,
sometimes within three months of onset.
Gold, penicillamine and *sulphasalazine* appear
to have a similar therapeutic efficacy, but
sulphasalazine is significantly the least toxic;
the *immunosuppressives* are more effective
and generally more toxic; the *antimalarials* are
less effective and less toxic.
● **Systemic corticosteroids** tend to be
reserved for cases with inflammation so
severe that it cannot be controlled by second
line drugs.

Relief of pain and muscle stiffness and suppression of inflammation

NSAIDs improve clinical indices of disease activity, e.g. joint swelling, but have no effect on
laboratory indices, e.g. plasma viscosity, or on its
outcome, e.g. joint destruction. When the disease
is mild, a reasonable course is to start with a
proprionic acid derivative, e.g. ibuprofen,
naproxen, since these drugs are less toxic to the
stomach than those with more prominent anti-
inflammatory action. It may be necessary to try
several within the group to find one which suits
an individual patient; any drug selected should
be used for 1–2 weeks before abandoning it (unless adverse effects are substantial). Paracetamol
may be added if additional analgesia is required.

When inflammation is more severe a NSAID
with more pronounced anti-inflammatory effect
(and more risk of adverse effects) is needed.
Some prefer aspirin (2–6 g/d) but the high dose
needed (just below that which induces tinnitus)
means that gastric intolerance is common. Alternatively, another major anti-inflammatory drug
such as indomethacin or piroxicam may be used.
If nocturnal pain or morning stiffness is a problem, indomethacin given either orally or as a
suppository the night before may benefit because
its duration of action is sufficiently long.

Modification of the disease process

Certain drugs improve both the clinical and
laboratory indices of inflammation, and probably
also the course of the disease, i.e. retard structural damage to joints; these are known as *second
line or disease modifying drugs*. The decision to embark on the treatment with such agents should
be undertaken only by a physician with special
experience of their use. Evidence indicates that
radiographic progression of the disease is slowed.
Gold or penicillamine are probably the most effective agents for preventing progression of the
arthritis, best results being obtained in early
cases. In the event of failure to respond to gold,
penicillamine should be tried and vice versa; 80%
of patients will respond to one or other.

Gold salts

These appear to reduce immune responsiveness
by inhibiting the migration of mononuclear cells
into areas of inflammation; they may also stabilise

lysosomal membranes and thus prevent the release of enzymes that damage cartilage. *Sodium aurothiomalate* by deep i.m. injection or *auranofin* by mouth is most commonly used. The oral form appears to be marginally less effective but causes fewer and less severe adverse reactions.

Distribution of gold is complex; it binds extensively to plasma albumin and is also distributed to inflamed synovium, kidney and liver. After a single dose the $t_{\frac{1}{2}}$ of auranofin is 400 h. Gold is eliminated mainly by the kidney and to a lesser extent in the faeces which it probably enters following biliary excretion. The plan of therapy is gradually to build up the amount of gold in the body to an effective concentration and then to deliver a maintenance dose until the disease becomes inactive. If there is no response within 4 months, it is probably best to change to another treatment.

Gold is used in patients with active, progressive disease, as shown by early deformities or radiological bone changes, in whom anti-inflammatory analgesics have failed and in whom it is wished to avoid beginning an adrenal steroid or to reduce steroid dosage.

Adverse effects occur in about one-third of patients and in some, gold may have to be discontinued. They include pruritus, dermatitis, glossitis and stomatitis, most commonly, and also blood disorders, hepatic and renal damage, peripheral neuritis and encephalopathy. Serious toxicity is rare when observation is careful (monthly blood counts and urinalysis) and the drug stopped at the earliest sign of harm. Any serious effect, or one which does not subside rapidly, should be treated with a chelating agent; dimercaprol is probably preferable to penicillamine.

Penicillamine (Distamine)

The precise mode of action of penicillamine in rheumatoid arthritis is unknown. Its action as a chelator of a number of metals (including gold), is valuable in poisoning (see Ch. 9 and hepatolenticular degeneration). Penicillamine is well absorbed following administration by mouth, then partly metabolised and partly excreted unchanged by the liver. After a single oral dose the

$t_{\frac{1}{2}}$ is 3 h but it is longer when chronic dosing is discontinued, suggesting that the drug is being released from a tissue store. The indications for using penicillamine are as for gold (above).

Adverse effects are frequent and up to one-third of patients may discontinue the drug; it is better tolerated if the dose is raised only at monthly intervals (with satisfactory blood counts and urinalysis). Patients may experience gastrointestinal upset, and dose-related impairment of taste is common. Thrombocytopenia is frequent but resolves when the drug is withdrawn unless it indicates the more serious aplastic anaemia which penicillamine may also cause. Allergic reactions (rashes, fever) tend to occur during the early stages of treatment. Proteinuria, if it is heavy, is a reason for stopping penicillamine for it may herald the development of the nephrotic syndrome.

Captopril (an angiotensin converting enzyme inhibitor) has a structural similarity to penicillamine and is being evaluated for treating rheumatoid disease.

Antimalarials

Antimalarials of the chloroquine group offer an alternative to gold, penicillamine and other immunosuppressive drugs as they are less toxic, but they are also less effective. They appear to stabilise lysosomes and inhibit collagen breakdown.

Chloroquine (see Ch. 13) may achieve a useful response in about 50% of patients after 4 weeks of therapy. It accumulates in many organs, including the eye where it can cause retinal damage that may be irreversible; this is the principal disadvantage to its use in rheumatoid disease which must necessarily be long-term. Serious ocular damage should be avoided if the dose of chloroquine is below 3.5 mg/kg (hydroxychloroquine 6.5 mg/kg) but patients should have an ophthalmological examination before starting, and every 6 months during therapy.

An attempt should be made to withdraw the drug slowly, in a year. Omission of the drug for 3 months every 4 to 6 months (drug holiday) may allow prolonged therapy safely. Hydroxychloroquine is an alternative which may cause fewer adverse effects.

Sulphasalazine

Radiographical evidence indicates that sulphasalazine delays the progression of rheumatoid arthritis, but its mode of action is unclear. Its therapeutic efficacy appears to equal that of gold; the doses necessary to achieve this are greater than those normally used for ulcerative colitis (see p. 539) and adverse effects, notably dyspepsia, can be troublesome. The safety profile of sulphasalazine is well established from experience in inflammatory bowel disease and treatment can be continued indefinitely.

Immunosuppressive drugs

Methotrexate is effective and, in a dose of 7.5 mg once weekly by mouth, is probably tolerated better than other second line agents. *Azathioprine* is as active as gold or penicillamine and like these drugs it can be used for its steroid sparing effect in patients who have received excessive steroid. Marrow suppression may develop and regular blood counts should be performed. Cyclosporin has similar therapeutic efficacy. *Cyclophosphamide* is more effective but carries a greater risk of toxicity and should be reserved for cases resistant to less toxic drugs. Radiographical evidence indicates that cyclophosphamide retards joint destruction.

Immunosuppressives are carcinogenic and the magnitude of this risk, particularly important in younger patients with a long life expectancy, is uncertain; they are also mutagenic and teratogenic so that precautions to avoid reproduction whilst taking the drugs are essential for both sexes.

Adrenal steroids

There is reluctance to start *systemic corticosteroid* for rheumatoid disease because of the danger of adverse effects but this course is justified in some circumstances.

- To provide interim relief of inflammatory symptoms during the weeks that it takes second line drugs to act.
- Spaced single enormous doses (pulse treatment), e.g. methylprednisolone 1 g monthly for 1–3 months, are sometimes used for rapid and sustained relief of flares of the disease.
- In extreme severity, prednisolone 20–40 mg/day, will very effectively suppress inflammation, e.g. with vasculitis or rheumatoid lung, and indeed prednisolone administered over a period of months may actually slow down aggressive (rapidly progressing) disease.
- Where second line drugs have failed or have produced intolerable adverse effects. The object is to reduce inflammation in affected joints at a dose which is sufficiently low to administer with safety over a long period. Usually the total daily maintenance dose should not exceed prednisolone 7.5 mg or its equivalent of other steroids and once-daily administration at 08:00 h may minimise adrenal suppression.

Intra-articular injection of corticosteroid (triamcinolone, hydrocortisone, prednisolone or dexamethasone) is very effective when one joint is more affected than others. Benefit from one injection may last many weeks (shorter in active cases). Aseptic precautions must be extreme, for the steroid will suppress inflammatory response and any introduced infection may spread dramatically. With repetition, enough may be absorbed into the blood to cause adrenal suppression. The placebo effect of intra-articular injection is great. Too frequent resort to corticosteroid injection may actually promote joint damage by removing the protective limitation conferred by pain; such injections in a single joint should not exceed 2 or 3 per year.

Other aspects of the treatment of this disease are important but are outside the scope of this book.

Rheumatic fever

Aspirin is so effective in relieving pain and inflammation in acute rheumatism that failure to respond within 48 h throws doubts on the diagnosis. From their introduction into therapeutics, adrenocortical steroids have also been used; they provide dramatic relief but should be reserved to replace aspirin in patients with severe carditis. Neither aspirin nor adrenal steroids prevents the development of late cardiac complications.

In the acute stage, oral Aspirin Tabs, Dispersible (a soluble form) in a dose of about 100 mg/kg/d should be given. In the adult a plasma salicylate of 250 mg/l is usually effective but in children, concentrations up to 350 mg/l may be required. Dose is adjusted according to the tolerance of the drug and relief of symptoms. In mild cases treatment is continued for 6 weeks.

When there is evidence of carditis (cardiac enlargement or pericarditis), a corticosteroid should be used instead of aspirin since the latter may precipitate cardiac failure. Prednisolone 10–15 mg/d (adult dose) is usually sufficient and specific therapy for cardiac failure may also be necessary.

A 10-day course of benzylpenicillin should be given to kill any streptococci. For prophylaxis see Chapter 12 (Infection of the throat).

Osteoarthritis

A NSAID is used, the choice being appropriate to the amount of pain and inflammation experienced by the patient, and on the tolerance of adverse effects. Evidence suggests that use of *strong* anti-inflammatory drugs may accelerate destruction of some joints, e.g. the hip, by inhibiting the synthesis of vasodilator prostaglandins which are essential for adequate perfusion with blood for the natural repair of joint structures.

There is no general case for using intra-articular corticosteroid in osteoarthritis but local injection of triamcinolone can provide relief for a single periarticular tender spot or for a knee joint that is acutely inflamed.

Anklyosing spondylitis

Indomethacin is effective and may also be needed at night to treat stiffness the next morning. Adrenal steroids are rarely used. Phenylbutazone is very effective, but toxic (see above). The value of radiotherapy is controversial. Physical methods of treatment including active exercises are of the first importance to prevent deformity.

DRUGS AND GOUT

Gout affects about 0.25% of the population of Europe and North America. Drugs are effective in management but some drugs can precipitate the disorder. Patients with gout but no visible tophi have a urate pool that is 2 or 3 times normal and since this exceeds the amount that can be carried in solution in the extracellular fluid, microcrystalline deposits form; patients with tophi have a urate pool that may be 15–26 times normal.

Urate is mainly excreted by the kidney and the following processes are relevant: it is freely filtered by the glomerulus and then reabsorbed from the tubule fluid, and also secreted from the blood into the tubular fluid; the urate that appears in the urine represents the excess of secretion over reabsorption which are both active, energy-requiring processes that can be affected by drugs.

Hyperuricaemia and gout have numerous causes (metabolic, neoplastic, renal disease, idiopathic) but all depend essentially on two processes, namely: underexcretion of urate and overproduction of urate. Drugs may contribute to these processes as follows:

Underexcretion of urate is caused by all diuretics except spironolactone, aspirin (in low dose, see p. 217), ethambutol, pyrazinamide, nicotinic acid, and alcohol (which increases urate synthesis and also causes a rise in blood lactic acid that inhibits tubular secretion of urate).

Overproduction of urate, due to excessive cell destruction releasing nucleic acids, occurs when myeloproliferative or lymphoproliferative disorders are treated by drugs.

Two phenomena are necessary for an attack of gout:

1. Crystals of monosodium urate are deposited

in the joints from hyperuricaemic body fluids.

2. There is a local inflammatory response to the presence of the crystals with phagocytosis (of the crystals).

Drugs that are effective in the management of gout

- *suppress the symptoms* (anti-inflammatory drugs), i.e. indomethacin, azapropazone, diclofenac, naproxen, piroxicam and sulindac; colchicine; adrenal steroids and corticotrophin
- *prevent urate synthesis*, i.e. allopurinol
- *promote elimination of urate* (uricosurics), i.e, probenecid, sulphinpyrazone.

Anti-inflammatory drugs

Except for colchicine, those listed above are described earlier in the chapter or elsewhere.

Colchicine

This is an alkaloid from the autumn crocus (colchicum). It is an antimitotic agent of little use in neoplastic disease, but valuable in gout, in which it relieves pain and inflammation in a few hours. Such rapid relief is considered to confirm the diagnosis because non-gouty arthritis is unaffected, though failure does not prove the patient has not gout. The curious specificity of colchicine in relieving the pain of gout is not fully explained but may be due to interruption of the inflammatory cycle by inhibition of leucocyte migration and metabolic activity in the inflamed area. A similar mechanism operates in the use of colchicine in recurrent hereditary polyserositis (familial mediterranean fever), including amyloid formation.

Colchicine is absorbed from the gut; some is metabolised in the liver and some is excreted unchanged in the bile and reabsorbed from the gut. This enhances its gut toxicity. The $t_{\frac{1}{2}}$ is 1 h.

In acute gout colchicine 1 mg may be given by mouth, followed by 0.5–1 mg 2-hourly until either relief or adverse effects ensue. Benefit is usually felt in 2 or 3 h and is marked within 12 h. The total needed is usually 3–6 mg and it is unwise to exceed 10 mg. Once the effective dose is known, patients can take this total at once when they feel an attack coming on, and then 0.5 mg hourly. Colchicine can prevent acute attacks (but see below).

Adverse effects may be severe, with abdominal pain, vomiting and diarrhoea which may be bloody, and probably due to inhibition of mitosis in the rapidly reproducing cells of the intestinal mucosa. Renal damage can occur, and, rarely, blood disorders. Large doses cause muscular paralysis.

Prevention of uric acid synthesis

Allopurinol (Zyloric) inhibits xanthine oxidase, the enzyme that converts xanthine and hypoxanthine to uric acid. Patients taking allopurinol excrete less uric acid and more xanthine and hypoxanthine in the urine; these compounds are both more readily excreted in renal failure and are more soluble than uric acid so that xanthine stones rarely form.

Allopurinol ($t_{\frac{1}{2}}$ 2 h) is readily absorbed from the gut, it is metabolised in the liver to alloxanthine ($t_{\frac{1}{2}}$ 25 h) which is also a xanthine oxidase inhibitor; it is excreted unchanged and as alloxanthine by the kidney.

Allopurinol is indicated where urate lithiasis has occurred or where tophi are extensive, in blood diseases where there is spontaneous hyperuricaemia, and during treatment of myeloproliferative disorders when cell destruction creates a high urate load. Allopurinol prevents hyperuricaemia due to diuretics. It can be combined with a uricosuric agent. A single daily dose of 300 mg by mouth is usually adequate but up to 600 mg or even more in total may be given in severe cases.

Adverse effects apart from the precipitation of acute gout (below) are rare and include allergies of various kinds: leucopenia, gut upsets, skin rashes and liver damage. Allopurinol prevents the oxidation of the active drug mercaptopurine to an inactive metabolite; if an ordinary dose of mercaptopurine be given to a patient whose gout is being treated with allopurinol, dangerous potentiation occurs.

Uricosurics

Probenecid (Benemid) inhibits the active transport of organic anions across the kidney tubule, preventing both reabsorption from the tubular fluid and secretion into it; inhibition of urate reabsorption increases its excretion in the urine. (Inhibition of tubular secretion of penicillin by probenecid is utilised when high plasma penicillin concentrations must be maintained after a single dose, e.g. in treating gonorrhoea.)

Probenecid is partly metabolised and partly excreted unchanged in the urine. The $t_{\frac{1}{2}}$ depends on dose and varies from 6–12 h.

To prevent gout, probenecid 0.5 g/d is taken by mouth for the first week, rising to 1–2 g/d total. As the initial loss is high, crystals of urate may appear in the urine unless it is maintained at pH 6 or above for the first month of probenecid (or any other uricosuric) administration, e.g. with Potassium Citrate Mixture 12–24 g/day with water or Sodium Bicarbonate Powder 5–10 g/day with water. A high fluid intake (2 l/day) should also be taken to avoid the dangers of mechanical obstruction or stone formation. Probenecid should not be used if there is severe renal impairment: it may be ineffective and may worsen renal damage.

Probenecid causes gastrointestinal upset in a few patients and allergy occasionally. It blocks renal tubular excretion of and prolongs the effect of organic acids including penicillins, cephalosporins, zidovudine, acyclovir, naproxen, indomethacin, methotrexate and sulphonylureas. Its uricosuric effect is blocked by aspirin.

Sulphinpyrazone (Anturan) is structurally related to phenylbutazone and acts like probenecid. It is a potent uricosuric and alkalinisation of the urine and high fluid intake (see above) are necessary at first to avoid crystalluria. Sulphinpyrazone causes gastric upset and is contraindicated in peptic ulcer.

Drug treatment of gout

Acute gout

NSAIDs (but not aspirin which in low dose causes urate retention) are highly effective, terminating the attack in a few hours. Early treatment is important. Indomethacin is a first choice and 25–50 mg may be given orally 3 times a day with a fourth (sometimes larger) dose at night, possibly taken as a suppository (100 mg). Naproxen, diclofenac, sulindac, piroxicam and azapropazone are effective alternatives. Colchicine is traditional and may be used when patients cannot tolerate NSAIDs. It may be the drug of choice in a *first* attack of severe monarticular arthritis, as a good response helps make the diagnosis, which can be difficult. If these drugs fail, prednisolone 40 mg/d may be used, reducing as quickly as symptoms allow.

Useless agents. It requires only a moment's thought to appreciate that uricosurics and allopurinol will not relieve an acute attack of gout.

Recurrent and progressive gout

This may be prevented by:

- persuading the patient to avoid chronic excess and acute debauchery (see below);
- allopurinol or a uricosuric drug if the serum urate consistently exceeds 0.6 mmol/l and the patient has had 3 or more attacks of acute gout.

Therapy should begin in a quiescent period. Allopurinol is preferred and is the treatment of choice if the patient has impaired renal function (see above). It may be combined with a uricosuric. Aspirin must not be taken concurrently with other uricosurics as it interferes with their action (tell the patient). Paracetamol may be used as an analgesic without interfering with therapy.

Colchicine also prevents gout, probably by suppressing acute attacks at their inception but prophylaxis with this alone is undesirable, for the plasma urate remains high allowing the disease process to continue (tophi, renal damage). But it, or indomethacin, may be used if an acute attack is expected, e.g. immediately after surgery.

Rapid lowering of plasma urate by any means may precipitate acute gout, probably by causing the dissolution of tophi. It is therefore usual to give prophylactic suppressive treatment with indomethacin during the first 2 months of allopurinol or uricosuric treatment. It can create an unfavourable impression if the patient, who has been told only that a drug will prevent gout, promptly has a severe attack.

Benefit from the lowered plasma urate will not be noticeable for some weeks. Medication should be adjusted to keep the plasma urate in the normal range. It can seldom be abandoned.

Chronic tophaceous gout. Tophi can sometimes be reduced in size and even removed by the prolonged use of allopurinol and uricosuric agents.

Precipitation of gout by diuretics. Any vigorous diuresis may precipitate acute gout by causing volume depletion which results in increased reabsorption of all substances that are normally partially reabsorbed in the proximal renal tubule, including urate. Furthermore most diuretics are organic acids that may compete with urate for secretion by the renal tubule. Diuretic-induced gout is of special importance in the elderly, in whom the presentation may be atypical. Spironolactone probably alone amongst the diuretics does not induce hyperuricaemia.

Aspirin and salicylic acid derivatives should be avoided in gout (the patient should be warned of the ubiquity of aspirin in proprietary preparations) because small doses inhibit urate secretion, causing urate to be retained.

Acute calcium pyrophosphate arthropathy (pseudogout) responds similarly to acute gout, though colchicine is likely to fail.

Diet, alcohol and gout

Dietary purines can be a significant contributory cause of hyperuricaemia and patients should avoid excesses of foods that contain purines, e.g. sweetbread, kidney, liver. Gouty patients tend also to be overweight and loss of weight lowers the plasma urate. Knowledge that alcohol induces acute gout is of long standing, and has been celebrated in verse:

A taste for drink, combined with gout,
Had doubled him up for ever.
Of *that* there is no manner of doubt –
No probable, possible shadow of doubt –
No possible doubt whatever.[4]

But the poet did not know of the mechanisms (see above).

---

[4] Don Alhambra's song in Act 1 of the Savoy opera, The Gondoliers or The King of Barataria. W. S. Gilbert (1836–1911).

GUIDE TO FURTHER READING

Bennett W M, DeBroe M E 1989 Analgesic nephropathy — a preventable renal disease. New England Journal of Medicine 320: 1269

Brooks P M, Day R O 1991 Nonsteroidal anti-inflammatory drugs – differences and similarities. New England Journal of Medicine 324: 1716

Editorial 1989 NSAIDs and gut damage: Lancet 2: 600

Editorial 1989 Topical NSAIDs: a gimmic or a godsend. Lancet 2: 779

Hamerman D 1989 The biology of osteoarthritis. New England Journal of Medicine 320: 1322

Harris E D 1990 Rheumatoid arthritis. Pathophysiology and implications for therapy. New England Journal of Medicine 322: 1277

Hawkey C J 1990 Nonsteroidal anti-inflammatory drugs and peptic ulcers. British Medical Journal 300: 278

Lewis R A et al 1990 Leukotrienes and other products of the 5-lipoxygenase pathway. Biochemistry and relation to pathobiology in human disease. New England Journal of Medicine 323: 645

Oates J A et al 1988 Clinical implications of prostaglandin and thromboxane A_2 formation. New England Journal of Medicine 319: 689 (part 1), 761 (part 2)

Scott J T 1989 Alcohol and gout. British Medical Journal 298: 1054

15

Central nervous system I: pain and analgesics, drugs in terminal illness, narcotic analgesics

SYNOPSIS

'But pain is perfect misery, the worst
Of evils, and, excessive, overturns
All patience.'
(John Milton, 1608–1674, Paradise Lost)

One of the greatest services doctors can do their patients is to acquire skill in the management of pain.

- Pain: The phenomenon of pain. Clinical evaluation of analgesics. Choice of analgesics. Treatment of pain syndromes. Patient controlled analgesia
- Drugs in terminal illness: Symptom control and quality of life. Pain.
- Narcotic or opioid analgesics: Agonists, partial agonists, antagonists. Morphine and opioids. Classification by analgesic efficacy. Other opioids. Opioids used during and after surgery. Opioid antagonists. Non-opioid analgesics useful for pain in opioid addicts

PAIN

Pain is an unpleasant sensory and emotional experience associated with actual or potential tissue damage, or described in terms of such damage.[1]

The word 'unpleasant' comprises the whole range of disagreeable feelings from being merely inconvenienced to misery, anguish, anxiety, depression and desperation, to the ultimate cure of suicide.[2]

- **Analgesic drug**: a drug that relieves pain due to multiple causes, e.g. aspirin, paracetamol, morphine. Drugs that relieve pain due to a single cause or specific pain syndrome only, e.g. ergotamine (migraine), carbamazepine (neuralgias), glyceryl trinitrate (angina pectoris), are not classed as analgesics; nor are adrenocortical steroids that suppress pain of inflammation of any cause.

- Analgesics are classed as **narcotic** (which act in the central nervous system and cause drowsiness, i.e. opioids) and **non-narcotic** (which act chiefly peripherally, e.g. aspirin).

- **Adjuvant drugs** are those used alongside analgesics in the management of pain; they are

---

[1] Merskey H et al. Pain terms: a list with definitions and notes on usage. Pain 1979; 6: 249.
[2] Melzack R, Wall P. The challenge of pain. London: Penguin. 1982.

not themselves analgesics, though they may modify the perception or the concomitants of pain that make it worse (anxiety, fear, depression[3]), e.g. psychotropic drugs, or they may modify underlying causes, e.g. spasm of smooth or of voluntary muscle.

The general principle that the best treatment of a symptom is removal of its cause applies. But this is often impossible to achieve and symptom relief of pain by analgesic drug is required.

Pain is the commonest symptom that takes patients to doctors, but the complaint does not mean that an analgesic is needed.

Optimal management of pain requires that the clinician should have a conceptual framework for what is happening to the patient in mind and body.

Acute pain is managed primarily (but not invariably) by analgesic drugs, but *chronic* pain often requires adjuvant drugs in addition as well as non-drug measures.

Analgesics are *chosen* according to the cause of pain and its severity.

THE PHENOMENON OF PAIN

It used to be thought that pain was due to tissue injury or disease activating specific pain receptors that passed impulses to a 'pain centre' in the central nervous system where they entered consciousness as pain.

This oversimple picture fails to recognise four points:

- Pain can occur without tissue injury or evident disease and can persist after injury has healed.
- Serious tissue injury can occur without pain.
- Emotion (anxiety, fear, depression) is an inseparable concomitant of pain and can modify both its intensity and the victim's behavioural response.
- There is important processing of afferent nociceptive (see below) and other impulses in the spinal cord and brain.

Appreciation that pain is both a sensory *and* an emotional (affective) experience has allowed clinicians to realise that automatically to meet a complaint of pain with a prescription alone is not an appropriate response, for 'There is always more to analgesia than analgesics';[4] and that pain that is not the subject of a simple analysis by the clinician (and explanation to the patient) may be inadequately relieved because of lack of understanding, which also causes lack of resoluteness and tenacity in management. That doctors often do not provide adequate relief of severe pain (post-surgical, terminal care of advanced cancer) by bad choice and by overusing and, also important, underusing drugs, and by defective relations with their patients, has been, and still is, a justified and shaming criticism.

The different aspects of pain

Pain is not simply a perception, it is a complex phenomenon or syndrome, only one component of which is the sensation actually reported as pain.

Pain has four major aspects present to varying extent in any one case:

1. *Nociception*[5] is a consequence of tissue injury (trauma, inflammation) causing the release of chemical mediators (p. 232) which activate nociceptors (chemosensitive endings) in the tissue. Nociceptors are specialised nerve endings serving their own afferent fibres (A-delta and C); nociception is not due to overstimulation of touch or other receptors.
2. *Pain sensation* is a result of nociceptive input *plus* a pattern of impulses of different frequency and intensity from other peripheral receptors, e.g. heat, and mechano-receptors whose threshold of response is reduced by the chemical mediators; and of their processing in the brain whence modulating inhibitory impulses pass down to regulate the

---

[3] Tricyclic antidepressants may reduce morphine requirement in terminal care without noticeably altering mood.

[4] Twycross R G. J R Coll Physicians Lond 1984; 18: 32.
[5] Latin: *noxa*: injury.

continuing afferent input. But pain can occur without nociception (some neuralgias[6]) and nociception does not invariably cause pain; pain is a psychological state though most pain has an immediately antecedent physical cause.

3. *Suffering* is a consequence of pain and of lack of understanding by patients of the meaning of the pain; it comprises anxiety and fear (particularly in acute pain) and depression (particularly in chronic pain), which will be affected by patients' personalities, and their beliefs about the significance of the pain, e.g. merely a postponed holiday, or death, or a future of disability with loss of independence. Depression makes a major contribution to suffering; it is treatable, as are the other affective concomitants of pain.

4. *Pain behaviour* comprises consequences of 1 to 3 above, it includes behaviour that is interpreted by others as signifying pain in the victim, e.g. such immediate and obvious aspects as facial expression, restlessness, seeking isolation (or company), medicine-taking, as well as, in chronic pain, the development of querulousness, depression, despair and social withdrawal.

The clinician's task is to determine the significance of these items for each patient and to direct therapy accordingly. Analgesics may, but not necessarily will, be the mainstay of therapy; adjuvant (non-analgesic) drugs may be needed, as well as non-drug therapy (radiation, surgery).

It is also useful to distinguish between *acute pain* (an *event* whose end can be predicted) and *chronic pain* (a *situation* whose end is commonly unpredictable, or will only end with life itself).

Acute pain (fast conducting A-delta fibres) with major nociceptive input (physical trauma, pleurisy, myocardial infarct, perforated peptic ulcer) is seen by patients as a transient, though sometimes severe threat and they react accordingly. It is a symptom that may be dealt with unhesitatingly and effectively with drugs, by in-

jection if necessary, at the same time as the causative disease is assailed. The accompanying anxiety will vary according to the severity of the pain, and particularly according to its meaning for the patient, whether termination with recovery will soon occur, major surgery is threatened, or there is prospect of death or invalidism. The choice of drug will depend on the clinician's assessment of these factors. Morphine by injection has retained a pre-eminent place for over 100 years because it has highly effective antinociceptive and antianxiety effects; modern opioids have not rendered morphine obsolete.

Acute pain without nociceptive (afferent) input (some neuralgias) is less susceptible to drugs unless consciousness is also depressed, and any frequently recurrent acute pain, e.g. trigeminal neuralgia, poses management problems that are more akin to chronic pain.

Chronic pain (slow conducting type C fibres) is better regarded as a syndrome[7] rather than as a symptom (see above). It presents a depressing future to the victim who sees no prospect of release from suffering, and poses long-term management problems that differ from acute pain. Suffering and affective disorders can be of overriding importance and the consequences of poor management may be prolonged and serious for the patient. Analgesics alone are often insufficient and adjuvant drugs as well as non-drug therapy gain increasing importance. Even when they are effective in chronic pain, the high-efficacy opioids (morphine, pethidine) alter mood and carry a substantial risk of dependence that will have adverse consequences in the long term. Continuous use of these drugs is best avoided in chronic pain, *except* that of terminal care. But the lower efficacy opioids (codeine, dextropropoxyphene) may often be needed and used. Sedation should be avoided and therapy should be oral if possible; regimens should be planned to avoid breakthrough pain. Antidepressants can often be useful.

---

[6] *Neuralgia* is pain felt in the distribution of a nerve.

[7] A set of symptoms and signs that are characteristic of a condition though they may not always have the same cause (Greek: *syn* together, *dramein* to run).

Sedative-hypnotic drugs, e.g. benzodiazepines, may be needed for anxiety but may induce depression.

Chronic pain syndrome is a term used for persistence of pain when detectable disease has disappeared, e.g. after an attack of low back pain. It characteristically does not respond to standard treatment with analgesics. Whether the basis is neurogenic, psychogenic or sociocultural it should not be managed by intensifying drug treatment. Opioid analgesics, which may be producing dependence, should be withdrawn and the use of psychotropic drugs, e.g. antidepressants or neuroleptics, and non-drug therapy, including psychotherapy, should be considered.

Mechanisms of analgesia

Endogenous opioid neurotransmitters (endorphins, dynorphins, enkephalins) in the spinal cord and brain constitute an inhibitory system that is activated by nociceptive and other input, including treatments such as transcutaneous nerve stimulation and acupuncture. Administered opioids produce analgesia via the specific opioid receptors of this system. The fact that there are several types of receptor (mu, delta, kappa, epsilon, sigma) explains the differing patterns of actions of opioids and gives hope that selective new high-efficacy analgesics free from the disadvantages of the existing opioids may be designed.

Naloxone (competitive opioid antagonist or receptor blocker) can oppose the effects of endogenous opioids, at least to some degree, and has been found, as expected, to worsen (dental) pain.[8] Naloxone does not induce hyperalgesia or spontaneous pain because the opioid paths are quiescent until activated by nociceptive and other afferent input. Interestingly, naloxone has been found (in some studies) to reduce placebo effect.

In addition to these opioid mechanisms, non-opioid mediated pathways, e.g. serotonin, are important in pain. There is suggestion that opioid pathways are more important in acute severe pain, and non-opioid paths in chronic pain, and that this may be relevant to choice of drugs.

When a tissue is injured (any cause), or even merely stimulated, *prostaglandin synthesis* in that tissue increases. Prostaglandins have two major actions: they are mediators of inflammation and they also sensitise nerve endings, lowering their threshold of response to stimuli, mechanical (tenderness of inflammation) and chemical, allowing the other mediators of inflammation, e.g. histamine, serotonin, bradykinin, to intensify the activation of the sensory endings.

Plainly, a drug that prevents the synthesis of prostaglandins is likely to be effective in relieving pain due to inflammation of any kind, and this is indeed how aspirin and other nonsteroidal anti-inflammatory drugs (NSAIDs) act. This discovery was made in 1971, aspirin having been extensively used in medicine since 1899.[9]

The mechanism by which NSAIDs relieve pain is by cyclo-oxygenase (prostaglandin synthase) inhibition.

With this mode of action it is evident that NSAIDs will relieve pain when there is some tissue injury with consequent inflammation, as there almost always is with pain. They also act in the central nervous system (prostaglandins are synthesised in all cells[10] except erythrocytes) and there is probably some central component to the analgesic effect of NSAIDs.

But, it has to be said that analgesic and anti-inflammatory effects are not parallel, e.g. aspirin relieves pain rapidly at doses that do not significantly reduce inflammation and the onset of its anti-inflammatory effect at higher doses may be slow. Paracetamol is an effective analgesic for mild pain but has little anti-inflammation effect

---

[8] Naloxone also appears to cause *pyrovats* (practitioners of religious firewalking ceremonies) to quicken their pace over the hot coals.

[9] Propagandists for complementary (alternative) medicine allege that orthodox scientific medicine will not recognise any therapy, e.g. complementary medicine, unless its mode of action is known. This is untrue. Validated empirical observation, i.e. scientific evidence, is and always has been accepted.
[10] Which shows the undesirability of naming substances with reference to their, often chance, mode of discovery.

in arthritis, though substantial effect on post-dental extraction swelling. Other NSAIDs show a different mix of action against pain and inflammation.

An account of individual nonsteroidal anti-inflammatory drugs will be found in Chapter 14.

Corticosteroids diminish inflammation of all kinds by preventing prostaglandin synthesis (the phospholipase A_2 that releases the arachidonic acid that is required for such synthesis is inhibited). Short-term use may be valuable; long-term use poses many problems (see Ch. 33); in general the corticosteroid should be withdrawn after one week if there is no benefit.

The pain threshold is lowered by anxiety, fear, depression, anger, sadness, fatigue, or insomnia, and is *raised* by relief of these (by drug or by non-drug measures) and by successful relief of pain.

Since emotion is such an important factor in pain, it is no surprise that dummy tablets or injections (placebos) have long been known to alleviate pain, giving relief usually to about 35% of cases, but with the added disadvantage that they rapidly lose effect with repetition.

The importance of *the meaning of pain* to its victim is illustrated by injuries of war and of civilian life:

To the wounded soldier who had been under unremitting shell fire for weeks, his wound was a good thing (it meant the end of the war for him) and was associated with far less pain than was the case of the civilians who considered their need for surgery a disaster.[11]

The desire for analgesics was less amongst victims of battle injuries than amongst comparable civilian injuries.[12] On the other hand, morphine has been found to be relatively ineffective against experimental pain in man, probably because it acts best against pain that has emotional significance for the patient.

New analgesics have been successfully developed by *animal testing*, possibly because the emotional response to experimental pain in an animal is akin to the human response to disease or accidental injury. This emotional response does not generally occur in a subject who has volunteered to undergo laboratory experiments that can be stopped at any time, and it probably accounts for the fact that a placebo gives relief in only 3% of these cases; also for the fact that experimental pain in man has proved to be of small value in assessing the clinical value of potential analgesics that may act on the psychic response.

CLINICAL EVALUATION OF ANALGESICS

Therapeutic trials in *acute pain* are often conducted on patients who have undergone abdominal surgery or third molar tooth extraction, and in *chronic pain* on chronic rheumatic conditions. Only the patients can say what they feel and pain is best measured by a *questionnaire* or by a *visual analogue scale*; a line, 10 or 20 cm long, one end of which represents pain 'as bad as it could possibly be' (which patients identify as 'agonising') and the other end 'no pain'; patients mark the line on the point they feel represents their pain between these two extremes. Such techniques are amazingly reproducible.

Adverse effects are, of course, simultaneously recorded and taken into account when deciding clinical utility. Since what is being measured is how patients *say* they feel, careful precautions must be taken if a reliable result is to be obtained. The trial must be double-blind, or made double-blind as soon as possible. Observers who interrogate the patients for relief (intensity and duration) and adverse effects must be constant and trained. It has been found, for example, that if asked by a personable young woman, a higher proportion of patients admit to pain relief than if the same question is put by a man.

Support for the reliability of these techniques comes from the fact that similar results are obtained with the same drugs in different centres and that workers have identified 'unknown' coded samples.[13]

[11] Beecher H K. Pharmacol Rev 1957; 9: 59.
[12] Beecher H K. JAMA 1956; 161: 1609.
[13] Beecher H K Pharmacol. Rev. 1957; 9: 59.

Despite all the activity of chemists producing new compounds and of physicians in testing them with increasing accuracy, the alkaloids of opium and aspirin (1899), remain pre-eminent in the treatment of pain.

THE CHOICE OF ANALGESICS
Ranking of analgesics for clinical efficacy[14]

Mild pain
- Non-narcotic (non-opioid) analgesics or NSAIDs, e.g. aspirin, ibuprofen, paracetamol.[15] Where these fail after using the full dose range, proceed to:

Moderate pain
- Narcotic (opioid) analgesics, low-efficacy opioids, e.g. codeine, dihydrocodeine, dextropropoxyphene, pentazocine.
- Combined therapy of NSAIDs plus low-efficacy opioid, *not* necessarily as a fixed-dose formulation, many of which have an inadequate dose of one or other ingredient (see below) so that separate administration is commonly preferable though less convenient. Where these fail proceed to:

Severe pain
- High-efficacy opioids, e.g. morphine, diamorphine, pethidine, buprenorphine.
- An added NSAID is useful if there is a substantial tissue injury component, e.g. gout, bone metastasis.

Overwhelming acute pain
- High efficacy opioid plus a sedative/anxiolytic (diazepam) or a phenothiazine tranquilliser, e.g. chlorpromazine, methotrimeprazine (which also has analgesic effect).

Note: adjuvant drugs (p. 242) may be useful in all grades of pain.

'Keeping it simple'[16]

The three basic analgesics are aspirin, codeine and morphine.[17] The rest should be considered alternatives of fashion or convenience. Appreciating this helps to prevent the doctor 'kangarooing' from analgesic to analgesic in a desperate search for some drug that will suit the patient better. If non-narcotic or weak narcotic preparations such as aspirin–codeine, paracetamol–dextropropoxyphene, fail to relieve, it is usually best to move directly to a small dose of morphine [the quoted author refers to chronic cancer pain] than, for example, to prescribe dihydrocodeine i.e. change to an analgesic of higher efficacy rather than to another of similar efficacy.

It is necessary to be familiar with one or two alternatives for use in patients who cannot tolerate the standard preparation. The individual doctor's basic analgesic ladder, with alternatives, should comprise no more than nine or ten drugs in total. It is better to know and understand a few drugs well than to have a passing acquaintance with the whole range.

Using two analgesics

Simultaneous use of two analgesics of different modes of action is rational, but two drugs of the same class/mechanism of action are likely to be unprofitable *unless* there is a difference in emphasis, analgesia versus anti-inflammatory action; or a patient taking a NSAID with a long $t_{\frac{1}{2}}$, e.g. naproxen (14 h), is benefited by having available an additional drug of shorter $t_{\frac{1}{2}}$ to be taken for an acute exacerbation, e.g. ibuprofen, aspirin. Aspirin plus paracetamol is widely used and although aspirin (certainly) and paracetamol (probably) act by blocking prostaglandin synthesis there are substantial (and unexplained) differences between them.

A *low*-efficacy opioid can reduce the action of a *high*-efficacy opioid by excluding the latter from receptors (by competition).

---

[14] Based on Twycross R G In: Saunders Cicely M, ed. The management of terminal disease. London: Arnold. 1978. The work of this author contributes much to this chapter.

[15] Paracetamol is sometimes not classed as an NSAID because its anti-inflammatory pattern differs substantially from most, i.e. its efficacy is weak in rheumatoid arthritis.

---

[16] Twycross R G. J Roy Coll Physicians Lond 1984; 18: 32. The author is a leading authority on pain control and the management of terminal disease.

[17] All three were introduced in the 19th century.

Partial agonist (agonist/antagonist) opioids will also antagonise the action of other opioids, e.g. heroin, and may even induce the withdrawal syndrome in dependent subjects.

Fixed-ratio (compound) analgesic combinations

Large numbers of these are available. They are particularly offered as bridging the efficacy gap between aspirin or paracetamol and morphine. Many have an inadequate dose of one or other ingredient, e.g. codeine 5 mg, caffeine 10 mg. Doctors should consider the formulae of these preparations before using them.

Caffeine has been shown to enhance the analgesic effect of aspirin and of paracetamol and to accelerate the onset of effect, but at least 30 mg and probably 60 mg are needed (a cup of coffee averages about 80 mg and tea averages about 30 mg).

Tablets containing paracetamol (325 mg) plus dextropropoxyphene (32.5 mg) (co-proxamol, Distalgesic), in a dose of 1-2 tablets, provide an effective dose of both drugs. There is controversy about the merit (benefit:risk) of this formulation, which has been extremely popular with both prescribers and patients. Clinical trials are inconclusive as to whether it has efficacy superior to either drug alone and its popularity may be influenced by a mild euphoriant effect of the opioid, to which dependence can occur. A major objection to it is that in (deliberate) overdose death may occur within one hour due to the rapid absorption of the dextropropoxyphene, and combination with alcohol appears seriously to add to hazard. There has been enormous debate about this popular product, the passion with which it is conducted demonstrating that reliable data are lacking. Regulatory authorities are in a position to tell the manufacturer to obtain definitive data, but they seem reluctant to do so.

We do not attempt to rank the many preparations available because comparative evidence is lacking.

TREATMENT OF PAIN SYNDROMES

In general, pain (acute or chronic) arising from *somatic structures* (skin, muscles, bones, joints) responds to analgesics such as aspirin and paracetamol (non-narcotic), which do not alter psychic function and do not induce serious dependence (addiction). But pain arising from *the viscera* is most readily reduced by morphine[18] (narcotic), which alters both the pain threshold and the psychic reaction to pain and induces dependence with prolonged use. This distinction is not, of course, absolute and a high-efficacy opioid is needed for severe somatic pain. Mild pain from any source may respond to the non-narcotic analgesics and these should always be tried first.

Spasm of visceral smooth muscle

Pain due to spasm of visceral smooth muscle, e.g. biliary, renal colic, when severe, requires a substantial dose of morphine, pethidine or buprenorphine. These drugs themselves cause spasm of visceral smooth muscle and so have a simultaneous action tending to increase the pain. Papaveretum may be less prone to do this as it contains other opium alkaloids. Phenazocine and buprenorphine are less liable to cause spasm. An antimuscarinic drug such as atropine or hyoscine may be given simultaneously to antagonise this effect.

Prostaglandins are involved in control of smooth muscle and colic can be treated with NSAIDs (diclofenac, indomethacin, i.m., suppository, oral).

Spasm of striated muscle

This is often a cause of pain, including *chronic tension headache*. Treatment is directed at reduction of the spasm in a variety of ways, including psychotherapy, sedation and the use of a centrally acting muscle relaxant as well as

---

[18] Surgeons are rightly concerned that diagnosis of the acute abdomen be not hindered by a large dose of morphine administered with humane intent by the primary care doctor who first sees the patient.

non-narcotic analgesics, e.g. orphenadrine plus paracetamol (Norgesic), baclofen, diazepam, meprobamate. Local infiltration with lignocaine is sometimes effective, as are alcoholic drinks.

Neuralgias

Post-herpetic neuralgia, trigeminal neuralgia, causalgia, tabetic pain, can present almost insoluble problems. Analgesics may play only a subsidiary part in their management. In severe cases very high doses of non-narcotic analgesics with low-efficacy opioid are often reached with little benefit and an almost inevitable demand for high-efficacy opioid follows, with the risk of serious dependence as well as of inefficacy at doses that leave consciousness unimpaired. Psychotropic drugs may be useful adjuvants.

It has been accidentally discovered that an antiepileptic, carbamazepine (Tegretol) (p. 307), is effective in *trigeminal neuralgia*, probably by reducing excitability of the trigeminal nucleus. It supplants other drug therapy. A start should be made with a low dose, which should be adjusted to suit individuals, who generally soon learn to alter it themselves during remissions and exacerbations. It is not used for prophylaxis. The daily dose is 200–1600 mg orally, in divided doses. It is sometimes possible to withdraw the drug gradually over several months without relapse.

In neuralgias, other drugs worth trying in resistant cases include phenytoin (it raises the threshold of nerve cells to electrical stimulation), baclofen and antidepressants or neuroleptics, which may potentiate analgesics and also have an independent effect.

• *Herpes zoster.* The pain of the acute condition is mitigated by NSAIDs and opioids.

• *Post-herpetic neuralgia* is not prevented by acyclovir. The established condition may be helped by drugs used for trigeminal neuralgia, including antidepressants. Conventional analgesics are ineffective.

• *Phantom limb pain* is commonly resistant to analgesics; clonazepam may be tried. Prolonged relief may follow transient changes in sensory input; *decrease* (local anaesthetic to sensitive spots in the stump); *increase* (vibration).

• *Thalamic pain* e.g. following a cerebrovascular accident, commonly fails to respond to analgesics. Chlorpromazine is worth trying, and carbamazepine, and other adjuvant drugs.

Other pain syndromes

• The pain of *inflammation* responds to NSAIDs (aspirin is a NSAID although some talk as though it is not), but it may need added low-efficacy opioid.

• *Arthritis*, see Chapter 14.

• The pain of *minor trauma*, e.g. many sports injuries, is commonly treated by local skin cooling (spray of chlorofluoromethanes) or counter-irritants (see index). NSAIDs are effective and some are available for topical use.

• The pain of *severe trauma including post-surgical pain* (p. 359) usually needs narcotic analgesics. NSAIDs reduce the inflammatory consequences of the injury and so relieve pain.

• The pain of *peripheral vascular insufficiency* should be treated with non-narcotic analgesics. Low efficacy opioids may be needed eventually. Vasodilator drugs may help but also may be quite ineffective.

• The pain of *malignant disease* requires the full range of analgesics *and* adjuvant drugs and procedures (see above, and terminal care, below).

• *Bone pain*, including cancer metastases, requires NSAIDs alone and with opioids.

• *Nerve compression* can be relieved by corticosteroid (prednisolone), nerve block (local anaesthetic); nerve destruction can be achieved by alcohol, phenol.

• *Dysmenorrhoea*, see p. 609.

• *Mastalgia* may benefit from gamolenic acid (in evening primrose oil), danazol and bromocriptine; or from combined contraceptive pill.

Headache

Headache originating inside the skull may be due to traction on or distension of arteries arising from the circle of Willis, or to traction on the dura mater. Headache originating outside the skull may be due to local muscle spasm[19] or arterial inflammation or distension or may be referred pain from, e.g., the teeth, neck or nasal sinuses. Treatment by drugs is directed to relieving the muscle spasm, producing vasoconstriction or simply administering analgesics, beginning, of course, with the non-narcotics, e.g. paracetamol and aspirin.

Migraine

Migraine (classic and common) is *triggered* by a variety of factors, including stress (exertion, excitement, anxiety, fatigue, anger) and by food containing vasoactive amines (chocolate, cheese), by food allergy and also by hormonal changes (menstruation and oral contraceptives) and hypoglycaemia. These precipitants may initiate release of vasoactive substances stored in nerve endings and blood platelets. Attention to triggering factors is crucial to management.

The acute migraine attack appears to begin in serotonergic and noradrenergic neurons in the brain. These monoamines affect the cerebral and extracerebral vasculature (which may have developed abnormal responses) and they also cause release of further vasoactive substances such as histamine, prostaglandins, substance P.

The migraine *aura* is no longer thought to be the consequence of constriction of intracerebral vessels, but the throbbing *headache* is due to dilatation of pain-sensitive arteries outside the brain, including scalp arteries.

The numerous known facts cannot yet be arranged in a coherent scheme, but the basis of rational therapy is emerging. It will be seen that drugs having a considerable variety of actions can be useful, as follows:

Drugs that are useful in acute migraine attacks

- serotonin receptor agonist and antagonist
- α-adrenoceptor agonist

- inhibitor of prostaglandin synthase (NSAIDs)
- antiemetic and/or activator of gastric motility
- sedative

In prophylaxis

- serotonin receptor antagonist
- β-adrenoceptor antagonist (though probably not acting by that mechanism)
- calcium entry blocker
- ACE inhibitor
- antidepressant

Acute attacks

The acute migraine attack should be treated as early as possible with an oral dispersible (soluble) analgesic formulation so that it may be absorbed before there is vomiting and accompanying gastric stasis with slow and erratic drug absorption. Aspirin (600 mg) is effective and its antiaggregatory action on the platelets may add to its advantage; paracetamol, ibuprofen and naproxen are alternatives.

Paracetamol plus isometheptene (an indirectly acting sympathomimetic) (Midrid) suits some patients.

Metoclopramide is a useful antiemetic that also promotes gastric emptying and has been shown to enhance aspirin absorption. But plainly, if vomiting and gastric stasis already exist, it may not be absorbed and should be given i.m. (10 mg). Prochlorperazine (rectally), cyclizine and buclizine are alternative antiemetics.

Sedation (with a benzodiazepine) is useful especially if the attack has been triggered by emotional stress, and sleep is an important remedy in migraine.

Efficient use of an analgesic, an antiemetic[20] and a sedative is adequate for 90% of acute attacks. The remaining 10% need ergotamine.

Severe migraine attacks require ergotamine, which, given early after the onset of headache, will benefit about 60% of those treated.

---

[20] Patients seem enthusiastic about combinations of antiemetic (metoclopramide or buclizine) plus aspirin or paracetamol, sometimes with small amounts of codeine or docusate sodium, e.g. Migraleve, Migravess, Paramax.

---

[19] As in *tension headache* or frontal headache from 'eyestrain.'

Ergotamine has α-adrenoceptor agonist (vasoconstrictor) and serotonin antagonist actions. It must be used cautiously.

Mild overdose causes nausea and vomiting and can worsen headache (ergot has the complex agonist/antagonist action characteristic of ergot derivatives, p. 610) and this can lead patients and incautious doctors to think the migraine is uncontrolled and to increase the dose, with disastrous consequences: see below.

Ergotamine constricts all peripheral arteries (an effect potentiated by concomitant β-adrenoceptor block), not just those affected by the migraine process, and overdose can cause peripheral gangrene; paraesthesiae in hands or feet give warning. Because ergotamine has complex actions on receptors to which its binding is relatively stable, vasoconstriction due to overdose is best antagonised by a non-selective vasodilator such as sodium nitroprusside (rather than by an α-adrenoceptor blocker). Subjects of vascular disease, coronary and peripheral, are particularly at risk from ergotamine.

Another reason for giving close attention to dosage is that, though ergotamine has a $t_{\frac{1}{2}}$ of 2 h, its effect on arteries (due to tissue binding) persists as long as 24 h, thus repeated doses lead to cumulative effects long outlasting the migraine attack.

Ergotamine may be given orally (to be swallowed: crush the tablets), sublingually (bypassing gastric stasis), rectally, or by inhalation.

With *enteral* forms of ergotamine, total dosage in an acute attack should not exceed 6 mg (if there is no benefit from the first 2 mg, see below, the likelihood of higher dose being effective is small), and the maximum in one week should not exceed 10 mg.

By *inhalation* (360 μg per puff of metered aerosol), a puff every 5 min for up to 6 puffs (2.2 mg in an attack), and in one week 15 puffs (5.4 mg) maximum. Efficient use of an inhaler requires instruction (use a demonstration inhaler, not the patient's).

In one case of overdose a doctor overprescribed ergotamine and the dispensing pharmacist did not query the prescription. A court of law found both doctor and pharmacist to have been negligent, i.e. to have failed to take reasonable care in circumstances where it was foreseeable that such failure was likely to cause injury. The court ordered doctor and pharmacist to share a payment of compensation to the patient, who had suffered peripheral gangrene.

Ergotamine is a powerful oxytocic and is dangerous in pregnancy. It may precipitate angina pectoris, probably by increasing cardiac pre- and afterload (venous and arterial constriction) rather than by constricting coronary arteries.

Caffeine enhances absorption of ergotamine (both speed and peak blood concentration) and is often combined with it (though it may prevent sleep).

Preparations of ergotamine for acute migraine

Tablet (to swallow, crushed) ergotamine 1 mg + caffeine 100 mg (Cafergot); two tablets at onset and then one every 30 min if necessary (maximum 4 in 24 h; no repeat for 4 d; maximum 10 in week).

Tablet (to swallow, crushed) ergotamine 2 mg + cyclizine 50 mg + caffeine 100 mg (Migril); one at onset then 30 min intervals (maximum 4 per attack; 6 in week).

Tablet (sublingual) ergotamine 2 mg (Lingraine); one tablet at onset and then one after 30 min if necessary (maximum 3 in 24 h; 6 in week).

Suppository ergotamine 2 mg + caffeine 100 mg (Cafergot); one at onset; 2 in 24 h; 5 in week.

Inhalation by metered aerosol (Medihaler ergotamine), for dose see above.

Ergotamine should not be used for prophylaxis.

Dihydroergotamine is less effective than ergotamine.

Sumatriptan (principally a 5HT-receptor agonist) may selectively constrict dilated cerebral and extracerebral arteries and is an alternative.

Carbon dioxide inhalation (cerebral vasodilator) can sometimes stop an attack if given during the aura (cortical vasoconstriction). The most convenient technique is to rebreathe into a bag until dyspnoea occurs.

Drug prophylaxis of migraine

This should be considered when, after adjustment of lifestyle, diet, etc. there are still two or more attacks per month. Benefit may be delayed for several weeks.

Options (which may help up to 60% of patients) include:

● *Aspirin* continuously, e.g. 300 mg × 2/d, which blocks synthesis of prostaglandins, including thromboxane (aggregatory factor) in platelets. Higher doses will also block synthesis of prostacyclin (platelet antiaggregatory factor) in arterial walls and may make migraine worse. *If* this is the true mode of action in prophylaxis, lower doses of aspirin may be effective. Naproxen and other NSAIDs are also effective.

● β-*adrenoceptor block* by propranolol(dl); (the d-isomer, which lacks β-blocking action though it has membrane stabilising effect, also prevents migraine), as do other pure antagonists (atenolol, metoprolol) but not partial agonists, see p. 417. It seems that β-adrenoceptor block is not the prime therapeutic action.

If ergotamine (for acute attack) is given to a patient taking propranolol for prophylaxis there is risk of additive vasoconstriction (block of β-receptor dilatation with added α-receptor constriction).

The effective dose of propranolol is variable, 80–240 mg/ day orally.

● *Calcium entry blockers*, e.g. verapamil, flunarizine, have been found to be effective.

● *Pizotifen* and *cyproheptadine* block serotonin (5-HT) receptors as well as having some H_1-antihistamine action; they can be effective.

● *Methysergide* (an ergot derivative) blocks serotonin receptors but it has a grave rare adverse effect, an inflammatory fibrosis, retroperitoneal (causing obstruction to the ureters), subendocardial, pericardial and pleural. Drug 'holidays', i.e. withdrawal for 1–2 months each 6 months, are a prudent safeguard. Because of this risk, methysergide cannot be a drug of first choice though it may be justified for a patient who is experiencing a sequence of severe attacks.

● *Feverfew* (*Tanacetum parthenium*, related to the chrysanthemum) has been shown to have efficacy, perhaps by blocking serotonin release.

● *Other drugs* for which efficacy has been claimed include tricyclic and MAOI antidepressants: benefit may be delayed for weeks.

Premenstrual migraine may respond to mefenamic acid or to a diuretic.

After six months it is worth trying slow withdrawal of the prophylactic drug.

Attention to detail in the treatment of migraine is well repaid. General aspects of treatment are often more important than are drugs, e.g. psychotherapy, modification of way of living.

Cluster headaches may be treated as for migraine, but use of ergotamine may need to be more prolonged. If used over weeks, 2 days in each week should be ergot-free to avoid toxicity. Since bouts of headache tend to be of limited duration, e.g. a few weeks, short courses of methysergide are justified in intractable cases; pizotifen can be beneficial, also sumatriptan.

Headache of intracranial pressure (cerebral oedema) responds to dexamethasone (10 mg i.v.; 4 mg 6-hourly for 2–10 days) which reduces the pressure; and to non-opioid analgesics (see also terminal illness).

PATIENT-CONTROLLED ANALGESIA

The attractions of enabling patients to manage their own analgesics rather than be dependent on others are obvious. In mild and moderate pain it is easy to provide tablets for this purpose, but in severe chronic and acute recurrent pain, e.g. post-surgical, obstetric, myocardial infarction and terminal illness, other routes are needed to provide speedy relief just when it is needed, and a range of apparatuses has been developed, from the familiar (in obstetrics) inhalation devices to patient-controlled pumps for i.v., i.m., s.c. and epidural routes.

There are obvious problems, e.g. training patients, supervision, preventing overdose, in achieving the objectives, i.e. patient satisfaction with reduced (or, at least, not increased) demand on nurses' time, especially when the objective is to allow the patient to die comfortably at home.

Inhalation via a demand valve of nitrous oxide and oxygen, as in obstetrics, may be used temporarily in other situations as, for instance, *urinary lithiasis*, *trigeminal neuralgia*, during *postoperative chest physiotherapy*, for changing painful dressings and in emergency ambulances.

DRUGS IN TERMINAL ILLNESS

SYMPTOM CONTROL AND THE QUALITY OF LIFE

It is a general truth that we are all dying; the difference between individuals is the length and quality of the time that remains.[21] Terminal illness means that period (generally weeks) when active treatment of disease is no longer appropriate and the emphasis of care is on providing the maximum quality of life during these final weeks. This means that symptom control becomes the priority because,

One cannot adequately help a man to come to accept his impending death if he remains in severe pain, one cannot give spiritual counsel to a woman who is vomiting, or help a wife and children say their goodbyes to a father who is so drugged that he cannot respond.[22]

As the scope of life contracts, so the quality of what remains becomes more precious. Symptoms should not be allowed to destroy it. Drugs are pre-eminent in symptom control.

A remarkable instance of success in terminal care is provided by

an elderly gentleman with obstructing carcinoma of the esophagus who was a keen gardener. He remained at home, free from pain, attended a garden show on Saturday, worked in his garden on Sunday, and died on Monday.[23]

He was treated with continuous subcutaneous heroin (diamorphine) infusion (heroin has a higher solubility than morphine and so is more suitable for such use). Whilst the randomised controlled trial provides a major basis for therapeutic advance, telling us what *generally does happen*, the clinical anecdote yet has value, telling us what *can* happen, and providing examples for us to emulate.

Such an ideal course as the above example is too much to expect always. But with intelligent use of drugs, which follows from informed analyses of objectives, doctors can enable their patients to depart from life in peace[24] and with dignity, i.e. *true euthanasia*.[25]

Whilst the skilful use of drugs can provide incalculable relief and deserves careful study, this must not hide the fact that the manner, attentiveness, and human feeling of the attendants are dominant factors once any grosser physical and mental aberrations have been controlled by drugs. The needs of the dying have been summarised as security, companionship, symptomatic treatment, and medical nursing and domestic care. Nearly half of the deaths in England and Wales occur in the patient's own home.

PAIN

The considerations already discussed apply, but there are some aspects that deserve special attention.

Analgesics should be given regularly (adjusted to the patient's need, often 3–4-hourly) to *prevent* pain and not only to suppress it. Suppression of existent pain requires larger doses, particularly where the pain has generated anxiety and fear. When it is certain that pain will return, it is callous to allow it to do so when the means of prevention exist.

It is kind to leave a dose of analgesic accessible to patients, especially at night, when unnecessary

---

21 Mack R M. Lessons from living with cancer. N Engl J Med 1984; 311: 1640. Recommended reading: a personal account by a surgeon who had lung cancer with metastases.
22 Dr. Mary Baines, St. Christopher's Hospice, London.
23 Russell P S B. N Engl J Med 1984; 311: 1634.

24 '. . .; and for many a time
I have been half in love with easeful Death,
Call'd him soft names in many a mused rhyme,
To take into the air my quiet breath;
  Now more than ever seems it rich to die,
To cease upon the midnight with no pain.'
(John Keats: 1795–1821).
25 *Euthanasia* (Greek: *eu* gentle, easy; *thanatos* death) is the objective of all. It does not mean deliberately killing people peacefully, which is *voluntary* euthanasia.

suffering may result from reluctance to call a nurse or disturb a relative. In terminal illness, the question of whether or not the patient will become dependent on opioids ceases to be of importance (but see below) and the ordinary precautions against dependence, low, widely spaced doses, need not be rigorously applied.

Control of severe pain without objectionable sedation can be achieved in terminal illness by morphine with adjuvant drugs (given orally) in up to 80% of patients. Oral use preserves patients' independence (they do not have to rely on another person to give the next dose) as well as reducing the unpleasantness of frequent injections and the use of nursing time.

Full relief can only be achieved by attention to detail. This is sadly, too often, neglected. We therefore provide a detailed account of morphine use in this most important area of medical care where thoughtful attention to detail is so rewarding to patients, families and indeed to doctors themselves.

Oral morphine for pain in terminal care

Most patients can be managed without injections, which limit independence, are unpleasant, prodigal of nursing time and are more difficult to provide at home where most patients will prefer to die.

- Use a *simple aqueous solution,*[26] the strength of which is adjusted to give a volume of 5–10 ml per dose, e.g. begin with 1 or 2 mg/ml (or begin with a sustained-release formulation: see below).
- The usual oral *starting* dose is 5–10 mg 4-hourly (2.5 mg in the frail elderly): it can be added to soft drinks (a 20 mg/ml solution is available for this purpose; measurement must be precise). Morphine may also be used by buccal or sublingual route (lower dose).

---

[26] Solutions of morphine deteriorate once they are opened (exposed to air), and if exposed to light (keep in dark) and heat, they lose potency over as few as 2–4 weeks; competent pharmaceutical advice and preparation is required; stable formulations have been developed (Oramorph). The taste of morphine is bitter and patients may choose an accompanying drink to mask it. Tablets may be used.

- Peak plasma concentration is reached in $1\frac{1}{2}$–2 h.
- If the *first dose* is not more effective than previous medication, increase the second dose.
- If the pain is not more than 90% controlled in the first 24 h *increase* the dose by 50%. After that adjust dose 24-hourly as below.
- *Dose:* most patients get satisfactory pain control at 5–30 mg 4-hourly (a few will need more than 200 mg, but rarely 500 mg dose has been required); arbitrary fixed dosage is inappropriate, since doses and frequency are adjusted to meet the patients' need.
- *Change to morphine from other high-efficacy opioids*; higher starting doses of oral morphine will be needed.
- A *larger dose at night* (1.5–2 × daytime dose) or an added hypnotic may allow the patient to pass the night without waking in pain (and so to omit one night dose).
- *Dosage increments* of oral morphine given 4-hourly:
  - below 15 mg, add 5 mg
  - up to 30 mg, add 10 mg
  - up to 90 mg, add 15 mg
  - up to 180 mg, add 30 mg
  - above 180 mg, add 60 mg

Sustained-release tablets (MST Continus: 10, 30, 60, 100 mg, coloured differently) are available; they are taken 12-hourly; special dose regimens apply.

- *Constipation will occur*, see below; it is essential to manage it.
- *Initial drowsiness* (a few days) and confusion (in the elderly) are common and usually pass off. This should be explained to the patient ('You may feel sleepy or a little muddled'): if unpleasant sedation persists then small doses of amphetamine may be added.
- *Initial nausea* and *vomiting* may occur: an antiemetic controls it (e.g. prochlorperazine 2.5–5 mg, orally, 6–8-hourly), and can generally be withdrawn after 4–5 days.
- *Myoclonus* may occur, perhaps promoted by concurrent use of antidepressants or neuroleptics.
- When there are *problems with 4-hourly* administration of the liquid preparation, a sustained-release oral formulation is an alterna-

tive (above), as are suppositories or buccal (sublingual) formulations (the latter route by-passes the first-pass or presystemic elimination and does not require such high doses as when swallowed).

- *Breakthrough pain*: an additional dose of morphine or other agonist opioid analgesic (*not* a partial agonist) provided for self-administration is valuable, not least because it gives the patient confidence. A NSAID can also be used.
- *Respiratory depression* is seldom a problem with morphine used in this way.
- *Dependence* need not be feared. Both physical and psychological occurs, but the latter to only a small degree compared with drug abuse or other chronic pain syndrome; the social, psychological and medical aspects of morphine use in terminal care are so different from that of drug abuse that comparisons are inappropriate. Dose reduction, when required, e.g. after relief of pain by palliative radiotherapy or nerve block, should, of course, be gradual, but abrupt withdrawal (accidental) has been found to cause only mild withdrawal syndrome.
- *Acquired tolerance* is dealt with by increasing the dose.
- *To transfer from oral to injected dose or infused* morphine or diamorphine (heroin) e.g. due to difficult swallowing, vomiting, the injected dose should be half the oral dose (4-hourly swallowed) (if heroin is substituted, then one-third).

Adjuvant drugs

Phenothiazines are antiemetic, antianxiety and sedative agents and they may change the affective response to pain (particularly methotrimeprazine).

Tricyclic antidepressants (and perhaps others) have a morphine-sparing effect even in the absence of an effect or mood.

Amphetamine elevates mood and enhances analgesia.

Routine addition to morphine solutions of other drugs *such as cocaine, chlorpromazine and alcohol* has no merit.

Where oral drugs fail morphine may be given *intrathecally* (where the skill and knowledge is available). Morphine may be supplemented and

replaced by appropriate nerve blocks and nerve destructive procedures.

Conduction anaesthesia

The full range of techniques of local and regional anaesthesia are used appropriately, including extradural and intrathecal morphine (p. 374).

Other symptoms

- *Anorexia* is common in patients with widespread cancer; prednisolone 15–30 mg daily and/or alcohol in the patient's preferred form before meals, may help, or carbonated or other drink for which the patient has a taste.
- *Confusion* may not need treatment unless it is accompanied by restlessness: haloperidol in emergency: thioridazine (does not cause much sedation): chlorpromazine (if sedation is desired): chlormethiazole for insomnia.
- *Constipation* is usual in dying patients, whether due to opioid analgesic (see above) or to inadequate intake of food and fluid,[27] and physical inactivity. It can be exceedingly troublesome and management should begin early to forestall the need for the major unpleasantness and humiliations of manual removal of faeces and the lesser ones of enemas. Dietary measures should be used where practicable. A stimulant laxative and faecal softener (danthron plus poloxamer: co-danthramer) is commonly effective; suppositories, e.g. glycerol or bisacodyl, are useful; also lactulose. Good advice from St. Christopher's Hospice (London): if the bowels have not been opened for three days, perform a rectal examination and if the rectum is found to be loaded insert a suppository.
- *Convulsions*: sodium valproate orally is preferred to phenytoin as the latter interacts extensively with other drugs; where oral use is

---

[27] It is normal and comfortable to die slightly dehydrated; full hydration leads to full urinary bladder (with discomfort, restlessness incontinence), salivary drooling and death rattle; it also increases heart failure (with dyspnoea which enhances death rattle); intravenous tubes make final embraces almost impossible (Lamerton R Lancet 1991; 337: 981).

impracticable use phenobarbitone i.m. (for status epilepticus see p. 306).

- *Cough*: see p. 503.
- *Diarrhoea*: see p. 535.
- *Dyspnoea*. Chronic dyspnoea (not due to respiratory failure) may be relieved by an opioid (respiratory centre depression reducing its sensitivity to chemical stimuli), but when there is respiratory failure due to pulmonary disease any sedation may cause serious respiratory depression. Oxygen is used as appropriate; a benzodiazepine reduces the anxiety of dyspnoea; dexamethasone reduces inflammation around obstructive tumours that cause dyspnoea. Accumulations of mucus that the patient is too weak to expel cause 'death rattle'; this terminal event, often more distressing to others than to the patient, may be eliminated by (further) drying up the secretions with an antimuscarinic drug (hyoscine or atropine 4- to 8-hourly).
- *Emergencies* such as major haemorrhage, pulmonary embolus, severe choking, fracture of large bone: give morphine 10 mg plus hyoscine 0.4 mg i.m.; this combination provides acute relief and some desirable short-term retrograde amnesia which, with luck, will extend to the whole unpleasant episode.
- *Hiccup* (due to diaphragmatic spasm): where this is intractable and exhausting, chlorpromazine (or other phenothiazine) or metoclopramide may help; also baclofen, nifedipine or sodium valproate.
- *Insomnia*: temazepam, or chlormethiazole (which may be less prone to cause confusion in the elderly).
- *Intestinal obstruction* can be managed without surgery[28] (which only adds to the distress of dying). It is done by giving loperamide (or diphenoxylate) and/or hyoscine (or atropine) sublingually or s.c., for colic; antiemetics (sometimes combining two having different sites of action); and a faecal softener (without added laxative, which would increase peristalsis) for as long as obstruction is incomplete; there may be an inflammatory element in tumour obstruction, which can be relieved by substantial doses of corticosteroid (prednisolone 15 to 30 mg/day). When obstruction is complete the patient may vomit once or twice a day without great distress, but oral therapy may become impracticable; to avoid injections in an emaciated patient, drugs may be given by suppository (opioid plus antiemetic).
- *Itch*: see p. 636.
- *Lymphoedema*, e.g. due to pelvic cancer, that causes pain may be helped by prednisolone (15–30 mg/day).
- *Mental distress* may be helped by alcohol-opioid mixtures, antidepressants or tranquillisers, according to circumstances. Patients may too easily be drugged into uncomplaining silence, but it does not follow that they are not still in deep distress:

. . . the grief that does not speak
Whispers the o'er-fraught heart, and bids it break.[29]

And this unpleasant way of ending life can be avoided by discerning choice and, particularly, careful dosage of drugs.

- *A mouth* that is dry and painful may be due to candidiasis (treat with nystatin), to dehydration (rehydrate the patient judiciously[27] where this can be done orally, otherwise the symptom can be managed by frequent small drinks or crushed ice to suck plus assiduous mouth hygiene to prevent unpleasant infection), or due to antimuscarinic drugs including some antidepressants (withdraw the drug or adjust its dose).
- *Nausea and vomiting*, whether due to disease or to opioid drug, cause great distress and can be more difficult to manage than pain; two drugs acting by different mechanisms may be needed when a single agent fails, e.g. phenothiazine plus antimuscarinic, or either plus metoclopramide. For vomiting of *hypercalcaemia*: use an antiemetic and treat the cause (p. 655).
- *Night sweats* can be distressing and cause insomnia: indomethacin helps.
- *Restlessness* in terminal illness that has no

---

[28] A detailed account is given by Baines M et al. Lancet 1985; 2: 90.

[29] William Shakespeare (1564–1616). Macbeth, Act 4, Scene 3.

obvious cause, e.g. pain, full bladder, may be treated with methotrimeprazine (a phenothiazine tranquilliser with analgesic effect) by injection: it may be combined with morphine (or diamorphine), which are tranquillisers as well as analgesics: diazepam is useful for muscle twitching.

● *Swallowing* of solid-dose forms may be difficult and these may stick in the oesophagus in weak recumbent patients, especially if adequate fluid is not taken with the dose (at least two big gulps or 100 ml with the patient's trunk vertical); potassium chloride tablet is known especially to ulcerate the oesophagus.

● *Urinary frequency, urgency and incontinence*: flavoxate, terodiline, oxybutynin (antimuscarinics) may be useful; they may cause retention of urine if there is anatomical obstruction. The pain of an indwelling catheter may be alleviated by diazepam.

● *Raised intracranial pressure* (see p. 239): dexamethasone may be used indefinitely; reduce dose to 5 mg/d if practicable.

● *Fungating tumours and ulcers* may smell distressingly due to anaerobic bacterial growth. Benefit may be gained by topical providone iodine or metronidazole gel.

NARCOTIC OR OPIOID[30] ANALGESICS

AGONISTS, PARTIAL AGONISTS, ANTAGONISTS

Among the remedies which it has pleased Almighty God to give to man to relieve his sufferings, none is so universal and so efficacious as opium.
                    Thomas Sydenham, physician, 1680.

It is not known when opium (the dried juice of the seed head of the opium poppy) was first procured and used as a drug, but it was certainly in prehistoric times, and medical practice still leans heavily on its alkaloids, using them as analgesic, tranquilliser, antitussive and in diarrhoea.

Crude opium alone was used in medicine until 1806, when the principal active ingredient was isolated by Friedrich Sertürner, who tested the separate fractions he extracted from it on animals and tried pure morphine on himself and three young men. He observed that the drug caused cerebral depression and spasms of the extremities and that it relieved toothache. He named it after Morpheus.[31]

Opium contains many alkaloids, but the only important ones are *morphine* (10%) and *codeine*; *papaverine* is occasionally used as a vasodilator. In general, morphine is used now where opium was used in the past; its effects differ little from those of opium. However, purified preparations of mixtures of opium alkaloids, e.g. papaveretum (Omnopon), are available; minus noscapine which is suspected of genotoxicity.

Mode of action

Endogenous opioid peptides (endorphins, dynorphins, enkephalins), discovered in 1975, have been termed 'the brain's own morphine'. At last the question why the brain had opioid receptors, when there were no opioids in the body had its answer. These peptides are neurotransmitters in complex pain-inhibitory systems. They attach to specific opioid receptors (four main types: mu, kappa, delta, sigma), and it is on these receptors that administered opioids also act (via neuronal K and Ca channels). Opioid drugs may be agonist to one class of opioid receptor, and antagonist (blocker) to another, which explains the differing patterns of action seen. A drug may also have dual agonist/antagonist (partial agonist) effect on a single receptor (which will result in a limited ceiling of therapeutic efficacy, and antagonism if it is given in the presence of a high

---

[30] The term opi*ate* has been used for the natural alkaloids of opium, and opi*oid* for other agents having similar action. The distinction is neither generally observed nor particularly useful. We here use *opioid* for all receptor-specific substances.

[31] In classical mythology Morpheus was son of Somnus, the infernal deity who presided over sleep. He was generally represented as a corpulent, winged boy holding opium poppies in his hand. His principal function seems to have been to stand by his sleeping father's black-curtained bed of feathers, on watch to prevent his being awakened by noise.

efficacy agonist, i.e. it will precipitate a withdrawal syndrome in subjects dependent on morphine or heroin). In addition, a weak (low-efficacy) agonist (codeine) will compete with a high-efficacy opioid for receptors and so reduce the receptor occupancy, and therefore the therapeutic efficacy of the latter, i.e. a weak agonist partially antagonises a strong agonist. It is no surprise that there are differences between opioids in emphasis or pattern of their many actions.

Some of the endorphins, dynorphins and enkephalins are about as active as morphine and some have higher efficacy; some are short and some are long-acting. The discovery of the role of natural opioid mechanisms in physiology and pathology opens up possibilities for major developments in pain management, and indeed, wider, for endogenous opioid mechanisms may play a role, e.g. in shock.

The continuing unravelling of opioid mechanisms has not yet provided an adequate explanation of opioid tolerance and dependence.

MORPHINE AND OPIOIDS IN GENERAL

Morphine will be described in detail and other opioid analgesics principally in so far as they differ from it.

The *principal actions* of morphine may be summarised:

On the central nervous system:
- *Depression*, leading to:
  analgesia
  respiratory depression
  depression of cough reflex
  sleep
- *Excitation*, leading to:
  vomiting
  miosis
  hyperactive spinal cord reflexes (some only)
  convulsions (very rare)
- *Changes of mood*: euphoria or dysphoria
- *Dependence*; affects other systems too.

Smooth muscle stimulation:
  Gastrointestinal muscle spasm (delayed passage of contents with constipation)
  Biliary tract spasm
  Bronchospasm
  Renal tract spasm: dubious, see below.

Cardiovascular system:
  Dilatation of resistance (arterioles) and capacitance (veins) vessels.

Morphine on the central nervous system

Morphine is the most generally useful high-efficacy opioid analgesic; it eliminates pain and also allows subjects to tolerate pain, i.e. the sensation is felt but is no longer unpleasant. It both stimulates and depresses the central nervous system. It induces a state of relaxation, tranquillity, detachment and well-being (euphoria), or occasionally of unpleasantness (dysphoria), and causes sleepiness, inability to concentrate and lethargy, always supposing that this pleasant state is not destroyed by nausea and vomiting, more common if the patient is ambulant. Excitement can occur but is unusual. Morphine excites cats and horses, though it is illegal to put this to practical use in horse or cat racing. Generally, morphine has useful hypnotic and tranquillising actions and there should be no hesitation in using it in full dose in appropriate circumstances, e.g. acute pain and fear, as in myocardial infarction or road traffic accidents.

Morphine *depresses respiration* (rate and depth), principally by reducing sensitivity of the respiratory centre to rise in blood CO_2 tension. With therapeutic doses there is a reduced minute volume due to diminished rate and tidal volume. With higher doses carbon dioxide narcosis may develop. In overdose the patient may present with a respiratory rate as low as 2/min.

Morphine is dangerous when the respiratory drive is impaired by disease, including CO_2 retention from any cause, e.g. emphysema, or raised intracranial pressure.

In *asthmatics*, in addition to the effect on the respiratory centre, it may increase viscosity of bronchial secretions, which, with depression of cough and bronchospasm (see below) will increase small airways resistance.

In postsurgical patients morphine may promote pulmonary atelectasis by discouraging deep breathing, but abdominal or thoracic pain discourages it also.

Morphine also suppresses *cough* by a central action. It stimulates the third nerve nucleus causing *miosis* (pin-point pupils are characteristic of poisoning, acute or chronic; at therapeutic doses the pupil is merely smaller): it can obscure valuable pupillary changes in changing neurological states, e.g. head injury.

The chemoreceptor trigger zone of the *vomiting centre* is stimulated, causing nausea (40%) and vomiting (15%), a side-effect which, in addition to being unpleasant, can be dangerous in patients who have had abdominal operations, a cataract removed, or myocardial infarction. A preparation of morphine plus an antiemetic, e.g. cyclizine (Cyclimorph) reduces this liability. Some spinal cord reflexes are also stimulated, causing myoclonus and so morphine is unsuitable for use in tetanus and convulsant poisoning; indeed, morphine can itself cause convulsions.

Morphine causes *antidiuresis* by releasing antidiuretic hormone, and this can be clinically important.

Appetite is lost with chronic use.

Morphine on smooth muscle

Alimentary tract. Morphine activates receptors on the smooth muscle of the stomach (antrum) and of both large and small bowel, causing it to contract. Peristalsis (propulsion) is reduced and segmentation increased. Thus, although morphine 'stimulates' smooth muscle, delayed gastric emptying and constipation occur, with gut muscle in a state of tonic contraction. The central action of the drug probably also leads to neglect of the urge to defaecate. Delay in the passage of the intestinal contents results in greater absorption of water and increased viscosity of faeces, which contributes to the constipation. The management of opioid-induced constipation is an important aspect of terminal care.

Morphine causes high intrasigmoid pressures, which in colonic diverticular disease may result in the diverticula blowing up and becoming obstructed and failing to drain into the colon. Pethidine neither produces these high pressures nor prevents drainage, and so is preferable for the pain of acute diverticulitis if it should be severe enough to demand a narcotic analgesic. Morphine may also endanger anastomoses of the bowel immediately postoperatively and it should not be given in intestinal obstruction (excepting in terminal care).

Intrabiliary pressure may rise substantially after morphine (as much as 10 times in 10 minutes), due to spasm of the sphincter of Oddi. Sometimes biliary colic is made worse by morphine, presumably in a patient in whom the dose happens to be adequate to increase intrabiliary pressure, but insufficient to produce more than slight analgesia. In patients who have had a cholecystectomy this can produce a syndrome sufficiently like a myocardial infarction to cause diagnostic confusion. The electrocardiograph may be abnormal. Naloxone may give dramatic symptomatic relief as may glyceryl trinitrate. Another result of this action of morphine is to dam back the pancreatic juice and so to cause a rise in the serum amylase concentration. Morphine is therefore best avoided in pancreatitis; but buprenorphine has less of this effect.

Urinary tract. Any contraction of the ureters is probably clinically unimportant. Retention of urine may occur (particularly in prostatic hypertrophy) due to a mix of spasm of the bladder sphincter and to the central sedation causing the patient to ignore afferent messages from a full bladder.

Bronchial muscle is constricted, partly due to histamine release, but so slightly as to be of no importance, *except in asthmatics* in whom morphine is best avoided anyway because of its respiratory depressant effect. *If given in a severe attack of asthma, morphine may kill.*

When morphine is used and the *smooth muscle effects are objectionable*, atropine may be given simultaneously to antagonise spasm. Unfortunately it does not always effectively oppose the rise of pressure induced in the biliary system, nor does it restore bowel peristalsis. Glyceryl trinitrate will relax morphine-induced spasm.

Uterus. Labour is prolonged, but this may be the result of central psychological effects reducing patient cooperation rather than to an action on the uterus.

Cardiovascular system

Morphine, by a central action, impairs sympathetic vascular reflexes (causing veno- and arteriolar dilatation) and stimulates the vagal centre (bradycardia); it also releases histamine (vasodilatation). These effects are ordinarily unimportant, but they can be beneficial in acute left ventricular failure (paroxysmal nocturnal dyspnoea), relieving mental distress by tranquillising, cardiac distress by reduction of sympathetic drive and respiratory distress by rendering the centre insensitive to afferent stimuli from the congested lungs, but the effect can sometimes be harmful in patients taking antihypertensives, in acute myocardial infarction and with low blood volume; excessive bradycardia can be blocked by atropine.

Other effects of morphine include sweating, histamine release pruritus and piloerection.

Tolerance

Chronic use of morphine and other opioids is marked by acquired tolerance to the depressant agonist effects, e.g. analgesic action and respiratory depression (the fatal dose becomes higher), but not to some stimulant agonist effects, e.g. constipation and miosis, which persist.

Opioids that have mixed agonist/antagonist actions (partial agonists) induce tolerance to the agonist but not to the antagonist effects; naloxone (a pure antagonist) induces no tolerance to itself.

There is a cross-tolerance between opioids. (For dependence and withdrawal see below).

Acquired tolerance develops over days with continued frequent use and passes off (variably for different actions) over a few days to weeks.

Pharmacokinetics

Given s.c. (particularly) or i.m., morphine is rapidly absorbed when the circulation is normal, but in circulatory shock absorption will be delayed and it is best given i.v. Oral morphine is subject to extensive presystemic or first-pass metabolism (conjugation; gut wall and liver) and only about 20% of a dose reaches the systemic circulation; the oral dose is about twice the injected dose. The buccal or the sublingual route are also practicable and there is no first-pass metabolism; these routes are comparable to i.m. injection.

Morphine in the systemic circulation is metabolised by both liver and kidney; the conjugated metabolites include the pharmacologically active morphine-6-glucuronide. Elimination of morphine (10%) and metabolites is largely renal, but data conflict on whether action is prolonged in renal failure; it probably is not.[32]

The $t_\frac{1}{2}$ is 2 h (active metabolites slightly longer) and the duration of useful analgesia is 4–6 h (shorter in younger than in older subjects).

Morphine crosses the placenta and depresses respiration in the fetus at birth.

Other routes of administration used by specialists are epidural (obstetrics) and intrathecal; very low doses are used.

Dosage. Given s.c., i.m. **morphine** 10 mg is usually adequate; with 15 mg unwanted effects increase more than does analgesia; i.v. slowly $\frac{1}{4}$–$\frac{1}{2}$ i.m. dose. For oral dosage see terminal care p. 241. Continuous pain suppression can be achieved by morphine orally 4-hourly and s.c. 3-hourly or by continuous s.c. infusion using a battery-powered pump attached to the patient, who may even be ambulant.

The important uses of morphine and its analogues

● To relieve *severe pain* (but beware of masking useful diagnostic signs, e.g. in the

---

[32] Woolner, D F et al Brit. J. Clin. Pharmacol 1986; 22 : 55.

acute abdomen and pupillary signs in neurology).

- To relieve *anxiety* in serious and frightening disease, e.g. circulatory shock, severe haemorrhage, accidents.
- To relieve *dyspnoea* in acute left ventricular failure (paroxysmal nocturnal dyspnoea).
- *Premedication* for surgery.
- Symptomatic control of acute non-serious *diarrhoea*, e.g. travellers' diarrhoea (codeine, loperamide).
- To suppress *cough*.
- To control *acute restlessness* (rarely).
- To produce *euphoria* as well as pain relief in the dying.

Any of the desired effects may be interfered with by opioid-induced nausea, vomiting and dysphoria.

Morphine and disease. Morphine has long been standard treatment for vascular stock due to trauma. It tranquillises and relieves suffering, fear and pain but there may be such intense peripheral vasoconstriction that s.c. absorption is delayed for hours. A second or even third dose may therefore be injected before the patient has absorbed the first and so lead to poisoning when the vasoconstriction passes off. In such cases morphine should be given i.m. or slowly i.v. If the blood volume is low morphine may cause serious hypotension.

In hepatic failure small doses can cause coma (see Drugs and the liver), and it may be dangerous in *hypothyroidism* (slow metabolism). Serious hypotension can occur in *myocardial infarction*, also vagal *bradycardia* (treatable by atropine 0.3–0.6 mg i.v.).

In *respiratory insufficiency* (emphysema, asthma, raised intracranial pressure) it is dangerous, see above; also in *diverticulitis*, pancreatitis and after *cholecystectomy*, see above.

Interactions. Morphine is potentiated by neostigmine, chlorpromazine (perhaps) and MAOIs and tricyclic antidepressants. Any central nervous system depressant will have additive effects; cimetidine inhibits pethidine metabolism; rifampicin accelerates methadone metabolism; dextropropoxyphene inhibits warfarin metabolism.

Severe hypotension may occur with antihypertensive drugs.

Adverse effects (type A) have been mentioned and discussed. Dependence and overdose are treated below. Opioid use in obstetrics requires special care (p. 376).

Opioid dependence[33]

Physical dependence begins to occur within 24 h if morphine is given 4-hourly, and after surgery some patients may be unwittingly subjected to a withdrawal syndrome that passes for general postoperative discomfort.

Acquired tolerance may rapidly reach a high degree, an addict taking morphine 600 mg (heroin equivalent 400 mg) or even more several times a day. An average addict is more likely to take about 300 mg. Duration of tolerance after cessation of administration is variable for different actions, from a few days to weeks. Thus, addicts who have undergone withdrawal and lost tolerance, and who later resume their opioid careers may overdose themselves inadvertently.

Morphine or heroin dependence is more disabling physically and socially than is opium dependence. (Treatment of pain in opioid dependent subjects, see p. 255.) Chronic exposure to opioids leads to adaptive changes in the endogenous opioid system and no doubt in receptor numbers, sensitivity and cellular response. The abrupt withdrawal of administered opioid would be expected to provoke rebound or a withdrawal syndrome. This consists largely of the opposite of the normal actions of opioids. Also, noradrenergic mechanisms are modulated by endogenous opioids and these mechanisms are depressed by continuous opioid administration. Abrupt withdrawal rebound can be described as 'noradrenergic storm'.

---

[33] There is evidence that opioid abuse in adults might stem partly from an imprinting process during birth when opioids, barbiturates and nitrous oxide (for >1 h) are given to the mother (Jacobsen B et al. Br Med J 1990; 301: 1067).

The acute withdrawal syndrome in opioid (morphine, heroin) dependence

When an addict misses his first shot, he senses mild withdrawal distress ('feels his habit coming on') but this is probably more psychological than physiological, for fear plays a considerable role in the withdrawal syndrome. At this stage a placebo may give relief. During the first 8–16 h of abstinence the addict becomes increasingly nervous, restless and anxious; close confinement tends to intensify these symptoms. Within 14 h (usually less) he will begin to yawn frequently; he sweats profusely and develops running of the eyes and nose comparable to that accompanying a severe head cold. These symptoms increase in intensity for the first 24 h, after which the pupils dilate and recurring waves of goose flesh occur. Severe twitching of the muscles (the origin of the term 'kick the habit') occurs within 36 h and painful cramps develop in the backs of the legs and in the abdomen; all the body fluids are released copiously; vomiting and diarrhoea are acute; there is little appetite for food and the addict is unable to sleep. The respiratory rate rises steeply. Both systolic and diastolic blood pressure increase moderately to a maximum between the third and fourth day; temperature rises an average of about 0.5°C, subsiding after the third day; the blood sugar content rises sharply until the third day or after; the basal metabolic rate increases sharply during the first 48 h. These are the objective signs of withdrawal distress which can be measured; the subjective indications are equally severe and the illness reaches its peak within 48–72 h after the last shot of the opioid, gradually subsiding thereafter for the next 5–10 days. Complete recovery requires from 3–6 months with rehabilitation and, if needed, psychiatric treatment. The withdrawal syndrome proper is self-limiting and most addicts will survive it with no medical assistance whatever (this is known as kicking the habit, 'cold turkey'). Abrupt withdrawal is inhumane, but with the development of such drugs as methadone, it is possible to reduce the distress of withdrawal very considerably.[34]

It is usual to cover the acute withdrawal period (about 10 days) of injected morphine or heroin with an opioid taken orally and having a long $t_{\frac{1}{2}}$, e.g. methadone $t_{\frac{1}{2}}$ 48 h, perhaps supplemented with chlorpromazine or a benzodiazepine. Clonidine (0.1 mg × 4/d, reducing over about 4 days) can reduce the effects of noradrenergic hyperactivity by its agonist action on central presynaptic α_2-adrenoceptors that results in inhibition of sympathetic autonomic outflow; hypotension may occur.

A withdrawal syndrome occurs in the *newborn* of dependent mothers.

Opioids with partial agonist actions precipitate a withdrawal syndrome in dependent subjects, as do the antagonists naltrexone and naloxone (it is unkind, because it is unnecessary, to use an antagonist as a diagnostic test in suspected addicts).

Therapeutic addiction. There is a risk of making patients seriously dependent if prolonged or frequent treatment of pain with a high-efficacy opioid is undertaken (the more widely the doses are spaced, the less the risk), e.g. for trigeminal neuralgia, migraine or recurrent urinary colic. Terminal care is an exception, see above. It is impossible to rule on how quickly a patient can become seriously dependent, but it is generally a matter of weeks or months, though detectable physical dependence can occur in a day if the drug is given intensively. Dependence is less severe with partial agonists.

Pharmacological aids to prevention of relapse of addicts: see methadone and naltrexone.

Overdose

Death from overdose (of all opioids, low and high efficacy; agonist or partial agonist) is due to respiratory failure. Blood pressure is usually well maintained, if the patient is supine, until anoxia causes circulatory failure. At this point the pupils, whose small size is a useful diagnostic indicator, may dilate (also if there is hypothermia). Correct diagnosis is vital, for naloxone is a selective competitive antagonist. The combination of miosis and bradypnoea is almost diagnostic of opioid overdose. Naloxone does not have any of the actions of morphine, i.e. it has no agonist effects (coma, respiratory depression, miosis). Therefore it is safe to give naloxone as a therapeutic test in

---

[34] From Maurer D W, Vogel V H. Narcotics and narcotic addiction. Springfield, I U.: Charles C. Thomas. 1962. Courtesy of the authors and Charles C. Thomas, publisher, Springfield, Ill.

an unconscious or drowsy patient suspected of opioid overdose. The t_2^1 of naloxone (1 h) is shorter than most opioids and repeated doses or infusion will be needed. The guide to therapy is the state of respiration, not of consciousness. Patients with opioid overdose should be watched for recurrence of ventilatory depression, which is an indication for further naloxone. (For details of naloxone use see p. 255.) Apart from naloxone the general treatment is the same as for overdose by any cerebral depressant.

Addicts often take overdoses, whether accidentally or not, and naloxone, as well as reversing the life-endangering respiratory depression, will induce an acute (noradrenergic) withdrawal syndrome. Close cardiovascular monitoring is necessary, with use of peripheral adrenoceptor blocking agents or perhaps clonidine (see above), according to need.

PREPARATIONS OF OPIUM AND MORPHINE

There is a large number of obsolescent and obsolete formulations of opium.

Small doses of opium can be used for the symptomatic control of the milder diarrhoeas, e.g. Kaolin and Morphine Mixture. These and other preparations may be used by those who have a mind to and they have the efficacy of the opium they contain.

The only preparation of opium that remains in widespread use is *papaveretum* (Omnopon), a mixture of purified opium alkaloids chiefly used in pre-anaesthetic medication.

Morphine salts are used by injection, and by the oral, buccal, sublingual and rectal routes. *Sustained-release formulations*, oral (MST Continus) and i.m. (Duromorph, a microcrystalline form), are available.

The opioids discussed below are considered in relation to morphine (t_2^1 does not necessarily indicate duration of useful analgesia, which is related to affinity of the opioid for receptors: but t_2^1 gives useful information on accumulation).

CLASSIFICATION OF OPIOIDS BY ANALGESIC EFFICACY

Low-efficacy for mild and moderate pain	**High-efficacy for severe pain**
codeine	*buprenorphine
dihydrocodeine	dextromoramide
dextropropoxyphene	diamorphine (heroin)
*nalbuphine	dipipanone
*pentazocine	levorphanol
	*meptazinol
	methadone
	morphine
	papaveretum
	pethidine (meperidine)
*Partial agonist	phenazocine

Notes:
- The division into 2 classes is not absolute and some drugs listed for moderate pain can be effective in severe pain by injection.
- Fentanyl, alfenatil and phenoperidine are high-efficacy opioids used for surgery/anaesthesia.
- *Etorphine* is a high-efficacy opioid used to immobilise animals in veterinary practice. The doses used in large animals are enough to kill a man if, in a struggle, the drug is splashed on skin or mucous membrane, or there is a needle scratch. A competitive antagonist, naloxone, or diprenorphine (supplied for veterinary use), is *urgently* required.

Partial agonists were developed in the unrealised hope of eliminating the potential for abuse whilst retaining analgesic efficacy; they include pentazocine, buprenorphine, meptazinol and nalbuphine; they may induce psychotomimetic reactions. They are indeed less liable to induce dependence and to cause respiratory depression than are the pure agonists, though they do have these effects. Their antagonist action is chiefly evident against large doses of agonist, e.g. in addicts.

OTHER OPIOIDS (see also general account above)

Codeine (methylmorphine)

A low-efficacy opioid, it has a $t_{\frac{1}{2}}$ of 3 h and 10% is converted to morphine. It lacks efficacy for severe pain and most of its actions are about one-tenth that of morphine. It also has a qualitative difference from morphine in that large doses cause excitement. Dependence occurs but much less than with morphine.

Its principal uses are for mild and moderate pain and cough (long-term use is accompanied by chronic constipation) and for the short-term symptomatic control of the milder acute diarrhoeas.

The dose of codeine alone is 10–60 mg orally 4-hourly: and by injection up to 30 mg. There are numerous formulations for cough (e.g. Codeine Linctus) and for pain, in which it is commonly combined with aspirin and/or paracetamol (Aspirin and Codeine Tabs, Co-codaprin; Aspirin, Paracetamol and Codeine Tabs).

Pethidine (meperidine, Demerol)

Pethidine was introduced in 1939. It was discovered during a search for smooth muscle relaxants acting like atropine. It is not obviously related structurally to either morphine or atropine, though it is said that cognoscenti can discern resemblances to both. When given to mice it caused the tail to stand erect (Straub phenomenon) a characteristic of morphine-like drugs caused by spasm of the anal sphincter. This attracted attention and pethidine was examined for analgesic effect.

Pethidine cannot relieve such severe pain as can morphine, i.e. it has lower therapeutic efficacy, but is effective against pain beyond the reach of codeine. Despite its substantial structural dissimilarity to morphine, pethidine has many similar properties including that of being antagonised by naloxone.

Pethidine differs from morphine in the following ways:

- It does not suppress cough usefully.
- It does not constipate, but its effect in the upper small intestine is similar to morphine and there is spasm of the sphincter of Oddi.
- It is less likely to cause, urinary retention and to prolong childbirth.
- It has little hypnotic effect.
- Duration of analgesia is substantially shorter (2–3 h).

Pethidine causes vomiting about as often as does morphine; it has atropine-like effects, including dry mouth and blurred vision (cycloplegia and sometimes mydriasis, though usually miosis). Overdose or use in renal failure can cause central nervous system stimulation (myoclonus, convulsions) due to the major metabolite norpethidine, which is excreted by the kidney.

There is disagreement on the extent to which pethidine depresses respiration. It is probable that in equianalgesic doses it is as depressant as morphine.

Pethidine dependence occurs, with some tolerance, especially to the side-effects, but its psychic effects are less constant and less marked than those of morphine. Pethidine has evident advantages over morphine for pain that is not very intense, and it is widely used. It is usually given orally (50–100 mg) or i.m. (25–100 mg), when its effects last 2–3 h. The solution is irritant and so it is not given s.c. Given i.v. (25–50 mg) it is used sometimes in anaesthetic practice to provide a state of 'general analgesia'. It is widely used in obstetrics because it does not delay labour like morphine; but it enters the fetus and can depress respiration at birth.

Pethidine ($t_{\frac{1}{2}}$ 3 h) is metabolised in the liver and 5% is excreted unchanged in the urine. The latter is substantially greater if the urine is acid but in overdose it is not worthwhile to acidify the urine since naloxone is convenient and immediately effective.

Methadone (Physeptone) (1946)

This is a synthetic drug structurally and pharmacologically similar to morphine. Vomiting is fairly common (though somewhat less than with morphine) especially if the patient is ambulant, and sedation is less: 5–10 mg are given 6–12 hourly, orally or s.c. But since it has a long $t_\frac{1}{2}$ of wide range, 20–80 h, accumulation will occur, especially in the aged. Analgesia may last for as long as 24 h. If used for chronic pain in terminal care (12-hourly) an opioid of short $t_\frac{1}{2}$ may be provided for breakthrough pain rather than an extra dose of methadone. Renal excretion is increased in acid urine, but naloxone is more convenient and quickly effective.

Dependence occurs but this is less severe (slower onset and less severe withdrawal syndrome, compatible with the long $t_\frac{1}{2}$) than with morphine and heroin, and addicts to these drugs (by injection) are often transferred to oral methadone as part of their treatment.[35] Addicts who are cooperative enough to take oral methadone will feel reduced craving and less 'kick/buzz/rush' from i.v. heroin or morphine, should they be unable to resist temptation, because their opioid receptors are already occupied by methadone and the i.v. drug must compete. Reports of deaths in addicts entering prescribed methadone substitution programmes have been attributed to the cardiovascular effects of a membrane stabilising action, unlike morphine (see naltrexone).

Methadone is also useful for severe cough. *Levorphanol* (Dromoran) is similar to methadone.

Diamorphine (heroin) (1898)

This semisynthetic drug was first made from morphine at St. Mary's Hospital, London in 1874. It was introduced in 1898 as a remedy for cough and for morphine addiction and is very effective against both. Some years passed, however, before it was appreciated that it 'cured' morphine addiction by substituting itself as the addicting agent. Since then it has become a popular choice with addicts and has achieved such a reputation that it is difficult now to discover whether abusers are attracted to it because it is pleasanter or because of its reputation, plus its ready availability from drug peddlers. It is rapidly (in minutes) converted to morphine in the body.

It is commonly stated that heroin is the 'most potent' of all dependence-producing opioids. Weight-for-weight it is certainly more effective than morphine, and this is of importance in illicit traffic as heroin takes up less space, but in so far as *efficacy* in inducing dependence is concerned there is doubt.

In almost every country the manufacture of heroin, even for use in medicine, is now illegal. The first to try this prohibition as a remedy for widespread drug addiction was the USA, which banned heroin manufacture in 1924, provoked by the magnitude of their addiction problem and not yet discouraged by their experience of this type of approach with alcohol prohibition (1919 to 1933).

An effort was made in 1953 to achieve a worldwide ban on heroin in medicine (so that any heroin, wherever it was found *must* be illegal) and most countries agreed. The UK did not agree because legitimate supplies for medicine were not then getting into illicit channels (it has since remained available but is not exported). A ban now would be pointless since illegal heroin is readily available worldwide.

Many clinicians have long thought and some have passionately believed that heroin has unique therapeutic properties (euphoria, analgesic efficacy, lack of adverse effects); but research, as opposed to clinical impressions, has shown these beliefs in the superiority of heroin to be unfounded, *except* that heroin is more soluble than morphine to a useful degree[36] when continuous

---

[35] In the UK a special *Methadone Mixture 1 mg/ml* (the concentration is part of the official title) is specially provided for the management of opioid addicts; it is coloured green and formulated to prevent injection. It has × 2½ the strength of Methadone Linctus, for cough (yellow or brown); they must not be confused.

[36] Solubility in water: morphine sulphate 1 in 21; heroin hydrochloride 1 in 1.6.

pain control in terminal care can no longer be achieved by enteral morphine (oral, buccal, suppository) for any reason. The greater solubility of heroin is then a real advantage in wasted subjects requiring multiple injections (or continuous infusion) of high doses. *Intravenous infusion* (by pump) of diamorphine is increasingly used in severe pain; it can be highly effective and patients may even remain ambulant; see also Patient-controlled analgesia, p. 239.

Pharmacokinetics

Diamorphine (heroin) given parenterally has a $t_\frac{1}{2}$ of 3 min, being metabolised to the two active substances 6-acetylmorphine and morphine ($t_\frac{1}{2}$ 3 h). When given orally heroin is subject to complete presystemic or first-pass metabolism and has all been converted to morphine by the time it reaches the systemic circulation. It has been pointed out that oral heroin is essentially a pro-drug and 'may be considered a relatively inefficient means of providing systemic morphine'.[37] The greater potency of heroin (1 mg heroin $\equiv$ 1.5 mg morphine) may be due to the metabolite 6-acetylmorphine and to the common use of morphine as sulphate and heroin as hydrochloride.

Uses. Heroin is used medicinally for *pain* and for severe *cough* (Diamorphine Linctus).

Pentazocine (Fortral, Talwin) (1967)

An opioid partial agonist, this can induce a withdrawal syndrome in addicts (antagonist effect); it can also induce psychological and physical dependence (agonist effect), and this can be severe. It has not proved to be the solution to separating the property of analgesia from that of producing dependence, as was thought initially, though it is a distinct advance.

Its *analgesic efficacy* approximates to that of morphine, but its *potency* (weight for weight) is about one-third of morphine. Its $t_\frac{1}{2}$ is 3 h.

---

[37] Inturrisi C E et al. N Engl J Med 1984; 310: 1213.

Adverse effects of this partial agonist include: nausea, vomiting, dizziness, sweating, hypertension, palpitations, tachycardia, central nervous system disturbances (euphoria, dysphoria, psychotomimesis), and all are more likely with the higher peak plasma concentrations achieved after injection.

Uses are those of morphine (excepting in diarrhoea), and also for lesser and chronic pain, for its liability to induce dependence is less than morphine.

> **Dosage:** Pentazocine Tabs, 25–100 mg, 3–4-hourly; Pentazocine Inj, 30–60 mg, i.m., 3–4-hourly.

Pentazocine compared with morphine

Dependence liability: less, but definitely occurs.
Effect on opioid dependence: induces withdrawal syndrome.
Respiratory depression and *sedation*: less.
Duration of action: shorter.
Psychotomimetic effects: more.
Overdose respiratory depression: naloxone effective against both.
Nausea and vomiting: similar.
Constipation: less.
Cardiovascular effects of high doses: (chiefly important in myocardial infarction)
  morphine: hypotension, bradycardia.
  pentazocine: hypertension (systemic and pulmonary), tachycardia; so avoid in cardiovascular disease.

Phenazocine (Narphen) is a high-efficacy agonist used particularly in biliary colic for it has less capacity than other opioids to cause spasm of the sphincter of Oddi.

Buprenorphine (Temgesic) is a high-efficacy partial agonist with a $t_\frac{1}{2}$ of 3 h and a duration of action of 6–8 h; it has high receptor affinity (tenacity of binding) so that respiratory depression is only partially reversed by naloxone, and a respiratory stimulant may be needed in overdose, or assisted respiration. It has less liability to induce dependence and respiratory depression than pure agonists; it has little effect on the cardiovascular system and may spare the sphincter of Oddi (from induced spasm).

Because of extensive presystemic elimination when swallowed, buprenorphine is given by the buccal (sublingual) route (200–400 μg) or by i.m., or slow i.v., injection (300–600 μg).

Dextropropoxyphene (Doloxene) is structurally close to methadone and differs in that it is less analgesic, antitussive, and less dependence-producing. Its analgesic usefulness approximates to that of codeine. It is rapidly absorbed and has a $t_\frac{1}{2}$ of about 12 h. In overdose the rapidity of absorption is such that respiratory arrest may occur within one hour and also hypotension (probably due to a membrane-stabilising or quinidine-like action causing cardiac dysrhythmia), so that many subjects die before reaching hospital. Combination with alcohol (common with self-poisoning) enhances respiratory depression. Some critics think this disadvantage outweighs the benefits of the drug and wish to see it withdrawn. Dextropropoxyphene is commonly combined with paracetamol (co-proxamol, Distalgesic) and with aspirin (Doloxene Cpd).

Dihydrocodeine (DF118) is a low-efficacy opioid, but, curiously, it can make postoperative dental pain worse. It is not known how many agonist opioids can make pain worse, but naloxone (antagonist) can do this. It may be that where endogenous opioid pathways are highly activated by afferent nociceptive input, a weak agonist, by competitively replacing the more active endogenous opioid, acts as an antagonist in this situation. Whatever the explanation, such observations remind us of the importance of placebo-controlled studies in real-life situations and that assumptions that one pain is like another and so will respond similarly to drugs cannot be trusted. The investigators in this study remarked that placebo-controlled studies have

been criticized on legal, ethical and practical grounds. In particular, critics have questioned the probity of investigators who subject patients to placebos when they anticipate that the active drug will be effective. When we embarked on this trial, we expected to observe an analgesic effect —

probably greater than aspirin or paracetamol — with dihydrocodeine. The demonstration of hyperalgesia would have been impossible without a placebo and vindicates our approach to clinical studies of the efficacy of analgesics.[38]

Dosage is 30 mg orally: 25–50 mg deep s.c.

Dextromoramide (Palfium) and *dipipanone* (Diconal is dipipanone plus cyclizine, an antiemetic) are less sedating and shorter acting than morphine; they are suitable for acute attacks of pain, e.g. breakthrough pain in terminal illness.

Meptazinol (Meptid) is a high-efficacy partial agonist.

OPIOIDS USED PARTICULARLY DURING AND AFTER SURGERY

Fentanyl (Sublimaze) has higher efficacy than morphine, analgesia lasts 30–60 min (single dose) and $t_\frac{1}{2}$ is 3 h; it is used i.v. for neuroleptanalgesia (see index). Fentanyl is also used in combination with *droperidol* (a butyrophenone neuroleptic; Thalamonal).

Phenoperidine (Operidine) ($t_\frac{1}{2}$ 30 min) is similar.

Alfenatil (Rapifen) ($t_\frac{1}{2}$ 1.5 h) given i.v., provides maximum analgesia in 90 s, which lasts about 10 min from a single dose; it is used for brief painful operations.

Nalbuphine (Nubain) is a partial agonist given by injection.

Opioids (non-analgesic) used for anti-motility effect on the gut include loperamide and diphenoxylate (p. 537).

OPIOID ANTAGONISTS

Naloxone

Naloxone (Narcan) is a (pure) competitive opioid antagonist at ordinary doses. It antagonises both agonist and partial agonist opioids (though it may not be sufficient alone in buprenorphine overdose since this drug binds particularly tenaciously to receptors) and induces an acute withdrawal syndrome in dependent subjects.

---

[38] Seymour R A et al. Lancet 1982; 2: 1425.

Naloxone has high presystemic elimination when swallowed and is not used by this route. Given i.v., reversal of opioid-induced respiratory depression begins in 1–2 min, reversal of other effects — analgesia, depressed consciousness — can be slower. A prompt marked improvement in respiration has diagnostic value in opioid overdose, but poor or no response may occur because insufficient has been given, or with buprenorphine (above) or due to cerebral hypoxia or to hypothermia in severe cases.

Naloxone acts for about one hour, which happens to be about the $t_{\frac{1}{2}}$, though the peak effect on depressed respiration may be as brief as 10 min (the $t_{\frac{1}{2}}$ and duration of action are not synonymous; $t_{\frac{1}{2}}$ is the same for all doses of a drug; the duration of action is dose-dependent). Opioid analgesics act for much longer than their $t_{\frac{1}{2}}$ (due to tissue uptake) and either repeated i.v. doses of naloxone will be needed or continuous i.v. infusion; given s.c. or i.m., the onset of action is slower and duration is longer.

> **Naloxone dose** in suspected opioid overdose is as follows: initially 0.4–1.2 mg (some advocate up to 2 mg) i.v.; the patient is closely observed (respiration, pupils, consciousness) for 3 min; if response occurs but is inadequate, give a second dose; if there is no response but the history of opioid overdose is strong (accident in hospital, known heroin abuser) then repeat doses until there is a response or until 10 mg has been given.
>
> Infusion i.v. may be up to 5 mg/hour and may be required for days with opioids having a long $t_{\frac{1}{2}}$ (methadone).

Naloxone is also used to counter excess opioid effects after surgical analgesia or childbirth.

Other uses. Now that it is known or suspected that physiological opioid mechanisms are not confined to analgesia, and may play a detrimental role in vascular shock (suppression of adrenergic responses) in non-opioid comas and in some psychological disorders, naloxone has been tried in a wide range of conditions, but in none has it yet found a definitive role.

Naltrexone is similar to naloxone but longer acting ($t_{\frac{1}{2}}$ 4 h: active metabolite 13 h) with duration of effect 1–3 days according to dose. It can be used orally in *ex*-opioid abusers who are *fully* withdrawn (otherwise it will induce an acute withdrawal syndrome). A lapse by the patient is without any 'kick' or euphoria. But naltrexone does not reduce craving as does the agonist methadone. This use of naltrexone requires careful selection and supervision of subjects.

NON-OPIOID ANALGESICS USEFUL FOR PAIN IN OPIOID ADDICTS

Nefopam (Acupan) is neither an opioid nor a NSAID; it is effective against moderate pain; its mode of action is unknown. Since it lacks the disadvantages of opioids (constipation, respiratory depression) and has greater efficacy than NSAIDs, it provides an alternative. It is useful for pain in opioid addicts.

Nonsteroidal anti-inflammatory drugs are effective as analgesics, see Chapter 14.

GUIDE TO FURTHER READING

Beecher H K 1960 Control of suffering in severe trauma. Journal of the American Medical Association 173: 534

Clough C 1989 Treating migraine: try stress reduction and simple analgesia first. British Medical Journal 299: 141

Controversies in therapeutics 1989 Pain relief in active patients with cancer. British Medical Journal
(i) Baines M Analgesic drugs are the foundation of management 298: 36
(ii) Lipton S The early use of nerve blocks improves the quality of life 298: 37

Foley K M 1985 The treatment of cancer pain. New England Journal of Medicine 313: 84

Herring R et al 1991 Abrupt outpatient withdrawal of medication in analgesic-abusing migraineurs. Lancet 337: 1442

Hockley J M et al 1988 Survey of distressing symptoms in dying patients and their families in hospital and the response to a symptom control team. British Medical Journal 296: 1715

Inturrisi C E et al 1984 The pharmacokinetics of heroin in patients with chronic pain. New England Journal of Medicine 310: 1213

Modell W et al 1958 Factors influencing clinical evaluation of drugs with special reference to the double-blind technique. Journal of the American Medical Association 167: 2190

Murphy J J et al 1988 Randomised double-blind placebo-controlled trial of fewer-few in migraine prevention. Lancet 2: 189

Säive et al 1985 Oral morphine in cancer patients. British Journal of Clinical Pharmacology 19: 495

Seymour R A et al 1982 Dihydrocodeine-induced hyperalgesia in postoperative dental pain. Lancet 1: 1425

Tokola R A et al 1984 Effect of migraine attacks on paracetamol absorption. British Journal of Clinical Pharmacology 18: 867

Wanzer S H et al 1989 The physician's responsibility toward hopelessly ill patients. New England Journal of Medicine 320: 844

16

Central nervous system II: sleep and hypnotics, anxiety and anxiolytics

SYNOPSIS

- Sleep and drugs that induce sleep (hypnotics). About 30% of adults have difficulty sleeping and half of them consider the problem to be serious
- Insomnia. Management involves detailed analysis of the particular circumstances. A drug is not always appropriate but, if required, should be chosen for its suitable pharmacokinetics and used briefly
- Anxiety afflicts about 30% of the population. Drugs are only an appropriate treatment for disabling symptoms
- Hypnotics and anxiolytic sedatives: benzodiazepines, trichloroethanol derivatives, barbiturates
- Drugs can affect driving and skilled tasks

SLEEP AND DRUGS THAT INDUCE SLEEP (HYPNOTICS)

Sleep is an active (not merely a passive) circadian, physiological depression of consciousness. It is characterised by cyclical electroencephalographic (EEG) and eye movement changes, measures of which are used to describe sleep stages because they are convenient and seem to correlate with the fundamental physiological changes in neurotransmitter (noradrenaline, dopamine, serotonin, acetylcholine) functions that are inaccessible to measurement in clinical situations. Since these neurotransmitters are involved in psychiatric disorders it is no surprise that sleep disturbances are associated with mental disease.

Normal sleep (categorised by eye movements) is of two kinds, alternating during the night:

- NREM (non-rapid eye movement) (orthodox) or slow-wave EEG sleep; awakened subjects state they were 'thinking': heart rate, blood pressure and respiration are steady or decline and muscles are relaxed; growth hormone secretion is maximal; sleep is 'restful'.
- REM (rapid eye movement) (paradoxical) or fast-wave EEG sleep; awakened subjects state they were dreaming: heart rate, blood pressure and respiration are fluctuant, cerebral blood flow increases above that during wakefulness, the penis is erect

(unless there is dream anxiety), skeletal muscles are profoundly relaxed though body movements are more pronounced; the brain is 'active'.

A normal night begins with a sleep latency period as the subject passes from wakefulness into NREM sleep. An initial hour of NREM sleep is followed by about 20 min REM sleep, after which cycles of NREM sleep (about 90 min) abruptly alternate with REM sleep (about 20 min) for the rest of the night (i.e. about 4 cycles). Both kinds of sleep seem to be necessary for health (REM sleep especially to alleviate fatigue).

Hypnotics in full doses can disrupt the normal sleep pattern, suppressing REM sleep, though tolerance may develop. Benzodiazepines and chloral do this least. No hypnotic can be said to induce natural sleep.

On *abrupt withdrawal* of a drug that has suppressed REM sleep there is a rebound increase as though the body requires to recover what has been lost; nightmares occur with severe rebound; abnormal sleep patterns may persist for weeks after withdrawal. It has not been conclusively shown that the kind of abnormality induced by hypnotics is harmful. But there is some evidence that deprivation of REM sleep may be responsible for emotional disorder so that hypnotics should not be used without good reason. That hypnotics are extensively prescribed, and indeed overprescribed, is 'not disputed'.[1]

Non-hypnotic drugs and sleep

A range of other drugs have effects *on eye movement pattern* similar to hypnotics, when given in sufficient dose, e.g. heroin, morphine, alcohol, tricyclic and MAOI antidepressants, amphetamine and other appetite suppressants (though not dexfenfluramine). But effects on onset and duration of sleep differ.

---

[1] ' . . . many times, reaching for the prescription pad and writing something out is a way the doctor says "Get lost! I don't want to hear you". It is a way of terminating the encounter.' Leo Hollister; Prof. of Medicine, Psychiatry and Pharmacology, Stanford University, USA.

Clinical evaluation of the effects of hypnotics

Details of effects of hypnotics that will concern prescribers are illustrated by guidelines (WHO Europe[2]) for clinical evaluation. Evaluation begins with single dose studies in healthy volunteers in the morning, after a normal night's sleep. Tests to evaluate alertness, cognitive function, manual dexterity, coordination, reaction time, memory, etc. are administered. Then the drug is given at night to assess nocturnal effects, and residual effects the next day (hangover). The drug is then used in patients suffering insomnia (this presents particular ethical problems since the most suitable patients are those with chronic insomnia, in whom the clinical objective is to get them off all drugs rather than to encourage them to take new drugs).

Assessment is by questionnaires, with particular interest in sleep latency (time taken to go to sleep), number of nocturnal awakenings, time of final awakening and quality of sleep (including dreaming); subsequent daytime effects (hangover) are of particular concern.

Sleep laboratory studies with EEG, eye movement and electromyographic (under the jaw) recording are conducted on a small number of subjects.

It is also desirable to determine whether tolerance, and/or dependence occur, whether the drug is safe in long-term use, interactions with other drugs (including alcohol) and dosage in the old and in subjects with impaired elimination.

Hangover

The effects of hypnotics, including ordinary doses of some benzodiazepines (e.g. nitrazepam) taken at ordinary bedtime carry over into the afternoon of the following day. Often patients are aware of drowsiness, but even when they are not, impaired psychomotor performance occurs as shown by reaction time, tapping speed, attentiveness, ability speedily to cross out all examples of a single letter

---

[2] Guidelines for the clinical investigation of hypnotic drugs. Copenhagen: WHO Regional Office for Europe. 1983.

on a printed page, and ocular flicker fusion. This is not surprising since the $t_{\frac{1}{2}}$ of nitrazepam is about 30 h. Discussion of drug effects on skilled tasks, especially car driving, is on p. 339. Patients who have accidents and who have not been warned of the hazards of sedation during the day are likely to have a valid claim for compensation for any injury due to the negligence of the prescriber.

Termination of action of a *single dose* of a drug having a long $t_{\frac{1}{2}}$ is often determined by distribution into tissues where it has no action, e.g. fat, muscle, rather than by metabolism or elimination, so that the duration of action of a single dose may be satisfactorily free from hangover despite a long $t_{\frac{1}{2}}$, e.g. nitrazepam. But when a drug with a long $t_{\frac{1}{2}}$ is used *nightly*, there will be accumulation (of drug or of active metabolites) until a steady state is reached (at about five half-lives) and daytime impairment of performance may then become unacceptable. Thus, knowledge of the $t_{\frac{1}{2}}$ is useful, but is not the only factor in determining duration of action; tissue concentrations and receptor binding (affinity) are also important.

As a general guide, nightly use of drugs with a $t_{\frac{1}{2}} < 8$ h may, and those with a $t_{\frac{1}{2}} > 16$ h will still have effects the following day.

But next-day amnesia occurs, particularly with triazolam although it has a short $t_{\frac{1}{2}}$.

Timing of hypnotic administration

Patients should be advised. Generally a hypnotic is best taken on going to bed or a few minutes before. In bed, the subject may read a suitable book that provides interest but no excitement (arousal), e.g. most biographies, a textbook. If the hypnotic was taken on an empty stomach, sleep latency will commonly be about 20 min. Some people are suited by taking the hypnotic, e.g. a slowly absorbed benzodiazepine, one hour before going to bed, but for others this can carry a risk of going to sleep prematurely and even in a potentially hazardous or unpleasant situation, e.g. in the bath.

Occasionally it is appropriate to advise a patient who suffers intermittent insomnia or is

being weaned from chronic drug use, to go to bed, read a suitable book (above) and to take a short half-life drug, e.g. lormetazepam, if still wakeful after 1 or 2 hours; the availability of a single dose at the bedside for use if needed, gives confidence and may itself increase the ability to do without it. (Availability of a bottle of tablets at the bedside traditionally carries risk of inadvertent repeated self-administration; the hazard of this is one reason why benzodiazepines replaced barbiturates).

Dependence

It can be assumed that all hypnotics induce tolerance and dependence, with abrupt withdrawal consequences ranging from insomnia even to convulsions (where dosage has been high and prolonged). *Withdrawal* from chronic users should always be gradual (see Benzodiazepine dependence); the longer the use the slower should be the withdrawal (over weeks, reducing both dose and frequency); if symptoms (anxiety, insomnia, nightmares) occur then consumption should be stabilised until the symptoms disappear (a β-adrenoceptor blocker may assist by allaying somatic symptoms of anxiety); obviously, withdrawal symptoms are less acute with drugs (and active metabolites) having a long $t_{\frac{1}{2}}$ (slow fall in drug concentration giving time for adaptation). The subject should be warned of the possibility of symptoms and counselled that they will pass away; if confidence is lost, withdrawal will be unsuccessful.

Overdose. A single heavy overdose of a hypnotic may be followed by disturbed sleep for weeks even in subjects not habitually taking hypnotics.

INSOMNIA

Insomnia deserves special attention because it is common and causes much distress to its subjects. Its successful management involves much more than merely prescribing drugs, which should be regarded as temporary expedients only (see also above). *Insomnia is defined* as a belief of patients that they are not getting enough sleep despite opportunity to sleep. It comprises:

- *failure to fall asleep* within 45 min or
- *difficulty in staying asleep* (6 or more awakenings per night, or less than 6 h sleep): either of these at least 4 nights a week.[3]

Poor sleepers tend to overestimate the time it takes them to fall asleep (sleep latency) and to underestimate the time they stay asleep. When awakened during NREM (orthodox) sleep, subjects who complain of insomnia may claim they were not asleep. But some studies have found that nurses are liable to overestimate patients' sleep.

Clinical types of insomnia

- Tense people who lie awake in bed for hours unable to relax, and then sleep well.
- Exhausted people who, because they sleep early in the evening, wake early in the morning. They probably need no drug, but a midday rest.
- People who wake repeatedly throughout the night, for no obvious reason.
- People who wake repeatedly from physical discomfort or pain and who need treatment of that condition plus a hypnotic (temporarily).
- Depression, in which sleep is shorter (early waking), less sound, interrupted and restless; patients need treatment for depression, not hypnotics.
- Caffeine can cause difficulty getting to sleep, which increases with age; alcohol, though it can help people to get to sleep, can cause early waking (rebound).
- Overuse of hypnotics with development of tolerance (3–14 days) and rebound insomnia when attempts to abstain are made.

Prescribing hypnotics

A hypnotic is most often needed in:

- Short-term, transient and situational insomnia that is severe and distressing, e.g. acute

emotional disturbance, bereavement, domestic conflict, noisy hotel, to help the patient cope with brief episodes.

- Long-term (> 3 weeks) persistent insomnia, which may have no apparent cause or may follow on after the passing of an acute situation (conditioned insomnia); it also occurs in states of chronic anxiety and unhappiness. A detailed analysis of the pattern and the potential causes is required. If it is decided that a hypnotic is required, then the objective is to restore the sleep habit by brief use of a drug. Where use is prolonged beyond a few days, insomnia due to withdrawal may be interpreted by patients as demonstrating a need to continue the drug, which can cause great difficulty, especially if the doctors have not adequately counselled the patients and got their own objectives clear. It is all too easy to follow the indulgent path of repeat prescriptions.

Thus in both the above situations there is danger that emotional and physical dependence on the drug will occur. It is important not to allow prescription of hypnotics and sedatives to become a means of evading the patient's real problem. 'Unfortunately, some patients use the sedative hypnotics as a crutch to help them in the struggle against the everyday pressure of living,'[4] and sadly, even the best doctor sometimes surrenders to patient demand, though believing that continued use of a hypnotic is not in the patient's interest.

A prescription for a hypnotic is justified for a few nights or up to 4 weeks to combat insomnia due to *anxiety, provided* there is good reason to expect the cause to be removed either by changes in environment or by treatment[5] (e.g. sedative antidepressant drug or electric convulsions or other non-drug treatment). But where there is persistent insomnia or a long-standing personality disorder a prescription is not justified because: 1. tolerance develops, 2. dependence is likely, 3. sleep is not natural.

---

[3] Kales J et al. Clin. Pharmacol Ther 1971; 12: 691.
[4] Friend D G. Clin. Pharmacol Ther 1960; 1: 5.
[5] Oswald I. Pharmacol Rev 1968; 20: 274.

At a very rough reckoning about one night's sleep in every ten in this country (UK) is hypnotic induced . . . . People seem to want to turn consciousness on and off like a tap . . . . While it is time-consuming to take a careful clinical history, to conduct a full clinical examination and to give wise advice, it takes only a moment to write a prescription and this does please and often satisfies the patient . . . . We do not always draw a clear distinction between the patients' *wants* and what we think are their *needs*, and it is regrettable how much we accede to the patients' demands in order to placate them and to save ourselves time and trouble.[6]

Jet lag (loss of wellbeing and insomnia after transmeridian flights) is related to the need to adapt to new circadian rhythms; it is more difficult to adapt after an eastward flight (shorter day) than after a westward flight (longer day). Where subjects have a substantial problem it can be appropriate to provide a medium $t_\frac{1}{2}$ hypnotic to enable them to get to sleep and stay asleep.

Choice of a hypnotic

The benzodiazepines are now overwhelmingly the first choice because they:

- alter sleep pattern least
- are safer than other drugs in overdose
- do not significantly induce drug metabolising enzymes that cause unwanted interactions.

There are numerous members to choose between. The principal factors that determine selection are pharmacokinetic:

- speed of absorption and passage into the central nervous system, i.e. lipid-solubility
- half-life of the drug
- presence of active metabolites
- half-life of any active metabolites.

Taking these factors into account, a choice may be offered as follows:

- *temazepam*: $t_\frac{1}{2}$ 13 h, inactive metabolites; insignificant accumulation with repeated daily use, but may sometimes be too

short-acting for subjects of early waking; next-day amnesia is little or absent.
- *lormetazepam*: $t_\frac{1}{2}$ 9 h with inactive metabolites; insignificant accumulation with daily use.

The above are all *absorbed* reasonably fast: lorazepam and oxazepam are absorbed rather too slowly for use when rapid onset is important.

- Benzodiazepines with long $t_\frac{1}{2}$ and/or with metabolites of long $t_\frac{1}{2}$, e.g. diazepam, nitrazepam, flurazepam, are satisfactory as hypnotics for single, but not for daily doses. The long $t_\frac{1}{2}$ drugs (and active metabolites) may be used if there is daytime anxiety. Speed of onset, duration of effect and incidence of hangover depend on the dose and on the patient almost as much as on the choice of drug.
Benzodiazepines are numerous. Those not discussed here may give satisfactory results, but clinicians should decide what they want to achieve and consider the kinetics of the drug and its metabolites before using it.

- *Barbiturates* are obsolete as hypnotics.

Warning. If insomnia is due to pain an analgesic is essential. A hypnotic alone may result in mental confusion and restlessness.

Safety of hypnotics

Benzodiazepines are the safest, i.e. minimal enzyme induction and minimal hazard in overdose, including hazard to inquisitive children imitating their parents'/grandparents' pill-swallowing proclivities. Other hypnotics are more hazardous in overdose.

Irritant drugs (chloral hydrate) are obviously unsuitable for peptic ulcer patients. In cases where it is especially desired to avoid any *respiratory depression*, e.g. in severe asthmatics or in head injury, even benzodiazepines in ordinary doses can impair ventilation.

Interactions. All hypnotics synergise with alcohol and other cerebral depressants.

Many non-benzodiazepine hypnotics are hepatic enzyme inducers. Benzodiazepines are

---

[6]Dunlop D. Br Med Bull 1970; 26: 236.

hypnotics of first choice in patients taking warfarin (a drug with a narrow therapeutic range and particularly prone to pharmacokinetic interaction).

Age and hypnotics

In the *elderly* it is normal for sleep requirement to become less, and nocturnal awakenings to become more frequent. An ageing person who complains of this should obviously not be treated with a hypnotic; any persistent demands should be resisted for the most likely result will be that they will spend the rest of their lives taking a hypnotic to no advantage and to potential disadvantage.

The elderly are less tolerant of hypnotics. They should generally not receive long $t_{\frac{1}{2}}$ drugs, and should start with half the usual dose.

The *old*, particularly those with organic brain failure, may become confused with hypnotics and an occasional patient becomes excited or has nightmares on a particular drug; a neuroleptic (promazine) may be used alone, or even cautiously with a hypnotic. Confusion is more likely if a patient who has taken a full dose of hypnotic is kept awake by pain; adequate analgesia should accompany the hypnotic. The need to micturate may result in drugged old people hazardously wandering around the house, and there is evidence of increased incidence of falls with fractured hip.

Children: a benzodiazepine, chloral hydrate, promethazine, trimeprazine or promazine is used.

Miscellaneous

Food as an aid to sleep.[7] A *small* meal of milk and cereal promotes less restless sleep and there is experimental support for the popular belief that milk-cereal drinks do the same. The effect persists into the later night, suggesting that the cause is not only psychological expectation resulting from folklore and advertising, though these doubtless assist. Since broken sleep in-

creases with age it may be worth recommending the adoption of a pre-bed snack or drink before prescribing hypnotics to older patients with mild insomnia.

Snoring implies a risk of obstructive sleep apnoea, from which the subject needs to wake up. Hypnotics are contraindicated.

ANXIETY

Anxiety in moderation is a normal, appropriate and even useful response to life events and situations provided it stimulates achievement that may mitigate or remove the cause. But inappropriate or excessive or chronic anxiety is disabling, especially where the cause cannot be removed.

Yet anxiety may also occur without apparent exogenous cause, and subjects of this free-floating anxiety need and deserve help. Non-drug therapy may be best for many, but drugs are often useful for patients having a high level of anxiety. Doctors should not be over-ready to prescribe drugs, but neither should they be over-timid, for anxiety can be a curse that destroys the quality of life.

Benzodiazepines now dominate anti-anxiety medication. But anxiety does not manifest itself only as a psychic or mental state, there are also *somatic or physical concomitants*, e.g. consciousness of the action of the heart (palpitations), tremor, diarrhoea, which are associated with increased activity of the sympathetic autonomic system. These symptoms are not only caused by anxiety, they also add to the feeling of anxiety (positive feedback loop). In patients whose complaints are primarily of somatic or autonomic symptoms of anxiety rather than of anxiety itself a *β-adrenoceptor blocking drug* can give benefit; but it will generally not help where there is, e.g. tachycardia that is not causing symptoms, although it will reduce this.

Somatic symptoms of sympathetic overactivity accompany the performance of stressful tasks such as car driving in busy traffic, public speaking, playing a musical instrument, surgery and sports requiring calm skill without maximum output of work, bowling, shooting and sitting examinations; β-adrenoceptor block allows the

---

[7] Brezinova V et al. Br Med J 1972; 2: 431.

subject to feel calmer and so can improve performance.

Even in experienced surgeons a rise in heart rate begins as soon as scrubbing-up for an operating session is begun. In one study (8 surgeons) mean *maximum* heart rates were 137/min with mean heart rate 121/min (peak rates above 150/min were reached by 2 surgeons) regardless of the nature of the operation and regardless of seniority. Tachycardia of this degree corresponds to physical work that cannot be sustained for more than 10 min without extreme fatigue. Those people who cannot conceal their emotional state will be interested to know that 'if anything, those surgeons who were outwardly the most calm experienced the highest heart-rates'.[8] The mean heart-rate of surgeons operating after taking a β-adrenoceptor blocking drug (oxprenolol 40 mg orally) was 84/min. But it has not been shown that the surgeons actually operated better or were less fatigued.

The principal disadvantages of drug therapy are dependence and the 'medicalising' of what is essentially a matter of interpersonal relationships or an environmental problem.[9]

Choice and mode of use of anxiolytic agents

- *Benzodiazepines*, e.g. diazepam, oxazepam, are a first choice.
- *A beta-adrenoceptor blocker*, e.g. propranolol, where there are somatic symptoms.
- *A sedative antidepressant* where there is depression *with* anxiety, e.g. amitriptyline.
- *Buspirone* may be considered where a two-week delay in effect is acceptable.
- Other agents, e.g. chlormethiazole, may particularly suit the aged and alcoholics.

Recurrent panic attacks may be prevented, sometimes completely, by antidepressant or buspirone (with the expected delay in onset of effect). The

antidepressant benzodiazepine, alprazolam, is quickly effective but has a particular risk of dependence with difficult withdrawal.

Use of low doses of neuroleptics, e.g. chlorpromazine, for anxiety, has been superseded by benzodiazepines. Neuroleptics can be effective but are liable to have too many autonomic side-effects.

Benzodiazepine use should be limited to 2–4 weeks in anxiety that is severe, disabling or seriously distressing (i.e. these drugs should *not* be used for short-term mild anxiety).

Benzodiazepines are liable to induce dependence and patients in acute high-level anxiety states should be counselled that treatment will be brief, even only a few days. But where chronic anxiety seriously impairs social coping capacities, particularly where the causes can be seen to be irremovable, long-term therapy may seem inescapable although there is evidence that brief non-specialised counselling is as effective. After the drug has been taken for 4–6 months, a serious effort should be made to withdraw it; but this can be impossible and indefinitely prolonged therapy sometimes becomes obligatory as the lesser of two evils. This is why counselling should be preferred to the use of a drug at the outset.

Some *tolerance* to benzodiazepines occurs but anxiolytic efficacy has been claimed to last 6 months, although it is hard to distinguish between resurgence of the condition and a rebound or withdrawal syndrome.

Benzodiazepines with a long $t_{\frac{1}{2}}$ (of parent drug and/or active metabolite) are preferred for smooth effect: either a single nocturnal dose (where there is also insomnia), which will give anxiolytic effect the next day, or small divided doses (to minimise peaks of effects) during the day. The less lipid-soluble oxazepam and lorazepam give particularly smooth effect (slower absorption and slower entry into the CNS).

Where there are somatic symptoms, a β-adrenoceptor blocker may be effective alone or in combination with a benzodiazepine.

---

[8] Foster SE et al. Lancet 1987; 1: 1323.
[9] Lader M H Rational drug therapy 1978; 21: No9.

Bereavement

In an unexpected bereavement it would be harsh to deprive a seriously distressed person of sedation and sleep. But drugs should not be necessary for less acute distress and there is reason to think that benzodiazepines may inhibit psychological adjustment to the loss.

HYPNOTICS AND ANXIOLYTIC SEDATIVES[10]

Benzodiazepines

Benzodiazepines were discovered by serendipity (p. 34). In the mid-1950s the clinical successes of chlorpromazine suggested that tranquillisers were more than just general cerebral depressants. Industrial chemists of Hoffman–LaRoche were encouraged to produce novel compounds that might have selective tranquillising effect and that would lend themselves to molecular manipulation. Chlordiazepoxide was synthesised, but, other problems seeming more important, the project lost priority and chlordiazepoxide was left untested for 2 years. When it was eventually studied in animals it was found to be superior to existing tranquillisers, including a marked taming effect in monkeys. Some 16 000 patients were soon treated and the drug was licensed for general use in 1960. Since then thousands of benzodiazepines have been synthesised, hundreds tested and many tens have been marketed.

Actions

Benzodiazepines have hypnotic, sedative, anxiolytic, anticonvulsant and (central) muscle relaxant actions. They attach to a specific site on the GABA receptor/chloride channel complex, potentiating the effect of GABA (gamma-aminobutyric acid), an important inhibitory transmitter in the CNS which acts by opening chloride ion channels into cells. There are several subtypes of benzodiazepine receptor, which raises the possibility of separating the various actions of the benzodiazepines by molecular manipulation so that, for example, anxiolytic effect may be achieved without concomitant sedation, which would be an important advance (there is some selectivity in this area between existing drugs).

Benzodiazepines may act chiefly on the brain reticular activating system (reducing sensory input), the limbic system (affect), the median fore-brain bundle (reward and punishment systems) and the hypothalamus.

Once receptor *agonists* have been made, *antagonists* follow, e.g. flumazenil, used for termination of agonist effect after use, e.g. endoscopies and to diagnose overdose (p. 269).

There are also benzodiazepines that have opposite (not merely blocking) actions, i.e. excitation, and these are called *inverse agonists* (see p. 75). The full possibilities for scientific discovery and therapeutic use of benzodiazepines in behaviour modification have yet to be explored.

Occasionally the agonist (sedative) compounds in current use cause *paradoxical effects* e.g. excitement, hostility and antisocial acts. Alteration of dose, up or down, may eliminate these (as may chlorpromazine in an acute severe situation).

Benzodiazepines shorten the time taken to go to sleep (sleep latency), decrease intermittent awakening and increase total sleep duration. Choice of drug as hypnotic is determined by *pharmacokinetic properties* (see, Choice of a hypnotic, above). The choice as anxiolytic sedative is also largely determined by pharmacokinetic properties (see Table 16.1, p. 266); slow absorption and long $t_{\frac{1}{2}}$ give smooth effect. Selectivity between anxiolytic and sedative effect is low, though some trials suggest it, e.g. clorazepate may be less sedative than diazepam for equal anxiolytic effect, but no definitive recommendations can be made. Diazepam remains the standard member of the group, having a $t_{\frac{1}{2}}$ of 30 h with an active metabolite (desmethyl-diazepam) with a $t_{\frac{1}{2}}$ of 80 h. A single dose before

---

[10] Sedative: a drug (or dose of a drug) that calms or soothes without inducing sleep though it may cause sleepiness: a small dose of a hypnotic or *tranquilliser* often suffices for this. The imprecise term tranquilliser implies a drug that will quieten a patient without significantly impairing consciousness. The ideal tranquilliser would allay pathological anxiety, i.e. be *anxiolytic*, and allay nervous tension without altering any other cerebral functions; especially it would not cause sleepiness; it would suppress mania and psychotic overactivity.

going to bed provides quick hypnotic effect and repeated doses give anxiolytic effect with less sedation throughout the next day. If a dose is needed during the day the rapid absorption of diazepam may cause undesirable sedation (which can be mitigated by using several small doses though that adds inconvenience). The more slowly absorbed oxazepam may be preferred.

As well as causing sedation and drowsiness, benzodiazepines impair memory (see below) and intellectual and psychomotor function.

Uses

Anxiety (without or with psychotic states), panic attacks, insomnia, alcohol withdrawal states, night terrors and somnambulism (children), muscle spasm due to a variety of causes, including tetanus and cerebral spasticity; epilepsy; anaesthesia and sedation for endoscopies and cardioversion.

Curiously, perhaps, benzodiazepines are extensively prescribed by primary care doctors for depression; but they are not antidepressant (except perhaps alprazolam when anxiety is dominant in a mixed anxiety/depression). The reason is obscure but may be related to complaints of side-effects from the usual antidepressants. Benzodiazepines are not appropriate for phobic and obsessional states.

Tolerance occurs with chronic use and there is cross-tolerance within the group.

Amnesia for events subsequent to administration occurs with high doses, i.v. for endoscopy, dental surgery (with local anaesthetic), cardioversion, and in these situations it can be regarded as a blessing.[11] But embarrassing amnesia can also occur with oral use: it is wise to warn travellers of this. High doses of triazolam particularly may cause amnesia.

Elderly and/or troubled people arrested for *shoplifting* frequently claim that their crime was caused by chronic benzodiazepine (or other)

therapy. Whilst it is natural to regard such claims with suspicion, those of us (not taking a benzodiazepine) who have nearly walked out of a self-service shop carrying goods we have neglected to present for payment will not be over-ready to dismiss the possibility (though amnesia selective for payment must arouse scepticism). A useful way of looking at the matter is to consider, not whether the drug caused an involuntary act of shoplifting (which is unlikely), but whether it might have made a contribution to absent-mindedness so that the necessary conscious intent to steal (required by criminal law) was not

---

Benzodiazepine doses as hypnotic (oral)

Temazepam Caps	10–30 mg orally
Lormetazepam Tabs	500 µg–1 mg orally

The elderly should be started on half the above doses. Sudden withdrawal can cause confusion.

Doses as anxiolytic sedative

Diazepam Tabs 2 mg × 3/day increasing to a total daily dose of 30 mg if really necessary (it may take 2 weeks to reach a steady state at each dose) *or* use 5–30 mg at night if there is insomnia and take advantage of anxiolytic efffect the next day.
Oxazepam Tabs 15–30 mg × 3/day.

Suppositories are available, e.g. diazepam (10 mg).

Injectable preparations

Intravenous formulations, e.g. diazepam 10–20 mg, given at 5 mg/min into a *large* vein (antecubital fossa) to minimise thrombosis: the dose may be repeated in 30–60 min for status epilepticus or in 4 h for severe acute anxiety or agitation: midazolam is a shorter acting alternative, e.g. for endoscopies. The dose should be titrated according to response, e.g. droping eyelids, speech, response to commands. *Intramuscular* injection of diazepam is absorbed erratically and may be slower in acting than an oral dose: lorazepam and midazolam are absorbed rapidly.
The elderly should receive half doses.

---

[11] Although one patient, normally a gentle man, believed he was being lied to when told the endoscopy had been performed. 'He assaulted his physician and was calmed only by a second endoscopy'. Later he was very embarrassed and apologised repeatedly. Lurie Y et al. 1990 Lancet 336: 576

Table 16.1 Data on some benzodiazepines (Long $t\frac{1}{2}$ drugs/metabolites are appropriate for anxiety. Short $t\frac{1}{2}$ drugs/metabolites are appropriate hypnotics)

Name	Plasma $t\frac{1}{2}$	Metabolites ($t\frac{1}{2}$h)	Remarks
Alprazolam (Xanax)	16	inactive	Has antidepressant activity
Bromazepam (Lexotan)	12	inactive	—
Chlordiazepoxide (Librium)	20	active (14 40) desmethyldiazepam (80) [see *note* 5]	Steady-state of effect about 3 days
Clobazam (Frisium)	35	active (42)	Used in epilepsy as well as anxiety
Clonazepam (Rivotril)	25	inactive	Used in epilepsy
Clorazepate (Tranxene)	prodrug	desmethyldiazepam (80)	—
Diazepam (Valium)	30	active (10) desmethyldiazepam (80)	High lipid solubility so quickly effective (orally): but slow i.m.
Flunitrazepam (Rohypnol)	29	active (minor)	—
Flurazepam (Dalmane)	prodrug (1)	active (6) desmethyldiazepam (80)	Effect depends on metabolites
Ketazolam (Anxon)	prodrug (1.5)	active (30) desmethyldiazepam (80)	Partly metabolised to diazepam
Loprazolam (Dormonoct)	7	active (7)	Insignificant accumulation
Lorazepam (Ativan)	20	inactive	Slowly absorbed and distributed (lower lipid solubility)
Lormetazepam (Lobramet, Noctamid)	9	inactive	Insignificant accumulation
Medazepam (Nobrium)	prodrug (1.5)	desmethyldiazepam (80)	—
Midazolam (Hypnovel)	3	inactive	Injected as adjunct in anaesthesia for endoscopies, dentistry etc.
Nitrazepam (Mogadon)	30	inactive	Superseded because of long $t\frac{1}{2}$
Oxazepam (Serenid)	7	inactive	Slowly absorbed and distributed (lower lipid solubility)
Prazepam (Centrax)	prodrug (1.5)	desmethyldiazepam (80)	Effect depends on metabolites
Temazepam (Euhypnos)	13	inactive	Insignificant accumulation
Triazolam (Halcion)	3	active (7)	Amnesia; excess of psychiatric reactions

Notes:
1. The use of official (generic) names to stress *similarity* and proprietary names to stress *difference* is well shown.
2. The $t\frac{1}{2}$ variability in individuals is very wide indeed though only a single figure is given in the table.
3. Formation of active metabolites does not necessarily mean they play a major role, especially with single doses.

4. Steady state will be reached in about $t_\frac{1}{2} \times 5$ of parent drug and active metabolites when present (but some active metabolites have only a minor role in clinical effect).

5. The principal active metabolite having a long $t_\frac{1}{2}$ (80 h, but with range 30–200) and common to many members is *desmethyldiazepam* (nordiazepam); drugs having this metabolite are suitable as anxiolytics. There is no point in changing a patient from one agent having desmethyldiazepam as a major metabolite to another drug of the same kind. Generally agents that are conjugated have inactive metabolites, and those that are oxidised have active metabolites.

6. Liver disease may prolong $t_\frac{1}{2}$ up to $\times 3$.

7. Duration of action is prolonged in the *elderly* (initial dose should be low) and additive effects with alcohol are important.

formed. When the circumstances of the particular case are known, the question may be asked whether it is safe to convict the person, i.e. that it is beyond reasonable doubt[12] that the drug was irrelevant. Many doubtful and pathetic instances are recorded in the newspapers; doctors are often asked to given evidence in Court; they will seek to be neither credulous nor callous.

Dependence, as shown by occurrence of *withdrawal symptoms*, is usual with therapeutic doses used beyond a few weeks, though it is commonly mild. Dependence occurs earlier with the short $t_\frac{1}{2}$ members but rebound or withdrawal symptoms are not so well correlated with $t_\frac{1}{2}$. Withdrawal symptoms begin after 2–3 days with alprazolam and lorazepam but may be delayed for 2–3 weeks with diazepam. They pass off over 2–4 weeks and are greatly affected by expectation and personality, i.e. the symptoms are passive-dependent traits.[13]

Symptoms include anxiety, agitation, irritability, confusion, delirium, depersonalisation, sleep disturbance, tremor, headache, muscle twitching or aches, sweating and diarrhoea. But patients have commonly been prescribed a benzodiazepine for similar symptoms and there is doubt in many cases just how much is a recrudescence of previous disorder and how much is evidence of true pharmacological dependence. After prolonged high doses abrupt withdrawal may cause confusion, delirium, psychosis and convulsions. Accounts of supposed withdrawal symptoms lasting for several months should be interpreted with caution.

Withdrawal of benzodiazepines should be gradual after as little as 3 weeks' use, but for long-term users it should be very slow, e.g. about 1/8 of the dose every 2 weeks, aiming to complete it in 6–12 weeks. Withdrawal should be slowed if marked symptoms occur (milder symptoms may be controlled by β-adrenoceptor block). Towards the end of the withdrawal of a short $t_\frac{1}{2}$ drug it may be useful to substitute a long $t_\frac{1}{2}$ drug (diazepam) to minimise rapid fluctuations in plasma concentrations.[14] Abandonment of the final dose may be particularly distressing. In difficult cases withdrawal may be assisted by concomitant use of a sedative antidepressant.

The occurrence of dependence will be minimised by critical prescribing using low doses for short periods or intermittently. Only in exceptional cases should use exceed a few weeks.

Interactions. There are additive effects with CNS depressants, including alcohol, which also speeds benzodiazepine absorption. Cimetidine may increase plasma concentrations of diazepam and chlordiazepoxide by as much as 50% (delayed metabolism and clearance); this does not happen with oxazepam and lorazepam. High caffeine intake reduces the anxiolytic effect.

[12] The criterion of proof used in English Courts of Law is:
Civil cases — balance of probabilities.
Criminal cases — beyond reasonable doubt.
Shoplifting is theft and is a criminal arrestable offence.

[13] The difficulty of assessing symptoms is shown by a study in which patients on long-term diazepam therapy experienced symptoms when they thought the drug was being withdrawn but in fact dosage remained the same. Tyrer P et al. Lancet 1983; 2: 1402.

[14] The BNF advises transferring the patient to diazepam at the start of withdrawal and gives the following equivalents. Diazepam 5 mg ≡ chlordiazepoxide 15 mg: lorazepam 1 mg: nitrazepam 5 mg: oxazepam 15 mg: temazepam 10 mg: triazolam 250 micrograms.

Overdose. Benzodiazepines are remarkably safe in acute overdose and the therapeutic dose × 10 induces sleep from which the subject is easily aroused. It is said that there is no reliably recorded case of death from a benzodiazepine taken alone by a person in good *physical* (particularly respiratory) health, which is a remarkable tribute to their safety (high therapeutic index); even if the statement is not absolutely true, death must be extremely rare. But deaths have occurred in combination with alcohol (which combination is quite usual in those seeking to end their own lives).

Flumazenil (p. 269) selectively reverses benzodiazepine effects and is useful in diagnosis, but is not generally used in treatment since its $t_\frac{1}{2}$ (1 h) is so short, and life-endangering CNS depression is so rare.

Benzodiazepines in pregnancy. The drugs are not certainly known to be safe, and indeed diazepam is teratogenic in mice.[15] The drugs should be avoided in early pregnancy as far as possible. It should be remembered that safety in pregnancy is not only a matter of avoiding prescription after a pregnancy has occurred, but that individuals on long-term therapy may become pregnant. Benzodiazepines cross the placenta and can cause fetal cardiac dysrhythmia, and muscular hypotonia and poor suckling in the newborn. Impairment of behavioural development in the months after birth has been proposed but not proved.

Social aspects of benzodiazepine use cause concern, and this is natural with up to 2% of the population taking the drugs chronically because they cannot sleep, feel anxious, worried, or unhappy. The enormous demand for these drugs (met by the medical profession) makes it hard to doubt that they relieve an immense amount of misery (as do tobacco and alcohol, which seem to be far more toxic both to the individual and to society). But increasingly there is criticism of lavish prescribing of these drugs and it is impossible to view with equanimity the continuous long-term use by numerous individuals of benzodiazepines over years. The possible social consequences of blunting of cognition and emotion remain undefined.

Adverse effects (see also above) include sleepiness and impaired psychomotor function and amnesia, causing hazard with car driving or operating any machinery (warn the patient). Dependence (see above).

Additive effects occur with alcohol, which is best avoided, though this will be a counsel of perfection in habitual alcohol users. Paradoxical behaviour effects (see above) and perceptual disorders, e.g. hallucinations, occur occasionally. Headache, giddiness, alimentary tract upset, skin rashes and reduced libido can occur. Extrapyramidal reactions, reversible by flumazenil, are rare.

Suggestions that long-term use can cause organic brain damage are not firmly substantiated.

Women, perhaps as many as 1 in 200, may experience sexual fantasies, including sexual assault, after *large doses* of benzodiazepine as used in dental surgery, and have brought charges in law against male attendants. Plainly a court of law has, in the absence of a witness, great difficulty in deciding who to believe. No such charges have yet been brought by a man against a woman.

Other benzodiazepines include brotizolam camazepam, clotiazepam, cloxazolam, delorazepam, estazolam, etizolam, halazepam, haloxazolam, mexazolam, nimetazepam, oxazolam, pinazepam, quazepam, tetrazepam.

It is such profusion that gives rise to criticism of both the pharmaceutical industry which produces the drugs (each company hoping that its product will indeed be an advance, but marketing it all the same if it is not) and regulatory bodies which permit this. It is good to have a choice, but there is such a thing as too much.

Three special benzodiazepines

Lorazepam differs from other members sufficiently to warrant description. It has a plasma $t_\frac{1}{2}$ of about 20 h which means that it is not

---

[15] Determined investigators can devise experiments in animals so that either fetal hazard or fetal safety is implied and it may not be obvious which predicts to man.

seriously accumulative. It is less lipid-soluble than others (diazepam) and penetrates and leaves the CNS more slowly so that onset and offset of effect are smoother. Lorazepam is metabolised (conjugated) to inactive metabolites, a process that is less influenced by age than is the oxidation of other members, e.g. diazepam. These properties render it more suitable as an anxiolytic than as a hypnotic. Unfortunately it appears to have a peculiar capacity to induce dependence and withdrawal of the drug can be particularly difficult, a substantial disadvantage.

Given i.v. as a sedative, e.g. in intensive care, and as premedication for surgery and endoscopies, the onset of effect (15 min) is slower than with diazepam and midazolam (2 min), which are more lipid-soluble; but it acts for longer and may induce more amnesia, for which many patients may be thankful.

Given i.m. it is absorbed more speedily than diazepam, which means that it is more suitable than diazepam for status epilepticus, when i.v. injection is impracticable.

Alprazolam (Xanax) may have useful antidepressant action as well as sedation in depression where anxiety is prominent; it also can benefit panic attacks, *but* it may be particularly difficult to complete withdrawal.

Triazolam (Halcion) (see Table 16.1, p. 266). Some regulatory bodies think the risks of adverse psychiatric effects outweigh its benefits.

Benzodiazepine antagonist

Flumazenil (Anexate) is a competitive antagonist at benzodiazepine receptors, and it may have some agonist actions, i.e. it is a partial agonist. It has a $t_{\frac{1}{2}}$ of 1 h (see Table 16.1 for $t_{\frac{1}{2}}$ of agonists) so that repeated i.v. doses or infusion may be needed in the clinical situation. Heavily sedated patients become alert within 5 minutes.

Clinical uses include reversal of benzodiazepine sedation after use for endoscopies, dentistry and in intensive care (recovery period needs supervision lest sedation recurs; if used in day surgery it is important to tell patients that they may *not* drive a car home). In self-poisoning flumazenil is chiefly useful in diagnosis; it does not oppose

depression due to non-benzodiazepines. Adverse effects of flumazenil include vomiting, brief anxiety, seizures in epileptics treated with a benzodiazepine and precipitation of withdrawal syndrome in dependent subjects.

Buspirone (Buspar)

Buspirone is structurally unrelated to other anxiolytics. It is a partial agonist at serotonin and dopamine receptors. It has no hypnotic, muscle relaxant or antiepileptic effect and it does not benefit benzodiazepine withdrawal symptoms.

Buspirone has a $t_{\frac{1}{2}}$ of 7 h and is metabolised in the liver; it has an active metabolite that may accumulate over weeks.

Anxiolytic efficacy is similar to or rather less than benzodiazepines. A disadvantage is that useful anxiolytic effect is delayed for 2 or more weeks. Buspirone causes little, if any depression of psychomotor function (unlike benzodiazepines) and does not, in modest doses, potentiate the effects of alcohol (unlike benzodiazepines).

Adverse effects include dizziness headache, nervousness, excitement, nausea, tachycardia and drowsiness.

Trichloroethanol derivatives

Chloral hydrate (1869)

The first synthetic hypnotic to be introduced was a welcome alternative to opium and alcohol. Chloral hydrate is a solid and is usually given orally in solution because it is so irritant to the stomach; it tastes horrible; a capsule is available.

Chloral induces sleep in about half on hour, lasting 6–8 h with little hangover. Chloral is a prodrug. It is rapidly metabolised by alcohol dehydrogenase into the active hypnotic trichloroethanol ($t_{\frac{1}{2}}$ 8 h). This is conjugated with glucuronic acid to an inert form. The ultimate metabolites are excreted in the urine and give a positive result in urine tests for reducing substances, but not, of course, for glucose oxidase (enzyme) tests. Chloral is dangerous in serious hepatic or renal failure, and aggravates peptic ulcer.

The oral hypnotic dose is 500 mg–2 g.

Interaction with ethanol is to be expected since chloral shares the same metabolic enzyme (alcohol dehydrogenase).

Trichloroethanol is a competitive inhibitor of the conversion of ethanol to acetaldehyde so that plasma ethanol concentration is higher than it would otherwise be; *thus ethanol is potentiated by chloral.*

If chloral has been taken for several days, ingestion of alcohol may induce vasodilatation, hypotension and tachycardia that cannot be explained by a simple potentiation.

Interaction with warfarin: effect enhanced.

Triclofos (Tricloryl) is a stable ester of trichloroethanol ($t_\frac{1}{2}$ 8 h).

Chloral betaine (Welldorm) is an alternative; it is preferred to dichloralphenazone which is a potent hepatic enzyme inducer (due to the phenazone).

Other hypnotics

Paraldehyde (1882) has had long use as a safe (little respiratory depression), oral hypnotic and by injection, for control of mania, alcohol withdrawal, status epilepticus and tetanus. But it has major disadvantages: it smells and tastes unpleasant and is partly excreted unchanged via the lungs (75% is metabolised; $t_\frac{1}{2}$ 5 h). It is an irritant (avoid in peptic ulcer) and causes painful muscle necrosis when injected i.m. When subject to light (store in darkness) and heat it decomposes to acetic acid and deaths due to corrosive poisoning by decomposed paraldehyde have occurred (do not use if the fluid is brown or smells of acetic acid). As the drug is used less, the hazard that stored drug is old and decomposed increases. For these reasons and because of the availability of benzodiazepines and phenothiazines, paraldehyde may be deemed obsolete (except in status epilepticus, p. 306). But it is cheap and may be chosen for that reason. The dose is 5–10 ml (diluted) orally or i.m. (larger doses should be divided between two sites), rectal or i.v. (dilute × 10 in 0.9% NaCl solution) administration. It dissolves plastic syringes.

Chlormethiazole (Heminevrin) is structurally related to vitamin B_1 (thiamine). It may act by altering dopamine function in the brain. It is particularly used in withdrawal from severe alcohol abuse (started at a high dose and withdrawn over 6 or 7 days; but not for patients who continue to drink) and in senile psychosis and confusion; it is a hypnotic, sedative and anticonvulsant (used in status epilepticus). It is comparatively free from hangover; it can cause nasal irritation and sneezing. Dependence occurs and use should always be brief. When taken orally, it is subject to extensive hepatic first-pass metabolism (which is defective in the old who get higher, as much as × 5, peak plasma concentrations), and the $t_\frac{1}{2}$ is 4 h (with more variation in the old than the young); it may also be given i.v.

Phenothiazines. Promethazine (Phenergan) is a useful long-lasting hypnotic ($t_\frac{1}{2}$ 12 h) especially in children. It is an antihistamine (H_1-receptor); other antihistamines having sedative action are also used as hypnotics. Trimeprazine (Vallergan) is used for short-term sedation and hypnosis in children.

Zopiclone (Zimovane) is a cyclopyrrolone with a $t_\frac{1}{2}$ of 5 h. Its efficacy is similar to benzodiazepines.

Hypnotics and anxiolytic sedatives of no particular merit include: meprobamate (Miltown), chlormezanone (Trancopal).

Barbiturates[16] (1903)

There is an increasing consensus that barbiturates are unsuitable as hypnotics because:

- barbiturates have a low therapeutic index, i.e. relatively small overdose (× 10 therapeutic dose) endangers life, with unconsciousness and respiratory depression;
- barbiturates illicitly obtained are popular drugs of social abuse;
- physical dependence occurs, with severe withdrawal syndrome sometimes including convulsions;

---

[16] Derivatives of barbituric acid, reputedly named by the original synthesiser after 'a charming lady named Barbara'. Miller LC JAMA 1961; 127: 27.

- barbiturates are potent inducers of hepatic drug metabolising enzymes and so are a source of unintended drug interactions.

But use, and abuse, continues. Therefore a general account is retained here. Knowledge of how to handle overdose remains important.

Actions

Barbiturates provide depression of the **central nervous system** ranging from *mild sedation* to *surgical anaesthesia* (see Ch. 20). For use as hypnotics and sedatives, depressant barbiturates have qualitatively similar actions; but they differ in the rate and method of disposal in the body, which has a bearing on their clinical use, and phenobarbitone and methylphenobarbitone have a greater *anticonvulsant* effect relative to the hypnotic effect. The *mode of action* may be similar to benzodiazepines, but with much less selectivity.

Pain. There is also evidence that barbiturates can antagonise analgesics and this may be borne in mind when they are used in patients with pain.

Respiration. A hypnotic dose of a barbiturate in a patient with marked respiratory insufficiency, e.g. severe pulmonary emphysema or asthma, will depress respiratory minute volume and arterial oxygen saturation. Benzodiazepines, paraldehyde and chloral are less objectionable in this respect.

Cardiovascular function. Barbiturates lower blood pressure at hypnotic and anaesthetic doses by reducing cardiac output; venous return to the heart is reduced due to peripheral venous pooling. Compensatory vascular reflexes are depressed.

Toxic doses may depress the myocardium and also reduce the peripheral resistance by blocking the sympathetic nerves.

Tolerance. When 18 former addicts were given 0.4 g pentobarbitone or quinalbarbitone daily for 90 days, tolerance began to develop within 14 days. They showed significant decrease in hours of sleep, in signs of clinical intoxication and in performance in psychomotor tests. Tolerance probably occurs to all hypnotics, but it is less marked than with opioids. With barbiturates and meprobamate the tolerance is at least partly due to *enzyme induction*.

Psychological and physical dependence occur with regular dosage of 0.4 g/day, or more, of barbiturate. If the dose exceeds 0.6 g/day the subject generally shows clinical signs of intoxication — impairment of mental ability, regression, confusion, emotional instability, nystagmus, dysarthria, ataxia and depressed somatic reflexes.

The withdrawal syndrome begins in 8–36 h and passes off over 8–14 days. It comprises, in approximate order of appearance, anxiety, twitching, intention tremor, weakness, dizziness, distorted vision, nausea; delirium and convulsions occur in severe cases.

Pharmacokinetics. Absorption after oral administration is rapid: plasma protein binding is variable, those with longer half-lives being less protein bound than those with shorter half-lives. Half-lives are the result of renal excretion and of metabolism in those used as hypnotics and sedatives.

Plasma $t_{\frac{1}{2}}$
    85 h: phenobarbitone
20–40 h: pentobarbitone, quinalbarbitone
          (secobarbital), amylobarbitone,
          butobarbitone

For those used as i.v. anaesthetics (see index), redistribution is a major factor in plasma half-life of initial doses.

Barbiturates *distribute* throughout the body.

Metabolism. For most barbiturates metabolism is chiefly hepatic. Barbiturates induce drug metabolising hepatic enzymes.

Excretion. The reason why there is little urinary excretion of unchanged barbiturate (except phenobarbitone, 25%) is not that they do not appear in the glomerular filtrate, but because barbiturate that appears in the glomerular filtrate, if un-ionised, diffuses back into the circulation through the renal tubule. This diffusion will be less if the drug is ionised, (see pH variation and kinetics, p. 87). This has been used successfully in the *treatment of overdose* by *phenobarbitone*, which has a pK_a of 7.2, and raising the urine pH to 7.5–8.5 (by sodium bicarbonate) achieves a substantial shift of un-ionised drug to the ionised and lipid-insoluble state. Urinary elimination may be more than doubled. Other barbiturates have higher pK_a (nearer 8) and so alkalinisation of the urine does not have useful effect.

Important features of severe overdose such as occurs with acute abuse, often i.v., include *prolongation of $t_\frac{1}{2}$* of the barbiturate with prolonged coma (days); *hypotension* due to CNS and cardiac depression leading to renal failure. This is treated by restoring central venous pressure and so cardiac output, by use of i.v. fluid and, if that fails, using a drug with cardiac inotropic effect (dobutamine); *elimination* of the drug is promoted by ensuring a good urine volume (e.g. 200 ml/h) and rendering it *alkaline* for phenobarbitone (see above); *active elimination* by haemoperfusion or dialysis may be needed in particularly severe and complicated cases; the use of a diuretic to enhance elimination makes management more difficult and risky without adequate benefit to compensate for this. *Respiratory stimulation* (doxapram) is only useful to sustain respiration until mechanical assistance can be set up. After overdose *sleep pattern* may be abnormal for weeks even in unhabituated subjects.

Contraindications to barbiturates. In severe pulmonary insufficiency, e.g. emphysema, even hypnotic doses of barbiturates depress respiration (see general account above).

Hepatic failure potentiates barbiturates (except barbitone, which is not metabolised).

Attacks of porphyria (see index) are induced in predisposed people.

The principal barbiturates have been listed under half-life, above: see also Anaesthesia for i.v. barbiturates, and Epilepsy.

Uses. Barbiturates are obsolete as hypnotics and sedatives, see above. The choice of drugs in *convulsive states* is discussed below.

For oral use the barbiturate or its more soluble sodium salt can be used; it matters little; but for parenteral administration a sodium salt is required. Soluble barbiturates may be injected i.m. when the dose is similar to that given orally. For i.v. injection the drug is given slowly (except thiopentone) and the dose judged by results. It is dangerous to give i.v. the more slowly metabolised and excreted drugs.

Acute adverse effects of barbiturates are almost entirely those of overdose: coma and respiratory and circulatory failure, leading to renal failure. Allergic reactions occur occasionally, particularly with phenobarbitone, rashes being the most common, but severe fatal reactions have rarely been recorded. See also Contraindications and Interactions, above.

Dependence and acute abuse with overdose is a serious social and medical problem: see above.

Bromides (1875) are handled in the body like chloride. They are now obsolete (not particulary effective and $t_\frac{1}{2}$ of 4 weeks) not only for epilepsy and as general sedatives but also for night screaming in children, townswomen who are going out of their minds, 'frightful imaginings' in late pregnancy, seasickness, somnambulism, nymphomania, and spermatorrhoea consequent on 'undue indulgence in bed'.[17]

DRUGS CAN AFFECT SKILLED TASKS AND CAR DRIVING

Many medicines affect performance, and not only the obvious examples, psychotropic drugs of all kinds, but also: antihistamines, antimuscarinics, analgesics including some NSAIDs, e.g. indomethacin, antiepileptics, antidiabetics (hypoglycaemia), some antihypertensives. *Alcohol* and *cannabis* are discussed on p. 339 and 349.

It is plain that prescribers have a major responsibility here, both to warn patients and, in the case of those who need to drive for their work, to choose medicines having minimal liability to cause impairment. One example must suffice. In a study[18] of two histamine H_1-receptor blockers, terfenadine did not impair car driving tests (weaving amongst bollards and 'gap acceptance') whereas triprolidine did. Subjects who were aware of drowsiness were yet unable to compensate, so that it is not enough to warn drivers to be more careful if they feel drowsy; they should not drive.

[17] Ringer S, Sainsbury H. A handbook of therapeutics. London: H K Lewis. 1897.
[18] Betts T et al. Br Med J 1984; 288: 281.

Patients who must drive when taking a drug of known risk (e.g. benzodiazepine) should be specially warned of times of peak impairment.

A patient who has an accident and who was not warned of drug hazard, whether orally or by labelling, may successfully sue the doctor in law. It is also necessary that patients be advised of the additive effect of alcohol with prescribed medicines.[19]

Car driving is a complex multi-function task that includes[20]

- visual search and recognition
- vigilance
- information processing under variable demand
- decision-making and risk-taking
- sensorimotor control.

It is evident that drivers may be more than usually accident prone without any subjective feeling of sedation or dysphoria: the fact that they feel OK does not mean that they are OK.

The criteria for safety in air-crew are more stringent than with car drivers.

Little is known of impairment and risk in skilled tasks other than driving. Concentration on psychomotor and physical aspects (injury) should not distract from the possibility that those who live by their intellect and imagination (politicians and even journalists may be included here) may suffer cognitive disability from thoughtless prescribing.

Resumption of car driving or other skilled activity after *anaesthesia* is a special case, and an extremely variable one. The following suggestions may serve.

After dentistry under local anaesthesia alone: 2 h.

Where a sedative (e.g. i.v. benzodiazepine, opioid or neuroleptic), or any general anaesthetic has been used: 24 h at least.

How the patient *feels* is not a reliable guide to recovery of skills.

GUIDE TO FURTHER READING

Batter M et al 1974 Cross-national study of the extent of anti-anxiety/sedative drug use. New England Journal of Medicine 290: 769

Bixler E O et al 1991 Next-day memory impairment with triazolam use. Lancet 337: 827

Brahams D 1990 Benzodiazepine and sexual fantasies. Lancet 335: 157

Controversies in therapeutics 1989 Risks of dependence on benzodiazepine drugs. British Medical Journal
(i) Tyrer P The importance of patient selection 298: 102
(ii) Ashton H A major problem of long term treatment 298: 103

Drew P J J et al 1985 The effects of acute beta-adrenoceptor blockade on examination performance. British Journal of Clinical Pharmacology 19: 783

Editorial 1985 Beta-blockers in situational anxiety. Lancet 2: 193

Gillin J C 1990 The diagnosis and management of insomnia. New England Journal of Medicine 322: 239, 324: 1735

Greenblatt D J et al 1989 Effect of gradual withdrawal on the rebound sleep disorder after discontinuation of triazolam. New England Journal of Medicine 317: 722

Lader M et al 1986 States of anxiety and their induction by drugs. British Journal of Clinical Pharmacology 22: 251

Nicholson A N et al 1986 Sleep after transmeridian flights. Lancet 2: 1205

---

[19] Nordic countries require that medicines liable to impair ability to drive or to operate machinery be labelled with a red triangle on a white background. The scheme covers antidepressants, benzodiazepines, hypnotics, drugs for motion sickness and allergy, cerebral stimulants, antiepileptics and hypotensive agents.

In the UK there are some standard labels that pharmacists are recommended to apply, e.g. No. 2: 'Warning. May cause drowsiness. If affected do not drive or operate machinery. Avoid alcoholic drink'. They are offered as 'a carefully considered balance between the unintelligibly short and the inconveniently long' (see BNF).

[20] In: Willett R E et al., eds. Drugs, driving and traffic safety. Geneva: WHO, 1983.

Prinz P N et al 1990 Geriatrics: sleep disorders and aging. New England Journal of Medicine 323: 520

Tyrer P 1989 Treating panic. British Medical Journal 298: 201

Tyrer P et al 1988 The Nottingham study of neurotic disorder: comparison of drug and psychological treatments. Lancet 2: 1988

17

Central nervous system III: drugs and mental disorder — psychotropic and psychoactive drugs

SYNOPSIS

Drugs are sometimes paramount in treatment but are often secondary to non-drug approaches.

In schizophrenia neuroleptic drugs, whose principal effect is to block dopamine receptors, are used; but they can exact a high price in adverse effects.

In depression, the monoamine hypothesis proposes that there is deficiency of noradrenaline and serotonin in the brain which can be modified by antidepressants.

Mania is associated with overactivity of brain noradrenergic transmission; it may be controlled and prevented by drugs.

- Drugs in mental disorder
- The schizophrenic syndrome and neuroleptic drugs
- Drugs for affective disorders: depression, mania (anxiety, see Ch. 16)
- Other psychological conditions: appetite, narcolepsy, attention deficit, nocturnal enuresis, organic brain syndromes and intellectual function, toxic confusional states, behaviour control, excessive sex drive in men, suicide and prescribed drugs
- Classification and dosage of psychotropic drugs
- Neuroleptics
- Antidepressants
- MAOIs
- Lithium
- Psychostimulants, appetite control
- Amphetamines
- Xanthines
- Ginseng

DRUGS IN MENTAL DISORDER

Writing prescriptions is easy, understanding people is hard.

(Franz Kafka, 1883–1924)

In the debate whether the basis for mental disorders is primarily physical or psychological it might seem that the two hypotheses are irreconcilable. But the ultimate experience of mental activity involves biochemical changes in transmission in the brain, and whether the initiating factors are primarily psychological or physical (biochemical) the use of a chemical to alter function beneficially can be appropriate. Most psychiatrists would seek for precipitating psychological and social events and endeavour to modify these as a part of therapy. They would do this despite their knowledge that there are important biochemical changes in the brain, but they would also seek to modify these with drugs.

Overreliance on drugs could lead to an undesirable reduction in the vital role of trained staff operating in a positive therapeutic environment, but neuroleptics can be a valuable means of enabling these staff to make psychological contact with and work alongside disturbed patients.

Drugs are cheaper to supply than are trained staff. But drugs are not a substitute for trained staff.

With the increasing recognition of mental illness as a major cause of unhappiness and disability, interest in the possibilities of drug therapy has increased. Medicinal chemists have responded by making analogues of endogenous neurotransmitters in the expectation that some of them will prove to be medicines. One snag is the difficulty of predicting therapeutic efficacy from the animal experiments that must necessarily precede clinical trial; another is how to determine by clinical trial whether a genuine therapeutic effect has occurred and, if so, whether it was in fact due to the drug or to environmental changes or to behavioural therapy, including any extra care by the physician.

Paul Ehrlich wrote that 'we must learn to aim, learn to aim with chemical substances'. But in order to aim we must have targets to aim at, and if benefits are to be obtained without unwanted effects, the targets must be precisely defined. In mental disorder the targets are increasingly being defined.

Though there have been many apparent breakthroughs, time and again they have been like elephants' footprints in the mud, making a large initial impression but quickly fading into the background.[1]

There is greater likelihood of therapeutic success from drugs in the *psychoses* in which behaviour differs from normal in kind, than in *psychoneuroses* in which it differs from normal mainly in amount.

Psychotropic drugs (drugs that alter mental function) act by altering endogenous chemotransmitter systems that pass nerve impulses at synapses, i.e. from the ending of one neuron across the synaptic cleft to the next neuron, e.g. noradrenaline, dopamine, serotonin, acetylcholine, gamma-aminobutyric acid (GABA), histamine, endorphins. Plainly the formation, storage, release and the occupation of receptors and post-receptor events caused by these active substances offer opportunities for intervention with appropriately designed chemicals (drugs). Research concentrates on these aspects.

Sites of action

Localisation of function (via these transmitters) within the brain, suggests three main anatomical sites of action[2] of drugs in mental disease:

- *reticular activating system*: attention, arousal, anxiety
- *limbic system*: affect or emotional content
- *hypothalamus*: control of autonomic nervous system: pituitary–endocrine control.

There is a complex range of interrelationships, e.g. the locus coeruleus interconnects the reticular formation, hypothalamus and cortex, also utilising these transmitters. But the transmitters are not confined to these sites, and so nonselective drugs will be expected to cause unwanted (adverse) effects, as indeed they do.

Schemes of drug action

Enough is now known to allow the formulation of provisional schemes of drug action and adverse reaction that begin to give the kind of understanding that may help clinicians to use psychotropic drugs more effectively than would be the case if they merely followed routine instructions as they do in cooking. What follows is *not* a definitive account; it cannot be, but it is offered to show the kind of approaches and interpretations that are currently being made.

Clinical evaluation

Clinical evaluation is done by recording changes in behaviour, performance of tasks and psychomotor tests, and opinions of the patient himself as well as of his family, nurses and doctors. There is a large number of rating scales, inventories, questionnaires and check lists to measure anxiety, depression, guilt, adverse effects, and they can be applied by observers or by the patient himself. The final court of appeal for efficacy and acceptability must always be the patient's clinical condition. Controlled trials in psychiatry also require to take into account important environmental factors and life events, e.g.

---

[1] Editorial. Lancet 1978; 1: 422.

[2] After Hollister L E Clinical pharmacology of psychotherapeutic drugs. 2nd edn. Edinburgh: Churchill Livingstone, 1983

attitudes of relatives, bereavement.

Not only is quantitative evaluation extraordinarily difficult in psychiatry, but there are also problems of diagnosis, which is less precise than that in most other branches of medicine.

Some of the hazards of uncontrolled studies have been demonstrated. In one case patients and hospital staff were told that two new drugs were to be tried, an 'energiser' and a 'tranquilliser'. The tablets were orange and yellow respectively, and were available in two sizes. Improvement was reported in 53% of patients taking the 'energiser' and in 80% of those taking the 'tranquilliser'. In fact both 'drugs' were lactose, made to taste bitter with quinine.[3]

Even where a careful double-blind technique is used successfully, bias due to the personality and beliefs of the physicians about the remedies can still affect the result. In a study on relief of anxiety by two active drugs and a placebo, the results varied according to which of two physicians was treating the patients.

Dr. A. was youngish in appearance, he expected no difference between the three treatments and his attitude to the patients was non-committal. No difference between the treatments was found.

Dr. B. had greying hair and a fatherly appearance and he expected that the pharmacologically active substances would prove superior to the placebo. Patients reported that he was 'helpful' and 'dependable'. A difference in favour of one of the active drugs appeared in his patients.

When both groups were added there was no significant difference.[4]

It is probable that effects of doctors' personalities and opinions can influence even the best conducted studies, and this may be more likely to happen where the drug is an adjuvant and not the mainstay of therapy. The fact that endeavours to eliminate bias are not invariably successful has been used as an argument against attempting controlled techniques in psychiatric comparisons. The logic of this is obscure.

Choice of drugs in mental and behavioural disorders

- Non-drug therapies are not discussed here. This is not because they are unimportant, but because they are outside the scope of a book on pharmacology.

Patients often get better without drugs, and sometimes in spite of them.

A patient with endogenous depression became very much better during 3 or 4 weeks following prescription of an antidepressant drug. The physician reminded her of the importance of continuing therapy despite the improvement. The patient smiled and said 'Oh, doctor, the tablets did not agree with me, so I stopped taking them after the first two or three days'.[5]

Note. 1. anti-depressants require about 10 days to produce benefit; 2. there is a great deal more to treatment than simply prescribing drugs; 3. when a patient improves following a prescription, it cannot be assumed that it is because of the prescription.

- Psychotropic drugs provide symptomatic or suppressive treatment only; they do not eliminate the disease but ameliorate the condition until recovery occurs. But it is possible that by reducing a symptom a vicious cycle may be broken so that recovery occurs sooner, and in severe cases drugs may allow the patient to re-establish contact with his environment and thus to become accessible to social and psychotherapy.

The effects of all drugs acting on mental processes vary greatly with the circumstances and the dose and the attitude of the prescriber.

- In **psychotic states** (severe *manic or depressive illness* and *schizophrenia*) neuroleptics or antidepressants (tricyclic or allies) are given in rapidly increasing doses at first, with longer intervals between increases later. Once the maximum long-term benefit is achieved the dose may be reduced gradually, even by as much as half, without loss of benefit; frequency of administration may sometimes be reduced to the convenient once a day.

Eventual withdrawal should also be gradual to

[3] Loranger A W et al. JAMA 1961; 176: 920.
[4] Uhlenhuth E H et al. Am J Psychiatry 1959; 115: 905.

[5] Merry J Lancet 1972; 1: 1175.

avoid sudden and dangerous relapse. Duration of treatment is impossible to predict; no attempt at withdrawal should be made until 6–8 weeks after apparent recovery from an acute episode and two-thirds of chronic cases need treatment for 3–4 years, in which case a long-acting i.m. formulation may be preferred.

The minimum effective dose should always be used, especially in patients in the community, and the need to continue therapy reviewed at least twice a year.

Resistant cases may be admitted to hospital to receive high doses. Severe intercurrent illness may reduce drug requirement.

• **In psychoneuroses** (anxiety, phobias, reactive depression, obsessive-compulsive disorders), the environment is relatively more important; drugs are best confined to short periods, to help patients over a bad phase of illness. *Prolonged drug therapy is seldom rewarding.* It must be admitted that this view is not unanimously held, some physicians believing that drug therapy is of great value in the routine treatment of psychoneuroses.

• **Combinations of psychotropic drugs** are sometimes useful. Initially at least, the drugs should be given separately, e.g. first an anti-anxiety agent and then a neuroleptic added and the dose adjusted to suit the patient. Fixed-dose combinations are unsatisfactory, chiefly because of this need to adjust the dose; but patients are less likely to take separate drugs reliably. Though there is evidence that mild-to-moderate mixed anxiety-depression (such as is seen in general practice and seldom finds a way to a psychiatrist) may benefit from, e.g. a mix of tricyclic + neuroleptic (Motival, Triptafen) or trycyclic + benzodiazepine. These preparations are frequently condemned by specialists but prescribed by family doctors; they should be further studied.

THE SCHIZOPHRENIC SYNDROME AND NEUROLEPTIC[6] DRUGS

Schizophrenia is associated with increased dopaminergic activity in the limbic structures of the brain. There is an increased number of dopamine-D_2 receptors in the brain and there may be receptor supersensitivity and over-production of dopamine, or reduced destruction due to enzyme abnormalities or deficiencies. It is not proved whether this is the primary defect in schizophrenia or whether it is a secondary or epi-phenomenon). Neuroleptic drugs that benefit schizophrenia, e.g. phenothiazines, butyro-phenones, thioxanthenes, are competitive antagonists of dopamine (dopamine-D_2 receptor blockers) and a precursor of dopamine, levodopa, predictably exacerbates symptoms of schizophrenia. D_1 receptors, postsynaptic and pre-synaptic (autoreceptors) are also involved, but it is not yet possible to present a coherent, clinically useful account.

Dopaminergic neurons are not confined to the limbic system. Dopamine-D_1 receptors, for example, also occur in the nigrostriatal (extrapyramidal) system and elsewhere, e.g. controlling hypothalamic hormone-releasing factors. Thus a non-selective dopamine antagonist (D_2 and D_1 receptors), e.g. chlorpromazine, would be expected to benefit schizophrenia but also to cause extrapyramidal movement disorders and endocrine changes, e.g. prolactin release. And this is indeed the case; all these effects occur with chlorpromazine. It also blocks *serotonin receptors* which may be relevant to its therapeutic effect. It has in addition alpha-adrenoceptor and cholinergic blocking activity. Indeed it was given the proprietary name 'Largactil' because it has such a large number of actions. Despite this lack of selectivity, chlorpromazine, the first (1951) neuroleptic or antipsychotic drug, was a major advance in therapeutics and it remains useful.

Neuroleptics are the most effective drugs and can greatly reduce *positive symptoms*, e.g. aggression, hyperactivity, delusions and hallucinations. But *negative symptoms*, e.g. apathy, respond less well.

Acute episodes may respond at once, but in chronic states response may be delayed for 3

---

[6] Neuroleptic: an imprecise term comprising the more powerful (major) tranquillisers used for antipsychotic effect. For definition of tranquilliser, see footnote on p. 264.

weeks or more. Additional treatments, e.g. an antidepressant (tricyclic) or electroconvulsive therapy (ECT), may be needed.

Maintenance therapy may be necessary to prevent relapse, especially if the patient's family is critical or otherwise unsupportive, as it often is, understandably.

The choice of drug is wide and may be illustrated as follows:

- Acute schizophrenic state: chlorpromazine or haloperidol
- Maintenance therapy: chlorpromazine or alternative phenothiazine or pimozide
- Long-term maintenance where patient compliance needs to be known with certainty: sustained-release or depot i.m. injection, e.g. fluphenazine decanoate 2–6 weekly.

Unfortunately neuroleptics have a capacity (variable between groups and members of groups) to induce serious extrapyramidal neuromuscular adverse effects, in particular a late onset (tardive) dyskinesia which may be irreversible (see below). But sulpiride and clozapine are relatively free from this.

Mechanism of adverse effects and treatment

Enough is now known to begin to explain the mechanism of the troublesome adverse effects of dopamine-receptor blocking neuroleptics (and antiemetics) and such knowledge is useful in management of patients. It may be summarised:

Neurological effects

Extrapyramidal motor disorders: tremor, dystonia, akinesia and/or a parkinsonian (or pseudo-parkinsonian) syndrome are to be expected. Idiopathic parkinsonism is due to underactivity or deficiency in dopaminergic neurons causing imbalance between dopaminergic and cholinergic systems (see Parkinson's disease). Evidently a dopamine receptor blocker will mimic this disease. Occurrence of the above effects may predict liability to tardive dyskinesia.

It is generally best to withdraw, or reduce the dose of the drug. But this may not be practicable since valuable benefit may be lost. In such cases it is necessary to treat the motor disorder with another drug. An antimuscarinic drug (procyclidine, benztropine) should be used, but routine prophylactic use is not justified. Many phenothiazines also have antimuscarinic effects and these are less liable to cause extrapyramidal disorders because they mitigate the dopaminergic/cholinergic imbalance.

Levodopa (converted to dopamine in the brain) is inappropriate because it will either be ineffective in the presence of a dopamine receptor blocker or if it is effective it will also antagonise the therapeutic effect in the limbic system.

Akathisia (extreme restlessness) occurs in about 20% of patients. It may respond to propranolol (a β-adrenoceptor blocker that enters the CNS); antimuscarinics are generally ineffective.

The above effects generally occur early in the course of treatment, but also may be tardive (late onset). Of the latter, one form is particularly prominent, as follows.

Tardive dyskinesia (from Latin *tardus*, slow or late-coming) is a disorder of involuntary movements (choreoathetoid movements of lips, tongue, face, jaws, and of limbs and sometimes trunk). It occurs generally after 2–5 years' use of a dopamine receptor blocker, though occasionally after a few months. It is due, paradoxically, to increase dopamine-sensitivity or activity due to changes in the receptors themselves and to upregulation (increase in numbers) of receptors characteristic of exposure to any blocking drugs. It particularly affects patients with organic brain disease and the elderly who should not be given these drugs if it can be avoided. It occurs in about 20% of treated schizophrenic patients, but in up to 40% of long-term institutionalised patients. Though generally mild, it may be severe and permanent.

Patients pass from a state of drug-induced reduction of dopaminergic activity to an indirectly drug-induced excess of dopaminergic activity. If this state continues then damage to the presynaptic membrane may result so that the presynaptic autoreceptors become supersensitive and the condition is irreversible.

If the neuroleptic is suddenly withdrawn, tardive dyskinesia may become worse because of the sudden accessibility to transmitter of the previously blocked but now more numerous receptors.

Also, antimuscarinics which are useful where there is a deficiency of dopaminergic activity (extrapyramidal disorders, above, and parkinsonism), since they restore the dopaminergic/cholingeric balance, will exacerbate tardive dyskinesia by increasing the imbalance that has already risen.

Rational management of tardive dyskinesia, if the dopamine sensitivity hypothesis is correct, implies:

- Use of minimum effective dose of neuroleptic.
- Alteration of neuroleptic dose (increase may, by blocking more dopamine receptors, cause transient improvement but may ultimately worsen the condition). Slow withdrawal of the drug is likely to be followed by recovery in early cases (occurring in the first year of therapy) but only half of later onset cases, who remain permanently affected. This is a serious matter.
- Change to a neuroleptic less likely to cause the condition, e.g. sulpiride, clozapine.
- Depletion of dopamine (catecholamine) stores, e.g. by tetrabenazine (p. 315).
- Increasing cholinergic activity by withdrawing any antimuscarinic drug being given against extrapyramidal reactions. Enhancement of cholinergic activity by giving precursors of acetylcholine, e.g. lecithin, has been only marginally effective; anticholinesterases have transiently modified the condition.
- Increase GABA-inhibitory action by using a benzodiazepine, baclofen or sodium valproate; there is a complex interrelation of GABA with dopaminergic/cholinergic balance.
- Miscellaneous: lithium and diltiazem may have benefited individuals.

- Drug holidays (1 month in 6) carry risk of therapeutic relapse; they may not help and there is even suspicion they may increase the risk.
- Early detection (by watching for developing tongue movements) when the condition is reversible is plainly important.

Other effects

Endocrine effects: hyperprolactinaemia due to block of the dopamine-mediated prolactin-inhibiting path in the hypothalamus, leading to galactorrhoea with amenorrhoea; also false positive pregnancy test. Increased libido may occur perhaps due to interference with normal conversion of androgens to oestrogens. But defective sexual function (impotence, amenorrhoea) can occur and constitute a hidden source of non-compliance.

Sedation is common.

Antimuscarinic effects, e.g. dry mouth, blurred vision.

Alpha-adrenoceptor block: hypotension.

Miscellaneous: hepatitis, blood disorders, corneal or lens opacities.

Neuroleptic malignant syndrome is a rare condition of uncertain cause but clinically similar to the genetically determined anaesthetic malignant hyperthermia. It usually occurs early in therapy, developing over about 2 days; it can be fatal.

The clinical state may not be distinguishable from a severe parkinsonian reaction, at least early in its development.

Treatment is urgent: withdrawal of the drug and administration of dantrolene and a centrally active dopamine agonist, e.g. bromocriptine. In extreme cases a competitive neuromuscular blocking agent is effective (unlike malignant hyperthermia). The syndrome may recur if neuroleptic administration is resumed.

The commonest precipitants may be fluphenazine and haloperidol, but it can also occur with antidepressants.

DRUGS FOR AFFECTIVE DISORDERS

DEPRESSION AND ANTIDEPRESSANTS

The first drug to be found effective in elevating mood in endogenous depression was amphetamine (developed in the late 1930s). But it was soon recognised as useful only in mild cases and to be prone to abuse. Amphetamines release noradrenaline stored in nerve endings and prevent its re-uptake into those same nerve endings by inhibiting the monoamine pump mechanism (see below).

In 1951, iproniazid (developed as an antituberculosis agent) was noticed to elevate mood, an effect associated with inhibition of the enzyme monoamine oxidase (MAOI). It was soon replaced in tuberculosis by isoniazid which did not inhibit MAO.

In 1954 reserpine (p. 423) was found to cause depression and to prevent the normal storage of noradrenaline (a substrate for MAO) in nerve endings.

Thus a drug that inhibited metabolism of monoamines (noradrenaline and serotonin) and allowed them to accumulate in nerve endings (iproniazid) relieved some cases of depression, and a drug that depleted nerve endings of their catecholamine stores (reserpine) was known to cause depression.

Research consequently was directed to monoamine metabolism, storage and release.

At about this time (1957) the development of further tricyclic neuroleptics derived from chlorpromazine led to the synthesis of a tricyclic iminodibenzyl derivative (imipramine), which, though it differed structurally only slightly from chlorpromazine, had no useful neuroleptic action but was found in clinical trials to have a useful antidepressant effect. When noradrenaline is released from a nerve ending into the synaptic cleft, its action on postsynaptic receptors is terminated not by destruction, as is the case with acetylcholine, but by diffusion away from the synaptic cleft and by re-uptake (by amine pump) into the nerve ending, where it is stored, and its metabolism is regulated by MAO (which is wholly inside the nerve ending). Tricyclics block the amine uptake pump.

The monoamine hypothesis

Thus drugs affecting depression are concerned with amine storage, release, or uptake. These observations are the basis of the *monoamine hypothesis of depression*, which proposes that endogenous depression is due to deficiency of CNS noradrenergic or serotonergic (5-HT) (monoamine) activity or transmission; MAOIs rectify this by preventing amine destruction, and tricyclics by preventing re-uptake (by inhibition of amine pump). Thus the concentration in nerve endings and at postsynaptic receptors is enhanced. Differences in clinical effect are attributed to differences in pattern of MAO inhibition (MAO-A or MAO-B) or by differences in the ratio of inhibition of noradrenaline to serotonin re-uptake.

But this *monoamine hypothesis* in its simplest form must be inadequate, for there are now in use antidepressants that inhibit the amine pump (cell uptake) for noradrenaline only (viloxazine), for serotonin only (clomipramine) and for neither (mianserin). But some drugs, e.g. mianserin and trazodone, may block a negative feed-back effect mediated by presynaptic adrenoceptors (autoreceptors),[7] so causing an increased release of transmitter.

Pharmacodynamic effect is immediate and the delay in onset of antidepressant effect (7–14 days) may represent the time needed to overcome compensatory feedback changes (if it is not due to inadequate initial dosage). Severe depression requires electroconvulsive therapy, which works quickly and may forestall suicide; it may work by increasing postsynaptic receptor response.

---

[7] An autoreceptor is a receptor anywhere on a neuron that responds to the transmitter released by that neuron. It usually mediates negative feedback. Presynaptic receptors are autoreceptors.

Treatment

Most cases of depression eventually recover spontaneously and most drugs take a week or two to act, so that careful controls are needed if credit for recovery is to be correctly attributed. Antidepressants can precipitate epilepsy in those with a family history of epilepsy, who have had previous ECT, or organic brain damage.

Endogenous depression: the tricyclic or allied group is the first choice, and a sedative or stimulant member is chosen according to individual need (see Table 17.3 p. 288). But ECT may be needed if depression is severe or if a quick effect is needed. A combination of a tricyclic and ECT may be ideal in severe cases, and the drug may reduce the number of shocks needed. Lithium may be added in resistant cases.

In very agitated depression a phenothiazine (chlorpromazine) may be a useful adjunct to a tricyclic antidepressant. Benzodiazepines are contraindicated (but see alprazolam).

It is important not to withhold ECT when a tricyclic fails. In one trial half the patients who failed to respond to imipramine in 4 weeks benefited from ECT.

At the first sign of overdose of antidepressant, the drug should be withdrawn and chlorpromazine given; but see mianserin.

Insomnia of depression (characteristically, early waking) may be relieved by an antidepressant drug and not require a hypnotic (though this may be kind in the period before the antidepressant effect occurs).

Reactive depression (exogenous), where drug therapy is necessary, is commonly associated with *anxiety* and is best treated by an anxiolytic sedative (though these are not antidepressants, except perhaps alprazolam), or a tricyclic antidepressant. A MAO inhibitor may be used if these fail.

Seasonal affective disorder (SAD) (winter depression) may respond to phototherapy (after 4 days); drug therapy (antidepressant, dexfenfluramine) is of uncertain benefit.

Prevention of endogenous depression
(a phasic or relapsing disorder)

When the oscillation is between normal mood and depression (unipolar depression) a tricyclic antidepressant may prevent relapse more effectively than lithium.

MANIA

Mania may be accompanied by overactivity of noradrenergic transmission, i.e. the opposite of depression, and drugs that enhance transmission can cause mania (MAOIs, tricyclics, levodopa). Lithium is effective; its exact mode of action remains uncertain. Because benefit is slow to develop (2–3 weeks) it is not suitable sole treatment of severe acute mania which will require a neuroleptic for control. Lithium is adequate for mild cases, but its chief use is prevention of relapse. Carbamazepine is also effective for prophylaxis.

Acute severe mania may be controlled by either promazine orally or by haloperidol (5–10 mg i.m.) repeated as necessary; lower doses are used for less urgent cases, and transfer to oral therapy for longer term management.

If the patient is in a single room, accompanied by a suitable nurse, smaller doses of neuroleptic drug will be needed, for excitement tends to subside sooner under these circumstances than it does in the presence of other patients, or if the patient is left entirely alone. Some manic patients are not quietened even by large doses of neuroleptic until they suddenly collapse with respiratory depression. Lithium can be used in milder cases where there is no haste.

Prevention of manic-depressive disorder

In this condition oscillation is between states both above and below normal mood (bipolar) and lithium is effective in prophylaxis of both the manic and depressive phases. Carbamazepine is used where lithium fails.

ANXIETY AND TENSION: see Chapter 16.

OBSESSIVE-COMPULSIVE DISORDER

Behavioural therapy may usefully be supplemented by an antidepressant that inhibits serotonin re-uptake into neurons (clomipramine, fluoxetine); sometimes by an anxiolytic sedative.

Severe chronic phobic anxiety that has resisted other treatment sometimes responds to an MAOI or to a tricyclic antidepressant despite the absence of overt depression.

OTHER PSYCHOLOGICAL CONDITIONS

Acute behavioural disturbances: a neuroleptic or a benzodiazepine orally or i.m.

Appetite disorders: anorexia and bulimia. Drugs are adjuvant to behaviour therapy. In anorexia nervosa chlorpromazine is useful, and cyproheptadine may be tried as an appetite stimulant if there is no bulimia.

In bulimia dexfenfluramine and fluoxetine may benefit. An antidepressant may sometimes help either condition even if there is no clinical depression; benefit may be transient.

Obesity: see p. 296.

Narcolepsy is benefited by activating noradrenergic mechanisms with amphetamine, dexamphetamine, methylphenidate, mazindol or caffeine. A tricyclic antidepressant may be tried.

Attention deficit disorder (hyperkinetic disorder) in children responds to adrenergic activation by dexamphetamine (or methylphenidate or pemoline). The child becomes more able to sustain attention and so less active. If these drugs fail, an antidepressant may be tried. Drug therapy should be as brief as possible (3 weeks–3 months) and confined to children above 5 years. There is risk that growth may be diminished by disruption of the sleep pattern and so of the circadian rhythm of growth hormone secretion. This is especially important at the period of closure of the epiphyses, when drugs should be withheld if possible.

There have been complaints, with seeming justification, that merely naughty active children who are a nuisance at school or in the home or whose behaviour is the result of parental problems are being misdiagnosed and made into drugged family scapegoats. There is virtually no situation in which an aggressive child or adolescent should be treated only pharmacologically.

Nocturnal enuresis in children can often be controlled by a tricyclic antidepressant (imipramine), but relapse on ceasing its use is usual. There is a very real hazard of accidental poisoning and parents must be made to understand the risk of leaving the drug accessible in the home of small children. Attractively tasty syrups are hazardous; tablets should be used; but only after non-drug approaches have failed, say after 7 years of age, not before.

Desmopressin (antidiuretic hormone) by intranasal metered aerosol has similar efficiency (15–40% completely dry *during use*). It has the advantage of being safer than antidepressant. Short-term use, e.g. for a holiday, is acceptable. Children above 9 years respond best.

Organic brain syndromes and senile dementias of Alzheimer type where patients are seriously uncooperative and disturbed are sometimes helped by a neuroleptic, promazine, thioridazine or haloperidol. Anxiolytic sedatives (benzodiazepines) are best avoided lest slightly agitated patients who can conduct their personal toilet are converted to tranquil patients who cannot. These patients are commonly intolerant of drugs and a low dose should be used initially. Nocturnal delirium may be made worse by hypnotics and helped by caffeine taken as strong tea.

Some benefit may occur with agents that enhance cholinergic function, e.g. the centrally-acting anticholinesterase tacrine (tetrahydroaminoacidine, THA) and the acetylcholine precursor lecithin. Benefit is confined to the equivalent of the deterioration which could be expected over a few months. Antimuscarinic drugs (as used in parkinsonism) aggravate the condition. Some apathetic patients have obtained a little benefit from selegiline.

Intellectual or cognitive function (nootropic[8] drugs: cognition enhancers). With ageing populations becoming more and more for-

---

[8] Drugs affecting the intellect (Greek: mind turning).

getful, investigators and drug developers are turning to the possibilities of improving cognitive function, especially age-associated memory impairment. Experiments on memory in rats are easy to do and numerous drugs appear to have some effect, e.g. endorphins and naloxone, corticotrophin and vasopressin (peptides), adrenergic and cholinergic agents. The locus coeruleus of the brain is known to be concerned with memory regulation, and these drugs can be shown to increase its neuronal firing.

No drugs have been shown reliably and substantially to improve impaired or normal memory in man over long periods.

But there is evidence of some effect for meclofenoxate, pemoline and co-dergocrine. It is unlikely that vasodilatation has any effect, and any benefit of such drugs is likely to be due to brain cell actions.

Prescribers who seek to help their senile or other patients' memories with drugs will do well to remember that whilst benefits will be limited at best, it is quite easy to impair the fragile intellectual function of the old with ill-chosen, uncritical, unmonitored prescribing.

Learning. Studies in animals have shown that drugs that modify cholinergic and adrenergic mechanisms in the central nervous system or alter the synthesis of RNA can enhance learning. It will be time to take this topic seriously in medicine when efficacy has been demonstrated in a resistant human population such as medical students.

Toxic confusional states, e.g. delirium tremens or post-surgical confusion, may be benefited by diazepam, chlorpromazine or chlormethiazole. Paraldehyde is also often satisfactory. Correction of any accessible biochemical, toxic or anoxic abnormality is of the first importance.

Behaviour control. The fact that drugs can be used to quell inconvenient behaviour of the mentally handicapped, the demented and psychotics, and as a cheap substitute for skilled staff in institutions, including prisons, is a matter for concern. Similar use on persons deemed by authority to be social or political deviants is also something to be feared; there is no doubt that it has occurred. Use of psychotropic drugs for 'problem children' is an area of particular concern, e.g. imipramine for school phobia.

Excessive sex drive in men may be reduced by oestrogen or by antiandrogen (cyproterone). The breasts may enlarge sufficiently to require surgical removal. These treatments may be indicated in abnormal personalities with pronounced sexual aggression. They raise particularly powerful ethical issues where the choice is between therapy with liberty, or loss of liberty, e.g. repeated sexual assaults on children. Benperidol (a butyrophenone) can also be effective.

Suicide and prescribed drugs. Sometimes it is necessary to prescribe drugs for potentially suicidal patients living at home. In such cases it is usual to prescribe minimal doses for short periods and, when the danger seems serious, to hand over the supply of drugs to a responsible person rather than to the patient. Benzodiazepines are the sedatives and hypnotics of choice in such patients as heavy overdose is most unlikely to kill the patient.

Some antidepressants, e.g. mianserin, may be less cardiotoxic in overdose than others.

An ingenious formulation of paracetamol containing enough methionine to protect the liver in overdose has been devised (Pameton).

Drug induced suicide: see reserpine and Table 17.3 (Note 1).

CLASSIFICATION OF PSYCHOTROPIC[9] DRUGS

So little is known about the biochemical basis of mental disorder that no definitive classification based on mechanisms of action can yet be offered. Drugs are classified provisionally according to the symptoms they are used to relieve and by chemical group.

1. Neuroleptics (antipsychotics) are drugs with therapeutic effect on schizophrenia and some other psychoses; they cause emotional quietening, indifference and psychomotor slowing; they also cause movement disorders. Such an imprecise definition illustrates how little is

---

[9] Psychotropic = affecting the mind.

known of the diseases and of how the drugs provide benefit.

- *Phenothiazines*: see Table 17.1.
- *Butyrophenones* are similar to class 3 phenothiazines (see Table 17.1). The group includes: benperidol (Anquil), droperidol (Droleptan), haloperidol (Serenace), trifluperidol (Triperidol).
- *Diphenylbutylpiperidines* are closely related to the butyrophenones: fluspirilene (Redeptin), pimozide (Orap).
- *Benzamide*: sulpiride (Dolmatil).
- *Dibenzodiazepine*: clozapine (Clozaril).
- *Thioxanthenes*: flupenthixol (Depixol), zuclopenthixol (clopenthixol is a racemic mixture) (Clopixol).
- *Indole derivative*: oxypertine (Integrin).

2. Anxiolytic sedatives and other drugs used in anxiety, see Chapter 16.

3. Antidepressants

- *Tricyclic* and related agents (see Table 17.3).
- *Monoamine oxidase inhibitors*: phenelzine (Nardil), isocarboxazid (Marplan), tranylcypromine (Parnate).
- Miscellaneous: L-tryptophan is a precursor of serotonin (5-HT); alprazolam is an antidepressant benzodiazepine.

4. Lithium and **carbamazepine** for mania and manic-depressive psychosis.

5. Psychostimulants increase the level of alertness and/or motivation.

- Amphetamines: methylphenidate (Ritalin), pemoline (Volital). This group is obsolete except for occasional special use.
- Caffeine.

6. Psychodysleptics (hallucinogens, psychedelics psychotomimetics) produce mental phenomena, particularly cognitive and perceptual (see non-medical drug use).

DOSAGE OF PSYCHOTROPIC DRUGS

Because of the difficulty in measuring responses in psychiatry, and the variability caused by en-

vironmental factors, drugs are commonly given in arbitrarily fixed or at least crudely adjusted doses. This militates substantially against precise clinical evaluation and against achievement of optimum therapeutic effect, unless plasma concentrations are measured and can be related to therapeutic effect.

In the case of *tricyclic antidepressants*, standard doses may produce steady-state plasma concentrations varying by a factor of 10 or more. The ideal therapeutic response may occur at intermediate plasma concentrations, falling off as the concentration rises above an optimum, i.e. there is a *therapeutic window*. It is plain that when a patient does not respond, knowledge of plasma concentration will be valuable in order to allow a decision whether this is a true therapeutic failure or whether the dosage is wrong. This information is at present seldom available.

Once-daily dosage (at night) is commonly satisfactory, with increments at intervals appropriate to the plasma $t_{\frac{1}{2}}$, which indicates when a steady state will have been reached, i.e. about $5 \times t_{\frac{1}{2}}$.

For *neuroleptics* (which are difficult to measure chemically) also, individual variation is great and drug $t_{\frac{1}{2}}$ ranges from 10 to 50 h. Injectable depot formulations, given at intervals of weeks, are widely used.

INDIVIDUAL DRUGS BY CLASS

NEUROLEPTICS (see Table 17.1)

Chlorpromazine

As a result of investigation of phenothiazine compounds for possible anthelminthic effect, first promethazine, the useful sedative and antihistamine, was discovered, and then chlorpromazine (1951).

Chlorpromazine has a large number of actions. It blocks dopamine, α-adreno-, muscarinic (cholinergic), serotonin and histamine-H_1 receptors. It has a quinidine-like effect on the heart and can cause cardiac dysrhythmias. Practical therapeutics might be better served if they were distributed amongst 3 or 4 drugs instead of being concentrated in one. They include:

Central nervous system. The term *neuroleptic* was introduced to describe the characteristic emotional quietening, indifference and psychomotor slowing induced by chlorpromazine.

There is evidence that chlorpromazine acts in the hypothalamus and brain-stem reticular formation. In animals chlorpromazine quietens wild and angry monkeys. Chlorpromazine has a remarkable ability to control hyperactive and hypomanic states without seriously impairing consciousness, and it modifies abnormal behaviour in schizophrenic states. It is ineffective against depression unless this is accompanied by agitation, and indeed may make it worse. Normal people often feel sleepy, apathetic and indifferent to the environment after taking chlorpromazine and it also induces some indifference to pain. In large doses chlorpromazine causes dystonias. In moderate doses it controls the muscle spasm of tetanus, but very large doses may make it worse. This is probably an effect on the reticular formation where stimulation of one area activates, and of another depresses, spinal reflexes. Chlorpromazine also reduces muscle spasticity due to other neurological lesions. Epilepsy may be precipitated in predisposed people, but the drug has been used with success in epileptics with schizophrenic illness.

Chlorpromazine is an *antiemetic* effective against both drug and disease-induced vomiting, but ineffective against motion sickness.

The *peripheral α-adrenoceptor blocking effect* is moderately strong, and postural hypotension may occur. The peripheral vasodilatation induced by this action of chlorpromazine causes heat loss, and body temperature may fall, as with other long-acting vasodilators, especially if the patient is anaesthetised or is old. Some central effect on the temperature regulating mechanism is also probable.

Potentiation of other drugs. Chlorpromazine potentiates all cerebral depressants including alcohol, analgesics, hypnotics, anaesthetics, and curare. These effects can have clinical importance, but usually only if the drugs are being used in large doses.

Miscellaneous actions. Chlorpromazine has weak antihistamine, ganglion-blocking and quinidine-like actions (it can produce ECG changes) (see also above). It is a local anaesthetic, but in solution it is very irritant.

Pharmacokinetics. Chlorpromazine has a $t_{\frac{1}{2}}$ of about 35 h; there is substantial hepatic first-pass effect and drug action is terminated by metabolism. However, therapeutic effect on behaviour may be delayed for as long as 4 weeks; benefit may last months after cessation, and hepatic metabolites may be excreted for months.

Uses. Chlorpromazine is used in mental disorders, as an antiemetic and to aid the production of hypothermia in anaesthesia. It is used in severe pain, both to potentiate other drugs and to induce indifference to pain by altering the emotional response. It is worth trying in persistent pruritis. It can be effective against intractable *hiccup*.

Table 17.1 Phenothiazines classed by clinical effects

Name	Sedation	Antimuscarinic effects	Extrapyramidal effects
Class 1			
Chlorpromazine (Largactil)			
Methotrimeprazine *Veractil*	strong	moderate	moderate
Promazine (Sparine)			
Class 2			
Pericyazine (Neulactil)			
Pipothiazine *Piportil*	moderate	pronounced	slight
Thioridazine (Melleril)			
Class 3			
Fluphenazine (Modecate)			
Perphenazine (Fentanyl)			
Prochlorperazine (Stemetil)	slight	slight	pronounced
Thiethylperazine (Torecan)			
Thiopropazate (Dartalan)			
Trifluoperazine (Stelazine)			

Note. Antimuscarinic action protects against extrapyramidal effects.

Phenothiazine neuroleptics should not be used for minor conditions.

Dosage varies widely. Starting doses may be 25 mg orally (preferably not i.m: local toxicity) 4- to 6-hourly; dosage may be increased every 3 to 4 days; see Table 17.2.

Adverse reactions include: drowsiness and lethargy (though the patient remains rousable), postural hypotension, hypothermia in the elderly, dry mouth; weight gain; disturbance of male sexual function.

For important neurological effects see p. 279.

Galactorrhoea (with amenorrhoea) is due to block of the dopamine-mediated prolactin-inhibiting path in the hypothalamus (plasma prolactin concentration is raised).

Blood disorders and rashes, sometimes photosensitive, occur, and with prolonged use there may be permanent pigmentation. Fits may occur and, rarely, lens opacities.

The most serious effect is cholestatic (obstructive) jaundice, in which cellular damage is generally trivial, the principal impact being on the bile canaliculi, which show cellular infiltration and biliary stasis. Jaundice most commonly occurs 2–4 weeks after starting therapy but relapse can occur at once on restarting it in a patient who has had chlorpromazine jaundice. This and its irregular occurrence suggest that it is an allergic reaction. Recovery is almost invariably complete within a few weeks, but permanent liver damage has been reported. Hepatic biopsy has revealed lesions in patients taking chlorpromazine who are free from jaundice. The possibility of liver damage or blood disorder is sufficiently high to make casual use of chlorpromazine reprehensible. The danger is particularly great if there is a history of alcoholism.

Cardiac dysrhythmias can occur. Chlorpromazine causes *contact dermatitis* and staff who inject it should take care; tablets should not be crushed.

Other phenothiazines. There is a great variety available. Although most of those advocated in psychiatry represent attempts to improve on chlorpromazine, none has been shown definitely to be an all-round improvement; but piperazine derivatives cause less hypotension.

Table 17.2 Some phenothiazine neuroleptics

Classification by side chain	Total oral daily dose in mg (1–3 doses)*
Aliphatic	
chlorpromazine	50–1000*
promazine	40–800*
Piperazine	
trifluoperazine	2–10*
perphenazine	12–24*
Piperidine,	
thioridazine	75–200*

*Milder cases treated as out-patients generally receive dosage at the lower end of this range. A single nightly dose may suffice sometimes. For agitation and restlessness in the elderly or debilitated: $\frac{1}{4}-\frac{1}{2}$ dose.

Their effects are similar to those of chlorpromazine although they differ in emphasis (see Table 17.1). They are classed by structural side chain (see Table 17.2).

Butyrophenones. Haloperidol ($t_{\frac{1}{2}}$ 18 h) is pharmacodynamically similar to phenothiazines (class 3 in Table 17.1).

Thioxanthenes are also pharmacodynamically similar to the phenothiazines. Flupenthixol particularly is used, often as a depot i.m. injection of the decanoate (in oil) every 2–4 weeks. It also has antidepressant action.

Benzamide: sulpiride (Dolmatil) benefits negative symptoms of schizophrenia when used at *low* dose. Extrapyramidal effects are less than with other neuroleptics.

Dibenzodiazepine: clozapine (clozaril) has shown efficacy in both positive and negative symptoms of schizophrenia resistant to other neuroleptics; it is selective for a dopamine receptor subtype. It has the particular advantage that extrapyramidal effects are ordinarily mild and transient. But it has the particular disadvantage that it causes agranulocytosis in 1–2% of patients. For this reason its use is confined to patients resistant to other neuroleptics or where benefit from these is marred by severe extrapyramidal effects, including tardive dyskinesia. Precautionary leucocyte counts are mandatory.

Injectable depot (sustained-release) neuroleptics

Since about 40% of schizophrenics do not take tablets prescribed and even in hospital 20% of patients may not actually swallow the tablet given to them, it is useful to have neuroleptics that can be given i.m. at long intervals (1–4 weeks) for maintenance therapy. Use of these preparations has three advantages. The default rate is halved, defaulters are identifiable, absence of hepatic first-pass metabolism (that accompanies oral use) may allow control that is unobtainable with the oral route.

The decanoates of fluphenazine (Modecate) flupenthixol (Depixol) and haloperidol (Haldol decanoate) are used.

A small test dose should precede regular use because response is variable and adverse effects, when they occur, will be prolonged.

Extrapyramidal syndromes are common (2 days after injection and lasting for 5 days) and can be controlled by antimuscarinic antiparkinsonian drugs, e.g. benzhexol, orphenadrine. Severe depression can occur, and sometimes excitement (flupenthixol).

Flupenthixol (Depixol) has been shown to have less depressant effects and in small doses is used as an antidepressant.

ANTIDEPRESSANTS[10]

Tricyclics and allies: amine pump inhibitors

Structurally related to the phenothiazines, tricyclics prevent the active re-uptake into neuronal stores of released noradrenaline (chiefly), and serotonin at high doses. This action probably contributes to their potentiating effect on injected adrenaline and noradrenaline (negligible with isoprenaline), and to their cardiotoxicity in overdose. They also have antimuscarinic effects. Therapeutic effect is delayed for 7–14 days. Allied drugs inhibit re-uptake of both monoamines

---

[10] Classification of drugs by therapeutic use can be misleading, e.g. antidepressants can be useful in some cases of anxiety, panic attacks, chronic pain and nocturnal enuresis.

Table 17.3 Tricyclic and other antidepressants

Name	Class	Remarks
Amitriptyline (Tryptizol)	tricyclic	Sedative: may be cardiotoxic (sudden death) rather more than other tricyclics
Amoxapine (Asendis)	tri-	Onset of effect may be quicker
Butriptyline (Evadyne)	tri-	Less sedative
Clomipramine (Anaframil)	tri-	Less sedative: 5-HT uptake inhibitor
Desipramine (Pertofran)	tri-	Less sedative
Dothiepin (Prothiaden)	tri-	Sedative
Doxepin (Sinequan)	tri-	Sedative
Fluoxetine (Prozac)	other	Non-sedative: 5-HT uptake inhibitor
Flupenthixol (Fluanxol Depixol)	thioxanthene	Antidepressant neuroleptic
Fluvoxamine (Faverin)	other	Non-sedative: 5-HT uptake inhibitor
Imipramine (Tofranil)	tri-	Less sedative
Iprindole (Prondol)	tri-	Less sedative: does not inhibit amine pump
Lofepramine (Gamanil)	tetra-	Less sedative
Maprotiline (Ludiomil)	tetra-	Less sedative
Mianserin (Bolvidon)	tetra-	Sedative:does not inhibit amine pump: less cardiac risk: agranulocytosis
Nortriptyline (Aventyl)	tri-	Less sedative
Paroxetine (Seroxat)	other	5-HT uptake inhibitor
Protriptyline (Concordin)	tri-	Stimulant
Sertraline (Lustral)	other	5-HT uptake inhibitor
Trazodone (Molipaxin)	other	Sedative
Trimipramine (Surmontil)	tri-	Sedative
Viloxazine (Vivalan)	bi-	Less sedative

Notes to Table 17.3:
1. **Warning**: abnormal behaviour, including violence to others and to self, can occur with antidepressants. Plainly, to distinguish between drug-caused and disease-caused events can be impossible.
2 Tolerance to sedation may occur.
3. Hypnotics and anxiolytic sedatives may be combined.
4. Another antidepressant or neuroleptic should not be combined without special reason.
5. Antimuscarinic side-effects are common and tolerance may develop with continued treatment.

in varying proportions; some are selective for serotonin (see Table 17.3).

Pharmacokinetics. Tricyclic antidepressants, given orally, are well absorbed and have a high apparent volume of distribution implying that they preferentially enter some tissues and indeed they have been found to be concentrated in the myocardium. Steady-state plasma concentrations show great individual variation but are correlated with therapeutic effect and so measurement of plasma concentration can be useful (though it is often not available), especially if there is apparent failure of response. Tricyclics are metabolised in the liver. The $t_{\frac{1}{2}}$ varies from 15 to 100 h, with imipramine at the lower end and protriptyline at the upper.

Adverse effects include those characteristic of antimuscarinic action (dry mouth, raised intra-ocular pressure, blurred vision, bladder neck obstruction in older males). Male sexual function may be impaired. There also occur: postural hypotension, tremors, hallucinations, confusion, excitement, and violence to others and to self; precipitation of mania and epilepsy (avoid if there is a history of these) ; there may be cardiac hazard (sudden death) in using tricyclics in patients with any cardiac disease and perhaps even in those with apparently healthy hearts (but see mianserin).

Overdose causes cardiac dysrhythmias, hypotension and convulsions, which are treated by antidysrhythmic drugs, α or β-adrenoceptor block and anticonvulsants, e.g. diazepam. Acidosis may occur and can be treated with sodium bicarbonate. Overdose should be taken extremely seriously, especially in children.

Physicians may find themselves in the curious position of giving warning of these hazards to patients who have expressed a desire to end their own lives, i.e. of the importance of keeping them in a place safe from children and of refraining from overdose to themselves. Nevertheless, the common antimuscarinic effects should be mentioned because they almost always occur and add to the burden of worry and so promote non-compliance in depressed patients if they are unaware of their origin and that they do not herald disaster.

Abuse is not a problem with tricyclics since their immediate effects are not noticeably pleasant, but some *dependence* does occur, see below.

Interactions. Catecholamines and other sympathomimetics are potentiated (but nor β_2-receptor agonists used in asthma). This is important and even the amounts of adrenaline or noradrenaline in dental local anaesthetics may produce a serious rise in blood pressure. Severe toxicity, resembling atropine overdose, can occur if full doses of tricyclic are combined with an MAO inhibitor. Such combination is sometimes used clinically, but great caution is needed.

Tricyclics potentiate most antihypertensives but they antagonise clonidine and antagonise adrenergic-neuron-blocking antihypertensives by preventing their uptake into the adrenergic nerve ending, which is their site of action. The tetracyclic, mianserin, does not do this.

Neuroleptics inhibit metabolism of tricyclics. Enzyme induction, e.g. anticonvulsants, can even halve plasma concentration of tricyclics, though the clinical importance of this is diminished by the activity of some of the metabolites.

Effects of alcohol may be increased.

Choice of tricyclic or allied antidepressant. Choice is largely made on secondary psychotropic actions: sedative, less sedative or stimulant members (see Table 17.3).

In the presence of cardiac disease and old age, mianserin or trazodone may be preferred as safer than others.

Use. Antidepressants are commonly given 2 or 3 times a day. But it is often satisfactory, particularly for the sedative drugs, to give a single evening dose; the half-lives of most are long enough to render this appropriate, and peak plasma concentrations occur during the night; the stimulant drugs may increase insomnia.

Dose. A general scheme[11] that takes account of the need for quick response as well as the accumulative properties (long $t_{\frac{1}{2}}$) of some tricyclics is as follows:

Amitriptyline single daily **dose** 3 h before bedtime, or imipramine in the morning:

Day 1	50 mg
Day 2	75 mg
Days 3–6	100 mg
Days 7–14	150 mg

After 14 days, if response is inadequate: add 25 mg increment every 2–3 days up to a maximum daily dose of 200 mg.

Day 28: re-evaluate; if no response, reconsider diagnosis or change to different drug.

Obviously, the patient will be closely supervised and the increments ceased or dosage lowered at any sign of intolerance. Comparable regimens can be devised for other drugs having different dose ranges. With such regimens there may be some accumulation of drug and once therapeutic effect is established the dose may be gradually lowered to the minimum that will maintain benefit.

There is evidence that tricyclic antidepressants have a therapeutic range of concentration both below *and* above which efficacy is lost. Thus if a patient does not respond, or loses response, it may be because the plasma concentration is too high or too low. This need not astonish, for drugs at high concentrations may antagonise their own actions by a variety of mechanisms, e.g. activating or blocking receptors for which affinity is low at low concentrations. This *therapeutic window* is of clinical importance, and plainly will complicate patient management.

Duration and withdrawal. Therapy may be continued for 3–6 months and the drug

---

[11] Based on Hollister, L E (1978) (1983) Clinical pharmacology of psychotherapeutic drugs. Edinburgh: Churchill Livingstone.

withdrawn over about 6 weeks (to avoid an unpleasant acute withdrawal syndrome of headache, nausea, anxiety and bad dreams) or else, if there is established cyclic (unipolar) depression, it may be continued at low dose for long-term prophylaxis (25–50 mg daily). Relapse of depression may be delayed for about 2 months, so follow-up of patients is essential.

Other uses include nocturnal enuresis and chronic pain. Pathological laughing and weeping such as occurs with bilateral forebrain disease, e.g. multiple sclerosis, may respond to low dose amitriptyline.

Other drugs listed in Table 17.3, p. 288, can give satisfactory results. They vary in minor respects and some may be less cardiotoxic in overdose, e.g. mianserin (below).

Warnings. Benefit from antidepressants may be delayed for 7–14 days and patients should be told this for it is quite time enough for a person who is already minded to end his life to take a firm decision and to act on it. Electroconvulsive therapy acts quicker and may be needed as initial therapy, and there need be no delay in starting the drug.

Epilepsy. Drugs of this group are liable to precipitate fits in people with a family history of epilepsy, or who have had previous electroconvulsive therapy or who have organic brain damage. Treated epileptics are likely to require higher doses to compensate for hepatic enzyme induction by the anticonvulsants.

Atypical antidepressants. *Mianserin* ($t_{\frac{1}{2}}$ 30 h) does not inhibit the amine pump; it may act via central α_2-adrenoceptors. It is a sedative, has little antimuscarinic effect and is less cardiotoxic than are tricyclics, especially in acute overdose, properties that render it particularly suitable for use in the elderly. But it has a greater capacity to cause allergic blood disorders, agranulocytosis and aplastic anaemia (type B adverse reaction) especially during early weeks of treatment when the blood count should be monitored (monthly for 3 months). Hepatitis occurs.

Iprindole: mode of action unknown.

Flupenthixol (Depixol) is an antidepressant neuroleptic (thioxanthene).

MONOAMINE OXIDASE INHIBITORS (MAOIs)

In 1951 iproniazid (related to isoniazid) was tested for clinical antituberculosis activity and it was noticed that it stimulated the central nervous system. Early trials in psychiatry proved negative, but in 1958 a favourable report of its effect in chronically regressed and withdrawn patients precipitated a flood of therapeutic trials.

Iproniazid inhibits monoamine oxidases, a group of enzymes present inside cells of the brain, in peripheral adrenergic and dopaminergic nerve endings, and in the liver and gut wall, and which is concerned in the breakdown of serotonin and catecholamines (adrenaline, noradrenaline, dopamine). Many compounds with this effect and less toxicity have since been made; the structure of non-hydrazines resembles that of amphetamine.

The group includes

Hydrazine: phenelzine (Nardil); isocarboxazid (Marplan).

Non-hydrazine: tranylcypromine (Parnate); the member most likely to cause hypertension: selegiline (deprenyl, Eldepryl) for parkinsonism. Jaundice is more common with the non-hydrazines.

Actions. Drugs of this group have been found to have, to varying degrees, the following actions.

- MAO inhibition (other enzymes too); inhibition is irreversible, i.e. they are 'hit and run' or 'suicide' drugs; reversible inhibitors are under development, e.g. moclobemide.
- Sympathomimetic effect by inhibiting noradrenaline re-uptake (tranylcypromine) (some only, see below).
- Sympathetic ganglion blocking effect.
- Selectivity for one of the two principal enzymes (MAO-A, MAO-B), see discussion under parkinsonism. Nonselective inhibitors are ordinarily used for depression.

Their actions and interactions are as complicated as is to be expected from these facts.

When monoamine oxidases are nonselectively inhibited, there is an increase of serotonin and catecholamines in the CNS. In man such increases have powerful mental effects, ranging from feelings of well-being and increased energy to frank psychosis.

The increase in catecholamine stores in adrenergic and dopaminergic nerve endings means that there will be *potentiation of sympathomimetics* that act *indirectly*, i.e. by releasing stored noradrenaline, and of orally administered sympathomimetics that are substrates for MAO (present in the gut wall and liver). Deaths have occurred due to amphetamine. But important potentiation of administered adrenaline, noradrenaline and isoprenaline is not to be expected since these substances are chiefly destroyed by catechol-O-methyltransferase in the blood.

It is plain, both from experimental pharmacological studies and from fatal accidents during therapy, that sympathomimetics can be highly dangerous to patients taking MAO inhibitors. Severe hypertension occurs if levodopa (p. 311) is given in the presence of MAO inhibition.

Some MAO inhibitors (tranylcypromine) also have sympathomimetic activity similar to that of amphetamine, i.e. releasing stored noradrenaline, unrelated to enzyme inhibition and inhibition of noradrenaline re-uptake into the nerve endings. Thus, *hypertensive attacks are to be expected*; when they occur, they resemble the hypertensive attacks of phaeochromocytoma.

MAO inhibitors can, by themselves, also cause hypotension by sympathetic ganglion block. The hypertensive interactions mentioned above will still take place in the presence of hypotensive effect, so that a patient might suffer from postural hypotension, eat a meal of cheese (see below) and die in a hypertensive crisis.

Symptoms and treatment of hypertensive crisis. Severe throbbing headache occurs with slow palpitation. If headache occurs without hypertension it may be due to histamine release.

The hypertension is due to vasoconstriction from activation of α-adrenoceptors as in a phaeochromocytoma. The rational and effective treatment is an α-adrenoceptor blocker (phentolamine, 5 mg, i.v.).

Should excessive tachycardia occur after the phentolamine, a β-adrenoceptor blocker may be added (given initially it may further raise the blood pressure by blocking the peripheral vasodilator β_2-receptors). A vasodilator is also effective, e.g. nifedipine (a reliable patient may be instructed in self diagnosis and use, as for an attack of angina pectoris).

Pharmacokinetics. MAO inhibitors are taken orally; they are *hit and run* drugs, i.e. their effects greatly outlast their detectable presence in the body because they inhibit the enzyme irreversibly and termination of effect is dependent on synthesis of fresh enzyme, which takes weeks. *Thus adverse interactions may occur as long as 2–3 weeks after therapy has been withdrawn.*

The hydrazine group (see above) is acetylated (like isoniazid) and the population is divided into slow and fast acetylators.

Warning patients. Patients must be warned not to indulge in *self-medication* of any kind for many trivial remedies sold direct to the public, e.g. for nasal congestion, coughs and colds, contain sympathomimetics (ephedrine, phenylpropanolamine). Unfortunately some foods contain substantial amounts of sympathomimetics, largely tyramine, which act by releasing tissue-stored noradrenaline. These substances are normally inactivated by MAO in the intestine wall and liver (presystemic elimination), where large amounts of enzyme occur. Patients taking an MAOI are therefore deprived of this protection, so that, as well as having larger stores in nerve endings (waiting to be released), they absorb more of the sympathomimetics.

The first food interaction with MAO inhibitors was reported in 1963 and concerned cheese. It might be thought that, as cheese has been known to contain tyramine for at least 60 years, the danger might have been predicted, but it was not, and the association of hypertensive headache with evening meals of cheese was made by clinical acumen of a pharmacist whose wife was taking an MAOI.

Responses are variable, but *any food subjected to autolysis or microbial decomposition* during preparation or storage may contain pressor amines resulting from decarboxylation of amino acids.

The following **foods** either can produce, or may be expected to be capable of producing, dangerous hypertensive effects: **cheese**, especially if well matured (the amines are produced from the amino acids of casein by bacteria, e.g. tyramine from tyrosine; the concentration is higher just beneath the rind and around fermentation cavities); some **pickled herrings**; **broad bean pods** (contain dopa, a precursor of adrenaline); **hydrolysed protein** (Marmite, Bovril). **Wines** (red or white), and **beer** including non- or low-alcohol varieties contain very variable but generally low amounts of tyramine; over-ripe **bananas, avocados, figs**; fermented bean curds including **soy sauce**; fermented sausage, e.g. **salami**; **shrimp paste**; flavoured textured **vegetable protein**.

This list may be incomplete and there is a large number of anecdotal case reports supposedly implicating a wide range of foods. Any partially decomposed food may cause a reaction. Milk and yogurt appear safe. It is plain that patients must receive detailed instructions about their diet. They may cautiously try some of the above items to discover whether they are safe for themselves, and, if they are, they should not assume that the same food from different sources is harmless.

Interactions with drugs other than sympathomimetics. The following substances that are not metabolised by MAO may be *potentiated*:

Other antidepressants: excitement with tricyclics and allied drugs, especially with those that act by inhibiting serotonin re-uptake (clomipramine, fluoxamine, fluoxetine) when a life-threatening 'serotonin syndrome' may occur (hyperthermia, tremor, convulsions).

Narcotic analgesics: if pethidine is given to a patient taking a MAO inhibitor there is liable to be respiratory depression, restlessness, even coma, and hypotension. This is probably due to inhibition of the hepatic enzyme that demethylates pethidine. Interaction with other opioids occurs but is milder. If an opioid analgesic is essential, start with one-tenth of the usual dose.

Central nervous system depressants: barbiturates, anxiolytic sedatives, antihistamines, alcohol (probably), antiparkinsonian drugs; but not inhalation anaesthetics, carbamazepine, buspirone. Because of the use of numerous drugs during and around surgery, a MAOI is best withdrawn 2 weeks before, if practicable.

Antihypertensives (but hypertension and excitement may occur with methyldopa).

Insulin and oral hypoglycaemics.

Bee venom (perhaps): an environmental hazard.

The mechanisms of many interactions are obscure, they are probably due to inhibition of other drug metabolising enzymes. Reactions can be very severe and even fatal.

Use of MAO inhibitors. It is plain that patients taking these drugs are at risk in a number of ways and that, in the absence of specific indications for them, as well as of any evidence that they are superior to tricyclic and allied antidepressants, they are not drugs of first choice, though they may be found to suit some patients best. They are more effective in reactive and atypical than in endogenous depression and have a place as adjuvants in severe phobic states (claustrophobia, agoraphobia) resistant to other forms of treatment, e.g. behaviour therapy. So numerous are the necessary precautions that patients taking a MAO inhibitor should be supplied with a printed card with appropriate warnings.

The *therapeutic effects* of MAO inhibitors occur in from 1–2 days to 2 weeks, and may persist for as long as 2–3 weeks after stopping treatment, (as does the capacity for adverse drug reactions).

Anxiety and agitation may be made worse and depressed patients may even become hypomanic. Chlorpromazine can reduce this, monitored carefully in low dose.

Adverse effects in addition to the vascular effects (above) include: irritability, apathy, sadness, insomnia, fatigue, ataxia, tremulousness, restlessness, impotence, difficult micturition, sweating, hyperthermia, gastrointestinal disturbances, leucopenia, oedema, rashes, convulsions, jaundice. Optic nerve damage occurs with some. Appetite may increase.

Overdose can cause hypomania, coma, and hypotension or hypertension. General measures are used as appropriate with minimal administration of drugs: chlorpromazine for restlessness and excitement; phentolamine for hypertension; no vasopressor drugs for hypotension, because of risk of hypertension (use posture and plasma volume expansion).

L-tryptophan

L-tryptophan is an essential amino acid precursor of serotonin; some efficacy in depression has been shown; it can be toxic (eosinophilia/myalgia syndrome), though this may be due to an impurity; its place in therapy, if any, is uncertain.

LITHIUM

In 1949, during a search for biologically active substances in the urine of manic patients by injecting it into guinea pigs, it was found that the animals were affected by the accompanying large amounts of urea. Lithium urate, which is highly soluble, was selected to conduct investigations into urate toxicity. It was found to be sedative and to protect against manic urine toxicity. The carbonate was tried in manic patients, was found to be effective in the acute state and, later, to prevent recurrent attacks.[12]

The *mode of action* of lithium is uncertain; it modifies receptor responses to neurotransmitter monoamines via cyclic AMP, and an effect on cyclic AMP may also account for its capacity to affect adversely both thyroid and kidney function (below).

Pharmacokinetics. Knowledge of *pharmacokinetics* of lithium is important for successful use since the therapeutic plasma concentration is close to the toxic concentration (low therapeutic index). Lithium is a small ion that, given orally, is rapidly absorbed throughout the gut. High peak plasma concentration can be avoided by using sustained-release formulations. At first the distribution is throughout the extracellular water, but with continued administration it enters the cells and is eventually distributed throughout the total body water with a somewhat higher concentration in brain, bones and thyroid gland. The apparent volume of distribution is about 50 l in a 70 kg person (whose total body water is about

---

[12] Cade J. F. J. The story of lithium. In Ayd F. J., Blackwell B, eds. Biological psychiatry. Philadelphia: Lippincott. 1970.

40 l) which is compatible with the above. Lithium is not bound to plasma or other proteins.

Lithium is easily dialysable from the blood but the concentration gradient from cell to blood is not great and intracellular concentration (which determines toxicity) falls slowly. Lithium enters cells about as readily as does sodium but does not leave as readily (mechanism uncertain).

Lithium ion is filtered at the glomerulus and reabsorbed in the renal tubule by diffusion at the same site as sodium. Intake of sodium and water are the principal determinants of lithium elimination. In sodium deficiency lithium is retained in the body, thus *concomitant use of a diuretic* can reduce lithium clearance by as much as 50%, and precipitate toxicity. Lithium toxicity is treated by giving sodium chloride and water.

With chronic use the $t_{\frac{1}{2}}$ of lithium is 15–30 h. With such a $t_{\frac{1}{2}}$ and the need to maintain a plasma concentration close to the toxic level it is important to avoid unnecessary fluctuation (peak and trough concentrations). Lithium is therefore usually given 12-hourly and reliable sustained-release formulations are welcome.

A steady-state plasma concentration will be attained after 4–5 $t_{\frac{1}{2}}$s, i.e. about 5–6 days in patients with normal renal function. Old people and patients with impaired renal function will have a longer $t_{\frac{1}{2}}$ so that steady state will be reached later and dose increments must be adjusted accordingly.

Uses. Lithium may be used alone to control mild mania, but benefit is delayed for days and in severe cases a neuroleptic will be needed for immediate effect.

Lithium is the most effective drug in prophylaxis of manic depressive disorder. It should not be used unless monitoring of plasma concentration can be done. Duration of use should best not exceed 3–5 years (renal toxicity) but indefinite use may be unavoidable. Criteria for safe, i.e. slow, withdrawal without relapse have not been precisely defined.

Adverse effects. Adverse effects become common as the plasma concentration exceeds 1.5 mmol/l. Over 2.0 mmol/l adverse effects begin to be serious (CNS) and require urgent treatment, and at 4.0 mmol/l dialysis should be considered. Maximum toxicity is delayed for 1–2 days after the toxic concentration is reached.

Early effects that may not interfere with treatment include nausea and mild diarrhoea. But diarrhoea that is severe enough to cause significant sodium loss increases the risk of toxicity.

As the plasma concentration rises, central nervous system effects become prominent (coarse tremor, drowsiness, giddiness, ataxia, tinnitus, blurred vision, dysarthria, muscle twitching) and now intervention is required. Oedema can occur. In severe overdose the patient may be unconscious and develop cardiac dysrhythmias, hypotension and renal failure.

Nephrogenic diabetes insipidus (at therapeutic plasma concentrations) can occur with even brief use; the distal renal tubule becomes refractory to antidiuretic hormone. Renal cellular injury may occur with use prolonged beyond 3–5 years and so may hypothyroidism due to interference with thyroxine synthesis.

Overdose is treated by diuresis with NaCl and water (alkalinisation with sodium bicarbonate adds somewhat to elimination); an osmotic diuretic is added as judgement counsels; dialysis is effective. Because lithium leaves cells slowly, plasma concentration may rise again after acute reduction; also due to continued absorption

---

Dose[13] of lithium: initially 0.2–2.0 g daily, adjusted to achieve a plasma concentration of 0.4–1.0 mmol Li+/l by measuring samples taken 12 h after the preceding dose on day 4 or 7 of treatment, then weekly until dosage has remained constant for 4 weeks; thereafter monthly. Sustained-release formulations are usually given ×2/day.

Because of variations in pharmaceutical bioavailability patients should always take a formulation made by the same manufacturer. If change must be made then weekly monitoring of plasma concentration should be reinstituted.

It is evident that lithium therapy requires as much attention as insulin. Patients should be given a special information card.

---

[13] Lithium carbonate 400 mg = 10.8 mmol : Lithium citrate 564 mg = 6 mmol Li+.

from sustained-release formulation. Sodium depletion during treatment *must* be avoided.

Precautions. Knowledge of renal and thyroid function is desirable before starting therapy. Patients should be warned of the common first symptoms of overdose, i.e. nausea, vomiting, diarrhoea, coarse tremor. They can then stop taking lithium immediately, and usually long before there is an opportunity to measure the plasma concentration. Abrupt withdrawal may be followed by relapse into mania in about 2 weeks. Prolonged use (years) should only be practised if it is certain that benefit warrants it. Patients should always use the same formulation. Plasma concentration monitoring is essential (see under dosage, above). The minimum dose that is effective should be used.

Lithium toxicity may be precipitated by water and sodium loss as by diuretics, diarrhoea, vomiting and renal disease.

Interactions. Neuroleptics are potentiated as are other CNS active drugs; diuretics, see above; prostaglandin synthase inhibitors (NSAIDs) potentiate lithium (reduced elimination).

Pregnancy. Lithium may cause fetal cardiac abnormality. If lithium must be used, close monitoring of plasma concentration is needed because of the physiological pregnancy changes in body water and electrolytes. The newborn infant may be hypotonic and have a goitre; breast feeding is best avoided.

PSYCHOSTIMULANTS, APPETITE CONTROL

AMPHETAMINES

Amphetamine (racemic) and dexamphetamine (dextro: the laevo-form is relatively inactive) are the principal psychostimulants; their use in depression is obsolete. Amphetamine will be described, and its allies only in the ways in which they differ.

Mode of action. Amphetamine acts by releasing noradrenaline stored in nerve endings in both the CNS and the periphery. As with all drugs acting on the central nervous system, the psychological effects vary with mood, personality and environment as well as with dose.

Subjects become euphoric and fatigue is postponed. Although physical and mental performance may improve, this cannot be relied on; subjects may be more confident and show more initiative, and be better satisfied with a more speedy performance that has deteriorated in accuracy. On the other hand there may be anxiety and a feeling of nervous and physical tension, especially with large doses, and subjects develop tremors and confusion, and feel dizzy. Time seems to pass with greater rapidity. The sympathomimetic effect on the heart, causing palpitations, may intensify discomfort or alarm.

Amphetamine increases peripheral oxygen consumption and this, together with vasoconstriction and restlessness, leads to hyperthermia in overdose, especially if the subject exercises.

Dependence on amphetamine and similar sympathomimetics occurs; it is chiefly psychological, but there is a withdrawal syndrome, suggesting physical dependence; tolerance occurs.

Mild dependence on prescribed amphetamines became common, particularly amongst people with unstable personalities, depressives, and tired, lonely housewives. In the 1960s, adolescents began to turn to amphetamines for occasional use to keep awake to have 'fun' and then as an aid to the challenges normal to that stage of life. Unfortunately, drugs provide only the temporary solution of avoidance and postponement of such challenges, retarding rather than assisting progress to maturity.

As well as oral use, i.v. administration (with the pleasurable 'flash' as with opioids) is employed. Severe dependence induces behaviour disorders, hallucinations and even florid psychosis which can be controlled by haloperidol. Withdrawal is accompanied by lethargy, sleep, desire for food and sometimes severe depression, which leads to an urge to resume the drug.

Pharmacokinetics. Amphetamine ($t_{\frac{1}{2}}$ 12 h) is readily absorbed by any usual route and is largely eliminated unchanged in the urine. Urinary excretion is pH dependent; being a basic substance, elimination will be greater in an acid urine.

Uses. Amphetamine has had multifarious uses, but its potential for abuse is such that it should only be used where essential, and this is rare:

- *Narcolepsy*: patients pass directly into REM sleep; amphetamine delays onset of REM sleep.
- In some *hyperactive children* with attention deficit disorder.
- Against *fatigue*: seldom justified.
- *Appetite suppression*: alternatives are preferable.
- *Use in sport* is *ab*use.

Interactions are as expected from mode of action, e.g. antagonism of antihypertensives; severe hypertension with MAOIs and β-adrenoceptor blocking drugs.

Acute poisoning is manifested by excitement and peripheral sympathomimetic effects; convulsions may occur; also, in acute or chronic overuse, a state resembling hyperactive paranoid schizophrenia with hallucinations develops. Hyperthermia occurs (see above), with cardiac dysrhythmias, vascular collapse and death. Treatment is chlorpromazine with added antihypertensive, e.g. labetalol, if necessary; these provide sedation and α- and β-adrenoceptor block, rendering unnecessary the enhancement of elimination by urinary acidification.

Chronic overdose can cause a psychotic state mimicking schizophrenia.

Dexamphetamine, methamphetamine, phenmetrazine, phentermine, diethylpropion, methylphenidate, and pemoline are similar to amphetamine.

Appetite suppression

It was noticed casually in 1937 that patients receiving amphetamine tended to lose weight. This was investigated in animals and man and found to be due to a reduction in voluntary food intake. Dogs would starve in the presence of food when given amphetamine, although they still showed interest in being fed and jealousy of the dog being fed before them. It was only when food was actually placed in their cage that enthusiasm abated.

Amphetamine-type sympathomimetics with pronounced psychostimulant effects (diethylpropion, phentermine) suppress appetite (hunger), but the effect is transient, being as short as 2–3 weeks; dependence occurs. *They should only be used briefly, if at all*; they do not improve the long-term outlook.

Dexfenfluramine

Dexfenfluramine (Adifax) replaces the racemic fenfluramine (Ponderax); it is structurally related to amphetamine, but it causes release of serotonin from nerve stores, rather than noradrenaline. It is sedative rather than stimulant to the CNS and it may induce satiety, i.e. the subject eats as frequently, but amount is less. There may be some elevation of mood at the outset of therapy; in overdose amphetamine-like stimulant effects occur. Blood pressure is reduced.

Dexfenfluramine also has some peripheral effects on carbohydrate and lipid metabolism and it is uncertain whether these promote weight reduction.

Use. Dexfenfluramine is probably the drug of choice for obesity (when a drug is needed), and certainly so in hypertensives. Weight loss begins in 2 weeks and lasts for 3 months. It should not be necessary to give drug therapy indefinitely for obesity, and it is likely to be ineffective anyway. Some dependence occurs and abrupt withdrawal can cause depression which is especially marked after 4 days; withdrawal should be gradual.

Adverse effects include sleepiness, depression, diarrhoea, impotence, and increased dreaming.

Dependence can occur, with depression on abrupt withdrawal.

Heavy overdose can cause central nervous system stimulation and cardiac dysrhythmias.

Interactions. Dexfenfluramine does not antagonise antihypertensive therapy as do the amphetamines, indeed there may be some potentiation. Hypertension may occur with MAOIs. Sedatives and antidiabetics may be potentiated.

Mazindol (Teronac) is a tricyclic, structurally unrelated to amphetamine. It inhibits re-uptake of monoamines into nerve endings and it potentiates sympathomimetics and reverses the effect of antihypertensives.

Fluoxetine (Prozac) is an antidepressant that inhibits 5-HT re-uptake into nerve endings; it has anorectic action; it may be effective in bulimia nervosa.

Biguanide antidiabetics reduce intestinal carbohydrate absorption and may induce weight loss without reducing blood glucose concentration. But their use is probably best confined to diabetics.

Bulk preparations, e.g. methylcellulose or sterculia, are used to fill the stomach with non-nutrient material and induce a feeling of satiety.[14] Their use is probably based on a wrong physiological concept (unless enormous amounts are taken). Animals eat for calories, not bulk; it is possible to feel hungry in the absence of a stomach. Patients might as well be invited to eat flavoured toilet paper.

Thyroxine (T_4) or tri-iodothyronine (T_3) has long history of misuse in obesity. It is probably beneficial only when a diet so restricted as to amount to starvation has diminished the normal conversion of T_4 to T_3, a rare situation. Otherwise administration of T_4 or T_3 suppresses normal hormone production by the familiar feedback mechanism, and should not be used in the usual weight-losing regimens.

Appetite stimulation

Cyproheptadine (Periactin) blocks serotonin and histamine H_1-receptors. It has the unusual effect of increasing appetite, probably via an action on serotonin receptors in the hypothalamus. It is sometimes used as adjuvant therapy in anorexia nervosa that is without bulimic episodes. In general, little or nothing is gained by seeking to stimulate appetite by drugs.

Cyproheptadine also reduces corticotrophin release by blocking the serotonergic path controlling corticotrophin releasing factor and growth hormone and it has been used with variable success in Cushing's syndrome and acromegaly. It may also benefit other symptoms caused by serotonin release, e.g. post-gastrectomy dumping syndrome and carcinoid tumour.

Insulin increases appetite by reducing blood glucose concentration.

Canabis may induce hunger.

XANTHINES

The three xanthines, caffeine, theophylline and theobromine, occur in plants. They are qualitatively similar but differ markedly in potency. *Tea* contains caffeine and theophylline. *Coffee* contains caffeine, and *cocoa* and *chocolate* contain caffeine and theobromine. The *cola nut* ('cola' drinks) contain caffeine. Theobromine is weak and is of no clinical importance.

Mode of action

Caffeine and theophylline have complex and incompletely elucidated effects on intracellular calcium, on adenosine (vasodilator) receptors (block) and on noradrenergic function. Their capacity to inhibit phosphodiesterase, the enzyme that breaks down cyclic AMP (formation of which is stimulated by adrenoceptor agonists), occurs significantly only at concentrations higher than those reached in therapeutic use. When theophylline is used alongside salbutamol in asthma their actions add up to increased *benefit* to the bronchi, but increased *risk* to the heart.

Pharmacokinetics

Absorption of xanthines after oral or rectal administration varies with the preparation used. It is generally extensive but erratic. Caffeine metabolism is dose-dependent (saturation kinetics) with a $t_{\frac{1}{2}}$ rising from 4 h to more than 10 h in heavy coffee drinkers who are prone to adverse effects (see Chronic overdose, below). Xanthines are metabolised (more than 90%) by numerous enzymes, including xanthine oxidase.

For further details on theophylline, see Asthma.

---

[14] This approach has been carried to the extreme of inflating a balloon in the stomach.

Actions on mental performance

Caffeine is more potent than theophylline, but both drugs stimulate mental activity where it is below normal; they do not raise it above normal; thought is more rapid and fatigue is removed or its onset delayed. The effects on mental and physical performance vary according to the mental state and personality of the subject. Reaction-time is decreased. Performance that is inferior because of excessive anxiety may become worse.

Caffeine can (like amphetamine) also improve *physical performance* both in tasks requiring more physical effort than skill (athletics) and in tasks requiring more skill than physical effort (monitoring instruments and taking corrective action in an aircraft flight simulator). It is uncertain whether the improvement consists only of restoring to normal performance that is impaired by fatigue or boredom, or whether caffeine (and amphetamine) can also enable subjects to improve their normal maximum performance. The drugs may produce their effects by altering both physical capacity and mental attitude.

There is insufficient information on the effects on learning to be able to give any useful advice to students preparing for examination other than that *intellectual performance* may be assisted when it has been reduced by fatigue or boredom.

Effects on *mood* vary greatly amongst individuals and according to the environment and the task in hand. In general, caffeine (and amphetamine) induce feelings of alertness and well-being, euphoria or exhilaration. Onset of boredom, fatigue, inattentiveness and sleepiness is postponed.

Overdose can cause anxiety, tension and tremors and will certainly reduce performance. The regular, frequent use of caffeine-containing drinks is part of normal social life and mild overdose is common. Habitual tea and coffee drinkers are seldom willing to recognise that they have a psychological drug dependence.

Other effects

Respiratory stimulation occurs with substantial doses.

Sleep. Caffeine affects sleep of older more than it does of younger people and this may be related to the fact that older people show greater catecholamine turnover in the central nervous system than do the young. Onset of sleep (sleep latency) is delayed, bodily movements are increased, total sleep time is reduced, there are increased awakenings. Tolerance to this effect does not occur, as is shown by the provision of decaffeinated coffee; the caffeine is extracted (most, but not all) [15] by trichloroethylene.

Skeletal muscle. Metabolism is increased, and this may play a part in the enhanced athletic performance mentioned above. There is significant improvement of diaphragmatic function in chronic obstructive pulmonary disease.

Cardiovascular system. Both caffeine and theophylline directly stimulate the myocardium and cause increased cardiac output, tachycardia and sometimes ectopic beats and palpitations. This effect occurs almost at once after i.v. injection and lasts half an hour. Theophylline relieves acute left ventricular failure. There is peripheral (but not cerebral) vasodilatation due to a direct action of the drugs on the blood vessels, but stimulation of the vasomotor centre tends to counter this. Changes in the blood pressure are therefore somewhat unpredictable, but 250 mg caffeine (single dose) usually causes a transient rise of blood pressure of about 14/10 mm Hg in occasional coffee drinkers (but no additional effect in habitual drinkers); this effect can be used advantageously in patients with *autonomic nervous system failure* who experience post-prandial hypotension (2 cups of coffee with breakfast may suffice for the day). In occasional coffee drinkers, 2 cups of coffee (about 160 mg caffeine) per day, raise blood pressure by 5/4 mm Hg which is enough to be significant in epidemiological studies of blood pressure. The cerebral circulation responds differently; the vessels constrict, with consequent reduction of blood flow. Increased coronary artery blood flow may occur but increased cardiac work counterbalances this in angina pectoris.

---

[15] The European Community regulations define 'decaffeinated' as coffee (bean) containing 0.3% or less of caffeine (normal content 1–2%).

When given i.v. (aminophylline) slow injection is essential because high peak concentrations are equivalent to acute overdose (below).

Smooth muscle (other than vascular muscle, which is discussed above) is relaxed. The only important clinical use for this action is in reversible airways obstruction (asthma) (theophylline). Therapeutic effect is variable but can be excellent.

Kidney. Diuresis occurs in normals chiefly due to reduced tubular reabsorption of Na; similar to thiazide action, but weaker.

Miscellaneous effects. Gastric secretion is increased by caffeine given as coffee (by decaffeinated coffee too) more than by caffeine alone, and the basal metabolic rate may increase slightly (see skeletal muscle, above).

Acute overdose, e.g. aminophylline (see p. 512) i.v., can cause convulsions, hypotension, cardiac dysrhythmia and sudden death. Chronic overdose, see below.

Preparations and uses of caffeine and theophylline:

Aminophylline

The most generally useful preparation is aminophylline which is a soluble, irritant salt of theophylline with ethylenediamine; see asthma.

Attempts to make non-irritant orally reliable preparations of theophylline have resulted in choline theophyllinate and numerous variants. Sustained-release formulations are convenient for asthmatics, but they cannot be assumed to be bioequivalent and repeat prescriptions should adhere to the formulation of a particular manufacturer. Suppositories are available.

The principal uses of aminophylline

- *Asthma.* In severe asthma when β-adrenoreceptor agonists fail (often given i.v.); and orally to provide a background bronchodilator effect.
- *Paroxysmal nocturnal dyspnoea* (i.v. for immediate effect), to terminate an attack.
- In *neonatal apnoea*; caffeine is also effective.

- *In the dying patient* aminophylline i.v. may cause brief and unrepeatable but socially useful recovery of consciousness and coherence.
- Caffeine is used as an additional ingredient in analgesic tablets; about 60 mg potentiates NSAIDs. Also to *enhance oral ergotamine absorption* in migraine; in hypotension of *autonomic failure*.

Xanthine-containing drinks (see also above)

Coffee, tea and cola drinks in excess can make people tense and anxious and exacerbate peptic ulcer. Small children are not usually given tea and coffee because they are thought to be less tolerant of the central nervous system stimulant effect, but cola drinks irrationally escape this prohibition. It is possible to make an imposing list of diseases which may be caused or made worse by caffeine-containing drinks, but there is no conclusive evidence to warrant any general prohibitions. High doses of caffeine in animals damage chromosomes and cause fetal abnormalities; but studies in man suggest that normal consumption poses no risk. Epidemiological studies are not conclusive but suggest either no or only slight increased risk ($\times$ 2–3) of coronary heart disease in heavy (including decaffeinated) coffee consumers (>4 cups/day). See Lipids, below.

Dependence and tolerance. Slight tolerance to the effects of caffeine (on all systems) occurs. Withdrawal symptoms, attributable to psychological and perhaps mild physical dependence occur in habitual coffee drinkers (5 or more cups/day) 12–16 h after the last cup; they include headache (lasting up to 6 days), irritability, jitteriness; they may occur with transient changes in intake, e.g. high at work, lower at the weekend.

Chronic overdose. Excessive prolonged consumption of caffeine causes anxiety, restlessness, tremors, insomnia; headache, cardiac extrasystoles and confusion; diarrhoea may occur with coffee and constipation with tea. The cause can easily be overlooked if specific enquiry into habits is not made; including children regarding cola drinks. Of coffee drinkers, up to 25% who complain of anxiety may benefit from reduction of caffeine intake. A heavy *adult* user may be defined as one who takes more than 300 mg caffeine/day, i.e. 4 cups of 150 ml of brewed coffee, each containing 80± 20 mg caffeine per cup or 5 cups (60 ± 20) of instant coffee. The equivalent for tea would be 10 cups at approx 30 mg caffeine per cup; and of cola drinks about 2.0 l. Plainly caffeine drinks brewed to personal taste of consumer or vendor must have an extremely variable concentration according to source of coffee or tea, amount used, method and duration of brewing. There is also great individual variation in the effect of coffee both between individuals and sometimes in the same individual at different times of life (see Sleep, above).

Decaffeinated coffee[15] contains about 3 mg per cup; cola drinks contain 8–13 mg caffeine/ 100 ml; cocoa as a drink, 4 mg per cup; chocolate (solid) 6–20 mg per 30 g.

In *young people* high caffeine intake has been linked to behaviour disorders and a limit of 125 mg/l has been proposed for cola drinks.

Blood lipids. Cessation of coffee drinking can reduce serum cholesterol concentration in hypercholesterolaemic men.

Drinking 5 cups of *boiled* coffee/day increases serum total cholesterol by up to 10%; this does not occur with coffee made by simple filtration.

Breast fed infants may become sleepless and irritable if there is high maternal intake.

Fetal cardiac dysrhythmias have been reported with exceptionally high maternal caffeine intake, e.g. 1.5 l cola drinks/day.

Fertility. Women who drink excess of coffee may have difficulty in conceiving, but causal attribution of the association is not conclusive.

GINSENG

Ginseng is the root of 2 plants of the same family (oriental, *Panax ginseng*; Siberian, *Eleutherococcus senticosis*). It contains a range of biologically active substances (ginsenosides).

It has been used as a tonic or stimulant for thousands of years. In animal studies ginseng doubles the time that mice placed in water can

swim before becoming exhausted; it appears to have anti-fatigue effects in various other tests in mice (climbing up a rope that is moving downwards) and it increases sexual activity. In man, ginseng has been claimed to benefit performance of (Russian) athletes and astronauts (fewer fatigue-caused errors), and to reduce absenteeism due to respiratory illness in mining and steel workers and truck drivers. Oriental soldiers at war have used ginseng.

Despite accumulating evidence and wide use by the public, the medical profession in Western countries remains sceptical of the value of this 'tonic'. A range of adverse effects is reported, including oedema, hypertension, rashes, diarrhoea, sleeplessness and oestrogen-like effects.

GUIDE TO FURTHER READING

Anonymous 1983 A schizophrenic describes his recovery. Lancet 2: 562

Ashton C H 1987 Caffeine and health. British Medical Journal 295: 1293

Bass C et al 1989 Rediscovering monoamine oxidase inhibitors. British Medical Journal 298: 345

Black D 1991 Psychotropic drugs for problem children. British Medical Journal 302: 190

Duncan A J et al 1988 Antidepressant drugs in the elderly: Are the indications as long term as the treatment? British Medical Journal 296: 1230

Eagger S et al 1991 Tacrine in Alzheimer's disease. Lancet 337: 989

Editorial 1990 5-HT blockers and all that. Lancet 336: 345

Forbes J A et al 1991 Effect of caffeine on ibuprofen analgesia in postoperative oral surgery pain. Clinical Pharmacology and Therapeutics 49: 674

Gelder M 1990 Psychological treatment for depressive disorder. British Medical Journal 300: 1087

Hollister L 1988 Psychopharmacology: The bridge between psychiatry and biology. Clinical Pharmacology and Therapeutics 44: 123

Levy M et al 1983 Caffeine metabolism and coffee-attributed sleep disturbances. Clinical Pharmacology and Therapeutics 33: 770

Nicholson A N et al eds 1987 Symposium. Psychotropic drugs and performance. British Journal of Clinical Pharmacology 18: Suppl.1

Sharp D S et al 1990 Pharmacoepidemiology of the effect of caffeine on blood pressure. Clinical Pharmacology and Therapeutics 47: 57

Thelle D S 1991 Coffee, cholesterol and coronary heart disease. British Medical Journal 302: 804

Tonks C M 1977 Lithium intoxication induced by dieting and saunas. British Medical Journal 2: 1396

Tyrer P 1988 Prescribing psychotropic drugs in general practice. British Medical Journal 296: 588

18

Central nervous system IV: epilepsy, parkinsonism and allied conditions

SYNOPSIS

Epilepsy, in one form or another, affects 4–10 per 1000 of general populations.

- Epilepsy and antiepilepsy drugs: principles of management, withdrawal of therapy, pregnancy, epilepsy in children
- Pharmacology of individual drugs: carbamazepine, phenytoin, sodium valproate, clonazepam

Parkinsonism affects about 1:200 of the elderly population.

- Objectives of therapy
- Drugs used to treat the disease (including the special problems of long-term levodopa therapy)

Other disorders of movement

Tetanus

EPILEPSY AND ANTIEPILEPSY DRUGS

Bromide (1857) was the first effective anti-epilepsy drug, but is now obsolete. When phenobarbitone was introduced in 1912 it was found to control patients resistant to bromides.

The next success was the discovery in 1938 of phenytoin (a hydantoin) which is structurally related to the barbiturates. Since then many drugs have been discovered, but phenytoin still remains a drug of choice in the treatment of major epilepsy.

Epilepsy comprises sudden, excessive depolarisation of groups of cerebral neurons, which may remain localised (focal epilepsy) or which may spread to cause a generalised seizure.

Mode of action. Antiepilepsy (anticonvulsant) drugs inhibit the neuronal discharge or its spread, and do so by altering cell membrane permeability to ions and by enhancing the activity of natural inhibitory neurotransmitters such as gamma-aminobutyric acid (GABA), which induces hyperpolarisation.

PRINCIPLES OF MANAGEMENT

- Educate the patient about the disease, duration of treatment and need for compliance.
- Treat causative factors, e.g. cerebral neoplasm.
- Avoid precipitating factors, e.g. alcohol, stress.
- Anticipate natural variations, e.g. fits may occur only at night or shortly after waking.
- Give antiepilepsy drugs.

General drug therapy

The decision whether or not to initiate drug therapy after a single major seizure remains controversial.

- Therapy should start with a single well-tried and relatively non-toxic drug. *The majority of patients can be and should be controlled on one drug.*
- Dosage should be adjusted according to known pharmacokinetic properties. Measurement of plasma (or saliva) concentrations (if practicable) is useful at the outset of therapy and where any problems of efficacy or adverse reactions arise (see below). In the absence of facilities for measurement of plasma concentration then it may be necessary to establish the *maximum tolerated dose.*
- Attention to detail, including measurement of plasma (or salivary) concentrations, allows 80% of patients, or more, to be managed on a single drug. Few patients benefit from more than 2 drugs.
- If the first drug fails to give complete control there is a choice between withdrawing it completely (*slowly*, if it has had any useful effect at all) and *substituting* concurrently a drug of a different chemical group; or else of *adding* a second drug of a different chemical group.
- *Abrupt withdrawal.* Effective therapy must never be stopped suddenly either by the doctor (carelessness) or by the patient (carelessness, intercurrent illness or ignorance), or status epilepticus may occur. But if sudden withdrawal is imposed by occurrence of toxicity, a substantial dose of another antiepileptic should be given at once.
- This trial of drug after drug should be continued *until the epilepsy is controlled,* or until there are no more drugs to try. Up to 3 months may be needed to try a drug thoroughly in an individual.
- In cases where fits are liable to occur at a particular time of day, dosage should be adjusted to achieve *maximal drug effect at that time.*
- The patient should keep a *diary* of seizures.

Dosage

Start with about one-third of the expected maintenance dose and increase it weekly to reach the maintenance dose in 3 to 4 weeks, by which time any enzyme induction will have occurred and a steady state reached after the most recent dose increment. If plasma concentration measurements are available, a blood sample, taken at the end of the longest interval between doses, i.e. trough or minimal concentration (usually, and inconveniently, early morning), provides useful background information for further dose adjustment.

If fits continue the dose should be adjusted upwards until fits cease or adverse effects occur (maximum tolerated dose).

Frequency of administration. In general, taking into account convenience as well as pharmacokinetics, 2 equal daily doses morning and evening are recommended for routine practice. It is practicable to use once-daily administration with some drugs (having regard to the $t_{\frac{1}{2}}$) but there will be higher peaks and lower troughs of plasma concentration, and the consequences of a forgotten dose will be greater; sustained-release formulations for once daily use are available.

Interval between dose increments. If fits are infrequent it is obviously difficult to adjust dosage by therapeutic response. With phenytoin, a useful plan is to get the plasma concentration into the therapeutic range (measure it 1–2 weeks after instituting therapy and make appropriate adjustment) or, where this is not available, raise the dose gradually at 1–2 week intervals until an unwanted effect (nystagmus, dysarthria, ataxia) occurs and then reduce it slightly (maximum tolerated dose); but control may be achieved below this dose.

A fit or series of fits in a known epileptic often presents to a doctor who has never seen the patient before. It is important to consider the cause, whether it is non-compliance (which can be due to intercurrent disease), an inadequate drug regimen or an advance in the severity of the disease. Obviously measurement of drug plasma concentrations will help. It is important to avoid casual or impulsive alterations of regimen of drugs, which take a week or more to reach a steady state (long $t_{\frac{1}{2}}$), in the absence of accurate diagnosis.

Plasma or saliva drug concentration monitoring

Routine monitoring is particularly useful with phenytoin (which shows saturation kinetics). It is seldom really useful with other drugs unless there is a specific problem to be solved. Unnecessary monitoring wastes expensive resources. Monitoring is useful in the following circumstances:

- 2–4 weeks after commencing therapy
- When fits occur with standard dosage: the patient may be non-compliant, or compliant and simply need more drug
- When adverse effects occur
- When sodium valproate is added to another drug (pharmacokinetic interaction)
- When another antiepilepsy drug is withdrawn in the presence of sodium valproate
- In pregnancy
- When there is hepatic or renal disease.

Note. Many patients are controlled by plasma concentrations *below* the lower limit of the therapeutic range, and substantial diurnal fluctuations may occur.

Results of drug treatment, duration, withdrawal

60–95% of patients with treatable epilepsies, i.e. patients with fits but who are otherwise normal, can be completely relieved within 1 year. Plainly it is undesirable in principle to continue drug therapy for the rest of the patient's life if it can be safely withdrawn for, apart from general concerns about long-term drug therapy, there is evidence suggestive of adverse effects on behaviour and cognitive function that must be a particular cause for disquiet during childhood (development and education).

After at least 2 years, and preferably 3 or 4 years, of complete freedom from attacks, withdrawal of medication should be considered. In adult epilepsy, drug withdrawal is associated with about 20% relapse during withdrawal and a further 20% relapse over the following 5 years, after which relapse is unusual.

Relapse is more likely when the epilepsy has been severe and prolonged, and with major than with minor epilepsies.

Withdrawal should be slow, over about 6 months. If a fit occurs, full therapy must be resumed again for 2–3 years. A daytime fit during or after the process results in loss of driving licence for at least a year; some patients may prefer not to risk this at all, or only after 5 years of freedom. Adverse effects of prolonged treatment can be a significant factor in the decision.

Car driving and epilepsy. The UK allows patients to drive a car (but not a truck or bus) if they have not had a daytime fit for 2 years (or for 3 years if subject to asleep fits).

Pregnancy and epilepsy

Pharmacokinetics

Pharmacokinetics are altered due to physiological changes, see p. 109. Since what is important therapeutically is the concentration of free drug, and what is measured is the concentration of the free plus bound drug (total drug), it is evident that acceptance of the total plasma concentration as a guide to therapy when protein binding has changed can be misleading. Hepatic drug metabolism may increase. Erratic fluctuations in plasma concentrations may occur. Drug concentration should be kept at the lower end of the therapeutic range.

In practice, the patient is closely watched clinically and the dose of drug increased if seizures occur more often than expected. After delivery the pharmacokinetics revert to pre-pregnancy state over a few days.

Antiepilepsy drugs pass into breast milk, but the total quantities ingested by the baby are small and breast feeding may be considered safe (except when taking phenobarbitone; $t_{\frac{1}{2}}$ 100 h). Though there is possibility of sedation of the baby the advantages of breast feeding outweigh this but if somnolence and poor suckling occur breast feeding may have to be abandoned.

Fetal abnormality

Children of mothers taking antiepilepsy drugs show an approximately × 2.5 increased rate of malformations at birth (above the background 1–2%), especially cleft palate and lip, and heart abnormalities. This is probably due to the drugs rather than to the disease. Withdrawal of effective therapy during early pregnancy cannot be recommended because seizures are dangerous to both the woman and the fetus (except perhaps in minor epilepsy, when consciousness is not lost). Women of reproductive age should be treated with the simplest possible regimen (one drug at minimum effective dose, which will be assisted by measuring plasma concentration). Folate deficiency due to altered folate metabolism also occurs with hydantoin and barbiturate anticonvulsants and is a suspected cause of fetal neural tube defects (spina bifida). Sodium valproate carries a definite risk of spina bifida (even as much as 1–2%); and carbamazepine perhaps less.

A folate supplement seems sensible in a woman who wishes to become, as well as who has become, pregnant.

Carbamazepine may be considered the drug of choice for women of childbearing potential. A curious multiple syndrome has been tentatively named *fetal hydantoin syndrome.*

Newborn babies of mothers taking antiepilepsy drugs sometimes have reduced clotting factors, remediable by giving vitamin K antenatally; it is attributed to the drugs, perhaps by enzyme induction.

Contraception

Because of induction of steroid metabolising enzymes by some antiepileptic drugs (carbamazepine, phenytoin, barbiturates) with possible failure of contraception, it is prudent either to prescribe the higher dose oestrogen-containing oral contraceptives (at a level that avoids breakthrough bleeding, e.g. oestrogen 50 µg,) or, perhaps better, use a different mode of contraception.

Epilepsy in children

Fits in children are treated as in adults, but children may respond differently and become irritable, e.g. with sodium valproate or phenobarbitone.

It remains uncertain whether antiepilepsy drugs interfere with later development and education and it is certainly unwise to assume they do not. The sensible course is to control the epilepsy with minimal doses and attention to precipitating factors, with drug withdrawal when it is deemed safe to attempt it (see above).

When a child has *febrile convulsions* the decision to embark on continuous prophylaxis is serious for the child and depends on an assessment of risk factors, e.g. age, nature and duration of fit. Prolonged drug therapy, e.g. with phenytoin or phenobarbitone has been shown to interfere with cognitive development, the effect persisting for months after the drug is withdrawn. Parents may be supplied with specially formulated rectal *solution* of diazepam (absorption from a suppository is too slow) for easy and early administration, and advised on managing fever, e.g. use paracetamol at the first hint of fever, and tepid sponging.

Post-traumatic epilepsy

Developed epilepsy after head injury is treated in the usual way. Prevention of epilepsy in the first week after severe head injury may be accomplished by phenytoin. No drug has been proved effective in prevention over longer periods.

Status epilepticus

Status epilepticus is a medical emergency. Treatments of choice are shown in Table 18.1. Diazepam may cause hypotension and respiratory depression if combined with other anticonvulsant or if the seizures are due to acute brain injury (when phenytoin is preferred). If i.v. injection of diazepam is impracticable, give a *solution* per rectum. Absorption from i.m. injection is slow and erratic. Duration of anticonvulsant effect of diazepam is short and it should be followed at once by phenytoin i.v. (monitor ECG) to avoid relapse. Alternative drugs include clonazepam, lorazepam, and chlormethiazole. Paraldehyde, which has little respiratory depressant effect, is still used where full resuscitation facilities are not

Table 18.1 Drugs of choice in treatment of epileptic seizures[4]

Seizure disorder	Drugs	Usual daily dosage Adults	Children	Usual therapeutic serum concentrations
Primary generalised tonic-clonic (grand mal)				
Drugs of choice:	Carbamazepine	600–1200 mg	20–30 mg/kg	6–12 µg/ml
	or			
	Phenytoin	300–400 mg	4–7 mg/kg	10–20 µg/ml
	or			
	Valproate	1000–3000 mg	15–60 mg/kg	50–100 µg/ml
Alternatives:	Phenobarbital	120–250 mg	3–5 mg/kg	15–35 µg/ml
	Primidone	750–1500 mg	10–25 mg/kg	6–12 µg/ml
Partial, including secondarily generalised				
Drugs of choice:	Carbamazepine	600–1200 mg	20–30 mg/kg	6–12 µg/ml
	or			
	Phenytoin	300–400 mg	4–7 mg/kg	10–20 µg/ml
Alternatives:	Phenobarbital	120–250 mg	3–5 mg/kg	15–35 µg/ml
	Primidone	750–1500 mg	10–25 mg/kg	6–12 µg/ml
Absence (petit mal)				
Drugs of choice:	Ethosuximide	750–2000 mg	20–40 mg/kg	40–100 µg/ml
	or			
	Valproate	1000–3000 mg	15–60 mg/kg	50–100 µg/ml
Alternative:	Clonazepam	1.5–20 mg	0.01–0.2 mg/kg	.013–.072 µg/ml
Atypical absence, myoclonic, atonic				
Drug of choice:	Valproate	1000–3000 mg	15–60 mg/kg	50–100 µg/ml
Alternative:	Clonazepam	1.5–20 mg	0.01–0.2 mg/kg	.013–.072 µg/ml

Status epilepticus Drugs of choice		Usual initial dose	Usual rate	Repeat doses PRN	Maximum 24 h
Diazepam, IV	Adults	5–10 mg	1–2 mg/min[3]	5–10 mg *q20–30* min	100 mg
	Children	0.25–0.4 mg/kg[2]		0.25–0.4 mg/kg[2] *q20–30* min	40 mg
Phenytoin, IV	Adults	15–20 mg/kg	30–50 mg/min	100–150 mg *q30* min	1.5 g
	Children	15–20 mg/kg	0.5–1.5 mg/kg/min	1.5 mg/kg *q30* min	20 mg/kg
Phenobarbital, IV	Adults	10–20 mg/kg	25–50 mg/min	120–240 mg *q20* min	1–2 g
	Children	20 mg/kg	25–50 mg/min	6 mg/kg *q20* min	40 mg/kg

[1] First choice if primary generalised tonic-clonic also present
[2] To a maximum of 5–10 mg
[3] Slower rates of administration should be used for children
[4] This table is reproduced by permission of The Medical Letter on Drugs and Therapeutics: NY: USA.

available. General anaesthesia with or without neuromuscular block may even be necessary. Once the emergency is over, exploration of the reason for the episode and reinstitution of therapy, guided if possible by plasma concentrations, is immediately required. Chlormethiazole i.v. is preferred for the fits of pre-eclamptic toxaemia of pregnancy where safety of the fetus is a priority (also phenytoin and magnesium sulphate i.m.).

PHARMACOLOGY OF INDIVIDUAL DRUGS

Carbamazepine

Carbamazepine (Tegretol) is structurally related to imipramine. Because another antiepileptic (phenytoin) is sometimes beneficial in *trigeminal neuralgia*, carbamazepine was tried in this condition, for which it is now the drug or choice. It has since become a drug of choice for generalised tonic-clonic and partial seizures. It impairs cognitive function less than does phenytoin.

Pharmacokinetics. The $t_\frac{1}{2}$ of carbamazepine falls from 35 h to 20 h over the first few weeks of therapy due to induction of hepatic enzymes that metabolise it as well as other drugs, including steroids (adrenal and contraceptive), theophylline and warfarin. Cimetidine and valproate inhibit its metabolism. There are *complex interactions* with other antiepilepsy drugs, which constitute a reason for monodrug therapy.

Standard tablets are taken twice a day.

Adverse effects include CNS symptoms (reversible blurring of vision, diplopia, dizziness) and depression of cardiac AV conduction. Also, gut symptoms, skin rashes, blood disorders and liver and kidney dysfunction. Osteomalacia by enhanced metabolism of vitamin D (enzyme induction) occurs over years; also folate deficiency.

Hydantoins: phenytoin

Phenytoin (diphenylhydantoin, Epanutin, Dilantin) (1938) alters ionic fluxes (Na, K, Ca) across cell membranes; its effect is described as membrane stabilising, which prevents the initiation and spread of repetitive neuronal discharges. Phenytoin orally is well absorbed but there have been pharmaceutical bioavailability problems in relation to the nature of the dilutent in the capsule; patients should always use the same formulation.

Phenytoin provides a major example of the importance of knowledge of **pharmacokinetics** for successful prescribing. The important aspects are plasma protein binding, saturation (zero-order) kinetics, hepatic enzyme induction and enzyme inhibition. Opportunities for *clinically important* unwanted interactions are extensive.

Phenytoin is 90% bound to plasma albumin so that quite small changes in binding, e.g. a drop to 80%, will have a major effect on the concentration of *free* drug. Simple displacement interaction is generally not clinically important when first-order kinetics applies (metabolism increases in proportion to the rise in free drug concentration) but when there is saturation and, in addition,

enzyme inhibition (see below), toxicity may result.

Phenytoin is hydroxylated in the liver and this process becomes saturated at about the doses needed for therapeutic effect. Thus phenytoin at low doses shows first-order kinetics but this changes to saturation kinetics or zero-order kinetics as the therapeutic plasma concentration is approached, i.e. smaller dose increments at longer intervals are needed to obtain the same proportional rise in plasma concentration.

A clinically meaningful single half-life can be quoted where a drug is subject only to first-order kinetics. At low doses, giving sub-therapeutic plasma concentrations, the $t_\frac{1}{2}$ of phenytoin is 10–15 h. But at higher doses, giving therapeutic plasma concentrations (the enzyme system has become saturated), the $t_\frac{1}{2}$ can be > 60 h. This has major implications for patient care, e.g. the time taken to reach a steady-state plasma concentration after a dose increment (about 5 half-lives) is 2–3 days at low dose and about 2 weeks at high doses. Thus *dose increments should become smaller and less frequent as dosage increases* (this is why there is a 25 mg capsule). Plainly serial plasma concentration measurement will help the prescriber.

Enzyme induction. Phenytoin is a potent inducer of hepatic metabolising enzymes affecting itself, other drugs and natural endogenous substances (including vitamin D and folate). The consequences of this are: a slight fall of steady-state phenytoin level over the first few weeks of therapy, though this may not be noticeable if dose increments are being given; enhanced metabolism of other drugs including other anticonvulsants, e.g. carbamazepine, warfarin, steroids (adrenal and gonadal), thyroxine, tricyclic antidepressants, antirheumatics, doxycycline; naturally this can also work in reverse, and introduction of other enzyme inducers may lower phenytoin concentrations when there is capacity for increase in enzyme induction, e.g. rifampicin, ethanol.

Inhibition of phenytoin metabolism either by competition for the enzyme or by direct inhibition of enzyme activity can occur; plasma concentration of phenytoin rises. Drugs that inhibit phenytoin metabolism include: valproate, cimetidine, co-trimoxazole, isoniazid, chloramphenicol, some NSAIDs, disulfiram. There is a considerable body of mediocre and contradictory data, the lesson of which is that *possible interaction should be in the mind wherever other drugs are prescribed to a patient taking phenytoin.*

Adverse effects of phenytoin, many of which can be very slow to develop, include a considerable variety of central nervous system effects. Recognition that there is impairment of cognitive function, especially in learning situations, has led many physicians to prefer carbamazepine and valproate. Other effects range from sedation to delirium to acute cerebellar disorder to convulsions; peripheral neuropathy; rashes (dose related); gum hyperplasia (perhaps due to inhibition of collagen catabolism) more marked in children and when there is poor gum hygiene; coarsening of facial features; hirsutism; Dupuytren's contracture, pseudolymphoma; megaloblastic anaemia that responds to folate (perhaps partly due to increased folate requirements, for folate is a co-factor in some hydroxylations that are increased as a result of enzyme induction by phenytoin); anaemia probably only occurs when dietary folate is inadequate, but some degree of macrocytosis is common. Osteomalacia due to increased metabolism of vitamin D occurs after years of therapy.

Overdose (cerebellar symptoms and signs, coma, apnoea) is treated according to general principles. The patient may remain unconscious for a long time because of saturation kinetics, but will recover if respiration and circulation are sustained.

Other uses. The membrane-stabilising effect of phenytoin is used in cardiac dysrhythmias and, rarely, in resistant pain, e.g. trigeminal neuralgia.

Preparations: capsules for oral use should be taken (in 2–4 doses/day) with at least half a glass (120 ml) of water (if nausea occurs, they should be taken with food); phenytoin is also available for i.v. injection; it should not be given i.m. if this can be avoided as the pH of the solution has to be high to render it soluble; the fall in pH in the muscle leads to precipitation of the drug with slow absorption.

Sodium valproate: valproic acid

Sodium valproate (Epilim) (valpromide) acts by inhibiting the enzyme responsible for the breakdown of the inhibitory neurotransmitter, GABA, i.e. it inhibits GABA transaminase.

Pharmacokinetics. Valproate is about 90% bound to plasma albumin. It is metabolised in the liver and has a $t_{\frac{1}{2}}$ of 13 h.

Valproate inhibits the metabolism of itself at *low* (but not at high) doses; and that of phenobarbitone, phenytoin and carbamazepine. It displaces phenytoin from plasma albumin but the rise in free phenytoin is accompanied by increased phenytoin elimination and so the total phenytoin plasma concentration falls, but the concentration of free phenytoin is not much changed (when first-order kinetics apply).

Valproate does not induce drug metabolising enzymes but its metabolism is enhanced by induction due to other anticonvulsants.

Adverse effects are generally minor, e.g. nausea, but can include: liver failure (risk maximal at 2–12 weeks); transient rise in liver enzymes without sinister import (but patients should be closely monitored until the biochemical measures return to normal); pancreatitis; coagulation disorder due to inhibition of platelet aggregation (coagulation should be assessed before surgery); increased alertness and appetite, with weight gain. A curious effect is change in hair colour and temporary hair loss following which regrowth may be curly:

We thought the change might be welcomed by the patients, but one girl preferred her hair to be long and straight, and one boy was mortified by his curls and insisted on a short hair cut.[1]

Ketone metabolites may cause confusion in urine testing in diabetes.

See Pregnancy and epilepsy, above.

Barbiturates (see index)

Anticonvulsant members include phenobarbitone (phenobartal) ($t_{\frac{1}{2}}$ 100 h), methylphenobarbitone

---

[1] Jeavons P M et al. Lancet 1977 1: 359.

and primidone (Mysoline), which is largely metabolised to phenobarbitone (i.e. it is a prodrug). Sedation is usual.

Clonazepam

Clonazepam (Rivotril) is a benzodiazepine used for routine control of a variety of epilepsies (see above); *clobazam* is an alternative. Other benzodiazepines have antiepileptic action, but only at doses causing unacceptable sleepiness. The $t_\frac{1}{2}$ is 25 h. For *status epilepticus* clonazepam may be given i.v. slowly (30 s); it should not be given i.m. lest absorption be as slow as diazepam i.m. when peak plasma concentration can be delayed as long as 2 h, which is useless for the urgent control needed in this medical emergency, and complicates any other therapy given in the interval. *Lorazepam*, i.m. is somewhat more rapidly absorbed.

Vigabatrin (Sabril) (1989) is structurally related to the inhibitory CNS neurotransmitter GABA and it acts by irreversibly inhibiting GABA-transaminase so that GABA accumulates. Vigabatrin is effective in generalised tonic–clonic and partial seizures which are not adequately controlled by other drugs. The $t_\frac{1}{2}$ of vigabatrin is 6 h, and GABA-transaminase is resynthesised over 6 days.

It is not metabolised and does not induce hepatic drug metabolising enzymes. Adverse effects on the CNS are similar to those of other antiepilepsy drugs and include confusion and psychosis.

Succinimides: ethosuximide (Zarontin) is used in absence seizures (petit mal); it has a $t_\frac{1}{2}$ of 55 h. Adverse effects include gastric upset, CNS effects and allergic reactions including eosinophilia and other blood disorders, and lupus erythematosus.

Acetazolamide (Diamox) is a carbonic anhydrase inhibitor that, by producing acidosis, sometimes benefits atypical absence and other seizures in children.

Lamotrigine is an antagonist of glutamate (an excitatory amino acid in the brain); its place in therapy is yet to be determined.

PARKINSONISM

OBJECTIVES OF THERAPY

Parkinsonism is due to brain nigrostriatal dopamine deficiency. Drugs do not cure, but can, if properly managed, greatly improve quality of life in this progressive disease. *Two balanced systems* are important in the extrapyramidal control of motor activity at the level of the corpus striatum and substantia nigra: in one the neurotransmitter is *acetylcholine*; in the other it is *dopamine*. In Parkinson's disease there is degenerative loss of nigrostriatal dopaminergic neurons and the symptoms of the disease are due to dopamine depletion.

The two approaches to restoring the dopaminergic/cholinergic balance

1. Reduce cholinergic activity by antimuscarinic (anticholinergic[2]) drugs
2. Enhance dopaminergic activity by dopaminergic drugs which may:

* *prolong* the action of dopamine through selective inhibition of its metabolism (selegiline);
* *replete* neuronal dopamine by supplying levodopa, which is its natural precursor. Administration of dopamine itself is ineffective as it does not pass into the brain from the blood;
* act as *dopamine agonists* (bromocriptine, lysuride, apomorphine);
* *release* dopamine from stores and inhibit re-uptake (amantadine).

Both approaches are effective in therapy and may usefully be combined. It therefore comes as no surprise that drugs which prolong the action of acetylcholine (anticholinesterases) or drugs which deplete dopamine stores (reserpine) or block dopamine receptors (neuroleptics, e.g.

---

[2] The term *antimuscarinic* is now preferred to anticholinergic (p. 389).

chlorpromazine) will exacerbate the symptoms of parkinsonism or induce a Parkinson-like state.

Other parts of the brain in which dopaminergic systems are involved include the medulla (induction of vomiting), the hypothalamus (suppression of prolactin secretion) and certain paths to the cerebral cortex. Different effects of dopaminergic drugs can be explained by activation of these systems, namely emesis, suppression of lactation (mainly bromocriptine) and occasionally psychotic illness. Neuroleptics used to manage psychotic behaviour act by blockade of dopamine receptors and, as is to be expected, they are also anti-nauseant, may sometimes cause galactorrhoea, and can induce parkinsonism. Neuroleptic-induced parkinsonism is alleviated by antimuscarinics, but not by levodopa or amantadine, because the neuroleptics block dopamine receptors via which these drugs act. But many neuroleptics also have some antimuscarinic activity; those with greatest efficacy in this respect, e.g. thioridazine, are the least likely to cause parkinsonism.

DRUGS USED TO TREAT PARKINSON'S DISEASE

Dopaminergic drugs

Levodopa and dopa-decarboxylase inhibitors

Levodopa is a natural amino acid precursor of dopamine. The latter cannot be used because, being poorly lipid-soluble, it is not well absorbed from the gut and it does not usefully penetrate the CNS. Levodopa is particularly effective against tremor and hypokinesia. It is absorbed from the upper small intestine by active transport and has a $t_{\frac{1}{2}}$ of 1.5 h. It can traverse the blood–brain barrier, and within the brain it is decarboxylated to the neurotransmitter dopamine. But a major disadvantage is that levodopa is also extensively decarboxylated to dopamine in peripheral tissues so that only about 5% of an oral dose of levodopa reaches the brain. (Dopamine formed in peripheral tissues does not readily enter the brain because it is not lipid soluble.) Thus large quantities of levodopa have

to be given. These inhibit gastric emptying, delivery to the absorption site is erratic and fluctuations in plasma concentration occur. The drug and its metabolites cause significant adverse effects by peripheral actions, notably nausea, but also cardiac dysrhythmia and postural hypotension. This problem has been largely circumvented by the development of *decarboxylase inhibitors*, which *do not enter the central nervous system*, so that they prevent only the *extracerebral* metabolism of levodopa. The inhibitors are given in combination with levodopa and there is a range of formulations comprising a decarboxylase inhibitor with levodopa in various proportions: *co-careldopa* (carbidopa + levodopa in proportions 10 mg/100 mg, 25/100, 25/250) (Sinemet); *co-beneldopa* (benserazide + levodopa in proportions 12.5 mg/50 mg, 25/100, 50/200) (Madopar).

The same brain concentrations are produced as with levodopa alone, but only 25% of the dose of levodopa is required with the combinations, use of which smooths the action of levodopa and reduces the incidence of adverse effects, especially nausea, from about 80% to less than 15%.

Interactions. With unselective MAOI, the monoamine dopamine formed from levodopa is protected from destruction; it accumulates and also follows the normal path of conversion to noradrenaline (by dopamine β-oxidase); severe hypertension results. The interaction with selective MAO-B inhibitor, selegilene, is therapeutic (see below). Tricyclic antidepressants are safe. Levodopa antagonises neuroleptics (dopamine receptor blockers). Antihypertensives enhance hypotensive effects of levodopa. Metabolites of dopamine interfere with some tests for phaeochromocytoma.

Dopa-decarboxylase is a pyridoxine-dependent enzyme and concomitant use of pyridoxine (e.g. in self-medication with a multivitamin preparation) can enhance peripheral conversion of levodopa to dopamine so that less is available to enter the CNS, and benefit is lost. This effect does not occur, of course, with the now usual levodopa-decarboxylase inhibitor combinations. Dopamine receptor agonists reverse benefit.

Adverse effects: Postural hypotension occurs. *Nausea* may be a limiting factor if the dose is increased too rapidly; it may be helped by cyclizine 50 mg taken 30 min before food and by domperidone (little of which enters the brain). Levodopa-induced *involuntary movements* may take the form of general restlessness or head, lip or tongue movements or choreoathetosis. *Mental changes* may be seen: these include depression, which is common (best controlled with a tricyclic antidepressant), dreams and hallucinations. *Agitation and confusion* occur but it may be difficult to decide whether these are due to drug or to disease. *Cardiac dysrhythmias* are a rare feature. Increased sexual activity may occur and may or may not be deemed an adverse effect. It is probably due to improved mobility and resulting enthusiasm rather than to a pharmacodynamic effect of levodopa.

Dosage. Levodopa alone and in combination (see above) is introduced gradually and titrated according to response, the dose being altered every 2–3 days. A compromise is reached between benefit and adverse effects (generally involuntary movements and mental changes).

Compliance is important. Abrupt discontinuation of therapy leads to dramatic relapse.

Amantadine is an antivirus drug which, given for influenza to a parkinsonian patient, was noticed to be beneficial. The two effects are probably unrelated. It appears to act by increasing synthesis and release of dopamine, and by diminishing neuronal re-uptake. It also has slight antimuscarinic effect. The drug is much less efficacious than levodopa, whose action it will slightly enhance. It is more effective than the standard antimuscarinic drugs, with which it has an additive effect. Advantages include simplicity of use (initial oral dose 100 mg daily, increasing to twice or thrice daily, but rarely more than this) and relative freedom from adverse effects, which, however, include ankle oedema (probably a local effect an blood vessels), postural hypotension, livedo reticularis and central nervous system disturbances — insomnia, hallucinations and, rarely, fits.

Bromocriptine (Parlodel) is a derivative of ergot that has *dopamine agonist* activity. It is commonly used with levodopa. The drug is rapidly absorbed; the $t_\frac{1}{2}$ is 5 h, so that its action is smoother than that of levodopa, which can be an advantage in patients who develop end-of-dose deterioration with levodopa. Dosing should start at 1.0 mg orally nightly, increasing at approximately weekly intervals and according to clinical response, usually in the range of 10–40 mg per day taken in 3 divided doses with food. This is much more than the dose that is necessary to suppress lactation. For other uses, see index.

Nausea and vomiting are the commonest adverse effects; these may respond to domperidone but tend to become less marked as treatment continues. Postural hypotension may cause dizziness or syncope. In high dose confusion, delusions or hallucinations may occur, and, after prolonged use, retroperitoneal fibrosis.

Lysuride (Revanil) ($t_\frac{1}{2}$ 2 h) and *pergolide* ($t_\frac{1}{2}$ 6 h) are similar to bromocriptine.

Apomorphine is a derivative of morphine having structural similarities to dopamine; it is a *dopamine receptor agonist*. It can be useful in parkinsonism to treat difficulty in emptying the urinary bladder and the on-off syndrome. Apomorphine has to be given by injection (patients can be taught self-injection s.c.) and may need to be accompanied by an antiemetic, e.g. domperidone (which does not cross the blood–brain barrier as does metoclopromide), to prevent its characteristic emetic action. Overdose causes respiratory depression; it is antagonised by naloxone. Apomorphine can induce penile erection (without causing sexual excitement) and it enhances the penile response to visual erotic stimulation.

Selegiline (Eldepryl) is a selective inhibitor of monoamine oxidase (MAO) type B; MAO enzymes have an important function in modulating the intraneuronal content of neurotransmitter. The enzymes exist in two principal forms, which have specific substrates, inhibitors and locations in particular tissues. MAO-A deaminates serotonin, noradrenaline, tyramine and dopamine and is present in the liver, intestine and lungs.[3]

---

[3] Clorgiline is a selective inhibitor of MAO-A; it has not found a clinical use.

MAO-B is chiefly in the brain (substantia nigra and corpus striatum), where its physiological role is the metabolism of dopamine. Selegiline, because it inhibits MAO-B, delays the breakdown specifically of nigrostriatal dopamine, prolonging its effect. Thus its principal therapeutic benefit is to extend the action of levodopa in those patients who experience end-of-dose akinesia rather than on-off swings. The claim that selegiline delays progress of the disease needs confirmation.

The importance of the distinction between type A and type B MAOIs becomes further apparent when potential adverse reactions are considered (p. 291–3).

Selegiline, because it is a MAO-B inhibitor, does *not* create the risk of a hypertensive 'cheese reaction', since tyramine is metabolised as it traverses the gut wall and liver by MAO-A, which is not inhibited. Levodopa, given to a patient who is receiving selegiline, does not cause a hypertensive crisis, as that fraction of the drug which is converted to dopamine and then noradrenaline is metabolised by MAO-A in the periphery, e.g. lungs, liver.

The oral dose of selegiline is 10 mg/day in 1–2 doses; as an irreversible enzyme inhibitor, dosage cannot be accurately titrated as with a competitive receptor agonist. Its adverse effects are those of increased dopamine activity (see above); insomnia (give in morning); interaction with pethidine (see p. 292).

Antimuscarinic (anticholinergic) drugs (see also p. 388)

Antimuscarinics benefit parkinsonism by blocking acetylcholine receptors in the central nervous system, thereby partially redressing the imbalance created by decreased dopaminergic activity. Their use originated when hyoscine was given to parkinsonian patients in an attempt to reduce sialorrhoea by peripheral effect, and it then became apparent that they had other beneficial effects in this disease. Synthetic derivatives are now used orally. These include benzhexol, orphenadrine, benztropine, procyclidine biperiden, methixene. There is little to choose between these. Antimuscarinics produce modest improvements in tremor, rigidity, sialorrhoea, muscular stiffness and leg cramps, but little in hypokinesia.

They are effective i.m. or i.v. in acute drug-induced dystonias.

Unwanted effects include dry mouth, blurred vision, constipation, urine retention, glaucoma, hallucinations, memory defects, toxic confusional states and psychoses (which should be distinguished from pre-senile dementia).

TREATMENT OF PARKINSON'S DISEASE

The main features that require alleviation are *tremor, rigidity,* and *hypokinesia.*

General measures

These include the encouragement of regular physical activity and specific help such as physiotherapy and speech therapy.

Drug therapy

Drugs play an important role in symptom relief. No drug has yet been proved to delay progress of the disease, though the suggestion has been made for selegiline. If and when such an action is confirmed, early diagnosis of the disease will become important.

Initial treatment. Drugs should be started only when symptoms interfere with activities that are important to the patient. Antimuscarinics benefit rigidity, tremor and sialorrhoea, but have little or no effect on hypokinesia. Antimuscarinic drugs should be avoided in patients with glaucoma, difficulty in micturition, constipation and psychiatric disturbance.

Amantadine may be effective in the early stages of the disease, either alone or in combination with an antimuscarinic.

Selegiline, by preventing cerebral dopamine breakdown, can postpone the need to use levodopa (with all its complications, see below).

Long-term treatment

But, sooner or later treatment will involve dopamine replacement with *levodopa* (combined with a decarboxylase inhibitor) to replace CNS dopamine.[4] Rigidity and hypokinesia respond best to this but the combination is less effective in relieving tremor. Levodopa restores normal or near-normal activity in more than 75% of patients. Indeed, failure to respond should prompt the physician to question whether the patient has another basal ganglia defect (multi-system atrophy, cerebrovascular disease) or whether other drugs, e.g. phenothiazines, are involved. Dosage is best increased gradually, every 3 or 4 days (3–4 doses/d) using the smallest quantity that is effective.[8] The optimum dose varies substantially from patient to patient and within each patient with passage of time. The preparation co-careldopa 25/100 contains a relatively large proportion of carbidopa to ensure that there is adequate decarboxylase inhibition when only a small dose of levodopa is required. The varying amounts of levodopa in the various preparations of co-careldopa and co-beneldopa (above) permit flexible dose adjustment; small alterations may be beneficial.

Eventually, after 2–5 years, the progress of the disease demands that the total dosage be increased to the level at which adverse effects become troublesome. It is then of advantage to reduce each individual dose and increase the frequency of administration. After 6 years, on average 25% of patients will still derive substantial or moderate benefit from levodopa and experience an almost normal life expectancy. About 50%, however, fail to sustain the effect or find they cannot tolerate its adverse effects.

Another major problem with long-term treatment is *fluctuation in response to levodopa*. This is often a gradual process beginning with:

- *early morning akinesia* progressing to
- *peak dose dyskinesia* and

- *end-of-dose deterioration*; then the most severe form
- *the 'on-off' phenomenon*: this describes random fluctuations from mobility to dyskinesia or to parkinsonian immobility.

Severe dystonic muscle cramps of hand or foot may accompany the dyskinesia. In some patients, fluctuations are related to the timing of drug administration, when peak plasma concentrations coincide with the dyskinetic phase and low plasma concentrations with immobility, but other patients swing between states of mobility and akinetic mutism without apparent relation to the timing of doses. After receiving levodopa for 10 years, over 50% of patients experience such swings.

Management of these tribulations is difficult; it may involve the following:

- Gradual partial substitution of levodopa with *selegiline*, which delays CNS dopamine breakdown (if it has not been used at the outset). This is effective for end-of-dose deterioration in about 40% of patients but does not alleviate severe on-off fluctuations.
- Shortening the interval between doses of levodopa to hourly or less (adding levodopa between the doses of the combination formulation). Timing of dose in relation to meals is important for these interfere with absorption of the drug, especially when the protein content is high.
- Use of a dopamine receptor agonist, e.g. bromocriptine, apomorphine.

Drug-induced parkinsonism

Parkinsonism due to dopamine-receptor blocking drugs should be distinguished from idiopathic Parkinson's disease. In one series[5] of 95 new cases of parkinsonism referred to a department of geriatric medicine, 51% were associated with prescribed drugs and half of these required hospital admission. The clinical features of the drug-induced disease were very similar to those of idiopathic parkinsonism. After withdrawal of the offending drug most cases resolved com-

---

[4] An alternative strategy to minimise the special problems of long-term levodopa therapy (see below) is to use low-dose levodopa plus a dopamine receptor agonist (e.g. bromocriptine) from the commencement of levodopa therapy.

[5] Stephen P J, Williamson J. Lancet 1984; 2: 1082.

pletely in 7 weeks. Amongst the neuroleptic phenothiazines the commonest agent was prochlorperazine (Stemetil), usually given for vague 'postural instability' and which no longer seemed indicated in any case.

One old lady who had received trifluoperazine (for a minor fright and anxiety) for 5 weeks, took 36 weeks to recover from the drug-induced parkinsonism but never managed to get home again.

Treatment is by an antimuscarinic drug.

OTHER DISORDERS OF MOVEMENT

Essential tremor is often, and with justice, called benign, but a few individuals may be incapacitated by it. *Alcohol*, through a central action, helps about 75% of patients but is plainly unsuitable for long-term use and a β-*adrenoceptor blocker* will benefit about 50%; *primidone* is sometimes beneficial.

Drug induced dystonic reactions are seen:

- As acute reaction, often of the torsion type, and occur following administration of dopamine receptor blocking neuroleptics and antiemetics. An antimuscarinic drug, e.g. benztropine, given i.v. or i.m. and repeated as necessary, provides relief.
- In some patients who are receiving levodopa for Parkinson's disease.
- In patients on long-term neuroleptic treatment, who develop *tardive dyskinesia* (see p. 279).

Hepatolenticular degeneration (Wilson's disease) is caused by a genetic failure to eliminate copper absorbed from food so that it accumulates in the liver, brain, cornea and kidneys. A negative copper balance is established (with some clinical improvement if treatment is started early) by chelating copper in the gut with penicillamine (p. 223) or trientine.

Chorea from whatever cause may be alleviated by dopamine receptor blocking neuroleptics; also tetrabenazine (Nitoman), which inhibits neuronal storage of dopamine and serotonin.

Involuntary muscle spasm: including tics, blepharospasm, hemifacial spasm and spasmodic torticollis. These may respond to a range of drugs including antimuscarinic, levodopa, dopamine agonist, neuroleptic, clonidine, benzodiazepine. *Botulinum toxin*, which irreversibly blocks release of acetylcholine from cholinergic nerve endings has been injected locally with success in facial spasm, squint, torticollis etc; its effect lasts about 3 months.

Spasticity results from lesions of various types and sites within the central nervous system. Drugs used include the GABA agonist baclofen and diazepam.

Myotonic states in which voluntary muscle fails to relax after contraction may be symptomatically benefited by drugs that increase muscle refractory period, e.g. procainamide, phenytoin, quinidine.

TETANUS

Objectives

- Immediately neutralise with antitoxin any bacterial toxin that has not yet become attached irreversibly to the central nervous system.
- Kill the tetanus bacteria by chemotherapy, thus stopping toxin production.
- Control the convulsions whilst maintaining respiratory and cardiovascular function (which latter may be disordered by the toxin, see below).
- Prevent intercurrent infection (usually pulmonary).
- Prevent electrolyte disturbances and maintain nutrition.

The acute control of the convulsive state will be considered here.

Treatment

Therapy for convulsions may be initiated with chlorpromazine (which has a powerful muscle relaxant effect and which neither paralyses nor causes loss of consciousness); it is given 4–8 hourly. Diazepam or phenobarbitone is added as necessary. The drugs may be given orally when the convulsions are mild and there is no dysphagia, then i.m. An excess of chlorpromazine may make the convulsions worse, probably by stimulating the brain-stem reticular formation. Opioids are contraindicated.

The dosage and route of administration can only be decided when confronted with the patient. A regimen which should control convulsions of almost any severity would be chlorpromazine 1–1.5 mg/kg 4–8 hourly plus diazepam 3.0 mg/kg/day or phenobarbitone 0.5 mg/kg intermittently (between the chlorpromazine doses), as required. It may be impossible to avoid abolishing consciousness at times.

An alternative, in severe cases, is to paralyse the patient with tubocurarine or gallamine (on theoretical grounds these are preferable to depolarising agents) and to provide artificial respiration and enough sedation to impair awareness and memory. This requires skill and much equipment, with facilities for measuring blood pH, electrolytes and gases as well as ability to understand the meaning of the results. Unfortunately these requirements limit its applicability, particularly in the countries where tetanus is common, so that it is especially difficult to know whether results are superior to the more conservative anticonvulsant regimens.

Paralysis and artificial respiration should be seriously considered in all cases with laryngospasm, respiratory failure, severe chest infection and spasms so severe that they can only be controlled by making the patient unconscious. The action of the toxin in the CNS may cause *overactivity of the sympathetic autonomic system* (tachycardia, hypertension), which may be sufficient to require administration of α- and β-adrenoceptor blocking drugs. Attacks of hypotension can also occur.

Anticonvulsant therapy may be needed for 2 weeks or more and so attention to nutrition and to body electrolytes is vital right from the start, as is care of the respiratory tract (to avoid pneumonia) and gentle nursing (to minimise convulsions).

GUIDE TO FURTHER READING

Agid E 1991 Parkinson's disease: pathophysiology. Lancet 337: 1321

Brodie M J 1990 Established anticonvulsants and treatment of refractory epilepsy. Lancet 336: 350

Clough C G 1991 Parkinson's disease: management. Lancet 337: 1324

Editorial 1989 Spasticity. Lancet 2: 1488

Editorial 1990 Valproate, spina bifida and birth defect registries. Lancet 2: 1404

Editorial 1991 Antiepileptic drug withdrawal — hawks or doves. Lancet 337: 1193

Farwell J R et al 1990 Phenobarbital for febrile seizures — effects on intelligence and on seizure recurrence. New England Journal of Medicine 322: 364

Hauser W 1990 Prevention of post-traumatic epilepsy. New England Journal of Medicine 323: 540

Hughes A J et al 1990 Apomorphine test to predict dopaminergic responsiveness in parkinsonian syndrome. Lancet 336: 32

Mardsen C D 1990 Parkinson's disease. Lancet 335: 948

Parkinson Study Group 1989 Effect of deprenyl [selegiline] on the progression of disability in early Parkinson's disease. New England Journal of Medicine 321: 1364

Porter R J 1990 New antiepileptic agents: strategies for drug development. Lancet 336: 423

Saunders M 1989 Epilepsy in women of childbearing age. British Medical Journal 299: 581

Schever M L 1990 The evaluation and treatment of seizures. New England Journal of Medicine 324: 1213 and subsequent correspondence

Shorvon S D et al 1985 Is there a place for placebo controlled trials of antiepileptic drugs? British Medical Journal 291: 1328

19

Central nervous system V: non-medical use of drugs

SOCIAL ASPECTS

The enormous social importance of this subject warrants detailed treatment here.

All the naturally occurring sedatives, narcotics, euphoriants, hallucinogens, and excitants were discovered thousands of years ago, before the dawn of civilisation . . . By the late Stone Age man was systematically poisoning himself. The presence of poppy heads in the kitchen middens of the Swiss Lake Dwellers shows how early in his history man discovered the techniques of self-transcendence through drugs. There were dope addicts long before there were farmers.[1]

The drives that induce a person more or less mentally healthy to resort to drugs to obtain 'chemical vacations from intolerable selfhood'[2] will be briefly considered here, as well as some account of the pharmacological aspects of drug dependence.

That humanity at large will ever be able to dispense with Artificial Paradises seems very unlikely. Most men and women lead lives at the worst so painful, at the best so monotonous, poor and limited that the urge to escape, the longing to transcend themselves if only for a few moments, is and has always been one of the principal appetites of the soul.[2]

The dividing-line between legitimate use of drugs for social purposes and their abuse is in-

---

[1] Huxley A. Ann N Y Acad Sci 1957; 67: 677.
[2] Huxley A. The doors of perception. London: Chatto and Windus, 1954.

317

distinct for it is not only a matter of *which* drug, but of *amount* of drug and of whether the effect is directed antisocially or not. 'Normal' people seem to be able to use alcohol for their occasional purposes without harm but, given the appropriate personality and/or environmental adversity, many may turn to it for relief and become dependent on it, both psychologically and physically. But drug abuse is not primarily a pharmacological problem, it is a *social problem with important pharmacological aspects.*

It has been persuasively proposed that drug users are those who possess limited inner resources to cope with psychological stress and that drugs are used to fill a moral and spiritual void and to meet intense emotional needs. The character traits and emotional conflicts of drug users may reflect, in Western societies particularly, changes in child rearing and family stability in recent generations.[3]

Abuse potential of a drug is related to its capacity to produce *immediate* satisfaction (e.g. amphetamine and heroin give immediate effect, tricyclic antidepressants do not), i.e. to its route of administration in descending order: inhalation/ i.v.; i.m./s.c.; oral.

Some terms used

- **Drug abuse**[4] implies *excessive* (in terms of social norms) non-medical or social drug use.
- **Non-medical drug use**, i.e. all drug use that is not on generally accepted medical grounds, may be a term preferred to 'abuse'. Non-medical use means the continuous or occasional use of drugs by the individual, whether of his own choice or under feelings of compulsion, to achieve his own well being, or what he conceives as his own well being (see motives below).

---

[3] Nicholi A M. New Engl J Med 1983; 308: 925.
[4] The World Health Organization adopts the definition of the United Nations Convention on Psychotropic Drugs (1971). Drug abuse means the use of psychotropic substances in a way that would 'constitute a public health and social problem'.

Drugs used for non-medical purposes are often divided into two groups, hard and soft.

- **Hard** drugs are those that are liable seriously to disable the individual as a functioning member of society by inducing severe psychological and, in the case of cerebral depressants, physical dependence. The group includes heroin and cocaine.
- **Soft** drugs are less dependence-producing. There may be psychological dependence, but there is little or no physical dependence except with heavy doses of depressants (alcohol, barbiturates). The group includes sedatives and tranquillisers, amphetamines, cannabis, hallucinogens, alcohol, tobacco and caffeine.

As with many attempts to make convenient classifications, this fails, for it does not recognise individual variation in drug use. Alcohol can be used in heavy doses that are gravely disabling and induce severe physical dependence with convulsions on sudden withdrawal; i.e. for the individual the drug is 'hard'. But there are many people mildly psychologically dependent on it who retain their position in home and society. Similarly, amphetamines can be used in ways that cause doubt whether they should be described as 'hard' or 'soft'.

- **Hard-use** where the drug is central in the user's life and **soft-use** where it is merely incidental, are terms of assistance in making this distinction, i.e. what is classified is not the drug but the effect it has or the way it is used by the individual.
- **Drug dependence** (see p. 321).
- **Addiction**. The term 'addict' or 'addiction' has not been completely abandoned in this book because it remains convenient. It refers to the most severe forms of dependence where the compulsive craving dominates the subject's daily life. Such cases pose problems as grave as dependence on tea-drinking is trivial. But the use of the term *drug dependence* is welcome, because it renders irrelevant arguments about whether some drugs, e.g. tobacco, are addictive or merely habit-forming.

Non-medical drug use has two principal forms:

1. *Continuous use*, when there is a true dependence, e.g. opioids, alcohol, benzodiazepines.
2. *Intermittent or occasional use* to obtain a recreational experience, e.g. LSD, cocaine, cannabis, solvents, or to relieve stress, e.g. alcohol.

Both uses commonly occur in the same subject, and some drugs, e.g. alcohol, are used in both ways, but others, e.g. LSD or cannabis, are virtually confined to (2).

Drives to non-medical (or non-prescription) drug use[5]:

- *Relief of anxiety*, tension and depression; escape from personal psychological problems; detachment from harsh reality; ease of social intercourse.
- *Search for self-knowledge* and for meaning in life, including religion. The cult of 'experience' including aestheticism and artistic creation, sex and 'genuine', 'sincere' interpersonal relationships, to obtain a sense of 'belonging'.
- *Rebellion* against or *despair* about orthodox social values and the environment.
- *Fear of missing something*, and *conformity* with own social subgroup.
- *Fun*, amusement, recreation, excitement, curiosity.

---

[5] Psychoactive drug use by medical professionals has been studied by questionnaire (USA). Responses by approx. 300 out of 500 approached in each group.
Use for recreation, self-treatment or to assist work or athletic performance (caffeine and alcohol excluded):
physicians 59%; pharmacists 46%; medical students 77%; pharmacy students 62%.
The results do not differ substantially from those of general urban populations. The trend of such use is upwards; the authors express concern. McAuliffe et al. New Engl J Med 1986; 315: 805.

REWARDS FOR THE INDIVIDUAL

Two claims for the non-medical use of psychotropic drugs deserve to be mentioned:

1. that there is such a thing as a drug culture;
2. that dugs provide mystical or religious experience.

The term **drug culture** implies that drugs can provide the spiritual, emotional and intellectual experiences and development that are the basis for a way of life that can be described as a 'culture'.

It is inherently unlikely that chemicals could be central to a constructive culture and no convincing support for the assertion has yet been produced. (That chemicals might be central to a destructive culture is another matter.) That like-minded people practising what are often illegal activities will gather into closely knit subgroups for mutual support, and will feel a sense of community, is to be expected, but that is hardly a 'culture'. Even when drug-using subgroups are accepted as representing a culture (or subculture), it may be doubted if drugs are sufficiently central to their ideology to justify using 'drug' in the title, i.e. drug use is a secondary associated, and not a primary phenomenon. But claims for value to the individual and to society of drug experience must surely be tested by the criterion of fruitfulness for both, and the judgement of the individual concerned alone is insufficient; it must be agreed by others. The results of both legal and illegal drug use do not give encouragement to press for a large-scale experiment in this field.

The other claim is that drugs provide **mystical experience** and that this has valid religious content, so that it has great value and importance for the individual. If mysticism is to be discussed it must be defined. *Mystical experience* is best defined by listing its characteristics; these are feelings of:

- *Unity*: a sense of oneness with nature and/or God.
- *Ineffability*: the experience is beyond the subject's power to express or describe.
- *Joy*, peace, sacredness.
- *Knowledge*: insight into truths of life and

values, illuminations, revelations of enormous significance.
- *Transcendence* of space and time.

Mystical states are both transient and passive (subjects feel their will is in abeyance).

When such states do occur there remains the question whether they tell us something about a reality outside the individual or merely something about the mind of the person having the experience.

Mystical experience is not a normal dose-related pharmacodynamic effect of any drug, its occurrence depends on many factors, the subject (personality, mood) and his environment, and any preparation he may have undergone. The drug *facilitates* the experience, it does not *induce* it; drugs can facilitate unpleasant as well as pleasant experiences. It is not surprising that mystical experience can occur with a wide range of drugs that alter consciousness:

... I seemed at first in a state of utter blankness ... with a keen vision of what was going on in the room around me, but no sensation of touch. I thought that I was near death; when, suddenly, my soul became aware of God, who was manifestly dealing with me, handling me, so to speak, in an intense personal, present reality ... I cannot describe the ecstasy I felt.[6]

This experience occurred in the 19th century with chloroform; a general anaesthetic obsolete because of cardiac depression and hepatotoxicity.

There is no good evidence that drugs can produce experience that passes the test of *results*, i.e. fruitfulness to the individual and to society.

Whether a single administration of a drug can be used to initiate or trigger experiences that may result in an individual gaining beneficial insight is unproved. If emotional shock is acceptable in religious conversion, as it seems to be, there seems no obvious reason why a drug should not also be used on a single occasion after careful preparation. Plainly there is a risk of the ex-

perience becoming an end in itself rather than a means of development.

It is interesting that the *double-blind controlled trial* has been attempted in the field of spiritual experience and knowledge where, it has been pointed out, the passion with which a belief is defended is commonly in inverse proportion to the strength of the evidence that can be adduced for it.

Twenty well-prepared Christian theological students received, by random allocation, either psilocybin (a hallucinogen) or nicotinic acid (as an 'active' placebo). They attended a Good Friday church service lasting $2\frac{1}{2}$ h and wrote accounts of their feelings, completed questionnaires and were interviewed to elicit evidence of mystical experience. It was concluded that psilocybin facilitated mystical experience.[7] While such work is of interest it may be remembered that religious experience

means the whole of life interpreted, rather than isolated feelings. A religious man is not one who has 'experiences' ... but one who takes all life in a religious way ... religious experience ... is not the isolated outbreak of abnormal phenomena in this or that individual (though to read some psychological treatments of religious experience one would suppose so).[8]

Conclusions on the value of non-medical use of psychotropic drugs

- *For relaxation*, recreation, protection from and relief of stress and anxiety; relief of depression: moderate use of some 'soft' drugs may be accepted as part of our society.
- For *spiritually valuable experience*: justification is extremely doubtful.
- *As basis for a 'culture'* in the sense that drug experience (a) can be, and (b) should be central to an individually or socially constructive way of life: a claim without validity.

[6] Quoted in James W. Varieties of religious experience. Harlow: Longmans, 1902. Many subsequent editions of this classic. See also Leary T. The politics of ecstasy. London: MacGibbon and Kee, 1970. Other editions USA.

[7] Pahnke W N In: Aaronson et al. eds. Psychedelics: the uses and implications of hallucinogenic drugs. London: Hogarth Press. 1970.
[8] Dodd C H. The authority of the Bible. London: Fontana. 1960.

General pattern of non-medical drug use

- Any age: alcohol; tobacco; mild dependence on hypnotics and tranquillisers, occasional use of LSD and cannabis.
- 20–35 years old: hard-use drugs, chiefly heroin, cocaine and amphetamine.
- Under 16 years: volatile inhalants e.g. solvents of glues, aerosol sprays, vapourised (by heat) paints, 'solvent or substance' abuse, 'glue-sniffing'.
- Miscellaneous: any drug or combination of drugs reputed to alter consciousness may have a local vogue, however brief, e.g. drugs used in parkinsonism and metered aerosols for asthma.

DECRIMINALISATION AND LEGALISATION OF DRUGS FOR NON-MEDICAL USE

The decision whether a drug is acceptable in medical practice is made after an evaluation of its safety in relation to its efficacy. The same principle should be used for drugs for non-medical or social use. But the usual scientific criteria for evaluating efficacy are hardly applicable. The reasons why people choose to use drugs for non-medical purposes are listed above. None of them carries serious weight if the drug is found to have serious risks to the individual[9] or to society, with either acute or chronic use. Ordinary prudence dictates that any such risks should be carefully defined before a decision on legalisation is made.

There is no doubt that many individuals think, rightly or wrongly, that private use of cannabis, if not of 'harder' drugs, is their own business and that the law should permit this freedom. The likelihood that demand can be extinguished by education or by threats appears to be zero. The autocratic implementation of laws that are not widely accepted in the community can lead to violent crime, corruption in the police, and alienation of reasonable people who would otherwise be an important stabilising influence in society.

But though written laws are so often inflexible and combine what would best be separated, informal judicial discretion under present law may be permitting more experimentation than would recurrent legislative debate leading to substitution of one written law for another written law. It is recognised that this untidy approach, which may be best for the time being, cannot satisfy the extravagant advocates either of licence or of repression.

A suggested intermediate course for cannabis, and perhaps even for heroin, is that penalties for possession of small amounts for personal consumption should be removed (i.e. decriminalisation as opposed to legalisation), whilst retaining criminal penalties for suppliers. Such an approach is increasingly and informally being implemented.

Nobody knows what would happen if the production, supply and use of the major drugs, cannabis, heroin and cocaine were to be legalised, as tobacco and alcohol are legalised. There are those who, shocked by the evils of illegal trade, consider that legalisation could only make matters better. The debate continues about what kinds of evils affecting the individual and society can be tolerated and how they can be balanced against each other.[10]

DRUG DEPENDENCE

Drug dependence is a state arising from repeated, periodic or continuous administration of a drug, that results in harm to the individual and sometimes to society. The subject feels a desire, need or compulsion to continue using the drug and feels ill if abruptly deprived of it (abstinence or withdrawal syndrome); for discussion of *abrupt withdrawal* of drugs in general see p. 15.

Drug dependence is characterised by:

- Psychological dependence: the first to appear; there is emotional distress if the drug is withdrawn.

---

[9] Hazard to the individual is not a matter for the individual alone if it also has consequences for society.
[10] Editorial. Your heroin, sir. Lancet 1991; 337: 402. Engelsman E L Drug misuse and the Dutch. Br Med J 1991; 302: 484.

- Physical dependence: accompanies psychological dependence in some cases; there is a physical illness if the drug is withdrawn.
- Tolerance.

Physical dependence

The mechanisms of physical dependence on drugs and development of tolerance are ill-understood. Physical dependence and tolerance imply that adaptive changes have taken place in body tissues so that when the drug is abruptly withdrawn these adaptive changes are left unopposed, resulting generally in a rebound overactivity. The discovery that the CNS employs morphine-like substances (endorphins) as neurotransmitters allows speculation that exogenously administered opioid may suppress endogenous production of endorphins by a feedback mechanism so that when administration of opioid is suddenly stopped there is an immediate deficiency of endogenous opioid, which thus causes the withdrawal syndrome.

Tolerance may result from a compensatory biochemical cell response to continued exposure to opioid. In short, both physical dependence and tolerance may result from the operation of homeostatic adaptation to continued high occupancy of opioid receptors. Changes of similar type may occur with GABA transmission, involving benzodiazepines. Tolerance also results from metabolic changes (enzyme induction) and physiological/behavioural adaptation to drug effects, e.g. alcohol.

Physical dependence develops to a substantial degree with cerebral depressants, but is minor or absent with excitant drugs.

The distinction between physical and psychological dependence is not always clear, for the mental misery of the deprived heavy tobacco smoker may manifest itself in physical symptoms, such as digestive disturbances and tremors.

There is commonly *cross-tolerance* between drugs of similar, and sometimes even of dissimilar, chemical groups, e.g. alcohol and benzodiazepines.

Although 'no drug possesses mysterious powers to subjugate a human being',[11] there is danger in personal experimentation. Or as a modern American addict has succinctly, put it, 'They all think they can take just one joy-pop but it's the first one that hooks you'.[11] Unfortunately the subject cannot decide for himself that his dependence will remain mild.

Psychological dependence

This may occur to any drug that alters consciousness however bizarre, e.g. muscarine (see index) and to some that, in ordinary doses, do not, e.g. non-narcotic analgesics, purgatives, diuretics; these latter provide problems of psychopathology rather than of psychopharmacology.

Psychological dependence can occur merely on a tablet or injection, regardless of its content, as well as to drugs substances. Mild dependence does not require that a drug should have important psychic effects, the subject's beliefs as to what it does are as important, e.g. purgative and diuretic dependence in people obsessed with dread of obesity. We are all physically dependent on food, and some develop a strong emotional dependence and eat too much; and sexual activity, with its unique mix of arousal and relaxation, can for some become compulsive or addictive.

Types of drug dependence

The World Health Organization recommends that drug dependence be specified by 'type' when under detailed discussion.

Morphine-type:
  psychological dependence severe
  physical dependence severe; develops quickly
  tolerance marked
  cross-tolerance with related drugs
  naloxone induces abstinence syndrome

Barbiturate-type:
  psychological dependence severe

---

[11] Maurer D W, Vogel V H. Narcotics and narcotic addiction. Springfield: Thomas. 1962.

physical dependence very severe; develops slowly at high doses

tolerance less marked than with morphine

cross-tolerance with alcohol, chloral, paraldehyde, meprobamate, glutethimide, chlordiazepoxide, diazepam, etc.

Amphetamine-type:
psychological dependence severe

physical dependence slight: psychoses occur during use

tolerance occurs

Cannabis-type:
psychological dependence some

physical dependence dubious (no characteristic abstinence syndrome)

tolerance slight

Cocaine-type:
psychological dependence severe

physical dependence absent (or slight)

tolerance slight (to some actions)

Alcohol-type:
psychological dependence severe

physical dependence with prolonged heavy use

cross-tolerance with other sedatives

Tobacco-type:
psychological dependence strong

physical dependence slight

Drug mixtures:
Barbiturate-amphetamine mixtures induce a characteristic alteration of mood that does not occur with either drug alone

psychological dependence strong

physical dependence occurs

tolerance occurs

Heroin-cocaine mixtures: similar characteristics.

Route of administration and effect

With the i.v. route or inhalation much higher peak plasma concentrations can be reached than with oral administration. This accounts for the 'kick' or 'flash' that abusers report and which many seek, likening it to sexual orgasm or better. As an addict over-dramatically said 'The ultimate high is death'[12] and it has been reported that when hearing of someone dying of an overdose, some addicts will seek out the vendor since it is evident he is selling 'really good stuff.'[12] Addicts who rely on illegal sources are inevitably exposed to being supplied diluted or even inert preparations at high prices. North American addicts who have come to the UK believing themselves to be accustomed to high doses of heroin, have suffered acute poisoning when given, probably for the first time, pure heroin at an official UK drug dependence clinic.

Supply of drugs to addicts

In the UK, supply of officially listed drugs (a range of opioids and cocaine) for the purpose of sustaining addiction is permitted under strict legal limitations. Addicts must be notified by the physician to the Home Office and in the case of some opioids and cocaine, the physician requires a special licence. By such procedure it is hoped to limit the expansion of the illicit market and its accompanying crime, and to sustain young (usually) addicts, who cannot be weaned from drug use, in reasonable health until they relinquish their dependence (often over about 10 years).

When injectable drugs are prescribed there is currently no way of assessing the truth of an addict's statement that he needs x mg of heroin (or other drug), and the dose has to be assessed intuitively by the doctor. This has resulted in addicts obtaining more than they need and selling it, sometimes to initiate new users. The use of oral methadone or other opioid for maintenance by prescription is devised to mitigate this problem.

Treatment of drug dependence

Treatment consists of:

1. **Withdrawal** of the drug, which, whilst obviously important, is only a step on what can be a long and often disappointing journey to

---

[12] Bourne P. Acute drug abuse emergencies. New York: Academic Press. 1976.

psychological and social rehabilitation, e.g. in 'therapeutic communities'. In the case of drugs that cause physical dependence, withdrawal may be gradual (over about 10 days or more) or sudden, provided that in the latter case steps are taken to control the abstinence syndrome.

This may be done by judicious use of the same drug, but some prefer to use alternative drugs, generally, though not always, of similar kind, having a longer duration of action, for instance a *heroin* addict can be given methadone, an *alcoholic* may be given chlormethiazole, diazepam or chlordiazepoxide. A *barbiturate* addict may be given phenobarbitone 30 mg for every 100 mg of other barbiturate used per day (with max dose 400 mg/day of phenobarbitone), and this withdrawn over 2–3 weeks. If a patient is in very poor physical condition, withdrawal should be postponed until he is better. Sympathetic autonomic overactivity can be treated with a β-adrenoceptor blocker (or clonidine).

2. **Maintenance and relapse**. Relapsed addicts who live a fairly normal life are sometimes best treated by supplying drugs under supervision. There is no legal objection to doing this in the UK (see above) but naturally this course, which abandons hope of cure, should not be adopted until it is certain that cure is virtually impossible. A less harmful drug by a less harmful route may be substituted, e.g. oral methadone for i.v. heroin. Addicts are often particularly reluctant to abandon the i.v. route, which provides the 'immediate high' that they find, or originally found, so desirable.

Drugs are adjuvant only in the prevention of relapse, e.g. the use of an opioid antagonist so that if, in a moment of weakness, the subject takes a dose of heroin, the 'kick' is blocked. Such treatment requires on the part of the subject the will to succeed.

Treatment of severe pain in an opioid addict presents a special problem. High-efficacy opioid may be ineffective (tolerance) or overdose may result; low-efficacy opioids will not only be ineffective but may induce withdrawal symptoms, especially if they have some antagonist effect e.g. pentazocine. This leaves as drugs of choice non-steroidal anti-inflammatory drugs (NSAIDs), e.g.

indomethacin, and nefopam which is neither opioid nor NSAID.

Mortality

Young illicit users by i.v. injection (heroin, barbiturates, amphetamine) have a mortality up to × 40 normal. They die of overdose and of septicaemia, endocarditis, hepatitis, AIDS, gas gangrene, tetanus and pulmonary embolism, from the contaminated materials used without aseptic precautions (schemes to provide clean equipment mitigate this). Smugglers of illicit cocaine or heroin sometimes carry the drug in plastic bags concealed by swallowing or in the rectum ('body packing'). There have been instances of the packages leaking, with fatal result.

Escalation

A variable proportion of subjects who start with cannabis eventually take heroin. This disposition to progress from occasional to frequent soft use of drugs through to hard drug use, when it occurs, is less likely to be due to pharmacological actions, than to psychosocial factors, although increased suggestibility induced by cannabis may contribute.

De-escalation also occurs as users become disillusioned with drugs over about 10 years.

'Designer drugs'

This unhappily chosen name means molecular modifications produced in secret for profit by skilled and criminally minded chemists. Manipulation of fentanyl has resulted in compounds of extraordinary potency.

In 1976 a too-clever 23-year-old addict seeking to manufacture his own pethidine 'took a synthetic shortcut and injected himself with what was later with his help proved to be two closely related byproducts; one was MPTP' (methylphenyltetrahydropyridine).[13] Three days later he developed a severe parkinsonian syndrome that responded to levodopa. MPTP selectively

---

[13] Williams A. Br Med J 1984; 289: 1402. Davis G C et al. Psychiatry Res 1979; 1: 249.

destroys melanin-containing cells in the substantia nigra. Further such cases have occurred from use of supposed synthetic heroin. MPTP has since been used in experimental research on parkinsonism.

What the future holds for individuals and for society in this area can only be imagined.

Volatile substance abuse

Seekers of the 'self-gratifying high'[14] also inhale any volatile substance that may affect the central nervous system, adhesives ('glue-sniffing'), lacquer-paint solvents ('huffing'),[14] petrol, nail varnish, any pressurised aerosol and butane liquid gas (which latter especially may freeze the larynx, allowing fatal inhalation of food, drink or gastric contents, or even itself flood the lungs); solids, e.g. paint scrapings, solid shoe polish, may be volatilised over a fire. These substances are particularly abused by the very young (schoolchildren), no doubt largely because they are accessible at home and in ordinary shops and they cannot easily buy alcohol.[15] CNS effects include confusion and hallucinations, ataxia, dysarthria, coma, convulsions, respiratory failure. Liver, kidney, lung and heart damage occur. Sudden cardiac death may be due to sensitisation of the heart to endogenous catecholamines. If the substance is put in a plastic bag from which the user takes deep inhalations, or is sprayed in a confined space, e.g. cupboard, there is particularly high risk.

A 17-year-old boy was offered the use of a plastic bag and a can of hair spray at a beach party. The hair spray was released into the plastic bag and the teenager put his mouth to the open end of the bag and inhaled . . . he exclaimed, 'God, this stuff hits ya fast!' He got up, ran 100 yards and died.[16]

Signs of frequent volatile substance abuse include peri-oral eczema and inflammation of the upper respiratory tract.

---

[14] Editorial. A-huffin' and a-puffin', a-sniffin' and a-suckin'. Lancet 1974; 2: 876.
[15] In the UK sale of alcohol to anyone under 18 years is illegal and the vendor may lose his valuable licence to trade if he is convicted of breaking this law.
[16] Bass M. Sudden sniffing death. JAMA 1970; 212: 2075.

DRUGS AND SPORT

The rewards of competitive sport, both financial and in personal and national prestige, are the cause of determination to win at (almost) any cost. Drugs are used optimistically to enhance performance though efficacy is largely undocumented. Detection can be difficult when the drugs or metabolites are closely related to or identical with endogenous substances, and when the drug can be stopped well before the event without apparent loss of efficacy, e.g. anabolic steroids. It will be interesting to see if the extensive and expensive resources currently being deployed to unmask the unsportsmanlike ultimately will prove to have been well spent.

Use of drugs

Drugs may be used in the following ways:

• For 'strength sports' in which body weight and brute strength are the principal determinants (weight lifting, rowing, wrestling): *anabolic steroids*. There is evidence that, taken together with a high-protein diet and exercise, they increase lean body weight (muscle) but not necessarily strength. It is claimed they allow more intensive training regimens. Rarely, there may be episodes of violent behaviour, known amongst athletes as ''roid [steroid] rage'.

High doses are used, with risk of liver damage (cholestatic, tumours) especially if the drug is taken long term, which is certainly insufficient to deter 'sportsmen'. They may be more inclined to take more seriously the fact the anabolic steroids suppress pituitary gonadotrophin, and so testosterone production. There seem to be no reliable data on women.

Growth hormone (somatrem, somatropin) is being used or, rather, abused; data are lacking.

• For events in which output of energy is explosive (100 m sprint) or prolonged at a high level (bicycling, marathon running): *stimulants* (amphetamine type). They have probably caused death in bicycle racing (continuous hard exercise with short periods of sprint) due to hyperthermia and cardiac dysrhythmia in metabolically stimulated and vasoconstricted subjects exercising maximally under a hot sun.

Erythropoietin is also used in endurance sports to enhance oxygen carrying capacity of the blood.

- For events in which steadiness is essential (pistol, rifle shooting): β-*adrenoceptor blockers*.
- For events in which body pliancy is a major factor (gymnastics): delaying puberty in child gymnasts by endocrine techniques.
- Minor injuries are usual during athletic training and these may be suppressed by drugs (corticosteroids, NSAIDs) to allow the training to proceed maximally.
- *Diuretics* are used to reduce weight, e.g. boxers, jockeys, and to flush out other drugs in the hope of escaping detection; severe volume depletion can cause venous thrombosis and pulmonary embolism.
- Generally, owing to recognition of natural biological differences most competitive events are sexually segregated. In many events men have a natural biological advantage and the (inevitable) consequence has been that women have been virilised (by administration of *androgens*) so that they may outperform their sisters.

It seems safe to assume that anything that can be thought up to gain advantage will be tried by competitors eager for immediate fame. Reliable data are difficult to obtain in these areas. No doubt placebo effects are important, i.e. beliefs as to what has been taken and what effects ought to follow.

The dividing line between what is and what is not acceptable practice is hard to draw.

Caffeine can improve physical performance and it illustrates the difficulty of deciding what is 'permissible' or 'impermissible'. A cup of coffee is part of a normal diet, but some consider taking the same amount of caffeine in a tablet, injection or suppository to be 'doping'. The International Olympic Committee issues guidance from time to time; currently it objects to more caffeine in the urine that can be the result of 2 or 3 cups in a day.

The problem raised by use of local anaesthetics, anti-inflammatory analgesics and adrenal steroids for strains, hormonal adjustment or sup-

pression of menstruation and drugs for anxiety, are ethical rather than medical, as is the use of *hypnosis* in the reported competition success of a swimmer who, it is alleged, had been persuaded under hypnosis into the belief that he was being pursued by a shark.

Problems in prescribing for athletes

Prescribers to athletes should remember that they may inadvertently get their athlete patients into trouble with sports authorities who test for drugs, if they (the prescribers) are not familiar with the rules of sport and drugs. Examples include the use of: codeine, dextropropoxyphene, morphine, phenylpropanolomine, ephedrine, propranolol, drugs for diarrhoea, pain, decongestion, anxiety etc.

TOBACCO

Tobacco was introduced to Europe from South America in the 16th century. Although its potential for harm was early recognised its use was taken up avidly in every society that met it.

Composition

The composition of tobacco smoke is complex (about 500 compounds have been identified) and varies with the type of tobacco and the way it is smoked. The chief pharmacologically active ingredients are *nicotine* (acute effects) and *tars* (chronic effects).

Smoke of cigars and pipes is alkaline (pH 8.5) and nicotine is relatively un-ionised and lipid soluble so that it is readily absorbed in the mouth. Cigar and pipe smokers thus obtain nicotine without inhaling (they also have a lower death rate from lung cancer; which is caused by non-nicotine constituents).

Smoke of cigarettes is acidic (pH 5.3) and nicotine is relatively ionised and insoluble in lipids. Desired amounts of nicotine are only absorbed if it is taken into the lungs, where the enormous surface area for absorption compensates for the lower lipid solubility. Cigarette smokers therefore inhale (they have a high rate of death from lung cancer). The amount of nicotine absorbed from tobacco smoke varies from 90% in those who inhale to 10% in those who do not.

Tobacco smoke contains 1–5% *carbon monoxide* and habitual smokers have 3–7% (heavy smokers as much as 15%) of their haemoglobin as carboxyhaemoglobin, which cannot carry oxygen. This is sufficient to reduce exercise capacity in patients with angina pectoris. The $t_{\frac{1}{2}}$ of carboxyhaemoglobin is about 4 h so that heavy smokers with angina pectoris who reduce their cigarette consumption by only a few cigarettes a day will not achieve any useful reduction in carboxyhaemoglobin. Chronic carboxyhaemoglobinaemia causes polycythaemia.

Substances (polycyclic hydrocarbons and N-nitroso compounds) *carcinogenic* to animals have been identified in tobacco smoke condensates from cigarettes, cigars and pipes. They are responsible for the hepatic *enzyme induction* that occurs in smokers.

TOBACCO DEPENDENCE

The immediate *satisfaction* of smoking is due to nicotine, and also to tars, which provide flavour.

Whilst there is no major *personality* difference between smokers and non-smokers, cigarette smokers tend to be more extraverted, less rigid and more prone to antisocial tendencies than non-smokers. Pipe smokers are notably introverted.

Psychoanalysts have made a

characteristic contribution to the problem. 'Getting something orally', one asserts . . . 'is the first great libidinous experience in life'; first the breast, then the bottle, then the comforter, then food and finally the cigarette,[17] or the pipe.

Sigmund Freud, inventor of psychoanalysis, was a life-long tobacco addict. He suggested that some children may be victims of a 'constitutional intensification of the erotogenic significance of

the labial region', which, if it persists, will provide a powerful motive for smoking.[18]

Starting to smoke may be linked with 'self-esteem and status need', but probably not to adolescent rebellion.[19]

There is no difference in intelligence between smoking and non-smoking children, but the former are less academically successful, as are university students who smoke. Criteria for determining whether an observed association is causal are discussed later in this chapter.

Initiation and progression of tobacco use[19]

In most cases, learning to smoke occurs in adolescence and the subject's smoking status is confirmed by age 20 years.

Initially the factors are psychosocial; pharmacodynamic effects are unpleasant. But under the psychosocial pressures the subject continues, learns to limit and adjust nicotine intake, so that the pleasant pharmacological effects of nicotine develop and tolerance to the adverse effects occurs. Thus to the psychosocial pressure is now added pharmacological pleasure. Consumption rises and inhalation deepens. With developing maturity the psychosocial aspects diminish in importance and the desire and need for nicotine become dominant. If the nicotine intake becomes high, the drive for avoidance of withdrawal symptoms produces the 'chain-smoker', whose objective is to maintain plasma nicotine ($t_{\frac{1}{2}}$ 2 h) concentration.

The extraordinary power of this 'pleasure-drug', nicotine, has been summed up,

And a woman is only a woman, but a good cigar is a Smoke.[20]

---

[17] Scott R B. Br Med J 1957; 1: 671.

[18] Quoted in R. Coll. Phys Smoking or health. London: Pitman. 1977.
In 1929 Freud posed for a photograph holding a large cigar prominently. 'He was always a heavy smoker — twenty cigars a day were his usual allowance — and he tolerated abstinence from it with the greatest difficulty'. Jones E. Sigmund Freud: life and work. London: Hogarth Press. 1953.
[19] US Dept. Health, Education and Welfare. Smoking and health. 1964.
[20] Rudyard Kipling (1865–1936).

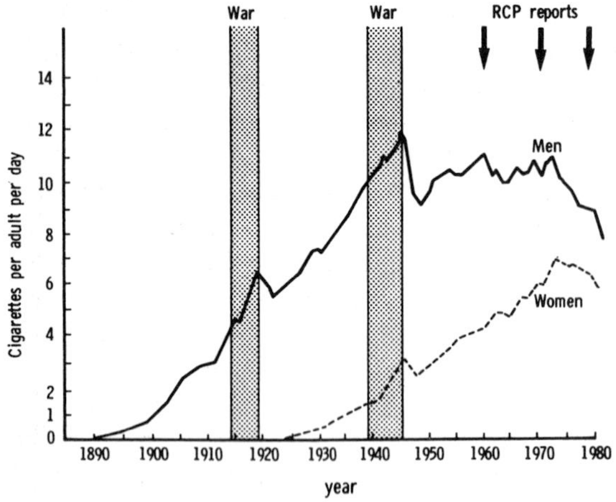

Fig. 19.1 Tobacco consumption in the UK, given as average number of cigarettes per adult per day for men and women separately, irrespective of whether they smoke or not. Since 1981 consumption for both men and women has declined, but only slightly.

The arrows indicate the dates of the 3 previous Royal College of Physicians (RCP) reports. Data from Tobacco Research (now Advisory) Council. By permission, R Coll Physicians Lond, from Health or smoking? London: Pitman, 1983

Types of smoking: summary

Non-pharmacological

- Psychosocial: uses symbolic value of the act to increase social confidence, status and self-esteem.
- Sensorimotor: to obtain oral, sensory and manipulatory satisfaction.

Pharmacological (plasma concentration of nicotine is adjusted automatically by changes in puffing rate and inhalation)

- Indulgent, the commonest: to obtain pleasure or to enhance an already pleasurable situation; frequency varies greatly.
- Sedative: to ease an unpleasant situation.
- Stimulant: to get a 'lift', to aid thinking or concentration, help with stressful situation, or help performance of monotonous task.
- Addictive: to avoid withdrawal feelings that occur as plasma nicotine ($t_{\frac{1}{2}}$ 2 h) concentration falls below a minimum, usually about 30 min after the end of the last smoke.

Characteristics of dependence

Psychological dependence is extremely strong and accounts largely for the difficulty of stopping smoking. Tolerance and some physical dependence occurs. Transient withdrawal effects include EEG and sleep changes, impaired performance in some psychomotor tests, disturbance of mood, and increased appetite, though it is difficult to disentangle psychological from physical effects in these last; also cardiovascular and gastrointestinal changes.

Acute effects of smoking tobacco

- *Increased airways resistance* occurs due to the non-specific effects of submicronic particles, e.g. carbon particles less than 1 μm across. The effect is reflex; even inert particles of this size cause bronchial narrowing sufficient to double airways resistance; this is insufficient to cause dyspnoea, though it might affect athletic performance. Four- to five-fold increase in resistance is necessary to cause noticeable dyspnoea and ten- to twenty-fold increase to cause severe dyspnoea such as can occur in asthma.

Pure nicotine inhalations of concentration comparable to that reached in smoking do not increase airways resistance.

- *Ciliary activity*, after transient stimulation, is depressed, and particles are removed from the lungs more slowly.
- *Carbon monoxide absorption* is physiologically insignificant in healthy young adults, but may be clinically important in the presence of coronary heart disease (see above).

NICOTINE PHARMACOLOGY

Pharmacokinetics

Nicotine is absorbed through mucous membranes in a highly pH-dependent fashion (see p. 326). The $t_{\frac{1}{2}}$ is 2 h. It is largrly metabolised to inert substances, e.g. cotinine, though some is excreted unchanged in the urine (pH dependent, it is un-ionised at acid pH). Cotinine is used as a marker for nicotine intake in smoking surveys because of its convenient $t_{\frac{1}{2}}$ (18 h).

Pharmacodynamics

Nicotine can both stimulate and depress nervous tissue function, depending on the dose and the interval between doses, and the psychological state of the subject; it can relieve anxiety or boredom.

No definitive statement can be made relating the pharmacodynamics of nicotine to the pleasure experienced by the smoker. Smokers who become more alert tend to take a lower dose of nicotine than do smokers who become more tranquil. In *doses used in smoking*, nicotine causes release of catecholamines in the CNS, also serotonin, and antidiuretic hormone, corticotrophin and growth hormone from the pituitary. The effects of nicotine on viscera are probably largely reflex, from stimulation of sensory receptors (chemo-receptors) in the carotid and aortic bodies, pulmonary circulation and left ventricle. Some of the results are mutually antagonistic.

In *large doses*[21] nicotine stimulates directly the ends of peripheral cholinergic nerves whose cell bodies lie in the central nervous system, i.e. it acts at autonomic ganglia and at the neuromuscular junction. This is what is meant by the term 'nicotine-like' or 'nicotinic' effect. Higher doses paralyse at the same points.

The central nervous system is stimulated, including the vomiting centre, both directly and via chemoreceptors in the carotid body; tremors and convulsions may occur. As with the peripheral actions, depression follows stimulation.

The following account tells *what generally happens* after one cigarette, from which about 1 mg nicotine is absorbed, although much depends on the amount and depth of inhalation and on the duration of end-inspiratory breath holding:

On the cardiovascular system the effects are those of sympathetic autonomic stimulation. There is vasoconstriction in the skin and vaso-dilatation in the muscles, tachycardia and a rise in blood pressure of about 15 mm Hg systolic and 10 mm Hg diastolic, and increased noradrenaline in the blood. Ventricular extrasystoles may occur. Cardiac output, work and oxygen consumption increase. Coronary vascular resistance decreases and blood flow increases in men aged 20–50 years. However if the resistance is fixed by atherosclerosis, flow does not increase, though work and oxygen consumption do. This may be a mechanism of tobacco-induced angina pectoris. It is possible that nicotine stimulates the myocardium by releasing noradrenaline stored in it, but at present it seems likely that this effect only occurs with higher doses.

Nicotine increases lipid concentrations in the blood, and also platelet adhesiveness, effects that may be clinically significant in atheroma and thrombosis.

On the gastrointestinal tract there are no important effects either on movement or secretion. Nausea and vomiting occur in the novice, probably due to stimulation of the vomiting centre.

Metabolic rate. Nicotine increases the metabolic rate, only slightly at rest,[22] but approximately doubles it during light exercise (occupational tasks, housework). This may be due to increase in autonomic sympathetic activity. The effect declines over 24 h on stopping smoking and accounts for the characteristic weight gain that is so disliked and which is sometimes given as a reason for continuing or resuming smoking. Smokers weigh 2–4 kg less than non-smokers (not enough to be a health issue).

Tolerance develops to some of the effects of nicotine, taken repeatedly over a few hours; a first experience commonly causes nausea and vomiting, which quickly ceases with repetition of

---

[21] Fatal nicotine poisoning has been reported from smoking, from swallowing tobacco, from tobacco enemas, from topical application to the skin and from accidental drinking of nicotine insecticide preparations. In 1932 a florist sat down on a chair, on the seat of which a 40% free nicotine insecticide solution had been spilled. Fifteen minutes later he felt ill (vomiting, sweating, faintness, and respiratory difficulty, followed by loss of consciousness and cardiac irregularity). He recovered in hospital over about 24 h. On the fourth day he was deemed well enough to leave hospital and was given his clothes which had been kept in a paper bag. He noticed the trousers were still damp. Within one hour of leaving hospital he had to be readmitted suffering again from nicotine poisoning due to nicotine absorbed transdermally from his still contaminated trousers. He recovered over three weeks, apart from persistent ventricular extrasystoles [Faulkner J M. JAMA 1933; 100: 1663].

[22] The metabolic rate at rest accounts for about 70% of daily energy expenditure.

smoking. Tolerance is usually rapidly lost; the first cigarette of the day has a greater effect on the cardiovascular system than do subsequent cigarettes.

Conclusion: the pleasurable effects of smoking are derived from a complex mixture of multiple pharmacological and non-pharmacological factors.

In this account *nicotine* is represented as being the major (but not the sole) determinant of tobacco dependence after the smoker has adapted to the usual initial unpleasant effects. But there remains some uncertainty as to its role, e.g. the failure of i.v. nicotine fully to substitute for smoking. Plainly it is important to analyse its exact place if less harmful alternatives to smoking, such as nicotine chewing gum, are to be exploited.

EFFECTS OF CHRONIC SMOKING

The Royal College of Physicians of London feels it has a duty to pronounce 'on a question of public health when action is required'. In 1725 it offered advice 'concerning the disastrous consequences of the rising consumption of cheap gin', and in 1962, 1977 and 1983, on the effects of smoking on health.[23] Its published reports are models of clarity and brevity.[24]

The US Public Health Service has published extensive reports.

The evidence for an association of smoking with various diseases consists of case control and cohort studies.

The detection of a statistical association does not prove a causal relationship. The causal significance of an association is a matter of judgement which goes beyond any statement of statistical probability. To *decide whether an observed association is causal*, several criteria, no one of which alone is sufficient, must be satisfied. These include:

- *Consistency* of association: diverse methods of approach should give the same answer.

- *Specificity* and *strength* of association: specificity means the precision with which the presence of, e.g. chronic bronchitis or lung cancer, can be used to predict that the victim smokes and vice versa; also the size of effect should be sufficient not to be obscured by any associated but non-causal factors, e.g. alcohol consumption; a correlation of effect (disease) with dose (amount smoked) is also important.

- *Temporal* association: the supposed cause, *smoking*, must operate before any evidence of the disease appears.

- *Coherence* of association: the associated event should fit in with all known facts of the natural history of the disease.

Mortality

The importance of finding out just what smoking does or does not do is shown below:

Percentage of men aged 35 who may expect to die before the age of 65

Non-smokers	15%
Smokers of 1–14 cigarettes a day	22%
Smokers of 15–24 cigarettes a day	25%
Smokers of 25 or more cigarettes a day	40%

- The average loss of life of a smoker of 25 cigarettes/day is about 5 years (UK and US studies).
- The time by which a habitual smoker's life is shortened is about 5 min per cigarette smoked.
- The extra risk of death (compared with that of life-long non-smokers) declines after a smoker ceases to smoke and returns to about that of non-smokers over 10–15 years.

The above applies to ordinary cigarettes.

Smoking and cancer

Bronchial carcinoma

Between 1920 and 1950 an epidemic of bronchial carcinoma occurred (rate in men increased × 20). Cigarette smoking satisfies the criteria for determining causation of an association (above) (lesser causes include exposure to a variety of industrial chemicals and atmospheric pollution).

---

[23] It is not intended to imply that the College was unconcerned about public health for over a century. This account relies heavily on these reports and on those of the US Public Health Service.

[24] We are grateful to the College for permission to use its Reports in the account that follows.

In men under 65 the death-rate is now falling, but it is still rising in women (except the youngest age group). These facts are compatible with the inevitable 20–40 year lag before changed habits affect the incidence of the disease. The risk of death from lung cancer is related to the number of cigarettes smoked and the age of starting, and is slightly reduced by use of filter-tipped cigarettes. Giving up smoking reduces the risk of death (see above and p. 353).

Pipe and cigar smokers suffer much smaller risks than cigarette smokers, probably because they inhale less.

Other cancers

The risk of smokers developing cancer of the mouth, throat and oesophagus is 5–10 times greater than that of non-smokers. It is as great for pipe and cigar smokers as it is for cigarette smokers. Cancer of the pancreas, kidney and urinary tract is also commoner in smokers.

Smoking can cause changes in DNA, and it seems likely that this effect is causally related.

Smoking and diseases of the heart and blood vessels

Coronary heart disease (CHD) is now the leading cause of the death in many developed countries. In the UK about 30% of these deaths can be attributed to smoking.

Under the age of 65 years smokers are about twice as likely to die of CHD as are non-smokers, and heavy smokers about $3\frac{1}{2}$ times as likely.

Sudden death may be the first manifestation of CHD and, especially in young men, is related to cigarette smoking. Smoking may induce chest pain on exertion (angina) from CHD and reduce ability to take vigorous exercise.

Smoking is especially dangerous for people in whom other risk factors (increased blood cholesterol, high blood pressure) are present, and they should be firmly warned of the consequences of smoking.

Atherosclerotic narrowing of the smallest coronary arteries is enormously increased in heavy and even in moderate smokers; the *increased platelet adhesiveness* caused by smoking increases the readiness with which thrombi form. The *carboxyhaemoglobinaemia* of habitual smokers (see p. 327) is enough to interfere with cardiovascular function in people who already have a problem of delivering oxygen to the heart. It also causes polycythaemia, which increases blood viscosity.

Stopping smoking reduces the excess risk of CHD in people under the age of 65, and after about 4 years of abstinence the risk approximates to that of non-smokers. Smokers who stop after a heart attack are less likely to have further attacks than those who go on smoking.

Hypertensives who smoke cigarettes are liable to develop an accelerated (malignant) phase which runs a rapid course.

Pipe and cigar smokers run little or no excess risk of CHD provided they are not heavy smokers and do not inhale. Heavy cigarette smokers who change over to pipe or cigar smoking often continue to inhale and thereby fail to reduce their risk.

Disease of the arteries of the leg is even more closely related to smoking, over 95% of patients with this condition, which causes pain on walking, being smokers. *Femoropopliteal vein grafts* survive less well in smokers. Death from *aneurysm of the aorta* is about 5 times commoner in smokers: there is also a positive association between smoking and *strokes*.

Smoking and chronic lung disease

The adverse effects of cigarette smoke on the lungs may be separated into two distinct conditions.

- *Chronic mucus hypersecretion*, which causes persistent cough with phlegm and fits with the original definition of simple *chronic bronchitis*. This condition arises chiefly in the large airways, usually clears up when the subject stops smoking and does not on its own carry any substantial risk of death.

- *Chronic obstructive lung disease*, which causes difficulty in breathing due to narrowing of the air passages in the lungs. This condition originates chiefly in the small airways, includes a variable element of destruction of peripheral lung units (emphysema), is progressive and largely irreversible and may ultimately lead to disability and death. The disease develops and progresses slowly in most smokers, but there appears to be a class of people who are peculiarly susceptible and who suffer rapid loss of lung function and who will die of this if they do not quit smoking.

Both conditions can co-exist in one person and they predispose to recurrent acute infective illnesses.

The obstructive syndrome is as specifically related to smoking as is lung cancer, and in a prospective survey of the effects of smoking on mortality amongst British doctors the relative risk for chronic obstructive lung disease was even more extreme than that for lung cancer. Despite this, in discussing the health effects of tobacco, there has generally been far more emphasis on lung cancer than on this more disabling, but equally fatal disorder.

The onset and progress of the disease, the mechanisms of which are multiple, is best characterised by patterns of change in the lung function test known as the one-second forced expiratory volume (FEV$_1$). These are outlined in Figure 19.2, where for simplicity FEV$_1$ is expressed as a percentage of what it would have been at age 25.

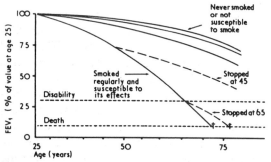

Fig. 19.2 Diagrammatic representation of decline in lung function with age based on actual data[25] and represented by percentage of one-second forced expiratory volume at age 25 in various population groups. The regular smoker who is susceptible (see text) to the damaging effects of cigarette smoke on the airways will show a rapid decline in function, though this can be slowed by stopping smoking. By permission, R Coll Physicians Lond: 1983: *ibid*

[25] Fletcher C M et al. Br Med J 1977; 1: 1645.

Other conditions

Gastric and duodenal ulcers are twice as common and twice as likely to cause death in smokers as in non-smokers, probably because smoking delays healing of the ulcers and increases the relapse rate. *Diseases of the teeth and gums* are also commoner in smokers.

Hepatic enzyme induction enhances metabolism of oestrogens (below) and androgens. Shrinkage of male genitalia is reported, but insufficient to constitute a real deterrent to smoking.

Cigarette smoke *depresses immunity* in animals and in man, and this may contribute to their increased liability to infection.

Pulmonary tuberculosis, certain skin rashes, and chest complications after surgical operations are commoner in smokers.

Tobacco amblyopia may be due to retinal damage by cyanide in the smoke; it is treated by *hydroxo*cobalamin.

General physical fitness is diminished by smoking, which impairs the function of the heart, lungs, and blood (above).

Interactions with drug therapy

Induction of hepatic drug metabolising enzymes by non-nicotine constituents of smoke causes increased metabolism of a range of drugs, including imipramine, oestrogens, theophylline, warfarin.

Women and smoking

Fertility

Women who smoke are more likely to be infertile or take longer to conceive than women who do not smoke. In addition, smokers are more liable to have an earlier menopause than are non-smokers. Increased metabolism of oestrogens may not be the whole explanation.

Complications of pregnancy

Smokers have a small increased risk of spontaneous abortion, bleeding during pregnancy and the development of various placental abnormalities. On the other hand, women who smoke have a lowered incidence of toxaemia of pregnancy though the advantages of this do not offset the disadvantages of smoking during pregnancy. The placenta is heavier in smoking than non-smoking women and its diameter larger. The enlarged placenta and placental abnormalities may represent adaptations to lack of oxygen due to smoking, secondary to raised concentrations of circulating carboxyhaemoglobin.

The child

The offspring of women who smoke are approximately 200 g lighter than the offspring of women who do not smoke. They have an increased risk of death in the perinatal period which is independent of other variables such as social class, level of education, age of mother, race or extent of antenatal care. The increased risk rises to twofold or more in heavy smokers and appears to be entirely accounted for by the placental abnormalities and the consequences of low birthweight.

Suggestions that the risk of congenital abnormalities is increased have not, in general, been confirmed. However, there is considerable evidence that the children of mothers who smoke may be disadvantaged even up to age 11 years. It is not clear whether this is due to the long-term effects of the mother smoking during pregnancy or are also the consequence of the mother or parents continuing to smoke as the child grows up. (see Passive smoking below).

Ex-smokers and women who give up smoking in the first 20 weeks of pregnancy have offspring whose birthweight is similar to that of the children of women who have never smoked.

The *placentas* of smokers show more abnormal DNA than those of non-smokers.

Contraception

Women who smoke tend to favour the Pill as a method of contraception and they too bear the brunt of its ill-effects. The risk of myocardial infarction, stroke and other cardiovascular diseases in young women is increased slightly by the combined Pill contraceptive or by smoking. But when the two are added the risks multiply together leading to an approximately tenfold increase in risk overall. This effect is unacceptably high ($\times$ 100) in heavy smokers (15/day or more) over 40 years of age. Only a light smoker under age 30 has a risk approximating to that of a non-smoking user.

STARTING AND STOPPING USE

Some children begin to smoke at 5 years of age, and it has been found that about one-third of adult regular smokers began before they were 9. About 80% of children who smoke regularly continue to do so when they grow up. The earlier in life a person starts to smoke regularly, the greater is the risk of early death.

Contrary to popular belief it is not generally difficult to stop, only 14% finding it 'very difficult'. But ex-smoker status is unstable and the long-term success rate of a smoking withdrawal clinic is rarely above 30%. The situation is summed up by the witticism, 'Giving up smoking is easy, I've done it many times'. That persons in upper economic social classes, and especially doctors, are most likely to stop suggests the importance of educated recognition of the health risks.

Though they are as aware of the risks of smoking as men, *women* find it harder to stop; they consistently have lower success rates. This trend crosses every age group and occupation. Women particularly dislike the weight gain (above).

There are *special aids*, including group therapy, snuff, graded cigarette holders, hypnosis, acupuncture and nicotine as chewing gum, transdermal patch or oral spray (it is better to take nicotine than tobacco smoke). None of them has a very high success rate and, apart from nicotine itself, no one emerges as strikingly more effective than any other. Nicotine formulation, when used casually without special attention to technique, has proved no better than other aids, but if used carefully and withdrawn as recommended, results are better. Various astringents are used in the mouth to make the smoke taste bad. All of these aids are capable of helping some smokers, but none is a substitute for the will and resolve of the individual to quit.

If the patient is heavily tobacco-dependent and severe anxiety, irritability, tension, headache, insomnia and weight gain (about 3 kg) and tension are concomitants of attempts to stop smoking, then an anxiolytic sedative (or β-adrenoceptor blocker) may be useful for a short time, but it is important to avoid substituting one drug-dependence for another.

In short, drugs have only a limited role, and 'the weaponry which may help the patient to hurdle his habit'[26] is divided between 'appeals to sense and the psyche' and so is beyond the scope of this book.

There is ample evidence to warrant strong advice against starting to smoke, but doctors are not consulted on this by individuals. The problem with, say, the elderly chronic bronchitic dependent on tobacco is different. Persuasion will be adapted to his personality but over-hasty and unreasonable prohibitions of patients' long-standing pleasures or vices do no good. The pliable patient is made wretched, but most are merely alienated, as was D G Rossetti (1828–82), who wrote,

> My doctor's issued his decree
> That too much wine is killing me,
> And furthermore his ban he hurls
> Against my touching naked girls.
> How then? Must I no longer share
> Good wine or beauties, dark and fair?
> Doctor, goodbye, my sail's unfurled,
> I'm off to try the other world.

Safer smoking

Plainly a safe cigarette that also satisfied the users' needs would solve the health problems of smokers, if not those of their neighbours. Some success has been achieved by filters that remove much of the tar, but some of the nicotine is dissolved in tar particles and smokers compensate by smoking or inhaling more; also CO production has been reduced. Current evidence is that 'safer' cigarettes are so little safer that policies to promote a non-smoking population should not be reduced.

To substitute a *smokeless way* of taking tobacco would eliminate respiratory disease. But fine cut or powdered tobacco (snuff) for nasal or oral use causes local cancers and periodontal disease. Society should 'not make the mistake of replacing the ashtray with the spittoon'.[27]

Passive (involuntary) smoking

Many non-smokers are exposed to tobacco smoke. At home, at work, on public transport and in public places, they can scarcely avoid breathing air contaminated by other peoples' smoke. This mode of smoke inhalation is not actively sought; it is *involuntary* or *passive smoking*.

It is difficult to measure the extent of the risk to health from passive smoke exposure, but evidence is accumulating of actual harm. Although the risks are, naturally, smaller, the number of people affected is large.

Mainstream and sidestream smoke

Smoke drawn through the tobacco and taken in by the smoker is known as mainstream smoke. Smoke which arises from smouldering tobacco and passes directly into the surrounding air, whence it may be inhaled by smokers and non-smokers alike, is known as sidestream smoke. Mainstream and sidestream smoke differ in composition, partly because of the different temperatures at which they are produced. Substances found in greater concentrations in undiluted sidestream smoke than in undiluted mainstream smoke include, nicotine ($\times 2.7$), carbon monoxide ($\times 2.5$), ammonia ($\times 73$), and some carcinogens (e.g. benzo-a-pyrene $\times 3.4$). However, whereas the smoker is exposed to undiluted mainstream smoke, the sidestream smoke, to which the passive smoker is exposed, is diluted by room air to a variable extent depending on distance from the smoking source and the amount of ventilation. Sidestream smoke con-

[26] Sprague H B. Monthly scientific publication of the American Heart Association, October 1964.

[27] Koop C New Engl J Med 1986; 314: 1020.

stitutes about 85% of smoke generated in an average room during cigarette smoking.

The concentration of *carbon monoxide* produced by smoking has been measured under experimental conditions in rooms of various size and in everyday social conditions. Smoke-free air contains about 2.0 parts per million (ppm) of carbon monoxide. Examples of concentrations found in smoky conditions include 7–9 ppm at parties, 8–33 ppm in a conference room, 40 ppm in a submarine, 15–60 ppm in an ordinary room, and 12–110 ppm in a car. The concentrations reached obviously depend on the degree of ventilation. Under ordinary social conditions with good ventilation, levels are usually below 10 ppm when smokers are present and below 3 ppm when they are not.

Unlike carbon monoxide, some of the *nicotine* derived from cigarette smoke will settle out of the air in a room. Nicotine (or its metabolites) concentrations in the blood and urine of people exposed experimentally to smoky atmospheres and in submarines are increased, but are much lower than those found in smokers. About half of the non-smokers living in cities have nicotine in their blood, and most have nicotine in their urine. The health consequences of this are unknown.

The balance of evidence on passive smoking in adults is that there are small causal effects on bronchial carcinoma, decrease in lung function tests and increased cardiovascular disease (relative risks 1.2–2.7).[28]

In *children*, especially those under 5 years and where the mother smokes, effects are greater. There is an increase in acute respiratory and in middle ear infections and effusions (glue ear), in chronic respiratory disease and a decrease in lung function. Children at 5 years are 1.0 cm shorter. But some disadvantages may persist even longer:

at the age of 11, intellectual performance as revealed by reading comprehension and mathematical ability is behind that of children of non-smoking mothers by a span of 6 to 7 months. It is not clear whether this is solely a consequence of parental smoking as the child grows up, or whether it could also be a delayed effect of maternal smoking during pregnancy.

The risk of all cancers (including leukaemia) combined may be increased by 30%.

Some of these matters remain controversial; epidemiological studies showing small risks are inevitably imprecise.

Medical students and smoking

Although medical students smoke less now than they did 10 years ago, male students smoke about the same as the general public of the same age and social classes, i.e. the decline in smoking is related to social class and not to specialised knowledge or to any feeling of obligation to set an example to others in this serious health issue. But, amongst women medical students, the smoking rate is only 50% that of the female general public of the same age and social class.

Hospital nurses are the sole studied health professional group in which smoking prevalence is not very much lower than in the general population.

ETHYL ALCOHOL (Ethanol)

The services rendered by intoxicating substances in the struggle for happiness and in warding off misery rank so highly as a benefit that both individuals and races have given them an established position within their libido-economy. It is not merely the immediate gain in pleasure which one owes to them, but also a measure of that independence of the outer world which is so sorely craved . . . We are aware that it is just this property which constitutes the danger and injuriousness of intoxicating substances . . .[29]

Alcohol is chiefly important in medicine because of the consequences of its misuse/abuse.

---

[28] A remarkable legal action has been conducted in the Federal Court of Australia. The Court sat for 90 days and heard international evidence. The judge concluded that there is compelling evidence that cigarette smoke causes in non-smokers, cancer, asthma attacks and, in children, respiratory disease. Whether or not the tobacco industry appeals successfully, this judgement is a 'major turning point in the worldwide efforts to reduce smoking related diseases': Chapman S et al. Brit Med J 1991; 302: 943.

[29] Freud S. Civilisation, war and death, Psycho-analytic epitomes, No. 4. London: Hogarth Press, 1939.

Alcohol misuse is a *social* problem with pharmacological aspects, which latter are discussed here.

The history of alcohol is part of the history of civilisation 'ever since Noah made his epoch-making discovery'.[30]

Pharmacokinetics

Absorption of alcohol taken orally is rapid, for it is highly lipid soluble and diffusible from the stomach and the small intestine. With moderate amounts, the highest blood concentration, as might be expected, is reached with stronger solutions.

However, solutions above 20% are absorbed more slowly because high concentrations of alcohol inhibit gastric peristalsis and cause pylorospasm, thus delaying the arrival of the alcohol in the small intestine, as does cigarette smoking. Large doses taken in very dilute solution are absorbed relatively slowly because of the large amount of water.

Absorption is delayed by food, especially milk, the effect of which is probably due to the fat it contains. Carbohydrate also delays absorption of alcohol and so alcohol in beer is absorbed more slowly than a simple solution. Habitual drinkers may absorb alcohol more rapidly than others.

There is an important *sex difference* in alcohol absorption and systemic bioavailability. Alcohol is subject to *gastric first-pass metabolism* (by alcohol dehydrogenases in the gastric but not in the intestinal wall); the liver, unusually, plays little role in presystemic elimination although it has a major role in its subsequent metabolism. The effect is enough to be clinically important. Gastric emptying time has a significant role in determining the exposure of alcohol to the effect (see above).

The stomach wall in *women* has less alcohol dehydrogenase and due to this, and to the lower volume of distribution (see below) alcohol attains higher concentration in systemic blood for the same dose, per kg, than in men. Alcoholics lose

[30] Genesis; 9: 21; Huxley A. Ann N Y Acad Sci 1957; 67: 675.

this protective mechanism. Cimetidine blocks it by enzyme inhibition.

After absorption, alcohol is rapidly *distributed* throughout the body water (dist. vol. 0.7 l/kg men: 0.6 l/kg women) and is not selectively stored in any tissue. If food is taken simultaneously alcohol disappears from the blood more rapidly than otherwise; it is not known how this happens.

Maximum *blood concentrations* after oral alcohol therefore depend on numerous factors including the total dose, sex, the strength of the solution, the time over which it is taken, the presence or absence of food, the time relations of taking food and alcohol and the kind of food eaten, as well as on the speed of metabolism and excretion. A single dose of alcohol, say 60 ml (48 g; equivalent to 145 ml whisky, 5–6 'whiskies', or *units*, see Figure 19.3), taken over a few minutes on an empty stomach will probably produce maximal blood concentration at from 30–90 min and will not all be disposed of for 6–8 h or even more. There are very great individual variations.

About 95% of absorbed alcohol is *metabolised*, the remainder being excreted in the breath, urine and sweat; convenient methods of estimation of alcohol in all these are available.

Alcohol follows first-order kinetics only after the smallest doses. Once the blood concentration exceeds about 10 mg/100 ml the enzymic elimination processes are saturated and elimination rate no longer increases with increasing concentration but becomes steady at 10–15 ml per hour in occasional drinkers. Therefore, as the blood concentration rises the $t_\frac{1}{2}$ gets longer, with potentially major consequences for the individual. Thus alcohol is subject to *dose-dependent kinetics*, *i.e. saturation* or *zero-order kinetics*. For further details of pharmacokinetics see p. 80.

Induction of hepatic drug metabolising enzymes occurs and this contributes to tolerance in habitual users. But there is also a tissue tolerance. Alcohol in the systemic circulation is *metabolised* (oxidised) by enzyme systems in the liver, first, by alcohol dehydrogenases into acetaldehyde and then to acetate, which is metabolised to carbon dioxide and water. At high concentrations, a second alcohol-inducible enzyme

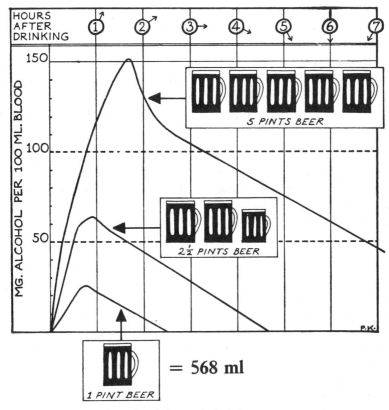

Fig. 19.3a Approximate blood concentrations after 3 doses of alcohol

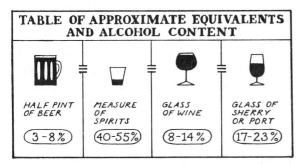

Fig. 19.3b Four standard units of drink (in which social consumption is measured); a unit contains approx. 10 ml (8 g) of alcohol. Knowledge of blood alcohol concentration does not allow a reliable estimate of how much has been consumed

system (dependent on cytochrome P_{450}) comes into play. Increased formation of metabolites is responsible for organ damage in chronic overconsumption, acetaldehyde in the liver and probably fatty ethyl esters in other organs, and also for the increased susceptibility to liver injury of heavy drinkers when exposed to anaesthetics, industrial solvents and to drugs. An *acute* substantial dose of alcohol inhibits hepatic drug metabolism. *Chronic use* of moderate amounts induces hepatic drug metabolising enzymes. Chronic use of *large amounts* reduces hepatic metabolic capacity by causing cellular damage.

Blood concentration of alcohol has great medicolegal importance. *Alcohol in alveolar air* is in equilibrium with that in pulmonary capillary blood and reliable, easily handled devices have been developed to measure it, for this avoids 'assaulting' the subject with a needle and can be used by police at the roadside on both drivers and pedestrians.

Pharmacodynamics

Alcohol acts on the **central nervous system** in the manner of general anaesthetics; it enhances

GABA-stimulated flux of chloride through receptor-gated membrane ion channels, a receptor subtype effect that may be involved in the motor impairment caused by alcohol, and to which the development of antagonists is possible.

It is not a stimulant; hyperactivity, when it occurs, is due to *removal of inhibitory effects*. The concept of higher levels of the central nervous system dominating lower levels is naive, and it is now known that there is a complex interdependence of the various parts, so that changes at one 'level' affect function at other 'levels', 'higher' or 'lower'. Alcohol, in ordinary doses, may act chiefly on the arousal mechanisms of the brain-stem reticular formation, inhibiting polysynaptic function and enhancing presynaptic inhibition. Direct cortical depression probably only occurs with high doses.

With increasing doses the subject passes through all the stages of general anaesthesia and may die of respiratory depression.[31] Psychic effects are the most important socially, and it is to obtain these that the drug is habitually used in so many societies, to make social intercourse not merely easy but even pleasant. They have been admirably described by Sollmann:

The first functions to be lost are the finer grades of judgement, reflection, observation and attention — the faculties largely acquired through education, which constitute the elements of the restraint and prudence that man usually imposes on his actions. The orator allows himself to be carried by the impulse of the moment, without reflecting on ultimate consequences, and as his expressions become freer, they acquire an appearance of warmth, of feeling, of inspiration. Not a little of this inspiration is contributed by the audience if they are in a similar condition of increased appreciation. . . . Another characteristic feature, evidently resulting from paralysis of the higher functions, is the loss of power to control moods.[32]

Environment, personality, mood and dose of alcohol are all relevant to the final effect on the individual.[33]

---

[31] Loss of consciousness occurs at blood concentrations around 300 mg/100 ml; death at about 400 mg/100 ml.

[32] Sollmann T. Manual of pharmacology. 8th ed. Philadelphia: Saunders. 1957.

[33] 'That which hath made them drunk hath made me bold.' Lady Macbeth in Macbeth, Act 2, Scene 2. W. Shakespeare.

These and other effects that are characteristic of alcohol, have been celebrated in the following couplets:[34]

> Ho! Ho! Yes! Yes! It's very all well,
> You may drunk I am think, but I tell you I'm not,
> I'm as sound as a fiddle and fit as a bell,
> And stable quite ill to see what's what. . . . .
>
> And I've swallowed, I grant, a beer of lot —
> But I'm not so think as you drunk I am. . . . .
>
> I shall stralk quite weight and not yutter an ell,
> My feech will not spalter the least little jot:
> If you knownly had own! — well, I gave him a dot,
> And I said to him, 'Sergeant, I'll come like a lamb —
> The floor it seems like a storm in a yacht,
> But I'm not so think as you drunk I am. . . . .
>
> I'm sorry, I just chair over a fell —
> A trifle — this chap, on a very day hot —
> If I hadn't consumed that last whisky of tot! —
> As I said now, this fellow, called Abraham —
> Ah? One more? Since it's you! Just a do me will spot —
> But I'm not so think as you drunk I am.

There is a good reason to believe that, in general, efficiency, both mental and physical, is reduced by alcohol in any amount worth taking for social purposes. There is an important exception; the person who is so disabled by anxiety or nervous tension that performance is gravely impaired may improve with the correct dose of alcohol. The alleviation of great anxiety may improve performance more than the alcohol depresses it. Such people, experiencing the immediate relief that alcohol brings, are more liable to become alcohol addicts. Another exception is a minority of introverted people.

Innumerable tests of physical and mental performance have been used to demonstrate the effects of alcohol. Results show that alcohol reduces visual acuity and delays recovery from visual dazzle; it impairs taste, smell and hearing, muscular coordination and steadiness and prolongs reaction time. It also causes nystagmus and vertigo. At the same time the subjects commonly have an increased confidence in their ability to perform well when tested and under-

---

[34] By Sir J C Squire (1884–1958). Quoted, by permission, R H A Squire.

estimate their errors, even after quite low doses. Attentiveness and ability to assimilate, sort and quickly take decisions on continuously changing information input, decline. This results particularly in inattentiveness to the periphery of the visual field, which is important in motoring. All these are evidently highly undesirable effects when a person is in a position where failure to perform well may be dangerous.

Car driving: alcohol

The effects of alcohol and psychotropic drugs on motor driving (Fig. 19.4) have been the subject of well-deserved attention, and many countries have made laws designed to prevent motor accidents caused by alcohol. The problem has nowhere been solved. In general it can be said that the weight of evidence points to a steady

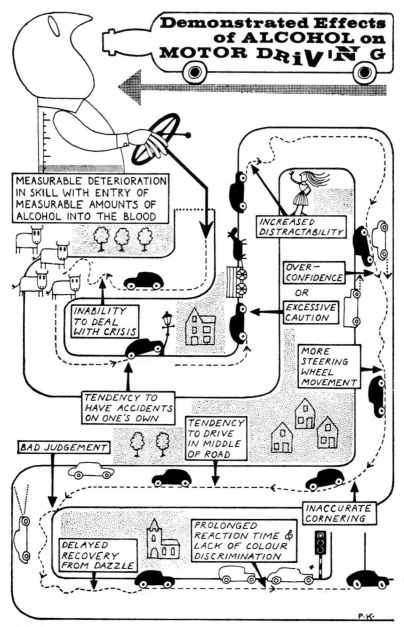

Fig. 19.4 Alcohol and driving

deterioration of driving skill and an increased liability to accidents, which begins with the entry of alcohol into the blood and steadily increases with blood concentration.

> Alcohol brings disaster on the road less because of lack of skill than because of *defective judgement in relation to skill.* . . . Furthermore, let us recognise that the danger may be less from the few who have imbibed a lot than from the many who have taken a little.[35]

Unfortunately it is not possible to observe and make measurements of driving skill in subjects who are both unaware that they are under observation and who are yet driving under normal traffic conditions. The undoubted tendency of alcohol to increase distractability, proneness to take risks and carelessness has not therefore been measured under normal conditions; in experimental conditions the well-known ability of users to 'pull themselves together' and to perform well temporarily when they know they are being tested will tend to give an unduly favourable picture of the effects of alcohol, but despite this, the evidence that its effects on driving are wholly evil is impressive.

In one study on city bus drivers, all of whom were recipients of awards for safe driving, it was found that even with these experienced professionals there was no 'safe' blood-alcohol level below which it was certain that no impairment of judgement would occur. Drivers attempted to pass through gaps less than the width of the bus.[36]

In another study using a motor driving trainer it was found that alcohol even in small doses caused drivers to move away from the kerb and to tolerate steering swings towards the road centre but not towards the kerb, also steering wheel movement increased and its timing became more faulty. Extraverts were not worried by the stress imposed by taking alcohol, they did not alter their speed greatly but were much less accurate. Introverts however appeared to try to compensate for the alcohol effect; they over-

reacted to the situation, moving the steering wheel more and changing speed, some slowing right down and others seemingly trying to show how quickly they could drive.[37]

Alcohol plays a huge part in causing motor accidents, being a factor in as many as 50%. For this reason, the compulsory use of a roadside breath test, followed if necessary by provision of a blood sample (or urine sample if the subject objects to blood being taken) is acknowledged to be in the public interest. But the breath test is now accurate enough to be sole evidence. In Britain a blood concentration exceeding 80 mg alcohol/100 ml blood (17.4 mmol/l)[38] whilst in charge of a car is a statutory offence. At this concentration, the liability to accident is about twice normal. Other countries set a more sensible 50 mg/100 ml, e.g. Yugoslavia, Nordic countries[39], some states of USA, Australia, Greece.

So clearly is it in the public interest that drunken driving be reduced that the privileges normally attaching to freedom of conscience as well as to personal eccentricity must take second place. In one instance[40] a follower of Mesmer[41] was convicted following refusal to provide a specimen after seeking to justify his position on the grounds of the presence in his blood of divine gifts; in another, an ingenious driver, having provided a positive breath test, offered a blood sample on the condition it should be taken from his penis; the physician refused to take it; the police demanded a urine sample; the subject refused on the ground that he had offered blood and that his offer had been refused. He was ac-

---

[35] Cohen J. In: Alcohol and road traffic. London: British Medical Association. 1963.
[36] Cohen J et al. Br Med J 1958; 1: 1438.

[37] Drew G C et al. B Med J 1958; 2: 993.
[38] Approximately equivalent to 35 µg alcohol in 100 ml expired air (or 107 mg in 100 ml urine). In practice, prosecutions are undertaken only when the concentration is significantly higher to avoid arguments about biological variability and instrumental error. Urine concentrations are little used since the urine is accumulated over time and does not provide the immediacy of blood and breath.
[39] In 1990 Sweden lowered the limit to 20 mg/100 ml, which has been approached by ingestion of glucose which is fermented by gut flora — the 'autobrewery' syndrome.
[40] Br Med J 1974; 2: 620.
[41] Friedrich Anton Mesmer (1733–1815) developed a theory that a healing occult force akin to magnetism permeated the universe, though concentrated in men and especially in himself.

quitted, but a Court has since decided that the choice of site for blood-taking is for the physician, not for the subject, and that such transparent attempts to evade justice should be treated as unreasonable refusal to supply a specimen under the law. The subject is then treated as though he had provided a specimen that was above the statutory limit. Another person refused venepuncture lest the needle infected him with AIDS. Yet another trick is to take a dose of spirits *after* the accident and *before* the police arrive. The police are told it was taken as a remedy for nervous shock. This is known as the 'hip-flask' defence.

Where blood or breath analysis is not immediately available after an accident, it may be measured hours later and 'back calculated' to what it would have been at the time of the accident. It is usual to assume that the blood concentration falls at about 15 mg/100 ml/h. Naturally, the validity of such calculations leads to acrimonious disputes in the courts of law.

There is also evidence that there is danger after alcohol has left the blood, during the 'hangover' period, perhaps due to irritability and fatigue.

Any reader who drives is urged to consult some of the references at the end of the chapter. They will prove interesting, and the knowledge gained may even save his, or more important, somebody else's life. Nor must the *intoxicated pedestrian* be forgotten.

Other drugs and driving

In road traffic accident fatalities 4.8% had taken a drug 'likely' to affect the CNS (chiefly older victims); 2.6% had taken drugs of abuse, chiefly cannabis; 35% had a detectable alcohol concentration (25% above the legal limit). Unfortunately accurate control figures are not available except in the case of epilepsy: 1.3% of fatalities had taken an antiepilepsy drug and the incidence of the disease in the general population is 0.4%.

Further effects of alcohol consumption

- Alcohol induces *peripheral vasodila-*

tation by depressing the vasomotor centre and this accounts for the feeling of warmth that follows taking the drug. Body heat loss is increased so that it is undesirable to take alcohol before going out into severe cold for any length of time, but it may be harmlessly employed on coming into a warm environment from the cold to provide quickly a pleasant feeling of warmth. In very cold places the overuse of alcohol can cause rapid hypothermia, e.g. drunks collapsed out of doors in winter. Alcohol does not usefully dilate the coronary blood vessels although it may relieve the pain of angina pectoris. An acute dose of 4–5 units raises the *blood pressure* which parallels the blood concentration: the mechanism is uncertain.

- Being a general anaesthetic, alcohol can be used as an ***analgesic and hypnotic*** when circumstances warrant it, e.g. for short periods in the elderly. As a sedative in status asthmaticus alcohol has much to commend it for it does not depress respiration in *therapeutic* doses, and may have some bronchodilator effect.

- Alcohol acts as a ***diuretic*** by inhibiting secretion of the antidiuretic hormone by the posterior pituitary gland. The reason it is useless as a diuretic in heart failure is that the diuresis is of water, not of salt. It also delays labour by *inhibition of oxytocin release* from the posterior pituitary.

- Alcohol ***injures the gastric mucosa*** with back diffusion of acid and increased cell shedding. It has little effect on gastric secretion (contrary to previous belief). After an acute binge the mucosa shows erosions and petechial haemorrhages (recovery may take 3 weeks) and up to 60% of chronic alcoholics show chronic gastritis. Alcohol has no proven important influence on peptic ulcer disease.

The ***vomiting*** which is so common an accompaniment of acute alcoholism is not primarily due to gastric irritation, for the incidence of vomiting at equivalent blood alcohol concentrations is similar following oral or i.v. administration, i.e. it is a CNS effect. This is not to deny that very strong solutions and dietary indiscretions accompanying acute and chronic alcoholism can cause vomiting by local gastric effects. That the emetic blood alcohol concentration is below that which induces coma may be one of the reasons for the rarity of deaths from acute alcoholism and for the fact that when death occurs, it is commonly due to suffocation from inhaled vomit.

Glucose tolerance: alcohol initially increases the blood glucose, due to reduced uptake by the tissues. This leads to increased *glucose metabolism*. A substantial dose of alcohol may cause slight hyperglycaemia due to activity of the sympathetic autonomic system.

Alcohol inhibits gluconeogenesis, and in a person whose hepatic glycogen is already low, e.g. a person who is getting most of his calories from alcohol or who has not eaten adequately for 3 days, this can result in *hypoglycaemia* that can be severe enough to cause irreversible brain damage. The hypoglycaemia is commonly at its maximum 6–18 h after taking the alcohol. It can be difficult to recognise clinically in a person who has been drunk, and this adds to the risk.

Hypoglycaemia is also enhanced by exaggeration of the normal insulin response to carbohydrate ingestion, and by exercise.

A variant in wealthy societies is the 'after lunch gin and tonic hypoglycaemia'.

Hyperuricaemia occurs (with precipitation of gout) due to accelerated degradation of adenine nucleotides resulting in increased production of uric acid and its precursors. Only at high alcohol concentrations does alcohol-induced high blood lactate compete for renal tubular elimination and so diminish excretion of urate. But heavy drinkers (>30 units/week) may stop having gout if they stop drinking alcohol.

Acute effects on sexual function. Nothing really new has been said since William Shakespeare wrote that alcohol 'provokes the desire, but it takes away the performance.' Performance in other forms of athletics is also impaired. Prolonged substantial consumption lowers plasma testosterone concentration at least partly as a result of hepatic enzyme induction; feminisation may be seen and men have been threatened with genital shrinkage.

As a *source of energy* (rather than a food) alcohol may be useful in debilitated patients. It is rapidly absorbed from the alimentary tract without requiring digestion and it supplies 7 calories[42] per gram as compared with 9 from fat and 4 from carbohydrate and protein. Heavy doses cause hyperlipidaemia in some people.

Tolerance to alcohol can be *acquired* and the point has been made that it costs the regular heavy drinker $2\frac{1}{2}$ times as much to get visibly drunk as it would cost the average abstainer.[43] This is probably due both to enzyme induction and to adaptation of the central nervous system. There are also racial differences in *natural tolerance*; whites are more tolerant than Mongolians.

Acute alcohol poisoning is a sufficiently familiar condition not to require detailed description. It is notorious that the behaviour changes, excitement, mental confusion, incoordination and even coma, which are characteristic, can be due to numerous other conditions and diagnosis can be extremely difficult if a sick or injured patient happens to have taken alcohol as well. Alcohol can cause severe hypoglycaemia (see above). Anyone who is liable to find himself called upon, especially by the police, to make a clinical diagnosis of drunkenness, or rather perhaps to exclude other causes as responsible for a person's behaviour, should consider the procedure very carefully. When applying clinical tests for drunkenness it is worth remembering that habitual physical skills can be retained to an advanced stage and that the results of performance tests cannot always be interpreted unambiguously.

An arrested man was told, in a police station, by a doctor, that he was drunk. The man asked, 'Doctor, could a drunk man stand up in middle of this room, jump into the air, turn a complete somersault, and land down on his feet?'

The doctor was injudicious enough to say, 'Certainly not' — and was then and there proved wrong'.[44] The introduction of the breathalyser, which only has a statutory role in road traffic situations, has largely eliminated such professional humiliations.

---

[42] 1 calorie ≈ 4.2 joules.
[43] Gaddum J H. In Lectures on the scientific basis of medicine, 1954–55. London: Athlone Press. 1956.
[44] Worthing C L. Br Med J 1957; 1: 643.

When a person is behaving in an excited or violent fashion due to alcohol it is dangerous to attempt to control him with sedatives or opioids because of the risk of inducing severe respiratory depression as a result of synergism of the drugs. But if sedation is essential, chlorpromazine, diazepam or paraldehyde in low dose are least hazardous. In patients who are comatose, the stomach may be emptied by tube; emesis, either therapeutic or due to the alcohol, is dangerous in any patient with impaired consciousness. Respiratory stimulants, e.g. doxapram, or controlled respiration are used as required: circulatory failure may occur. Alcohol dialyses well, but dialysis will only be used in extreme cases.

Large doses of *fructose* (laevulose)[45] i.v. enhance alcohol metabolism but also induce lactic acidosis. Claims that a dose of fructose swallowed during and/or at the end of an evening's drinking can render a subject who is unfit to drive, fit to do so, are dangerously misleading.

Acute hepatitis, which may be extremely severe, can occur with extraordinarily heavy acute drinking bouts. The serum transaminase rises after alcohol in alcoholics but not in others. The single case report that after a binge the cerebrospinal fluid tasted of gin remains unconfirmed.

Chronic alcohol consumption

The effects described above will occur but also, with heavy continuous drinking, there will be malnutrition (subjects take all the calories they need from alcohol, see above, and cease to eat adequately) with deficiency of B group vitamins particularly. The malnutrition complicates the long-term effects of alcohol itself.

Chronic *heavy* alcohol use is associated with **organ damage** due to metabolites of alcohol, *hepatic cirrhosis*, deteriorating brain function (psychotic states, dementia, seizures, Wernicke's encephalopathy, attacks of loss of memory); peripheral neuropathy and, separately, myopathy; *cancer* of the upper alimentary and respiratory tracts (many alcoholics smoke heavily, and this contributes), hepatic carcinoma and breast cancer in women; chronic pancreatitis; cardiomyopathy; bone marrow depression, including megaloblastosis (due to the alcohol and to alcohol induced folate deficiency); deficiency of vitamin K dependent blood clotting factors (due to liver injury); psoriasis; multiple effects on the hypothalamic/pituitary/endocrine system (endocrine investigations should be interpreted cautiously); Dupuytren's contracture.

Hypertension. Heavy chronic use of alcohol is an important cause of hypertension which should always be considered in both diagnosis and management. Cessation of use may be sufficient to eliminate or reduce the need for drug therapy.

Short-term rises in blood pressure occur with acute (binge) drinking and also with abrupt withdrawal. The mechanisms are uncertain.

In general, *reversal* of all or most of the above effects is usual in early cases if alcohol is abandoned. In more advanced cases, the disease may be halted (except cancer) but in severe cases it may continue to progress. Stopping drinking improves survival only in early cases. When wine rationing was introduced in Paris, France, in the 1939–45 war, deaths from hepatic cirrhosis dropped to about one-sixth the previous level; 5 years after the war they had regained their previous level. A similar, though lesser, effect was seen during alcohol prohibition in the USA (1919–33).

The claim that *moderate alcohol consumption* protects against coronary heart disease and stroke remains controversial as to causality, i.e. this negative association may be the consequence of various biases; but support for it increases.

Alcohol dependence syndrome[46] (**chronic alcoholism**): general aspects of dependence are discussed earlier in this chapter. Dependence varies between the social drinker for whom companionship is the principal factor, through individuals who take a drink at the end of a working (or indeed any) day, who feel a *need* and who

---

[45] Sucrose is hydrolysed to glucose and fructose in the intestine, but this takes time.

[46] A World Health Organization report prefers this term to 'alcoholism'.

would be reluctant to give it up, to the person who is overcome by need, who cannot resist and whose whole life is dominated by the quest for alcohol. The major factors determining physical dependence are *dose*, *frequency* of dosing, and *duration* of abuse.

Fluoxetine (serotonin antagonist) has been found to assist reduction of intake in problem drinkers.

Withdrawal of alcohol

Abrupt withdrawal of alcohol from an addict who has developed physical dependence, such as may occur when an ill or injured alcoholic is admitted to hospital, can precipitate withdrawal syndrome in 6 h and an acute psychotic attack (*delirium tremens*) and seizures (at 72 h), as well as agitation, anxiety and excess sympathetic autonomic activity.

Withdrawal is less unpleasant if the patient is sedated, e.g. with a benzodiazepine and a β-adrenoceptor blocker given for the symptoms of sympathetic overactivity. Chlormethiazole (Heminevrin), an anticonvulsant sedative, has a reputation as especially effective, but such a claim

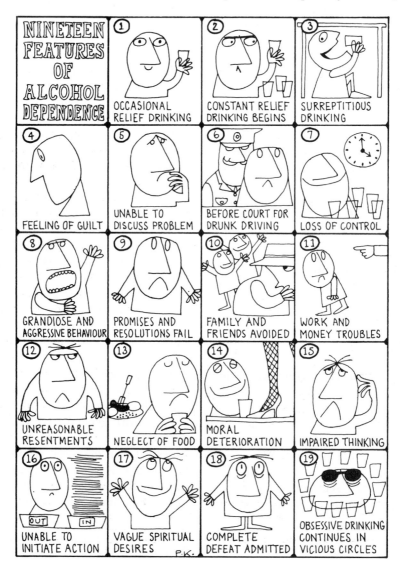

Fig. 19.5

is hard to prove. A butyrophenone neuroleptic may be needed for psychosis; not a phenothiazine, which may precipitate seizures. General aspects of care, e.g. attention to fluid and electrolyte balance, are important. Psychosocial therapy is more important than drugs, which are only of limited use.

The surprising beneficial effect of any therapy in the initial period of its trial is explained by the enthusiasm of the therapist combined with insufficient length to follow-up.[47]

It is usual to administer vitamins, especially thiamine, in which alcoholics are commonly deficient, and i.v. glucose unaccompanied by thiamine may precipitate Wernicke's encephalopathy.

Conclusion on the social use of alcohol. Alcoholism is a major scourge of the human race and the most dangerous property of alcohol is the readiness with which it produces dependence. Its acute effects and the rapidity of their onset and duration (due to its pharmacokinetic properties) allow users easily to adjust their intake to achieve the desired results; inability to abstain renders alcohol the menace to society that it is, as well as a genial social pleasure.

Knowledge of daily intake[48] is valuable to allow both prediction of disease and prevention, both by users and their medical advisers. Amounts suggested here relate to risk of *hepatic cirrhosis*, and not to acute effects. A *daily* consumption of 10 units (80 g) in *men* and 6 units (48 g) in *women* exposes the drinker to *serious* liver injury. But such injury may occur with 6 units (men) and as little as 2 units (women).[49]

If challenged by a patient to advise a safe upper limit (which, in fact, cannot be *accurately* defined), the doctor might reasonably reply: men, 3 units per day: women, 2 units per day. Anyone taking more than this should have 2 alcohol-free days per week.

Alcoholics with established cirrhosis have usually consumed about 23 units (184 g) daily for 10 years. It has long been thought that total consumption accumulated over time was the crucial factor for cirrhosis. Heavy drinkers may develop hepatic cirrhosis at a rate of about 2% per annum. The type of drink (beer, wine, spirits) is not significantly relevant to the health consequences.

A standard bottle of spirits (750 ml) contains 240 g of alcohol. A standard human cannot metabolise more than about 170 g per day. People whose intake is concentrated at the weekend allow their livers time for repair and have a lower risk of liver injury than do those who consume the same total on an even daily basis.

Drinking amongst medical students. In a questionnaire survey (350 students, 260 replies) the mean consumption was: males 20 units/week; females 14 units/week. Male consumption was similar to the matched general population, female consumption was higher. Of males 23% exceeded 35 units/week and 22% of women exceeded 21 units/week. Smoking was positively associated with heavy drinking. 'The results suggest that some medical students are compromising their future health and their academic performance through excessive drinking.'[50]

Indicator of heavy drinking. 50% of men who admit drinking above 450 g (56 units) a week have a raised plasma concentration of the enzyme gamma-glutamyltransferase (GGT >50 IU). The rise is due to hepatic enzyme induction by alcohol and perhaps also to cellular damage. The finding is not specific for alcohol, indicating only liver injury. Various other measures including aspartate aminotransferase, blood urate, triglyceride and raised mean corpuscle volume have been used as markers, though they are all non-specific. But taken together, these measures identify 75% of heavy drinkers; they return to normal rapidly on abstention (except mean corpuscular volume) which can be misleading. A skilfully worded questionnaire may yet be the most sensitive test of all.

[47] Kalant H. Quarterly Journal of Studies in Alcoholism 1962; 23: 52.

[48] For these and other data on alcohol, see Alcohol and disease. Br Med Bull 1982.

[49] Women appear to be more susceptible to liver injury than are men. This is not solely a matter of pharmacokinetics but may be also due to the greater occurrence of autoimmune reactivity that has been shown in women with alcoholic liver disease.

[50] Collier D J, Beales I L P. Br Med J 1989; 299: 19

There is a strong association between road traffic accidents in older car drivers and raised blood GGT concentration, suggesting that older problem drinkers (who often do not have an illegal blood concentration of alcohol at the time of the accident, as is characteristically the case with younger drivers) have an increased accident liability independent of recent alcohol consumption.

Pregnancy, the fetus and lactation

Pregnancy is unlikely to occur in severely alcoholic women (who have amenorrhoea secondary to liver injury). The spontaneous miscarriage rate in the second trimester is doubled by consumption of 1–2 units/day.

Fetal injury can occur in early pregnancy (fetal alcohol syndrome). It may be due to the metabolite, acetaldehyde, and so acute (binge) consumption is more hazardous than similar total intake on a daily basis. Plainly, disulfiram should not be used in a woman who is or might become pregnant.

The vulnerable period of pregnancy is at 4–10 weeks. Because of this, prevention cannot be reliably achieved after diagnosis of pregnancy (usually 3–8 weeks).

There is no level of maternal consumption that can be guaranteed safe for the fetus. But it is plainly unrealistic to leave the matter there, and it has been suggested that if the ideal of total abstinence is unachievable then two *small* drinks (< 2 units) per day should be the target, or, safer, 7 units per week. But *serious* risk requires consumption exceeding 10 units/week.

In addition to the fetal alcohol syndrome there is general fetal/embryonic growth retardation (1% for every 10 g alcohol per day) and this is not 'caught up' later.

Fetal alcohol syndrome includes the following characteristics: microcephaly, mental retardation with irritability in infancy, low body weight and length, poor coordination, hypotonia, small eyeballs and short palpebral fissures, lack of nasal bridge.[51]

---

[51] For pictures see Streissguth A P et al. Lancet 1985; 2: 85.

Children of about 10% of alcohol abusers may show the syndrome, with 13% having some alcohol-related abnormalities. In women consuming 12 units of alcohol per day the incidence may be as much as 30%.

Lactation. Even small amounts of alcohol taken by the mother delay motor development in the child; an effect on mental development is uncertain.

Pharmacological deterrence

Disulfiram (Antabuse). In alcoholics who are fairly well *and cooperative*, an attempt may be made to discourage drinking by inducing immediate unpleasantness. Disulfiram inhibits the enzyme aldehyde dehydrogenase so that acetaldehyde (toxic metabolite of alcohol) accumulates. This is so unpleasant that the patient does not wish to experience it again: disulfiram thus reinforces the perhaps otherwise ineffectual will-power which threat of delayed injury may not do. Such therapy by intimidation, whether self-administered or thrust on the patient (aversion), is not to be expected to play an major part in the treatment of alcoholism, a disease that is primarily a manifestation of psychological disorder. When patients are given disulfiram some have given a test dose of alcohol under supervision (after the fifth day), so that they can be taught what to expect and also to induce an aversion from alcohol. That this is not to be lightly undertaken is shown by the fact that, though rare, deaths have occurred following the 'test drink'. Such a test is now considered unwise except where full resuscitation facilities are available. A typical reaction of medium severity comes on about 5 min after taking alcohol and consists of generalised vasodilatation and fall in blood pressure, sweating, dyspnoea, headache, chest pain, nausea and vomiting; severe reactions include convulsions and circulatory collapse; they may last several hours. Disulfiram causes a similar reaction with paraldehyde and inhibits metabolism of warfarin, phenytoin and diazepam. The effect persists for 4 days after cessation of use.

It is clear that no patient should be given disulfiram without the fullest previous explanation and the certainty that the possible serious consequences of drinking a lot of alcohol in a few minutes are understood; even use of alcohol-based after-shave lotion has caused a reaction.

The disulfiram-alcohol interaction has long been known to workers in the rubber industry in which the substance is used, but it was not applied to therapeutics until after the chance experience of two Danish pharmacologists.[52]

Dr. Hald suggested that disulfiram could be employed as an anthelmintic . . . . The drug was tested on rabbits infected with worms and results were sufficiently encouraging to warrant clinical trial.

According to the custom in this house we never give a new drug to patients before we have taken at least double the recommended dose ourselves. During this routine procedure Dr. Hald and I discovered that we had developed an intolerance to alcohol. We compared symptoms and found them identical. The only thing we had in common was the tablets.

Further investigation disclosed the mechanism of the effect.

Emetics, administered after drinking, have been used in the 'aversion' treatment of alcoholism, to establish a conditioned dislike.

ALCOHOLIC DRINKS

The pharmacology of alcoholic drinks is not the same as the pharmacology of alcohol. The drinks contain other ingredients that may reduce the rate of absorption of alcohol (carbohydrate in beer), act as a carminative (essential oils), or diuretic (juniper oil in gin) or inhibit enzymes that are concerned in some drug metabolism. There is no conclusive evidence on this point, but there is reason to believe that the effects of ethanol in some drinks are prolonged by the presence of other substances, e.g. propyl to octyl alcohols, ethers, aldehydes, which delay ethanol metabolism by occupying the same metabolic paths (competition). These other ingredients are themselves hardly more toxic than ethanol. It should be remembered that when enough alcoholic drink has been taken to cause 'hangover', subjects have commonly debauched themselves

in other ways too. Dehydration (due to diuresis) is a prominent cause of 'hangover'; it may be usefully mitigated by drinking a substantial volume of water before going to bed.

During convalescence from *acute viral hepatitis* moderate alcohol consumption does not (as has long been supposed) lead to relapse or chronicity.

ALCOHOL AND OTHER DRUGS

All cerebral depressants (hypnotics, tranquillisers, antiepileptics, antihistamines) can either potentiate or synergise with alcohol, and this can be important at *ordinary* doses in relation to car driving. But, when supplies of hypnotics or tranquillisers are given to patients known to drink heavily, they should be warned to omit the drugs when they have been drinking. Deaths have occurred from these combinations.

Alcohol-dependent people with a physical tolerance are relatively tolerant of some other cerebral depressant drugs (hydrocarbon anaesthetics and barbiturates), but of course the synergism with these drugs still occurs. There is no significant acquired cross-tolerance with opioids.

Sulphonylureas (antidiabetics) cause a disulfiram-like reaction, as may metronidazole, griseofulvin, some cephalosporins and chloral.

Hepatic metabolism (see also Pharmacokinetics above). Substantial acute doses of alcohol depress hepatic hydroxylation and so increase the systemic bioavailability of drugs subject to high hepatic first-pass extraction to an extent that may have clinical importance.

Oral anticoagulants. Control may be disturbed by alcohol inhibiting hepatic metabolism directly, or enhancing it by enzyme induction; moderate drinking is unlikely to cause trouble.

Anticonvulsants can be metabolised faster due to enzyme induction and this contributes to its well-known adverse effect on epilepsy.

Miscellaneous uses of alcohol

In addition to those already mentioned, its use in strong solutions as an irritant has given alcohol a reputation as a restorative in fainting. When

---

[52] Dr. Erik Jacobsen. Personal communication.

such stimulation is indicated, a slap in the face is just as irritant, cheaper, always handy and cannot enter the lungs and cause pneumonia. Alcohol precipitates protein and is used to harden the skin in bedridden patients. Local application also reduces sweating and may allay itching. As a skin antiseptic 70% by weight (76% by volume) is most effective. Stronger solutions are less effective. Alcohol injections are sometimes used to destroy nervous tissue in cases of intractable pain (trigeminal neuralgia, carcinoma involving nerves).

OPIOIDS: HEROIN etc: see Chapter 15.

PSYCHODYSLEPTICS OR HALLUCINOGENS

These substances produce *mental changes that resemble those of some psychotic states.* They are used by people seeking a new experience or escape.

But psychiatrists also have used these drugs in supervised therapeutic sessions to encourage the release and reliving of unconscious material in the hope that, assisted by appropriate psychotherapy, the patient may gain insight and an improved ability to cope with his environment. Such use remains experimental and potentially dangerous (suicide, prolonged psychosis).

Experiences with these drugs vary greatly with the subject's expectations, existing frame of mind and personality and environment. Subjects can be prepared so that they are more likely to have a good 'trip' than a bad 'trip'.

EXPERIENCES WITH PSYCHODYSLEPTICS

The following brief account of experiences with **LSD** (lysergic acid diethylamide, lysergide) in normal subjects will serve as a model. Experiences with *mescaline* and *psilocybin* are similar:

Vision may become blurred and there may be hallucinations; these generally do not occur in the blind and are less if the subject is blind-folded. Objects appear distorted, and trivial things, e.g.

a mark on a wall, may change shape and acquire special significance.

Auditory acuity increases, but hallucinations are uncommon. Subjects who do not ordinarily appreciate music may suddenly come to do so.

Foods may feel coarse and gritty in the mouth.

Limbs may be left in uncomfortable positions.

Time may seem to stop or to pass slowly, but usually it gets faster and thousands of years may seem suddenly to go by.

The subject may feel relaxed and supremely happy, or may become fearful or depressed. Feelings of depersonalisation and dreamy states occur.

The experience lasts a few hours, depending on the dose; intervals of normality then occur and become progressively longer.

Somatic symptoms include nausea, dizziness, paraesthesia, weakness, drowsiness, tremors, dilated pupils, ataxia. Effects on the cardiovascular system and respiration vary and probably reflect fluctuating anxiety.

So disrupting to the individual are some of these drugs, particularly in respect of thought processes, that legal control is needed, perhaps especially in view of the possibility of their use in a 'person in a position of high authority when faced with decisions of great importance'.[53]

There is no shortage of accounts of experience with psychodysleptics, because there has been a vogue amongst intellectuals, begun by Mr. Aldous Huxley,[54] for publishing their experiences. Subsequent accounts are tedious to most except their authors and to those who would do the same; they have little pharmacological importance and reveal more about the author's egocentricity than about pharmacology. The same applies to published accounts of what it is like to be a drug addict.

INDIVIDUAL SUBSTANCES

Lysergide (LSD)

Lysergic acid provides the nucleus of the ergot alkaloids and it was during a study of derivatives

---

[53] Hoffer A. Clin Pharmacol Ther 1965; 6: 183.
[54] Huxley A. The doors of preception. London: Chatto and Windus, 1964.

of this in a search for an analeptic that in 1943 a Swiss worker investigating LSD (which structurally resembles nikethamide) felt queer and had visual hallucinations. This led him to take a dose of the substance and so to discover its remarkable potency, an effective oral dose being about 30 µg. The $t_\frac{1}{2}$ is about 3 h.

Tachyphylaxis (acute tolerance) occurs to LSD. Psychological dependence may occur, physical dependence does not.

LSD has been used in the dying; it induced analgesia and indifference. Its effect on the brain may partly be due to antagonism of serotonin at autoreceptors.

Serious adverse effects include: psychotic reaction (which can be delayed in onset) with suicide; teratogenic and mutagenic effects are speculative and the risk is small at worst.

LSD has curious effects in animals: green sunfish become aggressive, Siamese fighting fish float nose up, tail down, and goats walk in unaccustomed stereotyped patterns. The elephant exhibits episodically a form of sexual or delinquent behaviour known as 'musth'. LSD 100 µg/kg i.m. was given to an animal (the usual dose for man is up to about 2 µg/kg) to test whether this induced a similar state. The elephant developed laryngospasm and status epilepticus and died.[55] Badly planned experiments give useless results.

Mescaline is an alkaloid from a Mexican cactus (peyotl), the top of which is cut off and dried and used as 'peyote buttons' in religious ceremonies. Mescaline does not induce serious dependence and the drug has little importance except to members of some North and Central American societies and to psychiatrists and biochemists who are interested in the mechanism of induced psychotic states.

Tenamfetamine (MDA: methylenedioxymethamphetamine) is structurally related to mescaline as well as to amphetamine: it is popularly known as 'ecstasy': allied substances include STP (DOM) and DOB.

Phencyclidine (angel dust) was made in a search for a better intravenous anaesthetic. It is related to pethidine. It was found to induce analgesia without unconsciousness, but with amnesia, in man. However, the postoperative course was complicated by psychiatric disturbance (agitation, abreactions, hallucinations). As the interest of anaesthetists waned, so that of psychiatrists grew, and the drug has been used in experimental therapy. *Ketamine* originates from this work.

Psilocybin is derived from varieties of the fungus *Psilocybe* ('magic mushrooms') that grow in many countries. It is related to LSD.

Cannabis[56]

Cannabis is obtained from the annual plant *Cannabis sativa* (hemp) and its varieties *C. indica* and *C. americana*. The preparations that are smoked are called marihuana (grass, pot, weed, etc.) and consist of crushed leaves and flowers. There is a wide variety of regional names, e.g. ganja (India, Caribbean), kif (Morocco), dagga (Africa). The resin scraped off the plant is known as hashish (hash). The term cannabis is used to include all the above preparations. Since most preparations are illegally prepared it is not surprising that they are impure and of variable potency. The plant grows wild in the Americas,[57] Africa and Asia. It can also be grown successfully in the open in the warmer southern areas of Britain.

Pharmacokinetics

Of the scores of chemical compounds that the resin contains, the most important are the oily cannabinoids, including tetrahydrocannabinol (THC), which is the chief cause of the psychic action. Samples of resin vary greatly in the amounts and proportions of these cannabinoids according to their country of origin; and as the sample ages, its THC content declines. As a result, the THC content of samples can vary from almost zero to 8%.

Smoke from a cannabis cigarette (the usual

---

[55] Cohen S. Ann Rev Pharmacol 1967; 7: 301.

[56] We are grateful to Professor Sir William Paton for advice on cannabis.
[57] The commonest pollen in the air of San Francisco, California is said to be that of the cannabis plant, illegally cultivated.

mode of use is to inhale and hold the breath to allow maximum absorption) delivers 25–50% of the THC content to the respiratory tract.

THC ($t_{\frac{1}{2}}$ 4 d) and other cannabinoids undergo extensive biotransformation in the body, yielding scores of metabolites, several of which are themselves psychoactive. They are extremely lipid soluble and are stored in body fat from which they are slowly released.[58] Hepatic drug metabolising enzymes are inhibited acutely but may also be induced by chronic use of crude preparations.

Pharmacodynamics

Psychological reactions are very varied, being much influenced by the behaviour of the group. They commence within minutes of starting to smoke and last 2–3 h. Euphoria is common, though not invariable, with giggling or laughter which can seem pointless to an observer. Sensations become more vivid, especially visual, and contrast and intensity of colour can increase, although no change in acuity occurs. Size of objects and distance are distorted. Sense of time can disappear altogether, leaving a sometimes distressing sense of timelessness. Recent memory and selective attention are impaired; the beginning of a sentence may be forgotten before it is finished, and the subject is very suggestible and easily distracted. Psychological tests such as mental arithmetic, digit-symbol substitution and pursuit meter tests show impairment. These effects may be accompanied by feelings of deep insight and truth. Memory defect may persist for weeks after abstinence.

Once memory is impaired, concentration becomes less effective, since the object of attention is less well remembered. With this may go an insensitivity to danger or the consequences of actions.

A striking phenomenon is the intermittent wave-like nature of these effects which affects mood, visual impressions, time sense, spatial sense, and other functions.

The desired effects of cannabis, as of other psychodysleptics, depend not only on the expectation of the user and the dose, but also on the environmental situation and personality. Genial or revelatory experiences may indeed occur, e.g. 'Haschich Fudge'[59]

(which anyone can whip up on a rainy day). This is the food of Paradise . . . euphoria and brilliant storms of laughter, ecstatic reveries and extension of one's personality on several simultaneous planes are to be complacently expected. Almost anything St. Teresa[60] did, you can do better . . .

But this cannot be relied on.

The effects can be unpleasant, especially in inexperienced subjects, particularly timelessness and the feeling of loss of control of mental processes. Feelings of unease, sometimes amounting to anguish and acute panic occur as well as 'flashbacks' of previously experienced hallucinations, e.g. on LSD. There is also, especially in the habitual user, a tendency to paranoid thinking. High or habitual use can be followed by a psychotic state; this is usually reversible, quickly with brief periods of cannabis use, but more slowly after sustained exposures.

The effect of an acute dose usually ends in drowsiness and sleep. It is claimed that death has not occurred.

Tolerance, with continued heavy use, and a withdrawal syndrome occur (depression, anxiety, sleep disturbance, tremor and other symptoms), and many users find it very difficult to abandon cannabis use. In studies on self-administration by monkeys, spontaneous use did not occur, but once use was initiated, drug-seeking behaviour developed. Subjects who have become tolerant to LSD or opioids as a result of repeated dosage respond normally to cannabis but there appears to be cross-tolerance between cannabis and alcohol.

'Amotivational syndrome'. This term digni-

---

[58] When a chronic user discontinues, cannabinoids remain detectable in the urine for an average of 4 weeks and it can be as long as 11 weeks before 10 consecutive daily tests are negative (Ellis G M et al. Clin Pharmacol Ther 1986; 38: 572).

[59] From The Alice B. Toklas cook book. London: Michael Joseph. 1954. The author was companion to Gertrude (rose is a rose is a rose) Stein (1874–1946).
[60] St. Teresa of Avila (1515–82) was noted for her power of levitation.

fies an imprecisely characterised state, ranging from a feeling of unease and sense of not being fully effective, up to a gross lethargy, with social passivity and deterioration. It is difficult to assess, when personal traits and intellectual rejection of technological civilisation are also taken into account. Yet the reversibility of the state, its association with cannabis use, and its recognition by cannabis users make it impossible to ignore.

Escalation theory (see p. 324).

Cannabis and skilled tasks, e.g. car driving. General performance in both motor and psychological tests deteriorates, more in naive than in experienced subjects. Effects may be similar to alcohol, but experiments in which the subject is unaware that he is being tested (and so does not compensate voluntarily) are difficult to do, as with alcohol. Some scientists claim the effects are negligible but this view has been 'put in proper perspective' by a commentator[61] who asked how these scientists 'would feel if told that the pilot of their international jet taking them to a psychologists' conference, was just having a reefer or two before opening up the controls.'

Other effects. Cannabis smoked or taken by mouth produces reddening of the eyeballs (probably the forerunner of the general dilation of blood vessels and fall of blood pressure with higher doses), unsteadiness (particularly for precise movements), and tachycardia. The smoke produces the usual smoker's cough, and the tar from reefer cigarettes is as carcinogenic in animal experiments as cigarette tobacco tar. Increase in appetite is commonly experienced.

Cannabis is teratogenic in animals, but effect in humans is unproved, although there is impaired fetal growth with repeated use.

Management of adverse reactions to psychodysleptics ('bad trips')

Mild and sometimes even severe episodes can be managed by reassurance including talk, 'talking the patient down', and physical contact, hand holding, etc. (LSD and mescaline). The objective is to help the patient relate his experience to reality and to appreciate that his mental experiences are drug-induced and will abate. Because short-term memory is disrupted the treatment can be very time-consuming since the therapist cannot absent himself without risking relapse. But with phencyclidine such intervention may have the opposite effect, i.e. overstimulation. It is therefore appropriate to sedate all anxious or excited subjects with diazepam (or chlorpromazine or haloperidol). With sedation the 'premorbid ego' may be rapidly re-established.

If the 'bad trip' is due to overdose of an antimuscarinic drug, natural or synthetic, then diazepam is specially preferred, or a neuroleptic with no or minimal antimuscarinic effects, e.g. haloperidol. A dose of anticholinesterase that penetrates the central nervous system (physostigmine: tacrine) is effective in severe reaction to an antimuscarinic.

STIMULANTS

Cocaine

Cocaine (see also local anaesthetics) use is a widespread and ancient practice amongst South American peasants who chew coca leaves with lime to release the alkaloid. It is claimed to give relief from fatigue and hunger; and also from altitude sickness in the Andes, experienced even by natives when journeying by car or other 'fast' transportation; and also to induce a pleasant introverted mental state. Remarkable feats of endurance attributed to chewing coca leaves have been reported, but there is no sound scientific confirmation of them. A United Nations enquiry into coca-leaf chewing (1950) reported that there was psychological but no physical dependence. It also reported that its use caused physical exhaustion rather than the reverse, and advocated gradual suppression in the interest of the populations concerned. But what may have been (or even still may be) an acceptable feature of these ancient stable societies has now developed into a massive, criminal business, not for leaf chewing, but for the manufacture and export of purified cocaine to supply an eager and lucrative demand from unhappy but economically

---

[61] Dr G Milner.

richer societies where its use constitutes an intractable social problem. These economically developed societies, which cannot control social demand and importation, seek to eliminate the drug at its source in peasant societies that have come to rely on it for economic subsistence. When coca plantations are destroyed great distress ensues to local populations by a combination of economic deprivation and removal of the coca leaf, which, when used in the traditional way, helps to make tolerable lives of deprivation.

Cocaine (snow) is used as snuff (snorting), swallowed, smoked (below) or injected i.v. It is taken to obtain the immediate characteristic intense euphoria which is often followed in a few minutes by dysphoria. This leads to repeated use (10–45 min) during 'runs' of usually about 12 h. After the 'run' there follows the 'crash' (dysphoria, irritability, hypersomnia) lasting hours to days. After the 'crash' there may be depression ('cocaine blues') and decreased capacity to experience pleasure (anhedonia) for days to weeks.

Psychological dependence with intense compulsive drug-seeking behaviour is characteristic of even short-term use, but physical dependence is arguably slight or absent. Tachyphylaxis, acute tolerance, occurs.

The psychotropic effects of cocaine are similar to those of amphetamine (euphoria and excitement) but briefer and are due to blockade of the uptake of noradrenaline into adrenergic nerve endings, thus increasing its concentration at receptors; this information is relevant to treating overdose.

Intranasal use causes mucosal vasoconstriction, anosmia and eventually necrosis and perforation of the nasal septum.

Smoking involves converting the non-volatile HCl into the volatile 'free base' or 'crack' (by extracting the HCl with alkali); then vaporising it by heat (it pops or cracks) in a special glass 'pipe', or mixing it with tobacco in a cigarette. Inhalation with breath-holding allows pulmonary absorption that is about as rapid as an i.v. injection. It induces an intense euphoric state. The mouth and pharynx become anaesthetised.

Intravenous use gives the expected rapid effect (kick, flash, rush). Cocaine may be mixed with heroin (as 'speedball').

The $t_{\frac{1}{2}}$ of cocaine is 50 min; it is metabolised by plasma esterases.

Overdose is common amongst users (up to 22% of heavy users report losing consciousness). The desired euphoria and excitement turns to acute fear, with psychotic symptoms, convulsions, hypertension, tachycardia, dysrhythmias, hyperthermia; and coronary vasospasm may occur. Treatment is chosen according to the clinical picture (and the known mode of action), from amongst, e.g. haloperidol (rather than chlorpromazine) for mental disturbance: diazepam for convulsions: labetalol or a vasodilator for hypertension, and appropriate antidysrhythmic agents.

Fetal growth is retarded by maternal use, but teratogenicity is uncertain.

Amphetamine (p. 295) effects and use are similar to cocaine, but 'runs' are longer.

Caffeine, see p. 297.

Khat. The leaves of the khat shrub (*Catha edulis*) contain an alkaloid (cathinone) structurally similar to amphetamine. They are chewed fresh (for maximum alkaloid content) so that the habit was confined to geographical areas favourable to the shrub (Arabia, E. Africa) until modern transportation allowed wider distribution. Khat chewers (mostly male) became euphoric, loquacious, excited, hyperactive and even manic. As with some other drug dependencies subjects may give priority to their drug needs above personal, family and other social and economic responsibilities. Cultivation takes up serious amounts of scarce arable land and irrigation water.

GUIDE TO FURTHER READING

Ashton C H 1990 Solvent abuse: little progress after 20 years. British Medical Journal 300: 135

Benowitz N L 1988 Pharmacologic aspects of cigarette smoking and nicotine addiction. New England Journal of Medicine 319: 1318

Brooke O G et al 1989 Effects on birth weight of smoking, alcohol, caffeine, socioeconomic factors, and psychosocial stress. British Medical Journal 298: 795

Charness M E 1989 Ethanol and the nervous system. New England Journal of Medicine 321: 442

Collier D J et al 1989 Drinking among medical students: a questionnaire survey. British Medical Journal 299: 19

Dunbar J A et al 1987 Drinking and driving: choosing the legal limits. British Medical Journal 295: 1458

Editorial 1991 Nicotine use after the year 2000. Lancet 337: 1191

Fielding J E et al 1988 Health effects of involuntary smoking. New England Journal of Medicine 319: 1452: and, Angell M 1990 The interpretation of epidemiological studies. ibidem 323: 823

Forrest F et al 1991 Reported social alcohol consumption during pregnancy and infants' development at 18 months. British Medical Journal 303: 22

Gawin F H et al 1988 Cocaine and other stimulants: actions, abuse, and treatment. New England Journal of Medicine 318: 1173

Grunberg N E 1991 Smoking cessation and weight gain. New England Journal of Medicine 324: 768

Hallaghan J B et al 1989 Anabolic-androgenic steroid use by athletes. New England Journal of Medicine 321: 1042

Jackson R et al 1991 Alcohol consumption and risk of coronary disease. British Medical Journal 303: 211

Juntunen J et al 1988 Doctors' drinking habits and consumption of alcohol. British Medical Journal 297: 951

LaCroix A Z et al 1991 Smoking and mortality among older men and women in three communities. New England Journal of Medicine 324: 1619

Lieber C S 1988 Biochemical and molecular basis of alcohol-induced injury to liver and other organs. New England Journal of Medicine 319: 1639

Marc B et al 1989 Managing drug dealers who swallow the evidence. British Medical Journal 299: 1082

Rimm E B et al 1991 Prospective study of alcohol consumption and risk of coronary disease in men. Lancet 338: 464

Schenker S et al 1990 The risk of alcohol intake in men and women: All may not be equal. New England Journal of Medicine 322: 127

Tozun N et al 1991 Safety of alcohol after viral hepatitis. Lancet 337: 1079

Tzu-Chin Wu et al 1988 Pulmonary hazards of smoking marijuana as compared with tobacco. New England Journal of Medicine 318: 347

Wynder E L et al 1959 Cancer and coronary artery disease in Seventh-Day adventists. Cancer 12: 1016[62]

[62] This curious by-way is a study of lung cancer in Seventh Day Adventists, in the USA. It appears that members of this religious sect, which prohibits smoking, have an incidence of lung-cancer one-eighth of that of non-members. Indeed the only two men with lung cancer were converts who had smoked cigarettes until middle-age. In respect of cancer of sites not associated with smoking there was no difference from the control group, so that Seventh Day Adventists evidently have no general immunity from cancer. Therefore, to accommodate this evidence to the hypothesis of a genetic cause of both smoking and lung cancer, it would be necessary to stipulate that those born into the sect, but not those converted to it, inherit a low susceptibility to lung cancer.

'To many it will come as no surprise to learn that the benefits of religious observances are by no means restricted to the future life. But not often before can the evidence have been put on such a sure statistical basis.' (Editorial. A new angle on smoking. Br Med J 1959; 2: 1465.)

20

Anaesthesia and neuromuscular block

SYNOPSIS

General anaesthetics and neuromuscular blocking agents belong to the few classes of drugs whose actual administration is, by general consent, virtually confined to trained specialists. Nevertheless, anaesthesia as well as perioperative care must sometimes be conducted by non-specialists and their needs are particularly borne in mind in this chapter.

- General anaesthesia
- Pharmacology of anaesthetics
- Inhalation agents
- Intravenous anaesthetics
- Muscle relaxants: neuromuscular blocking drugs
- Local anaesthetics
- Obstetric analgesia and anaesthesia
- Anaesthesia in patients already taking drugs
- Anaesthesia in the diseased, old age and childhood; sedation in intensive therapy units

Acknowledgement: we are grateful to the World Health Organization for permission to quote WHO Model prescribing information: drugs used in anaesthesia (1989).

GENERAL ANAESTHESIA

Until the mid-19th century such surgery as was possible had to be done at tremendous speed. Surgeons did their best for terrified patients with alcohol, opium, hyoscine[1] and cannabis; occasionally by concussion with a wooden bowl or partial suffocation; the great French surgeon Dupuytren (1777–1835) prepared a patient for surgery by making a brutal remark which caused the subject to faint. With the introduction of general anaesthesia surgeons could operate for the first time with careful deliberation. The problem of inducing quick, safe and easily reversible unconsciousness for any desired length of time in man only began to be solved in the 1840s when the long-known substances nitrous oxide, ether, and chloroform were introduced in rapid succession.

The details surrounding the first use of surgical anaesthesia make unedifying reading at times for there were bitter disputes on priority following an attempt to take out a patent for ether.

Sir James Simpson, who was to popularise chloroform (1847), heard of the initial trials of ether in 1846 and wrote,[2] 'It is a glorious thought, I can think of naught else.' Just before

---

[1] A Japanese pioneer of about 1800 wished to test the anaesthetic efficacy of a herbal mixture including solanaceous plants (hyoscine-type alkaloids). His elderly mother volunteered as subject since she was anyway expected to die soon. But the pioneer administered it to his wife for, 'as all three agreed, he could find another wife, but could never get another mother' (JAMA 1966; 197: 10).

his death in 1870 he summarised the chief events of the introduction of anaesthesia in the USA.

It appears to me that we might correctly state the whole matter as follows:

1. That on the 11th December, 1844, Dr. Wells had, at Hartford, by his own desire and suggestion, one of his upper molar teeth extracted without any pain, in consequence of his having deeply breathed nitrous oxide gas for the purpose, as suggested nearly half a century before by Sir Humphrey Davy.

2. That having with others proved, in a limited series of cases, the anaesthetic powers of nitrous oxide gas, Dr. Wells proceeded to Boston to lay his discovery before the Medical School and Hospital there, but was unsuccessful in the single attempt which he made, in consequence of the gas-bag being removed too soon, and that he was hooted away by his audience, as if the whole matter were an imposition, and was totally discouraged.

3. That Dr. Wells' former pupil and partner, Dr. Morton of Boston, was present with Dr. Wells when he made his experiments there.

4. That on the 30th September, 1846, Dr. Morton extracted a tooth without any pain, whilst the patient was breathing sulphuric ether, this fact and discovery of itself making a NEW ERA in anaesthetics and in surgery.'

5 & 6. That ether was soon used in general surgery[3] and midwifery.

It should be chastening to modern drug developers that the first two effective general anaesthetics, nitrous oxide and ether, are still, when used together, after nearly 150 years, the *safest* choice for *unpractised* doctors who find themselves obliged by circumstances to administer a prolonged general anaesthetic.

The next important developments in anaesthesia were in the 20th century when the appearance of new drugs both as primary general anaesthetics and as adjuvants (muscle relaxants),

new apparatus, and clinical expertise in rendering prolonged anaesthesia safe, enabled surgeons to increase their range. No longer was the duration and kind of surgery determined by patients' capacity to endure pain.

Stages of general anaesthesia

Surgical anaesthesia using a single agent, e.g. ether, is classically divided into four *stages*, of which the third stage is subdivided into four *planes* (obviously, each merges with the next).

But the attainment of surgical anaesthesia (sleep, analgesia and muscular relaxation) with a single drug requires high doses that are liable to carry inconveniences and hazards, e.g. slow and unpleasant recovery, depression of cardiovascular function, and modern practice employs different drugs to attain each objective so that the classic stages no longer occur in visible succession.

Nevertheless, since these stages provide a background of understanding, and since the conveniences of sophisticated practice are not always available, an account is provided, as follows:

The procession of stages derives from descriptions of ether anaesthesia in unpremedicated patients, a slow unpleasant process. With modern techniques of i.v. anaesthesia and of premedicated inhalation, stages 1 and 2 may hardly be noticed by patient or anaesthetist.

Stage 1: analgesia. Analgesia is partial until stage 2 is about to be reached. Consciousness and sense of touch are retained and sense of hearing is increased.

Stage 2: delirium. The patient is unconscious, but automatic movements may occur. He may shout coherently or incoherently, become violent or leap up and run about. The prevention of these unpleasant manifestations lies in a skilful, smooth and quick induction in quiet surroundings. Sudden death, probably due to vagal inhibition of the heart or to sensitisation of the heart to adrenaline (endogenous or exogenous) by the anaesthetic agent, may occur in a violent second stage.

Stage 3: surgical anaesthesia. This is divided into four *planes* (see Fig. 20.1) and the

---

[2] Comrie J D. History of Scottish medicine, 2nd edn. London: Bailliére, Tindall and Cox, 1932, for Wellcome History of Medicine Museum.

[3] In December 1846 the first operation in England under ether (amputation of the leg of a butler from Harley Street) was conducted at University College Hospital, London. The surgeon, Robert Liston, after removing the leg in 28 s, a skill necessary to compensate for the previous lack of anaesthetics, turned to the watching students, saying, 'This Yankee dodge, Gentlemen, beats mesmerism hollow'. That night he anaesthetised his House Surgeon 'in the presence of two ladies'. (Merrington W R. University College Hospital and its Medical School: A history. London: Heinemann, 1976.)

required depth differs according to the kind of operation to be performed. Depth is determined by noting characteristic changes in respiration, pupils, spontaneous eyeball movements, reflexes and muscle tone.

Stage 4: medullary paralysis. Arrival at this stage constitutes an overdose.

Drugs in the practice of general anaesthesia

The practice of the anaesthetist has 3 main parts:

1. Before surgery, the assessment of the patient's psychological and physical condition including the relevance of any existing drug

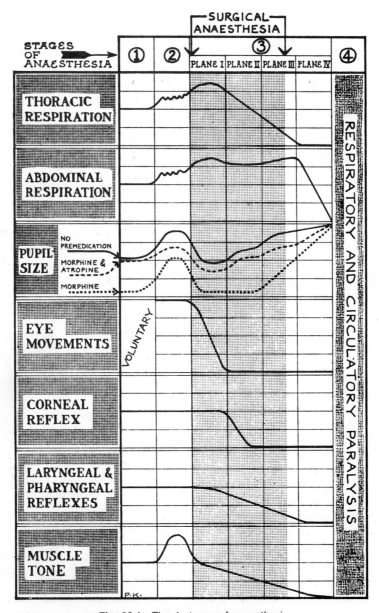

Fig. 20.1   The 4 stages of anaesthesia

therapy, all of which may influence the choice of the *premedication*, which may affect the choice of drugs in 2 below.

2. During surgery, the production of:

- unconsciousness
- analgesia
- muscular relaxation

Whilst these can be produced by a single drug, e.g. ether, thiopentone, to do so carries the disadvantages of heavy dosage (cardiac and respiratory depression, slow recovery), and professional anaesthetists employ a drug for each purpose from the wide range available.

3. After surgery, recovery, i.e. reversal of anaesthesia and neuromuscular block, and relief of pain and other aspects of postoperative care.

These 3 components are interdependent, the choice of drugs to be used at any one point affecting the choice of drugs both before and after; for instance drugs used in premedication may reduce both the amount of general anaesthetic and the postoperative medication required. Safety and comfort for the patient are paramount, and good operating conditions for the surgeon are also in the interest of the patient; but the provision of one may compromise the others. The problem may be approached in many different ways, using different combinations of the wide array of drugs that is available.

Simplicity enhances safety, for it is much easier to reach a clear diagnosis when few drugs have been given than when many drugs have inevitably confused the picture. With drugs, safety does not lie in numbers.

The anaesthetists' job is nowadays complicated by the fact that they are often presented with patients already taking drugs affecting the central nervous and cardiovascular systems.

The techniques of administration of anaesthetic drugs and the physical control of respiration are of great importance, but are outside the scope of this book. Premedication is treated relatively extensively as non-anaesthetists are more likely to find themselves concerned with it than with surgical anaesthesia.

Before surgery (premedication)

The principal aims are to provide:

- **Sedation and amnesia**. A patient who is going to have a surgical operation is naturally apprehensive, and it is kind to attempt to reduce this by explanation, reassurance and drugs. In one study a reassuring talk with the anaesthetist was found to have a greater calming effect than a barbiturate. But it cannot be assumed that all anaesthetists will be so successful. Preoperative preparation (which may commence on arrival in hospital for planned surgery, e.g. tranquillisers, and not merely 1 h before operation) is not solely humanitarian, for the discharge of adrenaline from the suprarenal medulla and the increased metabolic rate, which are concomitants of anxiety, render the patient both more difficult to anaesthetise and more liable to cardiac dysrhythmias with some anaesthetics.

Benzodiazepines promote desirable amnesia for the immediate postsurgical period.

Stress-induced increase in plasma cortisol is suppressed by adequate premedication.

Diazepam (oral, rectal, i.v.) is appropriate in adults; promethazine or chloral in children.

- **Analgesia** (an opioid), when there is existing pain or as a supplement to an anaesthetic agent having low analgesic effect, e.g. nitrous oxide, thiopentone. However, if postoperative pain is expected an analgesic may be given both before and at the end of the operation without waiting for the patient to complain of pain. This helps to avoid the postoperative restlessness that occurs if only sedatives were used preoperatively. Subanaesthetic doses of barbiturates actually have an anti-analgesic effect.

- **Inhibition of the parasympathetic autonomic system (antimuscarinic agent):**

to reduce bronchial and salivary secretions, which are liable to be profuse with the irritant ether and with ketamine; and to reduce any tendency to bronchospasm.

to reduce reflex bradycardia and hypotension using *atropine, hyoscine or glycopyrronium*.

Hyoscine can cause confusion in the old; Glycopyrronium does not readily enter the brain. The usual doses do not affect glaucoma adversely.

- There is a tendency nowadays to use lighter premedication and to adjust it to the expected needs of the patient and of the procedure to be undertaken.

Premedication should be chosen in the light of knowledge of patients' temperaments and of the way they react to the approaching ordeal, of their age, disease and medical history, the duration of surgery and whether it will be followed by severe pain, and of the anaesthetic agents that it is intended to use.

- **Routes of administration** are chosen according to general principles.
- **Timing**. Premedication is generally given 1 h before surgery.

- **The stomach**. A single dose of *a gastric ant-acid*, e.g. sodium citrate, may be given before a general anaesthetic as prophylaxis against aspiration of acid gastric contents (acid aspiration pneumonitis or Mendelson's syndrome); a histamine H_2-receptor blocker, e.g. ranitidine, is an alternative, to reduce gastric secretion volume as well as acidity. *Metoclopramide* hastens gastric emptying, usefully increases the tone of the lower oesophageal sphincter and is an antiemetic.

During surgery

The modern trend is to induce *unconsciousness, analgesia* and *muscular relaxation* with separate drugs. This triad can be produced with a single drug in large doses but the consequences of the resulting deep anaesthesia are unpleasant and may be dangerous.

A typical general anaesthetic consists of:

- *Induction*: thiopentone, i.v. (with suxamethonium if intubation is intended).
- *Maintenance*:
1. with nitrous oxide plus a volatile agent, e.g. halothane or ether, if the patient is to breathe spontaneously;
2. with nitrous oxide plus i.v. analgesic, e.g. fentanyl, morphine, pethidine, plus a competitive

neuromuscular blocking agent if muscle relaxation is needed for abdominal surgery (respiration will necessarily have to be provided by the anaesthetist); where neuromuscular block is used there is risk of a paralysed patient regaining consciousness (see Awareness under anaesthesia, p. 370).

If a neuromuscular blocking drug is not used, muscle relaxation can be provided by deep anaesthesia with an inhalation agent, e.g. ether, enflurane, but not halothane, though this is not easy; or by nerve block with a local anaesthetic, according to circumstances.

In addition, special techniques such as the production of hypotension or hypothermia may be required.

After surgery

The anaesthetist ensures that the effects of neuromuscular blocking agents and opioid-induced respiratory depression have either worn off adequately or have been reversed by an antagonist; the patient must never be left alone until conscious, with protective reflexes restored and stable circulation.

After operation the patient, who has already been submitted to preoperative medication and anaesthesia, may receive antibiotics; analgesics, sedatives and tranquillisers; purgatives and enemas; hypotensive or hypertensive agents; anticoagulants; cardiac stimulants or depressants; steroids, diuretics, and bronchodilators; and parenteral blood-volume expanders. To eliminate unnecessary drugs and reduce the use of others would be an act of clemency besides a welcome economy.[4]

Drug elimination may increase in the postoperative period, e.g. increased hepatic metabolism. Reduced gut motility may delay absorption of drugs.

Relief of pain after surgery presents many problems. Morphine and its derivatives are commonly used (usually intermittently, but sometimes by continuous i.v. infusion or intra or extradurally), but since opioids constipate, may cause vomiting, and depress cough and respiration, it will be appreciated that they have dis-

---

[4] Editorial Lancet 1961; 2: 589.

advantages, e.g. after operations on the bowel and chest and for day case surgery. Pethidine neither constipates nor suppresses spontaneous cough significantly, although it can be useful, given i.v., to reduce cough from an endotracheal tube. There is a wide choice from amongst the opioids and NSAIDs. Inhalation of nitrous oxide/oxygen mixture (Entonox) is also effective (see nitrous oxide) for brief analgesia, e.g. defaecation after haemorrhoidectomy.

Postoperative *vomiting* is largely preventable by skilled technique including avoidance of drugs that are particularly liable to cause it (ether, cyclopropane). Antiemetics can be effective.

Some special techniques related to general anaesthesia

- *Dissociative anaesthesia*; i.e. a state of analgesia and light hypnosis (the eyes may remain open), see ketamine. It is particularly useful where modern equipment and the necessary trained staff are lacking; also at scenes of major accidents and in war.
- *Neuroleptanalgesia*, in which the patient is in a state of analgesia but is cooperative. It is produced by a combination of a neuroleptic, e.g. droperidol, and a high-efficacy opioid analgesic, e.g. fentanyl or alfenatil. It is also used as a supplement to general anaesthesia, e.g. with nitrous oxide (*neuroleptanaesthesia*).
- *Sedation and amnesia* without analgesia is provided by diazepam and midazolam i.v. They can be used alone for procedures causing discomfort but not pain, e.g. endoscopy, and with a local anaesthetic where pain is expected, e.g. removal of impacted wisdom teeth. Anterograde amnesia is characteristic; the patient remains cooperative. For a general account of benzodiazepines and the competitive antagonist flumazenil, see Ch. 16.

Respiratory depression and apnoea can occur with the above especially in the elderly with cerebral atherosclerosis and patients with respiratory insufficiency. Laryngeal reflexes are not spared and inhalation of oral secretions or dental debris can occur.

- *Patient-controlled analgesia*, e.g. with nitrous oxide/oxygen mixtures (Entonox), is effective for brief procedures. Apparatus to allow patient control of intravenous analgesics has been developed.

PHARMACOLOGY OF GENERAL ANAESTHETICS

All the successful general anaesthetics are given i.v. or by inhalation because these routes allow closest control over blood levels and so of brain concentrations.

Mode of action

How anaesthetics quickly produce complete, controllable, reversible loss of consciousness remains uncertain.

General anaesthetics act on the brain, primarily on the midbrain reticular activating system and the cortex. A principal site of action (of both general and local anaesthetics) seems to be along the *neuronal lipid bilayer membrane*, which is disordered by the drugs so that cation (Na, K) movements through the protein pores (ion channels) which are associated with action potentials, are obstructed. The fact that increased atmospheric pressure can reverse anaesthesia is held to be compatible with this hypothesis. Other sites of action include neurotransmitter release and effects on postsynaptic membranes.

Many anaesthetics are very *fat-soluble* and there is good correlation between this and anaesthetic potency; the more fat-soluble tend to be the more potent anaesthetics, but such a correlation is not invariable. Some anaesthetic agents are not fat-soluble and many fat-soluble substances are not anaesthetics. There are no properties common to every agent and it is likely that there are several modes of action.

Clinical trials

Comparisons of general anaesthetics under routine clinical conditions are difficult to arrange, but they can be done.

Now that existing techniques of anaesthesia are so safe it is hard to expect a patient undergoing the anxiety of approaching surgery to consent to an experimental trial of a new drug, and to administer the drug, in however cautious a fashion, without the patient's (informed) consent is certainly immoral and assuredly illegal. In at least one country (USA) the problem has been approached by paying volunteers to undergo careful administration of graduated doses in a laboratory, with extensive monitoring of cardiovascular, respiratory and central nervous functions.

Comparison of potency of inhalation drugs both for efficacy and adverse effects, e.g. cardiac depression, may be made by measuring the minimum alveolar concentration (MAC) required to prevent reflex response to a surgical skin incision in 50% of subjects (MAC_{50}), or the MAC that prevents response in 95% of subjects (MAC_{95}), which is closer to real life clinical practice. A second point on the dose-response curve can be obtained for the MAC that just allows response to a spoken command. For non-volatile i.v. anaesthetics of which a dose can be accurately administered as a bolus or infusion, the equivalent is the anaesthetic dose (AD) that prevents movement in response to the noxious stimulus (AD_{95}); or the minimum infusion dose (as for MAC).

INHALATION AGENTS

Preferred agents

The preferred inhalation agents are those that are minimally irritant and non-flammable and comprise nitrous oxide and the fluorinated hydrocarbons, i.e. halothane and its allies. But the irritant, explosive ether retains a place because it is cheap and relatively safe in unskilled hands.

Pharmacokinetics of inhalation anaesthetics (volatile liquids, gases)

The level of anaesthesia is correlated with the tension (amount) of anaesthetic drug in the brain tissue and this is dependent on the development of a series of tension gradients from the high partial pressure delivered to the alveoli and decreasing through the blood to the brain and other tissues. These gradients are dependent on

the physical properties of the anaesthetic and the tissues, as well as on physiological functions (ventilation, blood flow).

It is not appropriate to discuss the detailed pharmacokinetics of anaesthetics here as they are chiefly important to professional anaesthetists, but some points of general interest are mentioned below.

An anaesthetic that has *high solubility* in blood (ether) will, if given at a steady concentration, provide a *slow induction*. This is because the blood acts as a reservoir (store) for the drug so that it does not enter the brain easily until the blood reservoir has been filled. A rapid induction can be obtained by increasing the concentration of drug inhaled initially and by hyperventilating the patient. This is difficult to do with ether because it is so irritant, and dangerous to do with agents that depress the cardiovascular system.

Agents that have *low solubility* in blood (nitrous oxide, cyclopropane, halothane), on the other hand, provide a *rapid induction* of anaesthesia because the blood reservoir is small and gas is available to pass into the brain sooner.

During *induction* of anaesthesia the blood is taking up anaesthetic gas selectively and rapidly and the resulting loss of volume in the alveoli leads to a flow of gas into the lungs that is independent of respiratory activity. When the anaesthetic is withdrawn the reverse occurs and there is a diffusion flow of gas from the blood into the alveoli, which, in the case of nitrous oxide, can account for as much as 10% of the expired volume and so can significantly lower the alveolar oxygen concentration. Thus mild clinical anoxia occurs, and it may last for as long as 10 min, and, though harmless to most, it may be a factor in cardiac arrest in patients with reduced pulmonary and cardiac reserve, especially when administration of the gas has been at high concentration and prolonged, when the outflow is especially vigorous. Oxygen should therefore be given to such patients during the last few minutes of anaesthesia and the early postanaesthetic period.

This phenomenon, *diffusion hypoxia*, occurs with all gaseous anaesthetics, but is most prominent with gases that are relatively insoluble in blood, for they will diffuse out most rapidly when the drug is no longer inhaled, i.e. just as induction is faster, so is elimination. Nitrous oxide is specially potent in this respect. Highly blood-soluble agents will diffuse out more slowly, so that recovery will be slower just as induction is slower, and with them diffusion anoxia is insignificant.

Nitrous oxide

Nitrous oxide (1844) is a gas with a slightly sweetish odour. It is neither flammable nor explosive. It produces light anaesthesia without demonstrably depressing the respiratory or vasomotor centre provided that normal oxygen tension is maintained.

Advantages. Nitrous oxide reduces the requirement for other more potent and intrinsically more toxic anaesthetic agents. It has a strong analgesic action. Induction is rapid and not unpleasant although transient excitement may occur. Recovery time rarely exceeds 1–4 min even after prolonged administration.

Disadvantages. Nitrous oxide is expensive to buy and to transport. It must be used in conjunction with more potent anaesthetics and muscle relaxants to produce a state of full surgical anaesthesia.

Uses. Maintenance of surgical anaesthesia in combination with other anaesthetic agents (halothane, ether, thiopentone or ketamine) and muscle relaxants. In subanaestheic dose, to provide analgesia for obstetric practice, for emergency management of injuries, during post-operative physiotherapy and for refractory pain in terminal illness.

Dosage and administration. For the maintenance of anaesthesia, nitrous oxide must always be mixed with at least 30% oxygen.

For analgesia, a concentration of 50% nitrous oxide with 50% oxygen usually suffices.

Contraindications. Any closed gas-filled space tends to expand during administration of nitrous oxide. It is therefore contraindicated in patients with: demonstrable collections of air in the pleural, pericardial or peritoneal space; intestinal obstruction; occlusion of the middle ear; arterial air embolism; decompression sickness; chronic obstructive airway disease; or emphysema.

Precautions. Continued administration of oxygen may be necessary during recovery especially in elderly patients (see Diffusion hypoxia above).

Adverse effects. The incidence of nausea and vomiting increases with the duration of anaesthesia. Because prolonged and repeated exposure may be associated with bone-marrow depression and a teratogenic risk, precautions should be taken to minimise ambient concentrations in operating theatres and intensive therapy units.

Drug interactions. Addition of 50% nitrous oxide/oxygen mixture to another inhalational anaesthetic reduces the required dosage of the latter by about 50%.

Storage. Nitrous oxide is supplied under pressure in cylinders, which must be kept below 25°C.

Cylinders containing premixed oxygen 50% and nitrous oxide 50% (Entonox) are available for analgesia. However, the constituents separate out at −6 °C, in which case adequate mixing must be assured before use (store at > 5°C for 24 h and invert the cylinder several times before use).

Halogenated agents: halothane

Halothane (1956) is a valuable agent in trained hands. It is a colourless, volatile, non-irritant liquid with a sweet odour. It is neither flammable nor explosive. In anaesthetic dosage it depresses both cerebral function and sympathetic activity and produces little, if any, preliminary excitement.

Advantages. Halothane is a potent non-flammable inhalational anaesthetic. Induction is smooth and rapid and surgical anaesthesia can be produced in 2–5 min. It does not augment salivary or bronchial secretions and coughing is less readily provoked than with ether. The recovery time is rapid and the incidence of postoperative nausea and vomiting is low. It does not react with soda lime and can be used in a closed-circuit system.

Disadvantages. Severe hepatitis, which may be fatal, is a recognised complication of halothane anaesthesia with incidence of 1:50 000. It is more likely to occur in patients who are repeatedly anaesthetised with halothane within a short period.

Little margin exists between the doses needed to produce respiratory and vasomotor depression. Because of its cardiodepressant effect halothane is usually combined with another inhalational agent, such as nitrous oxide or trichloroethylene, to produce surgical anaesthesia. Muscle relaxants are additionally required to prepare the patient for abdominal surgery.

Although it suppresses endogenous sympathetic activity halothane sensitises the heart to the dysrhythmic effects of catecholamines (endogenous and exogenous).

About 20% of halothane is metabolised and it induces hepatic enzymes, including those of anaesthetists.

Contraindications: a history of unexplained jaundice following previous exposure to halothane; a family history of malignant hyperthermia; raised cerebrospinal fluid pressure.

Precautions. The patient's anaesthetic history should be carefully taken to determine previous exposure and previous reactions to halothane, e.g. unexplained fever or jaundice.

At least 3 months should be allowed to elapse between each re-exposure to halothane. Repeated and frequent administration increases the risk of liver damage.

Adverse effects. Cardiac dysrhythmias may be induced, in particular atrioventricular dissociation, nodal rhythm and ventricular extrasystoles.

Hepatic damage occurs in a small proportion of exposed patients. Typically fever develops 2 or 3 days after anaesthesia accompanied by anorexia, nausea and vomiting. In more severe cases this is followed by transient jaundice or, very rarely, fatal hepatic necrosis.

Drug interactions. Halothane potentiates the response to antihypertensive agents. Premedication with atropine reduces the risk of hypotension and bradycardia. Interaction occurs with adrenaline (see above).

Enflurane (1966) is similar to halothane. Its isomer, *isoflurane* (1982), also may be an improvement. Both are metabolised less than halothane and are safer regarding the liver, and sensitisation to adrenaline.

Trichloroethylene (1934) is similar to the obsolete chloroform but is less toxic. It is nonflammable, cheap and retains a place in general anaesthetics for the latter reason. Its hypnotic effect is relatively weak but it is a potent analgesic. It causes tachypnoea and cardiac dysrhythmias like halothane (above). It has been used in a special inhaler for self-administration in childbirth.

Other agent: cyclopropane

Cyclopropane (1929) provides rapid induction and recovery (low solubility in blood), but it is explosive.

Ether (diethyl ether)

Although professional anaesthetists rarely use ether, it remains the safest inhalational agent in untrained hands. Though obsolete in the more wealthy countries, it still retains a place worldwide because of its low cost.

Ether is a colourless, highly volatile and flammable liquid.

Advantages. Ether is a reliable and potent anaesthetic that is particularly useful when elaborate apparatus is not available and cost is an important consideration. It may be used safely in closed circuits containing soda lime. The vasomotor centre is resistant to the doses required for full surgical anaesthesia. Because it is highly soluble in body tissues induction is slow and follows the classic stages of general anaesthesia. Full muscle relaxation is achieved in deep anaesthesia. Although irritant to the upper airway, ether is a bronchodilator and it can be of value in treating bronchospasm resistant to other drugs. It does not potentiate the dysrhythmic effect of sympathomimetic agents as much as other potent inhalational anaesthetics.

Disadvantages. Because ether is both flammable and explosive it can be used in hot dry climates only when special precautions are taken to prevent sparking and combustion; diathermy is contraindicated when ether is used with oxygen. Premedication with atropine is essential to avoid excessive bronchial and salivary secretion. Laryngeal spasm may occur during induction and intubation. Localised capillary bleeding can be troublesome. Postoperative nausea and vomiting are frequent and recovery time is slow, particularly after prolonged administration.

Uses. Induction and maintenance of anaesthesia during surgery. It is not metabolised.

Dosage and administration. Ether may be administered from many types of vaporiser. In emergency it may be dropped on to an open mask.

Premedication, see above.

When supplementary oxygen is used it can be fed under an open mask or into an open-ended T-piece connected to a drawover vaporiser.

Administration from vaporisers. Concentrations of ether vapour in the inspired gases should not exceed 15% during induction and should subsequently be reduced during maintenance of anaesthesia. Light anaesthesia (with or without muscle relaxants) can be sustained using 3–5% in air. Deep anaesthesia requires concentrations of up to 10%.

Open drop technique. This technique should be used only when no other means of delivering a general anaesthetic is available.

Ether is applied from a drop bottle to an open mask covered with multilayered gauze. During induction 12 drops/min are applied for 2 minutes, then 1 drop/s until the patient loses consciousness (usually within 5 minutes). The rate is subsequently adjusted to provide the required depth of anaesthesia. Deep levels of surgical anaesthesia cannot be achieved with this technique in less than 20–30 minutes.

Contraindications. Severe liver disease: raised cerebrospinal fluid pressure.

Precautions. In febrile children exposure to ether increases the risk of potentially fatal convulsions. If convulsions occur, ether should immediately be withdrawn, and the child's body temperature reduced by sponging with tepid water. Small doses of diazepam or thiopentone should be administered intravenously until convulsions cease.

Diathermy must not be used when ether/oxygen mixtures are in use and the operating theatre and its equipment should be designed to minimise the risk of static discharge, particularly in hot, dry climates. Electrical sockets and switches situated within 1 metre of the floor should be spark-proof. No potential source of combustion or sparking should be allowed within 30 cm of an expiratory valve emitting ether vapour.

Use in pregnancy. Ether should be used during pregnancy only when the need outweighs any possible risk to the fetus.

Low concentrations (no more than 4%) should be employed in obstetric procedures to avoid loss of uterine tone, excessive postpartum haemorrhage and respiratory depression in the neonate.

Adverse effects. Laryngeal spasm is common during induction.

Severe nausea, vomiting and bronchopneumonia are liable to occur postoperatively, particularly after prolonged, deep anaesthesia.

Transient postoperative effects include impairment of liver function and leukocytosis.

Dependence can occur in individuals who are repeatedly exposed to ether, e.g. operating theatre staff.

Drug interactions. The action of non-depolarising neuromuscular blocking agents is potentiated. In patients receiving β-adrenoceptor blocking agents such as propranolol, ether may cause myocardial depression.

Overdosage leads to severe central depression, characterised first by respiratory failure and later by cardiac arrest.

Spontaneous respiration is usually restored if intermittent positive pressure ventilation with oxygen is instituted promptly.

Storage. Ether should be stored is sealed containers protected from light, below 25°C.

Oxygen in anaesthesia

Oxygen should be added routinely to inhalational agents, even when air is used as the carrier gas, to protect against hypoxia. This is an essential precaution whenever halothane is used. When oxygen is not available, ether is the safest agent for maintenance of anaesthesia.

The concentration of oxygen in inspired anaesthetic gases should never be less than 21% (the concentration in air). It may be administered with the anaesthetic gases, or from a face mask or via a nasal catheter.

Combustion or sparking creates a danger of fire or explosion at high oxygen tensions. Use of cautery is contraindicated whenever oxygen is used in combination with ether. Reducing valves should not be greased, since this creates a danger of explosion.

Oxygen should not be used for longer or at a greater concentration than is necessary to prevent hypoxaemia.

After prolonged administration, concentrations greater than 80% at atmospheric pressure have a toxic effect on the lungs, which presents initially as a mild substernal irritation progressing to pulmonary congestion, exudation and atelectasis.

Use of unnecessarily high concentrations of oxygen in incubators has led to the development of retrolental fibroplasia and permanent blindness in premature infants.

Oxygen is supplied under pressure in cylinders, which must be kept below 25 °C.

Cylinders containing premixed oxygen 50% and nitrous oxide 50% are available for analgesia in some countries. However, the constituents separate out at −6 °C, in which case adequate mixing must be assured before use. When the two components are supplied from separate cylinders a safety device must be installed that cuts off the flow of nitrous oxide should the oxygen pressure fall.

Atmospheric pollution of operating theatres

Pollution by inhalation anaesthetics and other volatile substances (skin cleansers) has been suspected of being harmful to theatre personnel. An anaesthetist working with halothane can accumulate in 3–4 h amounts that will not be eliminated completely by the following morning.

Epidemiological studies have raised questions relating to excess of fetal malformations and miscarriages, hepatitis and cancer in operating theatre personnel. It was reported in 1972[5] that anaesthetists in the USSR had applied for a 15% salary bonus for working in a hazardous atmosphere. But it would seem a better solution to spend money on eliminating risk than on paying people to accept it. Sensible use of preventive measures probably renders the risks negligible, e.g. use of circle systems that allow low fresh gas flows, scavenging systems, improved ventilation of theatres (a minor contribution), filters that absorb volatile agents though not nitrous oxide; by using regional anaesthesia or total i.v. anaesthesia, i.e. no vapours or gases used, in preference to inhalation wherever feasible.

Precautions against atmospheric pollution, e.g. by frequent use of nitrous oxide, are also necessary in intensive therapy units.

INTRAVENOUS ANAESTHETICS

General pharmacokinetics of intravenous anaesthetics

While intravenous anaesthetics allow an extremely rapid induction because the blood concentration can be raised rapidly, there is no channel of elimination that can compete with the lungs for speed. The metabolic breakdown of many useful agents does not occur fast enough for really quick recovery and so reliance is put on rapid distribution of the drug, e.g. thiopentone, which can only be satisfactory for brief operations. With prolonged use, recovery from thiopentone must be slower, for the body is storing more and more of the drug and with repeated doses recovery depends on the mass of the storage tissues (muscle, fat), the blood flow through them, and the rate of metabolism and excretion of the drug. Attempts to use thiopentone i.v. as a sole anaesthetic agent in war casualties led to its being described as an ideal form of euthanasia.[6]

---

[5] Editorial. Anaesthesia 1972; 27: 1.
[6] Halford J J. A critique of intravenous anaesthesia in war surgery. Anesthesiology 1943; 4: 67.

Therefore substances rapidly absorbed and rapidly excreted through the lungs still offer the best prospect of precise control (with continuous administration) even in the presence of pulmonary disease, except perhaps severe emphysema. Elimination of inhaled anaesthetics can be hastened by inducing hyperventilation. There is no quick method of eliminating drugs whose action is normally terminated by metabolism or by redistribution. For the present it is usual to approach the ideal by using a combination of drugs in such a way that the disadvantages of each are less prominent.

But the need to reduce atmospheric pollution by inhalation anaesthetics (including nitrous oxide) and the apparently increasing problem of awareness (consciousness) of paralysed patients under nitrous oxide maintenance have been accompanied by a revival of interest in the use of i.v. drugs as sole anaesthetic agents (*total intravenous anaesthesia*). The requirements for prompt and complete termination of anaesthesia are stringent, but they are increasingly being met by the newer agents.

Thiopentone (thiopental)

Thiopentone is a very short-acting barbiturate which, administered parenterally, rapidly induces hypnosis and anaesthesia without analgesia. It is extensively bound to plasma albumin and is initially distributed most extensively in the highly vascular tissues of the brain and other organs. It subsequently diffuses selectively into fatty tissues where it is pharmacologically inactive (this process terminates the effect of an initial dose). It is slowly but almost entirely metabolised in the liver. The $t_\frac{1}{2}$ in the *distribution* phase is 2.5 min: after equilibration it is 10 h.

Advantages. Thiopentone usually exerts its cerebral depressant effect within 30 seconds and it persists for about 4–7 min. Anaesthesia is induced rapidly, pleasantly and without excitement.

Disadvantages. Thiopentone has insignificant analgesic action. Any muscular relaxation that occurs is too short to be of practical value. In contrast to ketamine, it cannot be used alone as an anaesthetic agent because the large and

repeated doses required accumulate in fatty tissues and are subsequently only slowly released; this results in prolonged anaesthesia and delayed recovery characterised by somnolence and respiratory and circulatory depression.

Uses. Induction of anaesthesia prior to administration of inhalational and other anaesthetics.

> **Thiopentone dosage and administration.**
> Adults and children: 3–5 mg/kg given by slow intravenous injection over 10–15 seconds and repeated, if necessary, after 20–30 seconds.
>
> Dosage requirements vary; they are reduced in the elderly, in hypovolaemic patients, and in patients heavily premedicated with narcotics or other cerebral depressants.
>
> The injection should be administered slowly until the patient becomes unconscious. Recovery after a *single* dose is rapid because of redistribution of the drug from the central nervous system into other tissues.

Contraindications. Thiopentone should not be used: if there is doubt that a clear airway can be maintained or if there is allergy to barbiturates; severe cardiovascular disease or hypotension; dyspnoea or obstructive respiratory disease; status asthmaticus; Addison's disease; hepatic dysfunction; myxoedema; a history of acute intermittent or variegate porphyria.

Precautions. Thiopentone should, whenever possible, be administered under the supervision of an experienced specialist anaesthetist.

Equipment for resuscitation and endotracheal intubation should be immediately available and ready for use.

The patient must always lie supine as even a small overdose can cause hypotension.

Concentrations greater than 25 mg/ml are liable to cause thrombophlebitis. Local extravasation can result in extensive necrosis and sloughing. Intra-arterial injection causes intense pain and may result in arteriospasm necessitating local use of vasodilators, supplemented, if necessary, by branchial plexus block and anticoagulation.

Adverse effects. A short period of apnoea may follow intravenous injection.

Rapid injection may result in severe hypotension and hiccoughs. Coughing, sneezing or laryngeal spasm may occur during induction.

Drug interactions. Other cerebral depressants may augment the action of thiopentone. Antihypertensives or diuretics may augment the hypotensive effect.

Overdosage. Serious overdosage results in respiratory depression necessitating assisted ventilation with oxygen, and hypotension progressing to circulatory collapse. In the latter event the head of the table must immediately be tilted down. Plasma expanders and pressor agents may be of value in patients who are unresponsive to this measure.

Methohexitone is a barbiturate similar to thiopentone.

Propofol (a phenol derivative) is notable for quick induction (30s) and for quick recovery (4 min) from a single dose: it is used both for induction and maintenance for procedures lasting up to about 1 h. The effect of a single dose is terminated by distribution; the elimination $t_{\frac{1}{2}}$ is 4 h.

Ketamine

Ketamine (1965) is a phencyclidine (hallucinogen) derivative. In anaesthetic doses it produces a trance-like state known as *dissociative anaesthesia*.

Advantages. Anaesthesia persists for up to 15 min after a single intravenous injection and is characterised by profound analgesia. Ketamine may be used as the sole agent for diagnostic and minor surgical interventions. It is less likely than other anaesthetic agents to induce vomiting. Since it does not induce hypotension the patient does not have to remain supine and its sympathomimetic effects are of particular value in patients who are shocked, severely dehydrated or severely anaemic. Because pharyngeal and laryngeal reflexes are only slightly impaired, the airway may be less at risk than is the case with other general anaesthetic techniques. It is of particular value in children and poor-risk patients, and also in asthmatic patients, because it rarely induces

bronchospasm. See also Dissociative anaesthesia, p. 360.

Disadvantages. Ketamine produces no muscular relaxation. It tends to raise heart rate and intracranial and intraocular pressure. In hypertensive patients it may raise blood pressure unduly. Hallucinations can occur during recovery (although rarely in children), but they are avoided if ketamine is used solely as an induction agent and followed by a conventional inhalational anaesthetic. Their incidence may also be greatly reduced by administration of diazepam both as a premedication and after the procedure.

Uses. Subanaesthetic doses of ketamine may be used to provide analgesia for painful procedures of short duration such as the dressing of burns, radiotherapeutic procedures, marrow sampling and minor orthopaedic procedures.

Ketamine may be used for induction of anaesthesia prior to administration of inhalational anaesthetics, or for both induction and maintenance of anaesthesia for short-lasting diagnostic and surgical interventions, including dental procedures, that do not require skeletal muscle relaxation. It is of particular value for children requiring frequent repeated anaesthetics.

Dosage and administration. Administration of ketamine (i.m. or i.v.) should always be preceded by premedication with atropine to reduce salivary secretions.

Premedication with diazepam reduces the subsequent requirement for ketamine and the incidence of emergence reactions but in this case there is a need for endotracheal intubation.

Induction. Intravenous route: 1–2 mg/kg by slow intravenous injection over a period of 60 seconds. More rapid administration may result in respiratory depression or apnoea and an enhanced pressor response. A dose of 2 mg/kg produces surgical anaesthesia within 1–2 min which may be expected to last 5 to 10 min.

Intramuscular route: 6–8 mg/kg by deep intramuscular injection. This dose produces surgical anaesthesia within 3–5 min and may be expected to last up to 25 min.

Maintenance. Following induction, as above, serial doses of 50% of the original intravenous dose or 25% of the intramuscular dose are administered as required. The need for supplementary doses is established largely by movement in response to surgical stimuli.

Tonic and clonic movements resembling seizures occur in some patients. These are not indicative of a light plane of anaesthesia or of a need for additional doses of the anaesthetic.

As an analgesic. 500 micrograms/kg i.m. or i.v. followed, if necessary, by a dose of 250 micrograms/kg.

Recovery. Return to consciousness is gradual. Emergence reactions with delirium may occur. Their incidence is reduced if unnecessary disturbance of the patient is avoided during recovery (although vital signs may be monitored) and they are unlikely to occur if diazepam is administered preoperatively and supplemented, if necessary, by a further 5–10 mg i.v. at the end of the procedure. Hypnotic doses of thiopentone (50–100 mg i.v.) may be required to suppress overt reactions but this will considerably prolong the recovery period.

Contraindications include: moderate to severe hypertension, congestive cardiac failure, or a history of cerebrovascular accident; acute or chronic alcohol intoxication; cerebral trauma, intracerebral mass or haemorrhage or other causes of raised intracranial pressure; eye injury and increased intraocular pressure; psychiatric disorders such as a schizophrenia and acute psychoses.

Precautions. Ketamine should, whenever possible, be used under the supervision of an experienced specialist anaesthetist who is confident of intubating the patient should this become necessary.

Pulse and blood pressure should be closely monitored. Mechanical stimulation of the pharynx should be avoided unless muscle relaxants are used.

Supplementary analgesia is often required in surgical procedures involving visceral pain pathways. Morphine may be used but the addition of nitrous oxide will often suffice.

During recovery, patients must remain undisturbed and under observation.

Use in pregnancy. Ketamine is contraindicated in pregnancy before term, since it has oxytocic activity. It is also contraindicated in patients with eclampsia or pre-eclampsia. it may be used for assisted vaginal delivery by an experienced anaesthetist. It is better suited for use during caesarean section; ketamine results in less fetal and neonatal depression than do other anaesthetics and the short exposure required has not been associated with emergence reactions when diazepam is used concomitantly.

Adverse effects: see above.

Neuroleptanalgesia/anaesthesia: see p. 360.

MUSCLE RELAXANTS: NEUROMUSCULAR BLOCKING DRUGS

A lot of surgery, especially of the abdomen, requires that voluntary muscle tone and reflex contraction be inhibited. This can be attained by deep general anaesthesia which carries hazard, e.g. cardiovascular depression, respiratory complications and slow recovery: also by nerve blocks, which can be difficult to do, or impracticable. Selective relaxation of voluntary muscle with neuromuscular blocking drugs allows surgery under light general anaesthesia and analgesia; it also facilitates tracheal intubation, quick induction and quick recovery. But it requires artificial respiration and great technical skill.

Neuromuscular blocking agents should be given only after induction of anaesthesia.

Neuromuscular blocking agents first attracted scientific notice because of their use as arrow poisons by the natives of South America, who used the most famous of all, curare, for killing food animals as well as enemies. In 1811 Sir Benjamin Brodie smeared 'woorara paste' on wounds of guinea-pigs and noted that death could be delayed by inflating the lungs through a tube introduced into the trachea. Though he did not continue until complete recovery, he did suggest that the drug might be of use in tetanus.

Despite attempts to use curare for a variety of diseases including epilepsy, chorea and rabies, the lack of pure and accurately standardised preparations as well as the absence of convenient routine techniques of artificial respiration if overdose occurred, prevented it from gaining any firm place in medical practice until 1942, when these difficulties were removed.

Drugs acting at the myoneural junction produce complete paralysis of all voluntary muscle so that movement is impossible and artificial respiration is needed. Attempts to achieve selective relaxation, sparing respiration, in the treatment of convulsions and disorders of muscle tone, have been unsuccessful.

The necessity for artificial respiration no longer deters anaesthetists, who are now quite accustomed to taking over respiration from the patient as a routine. It is plainly important that a paralysed patient should be in a state of full analgesia *and* unconscious during surgery (see below).

Neuromuscular transmission and its modification by drugs

When an impulse passes down a motor nerve to voluntary muscle it causes release of acetylcholine from the nerve endings into the synaptic cleft. This activates receptors on the membrane of the motor end-plate, a specialised area on the muscle fibre, opening ion channels for momentary passage of sodium which depolarises the end-plate and initiates muscle contraction.

Neuromuscular blocking agents used in clinical practice interfere with this process. However, substances that prevent the release of acetylcholine at nerve endings exist, e.g. *Cl. botulinum* toxin (see p. 315) and some venoms.

Principal mechanisms

There are two principal mechanisms by which drugs used clinically interfere with neuromuscular transmission:

1. **By competition** with acetylcholine (tubocurarine, gallamine, pancuronium, alcuronium, vecuronium, atracurium). These drugs are competitive antagonists of acetylcholine. They do not cause depolarisation themselves but they protect the end-plate from depolarisation by acetylcholine. The result is a flaccid paralysis.

Reversal of this type of neuromuscular block can be achieved with anticholinesterase drugs, such as neostigmine, which prevent the destruction by cholinesterase of acetylcholine released at nerve endings, allow the concentration to build up and so reduce the competitive effect of a given concentration of blocking agent.

2. **By depolarisation** of the motor end-plate (suxamethonium). Such agonist drugs activate the acetylcholine receptor on the motor end-plate and at their first application voluntary muscle contracts; but, as they are not destroyed immediately, like acetylcholine, the depolarisation persists. It might be expected that this prolonged depolarisation would result in muscles remaining contracted, but this is not so (except in chickens). However, with prolonged administration a depolarisation block changes to a competitive block (dual block). Because of the uncertainty of this situation a competitive blocking agent is preferred for anything other than short procedures.

Competitive antagonists of acetylcholine at the neuromuscular junction: non-depolarising neuromuscular blocking agents

The introduction of **tubocurarine** into surgery made it desirable to decide once and for all whether the drug altered consciousness. Doubts were resolved in a single experiment.[7] A normal subject was slowly paralysed (curarised) after arranging a detailed and complicated system of communication. Twelve minutes after beginning the slow infusion of curare, the subject, having artificial respiration, could move only his head. He indicated that the experience was not unpleasant, that he was mentally clear and did not want an endotracheal tube inserted. After 22 min, communication was possible only by slight movement of the left eyebrow and after 35 min paralysis was complete and direct communication lost. An airway was inserted. The subject's eyelids were then lifted for him and the resulting inhibition of alpha rhythm of the electroencephalogram

---

[7] Smith S M et al. Anesthesiology 1947; 8: 1. Note: a randomised controlled trial is not required for this kind of investigation.

suggested that vision and consciousness were normal. After recovery, aided by neostigmine, the subject reported that he had been mentally 'clear as a bell' throughout, and confirmed this by recalling what he had heard and seen. The insertion of the endotracheal airway had caused only minor discomfort, perhaps because of the prevention of reflex muscle spasm. During artificial respiration he had 'felt that (he) would give anything to be able to take one deep breath' despite adequate oxygenation. In another study curare was excluded from one arm by an inflated cuff so that the subject could make finger signals,[8] and this isolated forearm technique can be used to detect wakefulness in clinical anaesthesia.

Awareness. It is essential to ensure that paralysed patients do not regain awareness unnoticed during surgery. That this is not merely a theoretical risk is shown by the occasion when an anaesthetist, visiting his patient the day after the operation, was horrified when she sympathetically remarked, 'I had no idea you doctors were so badly paid.' He had discussed the inadequacy of his salary with a colleague during the operation. The patient had felt her bowels being manipulated but no pain.

However, pain can occur on such occasions, and both anaesthetists and patients will wish to avoid them. Awareness is most likely when nitrous oxide and oxygen are being used with neuromuscular block, and reflex signs suggestive of pain include bronchospasm, sweating and response of the pupil to light, as well as movement; but awareness can occur without these accompaniments.

In addition to its neuromuscular blocking effect tubocurarine blocks autonomic ganglia (acetylcholine antagonism) and causes tissue *histamine release*. Both these effects may cause an initial transient drop in blood pressure, and the latter may induce bronchospasm.

Curare is *insignificantly absorbed from the alimentary tract*, a fact known to the South American Indians, who use it to procure food.

Tubocurarine dose: after an i.v. *injection* the action is maximal in 4 min and lasts *usefully* for

---

[8] Campbell E J M et al. Clin Sci 1969; 36: 323.

30 min (the $t_{\frac{1}{2}}$ for *effect* is about 50 min). Use is declining in favour of gallamine.

Gallamine differs from tubocurarine in that it acts a little sooner (2 min) and does not release histamine, both desirable properties. It causes tachycardia (vagal block) and crosses the placenta, unlike other competitive antagonists; 80% is eliminated by the kidney and 20% is metabolised.

Alcuronium, pancuronium, pipecuronium and **vecuronium** are alternatives that differ in detail.

Atracurium is unique in that it is altered spontaneoulsy in the body to an inactive form ($t_{\frac{1}{2}}$ 30 min) by a passive chemical process (Hofman elimination). Duration of action (15–35 min) is thus uninfluenced by the state of the circulation, the liver or the kidneys, a real advantage in patients with hepatic or renal disease and in the aged. It is suitable for Caesarian section. Like tubocurarine it causes histamine release.

Antagonism of competitive neuromuscular block

The action of competitive acetylcholine blockers is *antagonised* by anticholinesterase drugs which allow accumulation of acetylcholine. Neostigmine (p. 385) is usually given i.v., preceded by atropine or glycopyrronium to prevent the parasympathetic autonomic effects of the neostigmine (especially the vagal bradycardia). It acts in 4 min and lasts for about 30 min so that the patient may relapse into paralysis again and so must be carefully watched. Too much neostigmine can cause neuromuscular block by depolarisation, which will cause confusion unless there have been some signs of recovery before neostigmine is given. Progress can be monitored with a nerve stimulator.

Neuromuscular blocking agents acting by depolarisation

Suxamethonium (succinylcholine) (Scoline) paralysis is usually preceded by muscular fasciculation, and this may be the cause of the muscle pain lasting 1–3 days that is a common sequence of its use and which can rarely simulate meningeal irritation. The pain can be largely prevented by preceding the suxamethonium with a small dose of a competitive blocking agent. Suxamethonium total paralysis lasts up to 4 min with 50% recovery ($t_{\frac{1}{2}}$ for effect) of about 10 min. It is particularly useful for brief procedures such as tracheal intubation or electroconvulsion therapy. Suxamethonium is destroyed by plasma pseudocholinesterase and so its persistence in the body is increased by neostigmine, which inactivates that enzyme, and in patients with hepatic disease or severe malnutrition whose plasma enzyme levels may be lower than normal. Procaine and amethocaine also are destroyed by plasma pseudocholinesterase and so, by competing with suxamethonium for the enzyme, may prolong its action and vice versa (lignocaine and prilocaine are metabolised differently). In addition there are individuals (about 1 in 2500 of the population) with hereditary defects in amount or kind of enzyme, who cannot destroy the drug as rapidly as normals.[9] Paralysis then lasts for hours; there is no effective way of restoring the enzyme or of eliminating the drug. Treatment consists in ventilating until recovery.

Repeated injections of suxamethonium can cause bradycardia, extrasystoles, other cardiac irregularities and even ventricular arrest. These are probably due to activation of cholinoceptors in the heart and are prevented by atropine. High doses stimulate the pregnant uterus and can cause premature labour. It can be used in Caesarian section as it does not readily cross the placenta.

Suxamethonium depolarisation causes a release of potassium from muscle which can be enough to cause cardiac arrest in patients who already have raised plasma potassium (burns, muscle trauma).

Uses of neuromuscular blocking agents

Neuromuscular blocking agents should only be employed by those who can intubate and ventilate.

- In surgery and in intensive therapy units they are used to provide muscular relaxation.
- In convulsions, e.g. electroconvulsion therapy, they are used to prevent injury due to the violence of the fit. In status epilepticus, tetanus or convulsant drug poisoning, neuromuscular blocking agents with mechanical respiration are used when lesser means are insufficient.

Other muscle relaxants

Drugs that provide muscle relaxation by an action on the central nervous system or on the muscle itself are not useful for this purpose in surgery; they are insufficiently selective and full relaxation, even if achievable, is accompanied by general cerebral depression.

But there is a place for drugs that reduce spasm of the voluntary muscles without impairing voluntary movement. Such drugs can be useful in *neurological spastic states, low back syndrome* and *rheumatism* with muscle spasm.

Baclofen (Lioresal) is a derivative of gamma-aminobutyric acid (GABA), an inhibitory central nervous system transmitter. It reduces spasticity and flexor spasms, but as it has no action on voluntary muscle power, function is commonly not improved. Ambulant patients may need their leg spasticity to provide support and reduction of spasticity may expose the weakness of the limb. It benefits some cases of trigeminal neuralgia. Baclofen is given orally and has a $t_{\frac{1}{2}}$ of 3 h.

Dantrolene (Dantrium) acts directly on muscle and prevents the release of calcium from sarcoplasm stores, see malignant hyperthermia (index).

Alternative centrally acting muscle relaxants include orphenadrine (Norflex), diazepam (Valium), carisoprodol (Carisoma), chlormezanone (Trancopal) and methocarbamol (Robaxin). Most are prone to cause objectionable sedation. See also quinine.

Allergic and pseudo-allergic reactions in general anaesthesia

Anaphylactic type allergic and pseudo-allergic reactions occur particularly to intravenous anaes-

---

[9] When cases are discovered the family should be investigated (plasma cholinesterase) and abnormal individuals warned.

thetics and muscle relaxants, and particularly during induction. They may be fatal. Treatment is as for anaphylactic shock (p. 125).

LOCAL ANAESTHETICS

Cocaine (see also p. 351) was the first local anaesthetic discovered. It was suggested as a local anaesthetic for clinical use in 1879. Nothing however was done until 1884 when Dr. Sigmund Freud in Vienna was reinvestigating the alkaloid, and invited Dr. Carl Koller to join him. The latter had long been interested in the problem of local anaesthesia in the eye, for general anaesthesia has disadvantages in ophthalmology. On observing the numbness of the mouth caused by taking cocaine orally he realised that this was a local anaesthetic effect. He tried cocaine on animals' eyes and introduced it into clinical ophthalmological practice, whilst Freud was on holiday. Freud had already thought of this use and discussed it, but, appreciating that sex was of greater importance than surgery, he had gone to see his fiancée. The use of cocaine spread rapidly and it was soon being used to block nerve trunks. Chemists then began to search for less toxic substitutes, with the result that procaine was introduced in 1905.

Desired properties. Innumerable compounds have local anaesthetic properties, but few are suitable for clinical use. Useful substances must be water-soluble, sterilisable by heat, have a rapid onset of effect, a duration of action appropriate to the operation to be performed, be non-toxic both locally and when absorbed into the circulation, and leave no local after-effects.

Mode of action. Local anaesthetics act on all nervous tissue to prevent the nerve impulse from arising and from propagating. They do this by reducing the passage of sodium through voltage-gated Na ion channels raising the threshold of excitability. They paralyse afferent nerve endings, sensory and motor nerve trunks and the central nervous system, although they may excite the latter first.

The fibres in nerve trunks are affected in order of size, the smallest (autonomic, sensory) first, probably because they have a proportionately high surface area, and then the larger (motor) fibres.

Pharmacokinetics. *By injection or infiltration* local anaesthetics are usually effective within 5 min and have a useful duration of effect of 1–1.5 h, which may be doubled by adding a vasoconstrictor (below). Obviously, *half* time of effect is of less interest to patients undergoing painful procedures than is the duration of *full* effect.

Most local anaesthetics are used in the form of the acid salts, as these are both soluble and stable. The acid salt (usually HCl) must dissociate in the tissues to liberate the free base, which is biologically active. This dissociation is delayed in abnormally acid, e.g. inflamed, tissues. The risk of spreading infection also makes local anaesthesia undesirable in infected areas.

Absorption from *mucous membranes* on topical application varies according to the compound. Those that are well absorbed are used as surface anaesthetics (cocaine, lignocaine, prilocaine). Absorption of topically applied local anaesthetic can be extremely rapid and give plasma concentrations comparable to those obtained by injection. This had led to deaths from overdosage, especially via the urethra.

For topical effect on *intact skin* for needling procedures a eutectic[10] mixture of bases of prilocaine or lignocaine is used (Emla = *e*utectic *m*ixture of *l*ocal *a*naesthetics). Absorption is very slow and a cream is applied under an occlusive dressing for at least 1 h.

Ester compounds (cocaine, procaine, amethocaine, benzocaine) are hydrolysed by liver and plasma esterases (and their effects may be prolonged where there is genetic deficiency).

Amide compounds (lignocaine, prilocaine, cinchocaine, bupivacaine) are dealkylated in the liver.

It is evident that defective liver function, whether due to primary cellular insufficiency, or to low liver blood flow in cardiac failure or due to β-adrenoceptor block, may both prolong the $t_\frac{1}{2}$ and allow higher peak plasma concentrations

---

[10] A mixture of two solids that becomes a liquid that melts and solidifies at one temperature.

of both types of local anaesthetic. But this is likely only to be important with large or repeated doses or infusions.

The *distribution* $t_{\frac{1}{2}}$ of a single dose of a local anaesthetic is a few minutes, determined by diffusion into tissues with concentrations approximately in relation to blood flow. But when an i.v. infusion is used, an equilibration with all body tissues has been achieved (steady state) then the $t_{\frac{1}{2}}$ is determined solely by elimination (above) and is longer, e.g. lignocaine 1.5 h. These considerations are plainly important in the management of cardiac dysrhythmias (p. 442).

Prolongation of action by vasoconstrictors

The effect of a local anaesthetic is terminated by its removal from the site of application. Thus anything that delays its absorption into the circulation will prolong its local action and can reduce its systemic toxicity where large volumes are used. Adrenaline or noradrenaline generally (1 : 200 000–1 : 400 000) are commonly used (dentists use 1 : 80 000) and they double the duration of effect, e.g. from 1 to 2 h. A vasoconstrictor should *not* be used for nerve block of an extremity (finger, toe, nose, penis). For obvious anatomical reasons, the whole blood supply may be cut off by intense vasoconstriction so that the organ may be damaged or even lost. In dentistry particularly it is sometimes useful to terminate local anaesthesia promptly when the operative job is done. This can be achieved by reversal of adrenaline vasoconstriction by injecting an α-adrenoceptor blocker (phentolamine) into the site.

Enough adrenaline or noradrenaline can be absorbed to affect the heart and circulation and reduce the plasma potassium. This can be dangerous in cardiovascular disease, with general anaesthetics that sensitise the heart to catecholamines (halothane) and with tricyclic antidepressants and potassium losing diuretics. An alternative vasoconstrictor is *felypressin* (synthetic vasopressin), which, in the concentrations used, does not affect the heart rate or blood press-

ure and may be preferable in patients with cardiovascular disease. There is no significant added hazard to the use of catecholamines in patients taking an MAOI, except perhaps where there is cardiovascular disease, and felypressin is preferable in these patients in any case.

Other effects

Local anaesthetics also have the following clinically important effects in varying degree:

- Excitation of parts of the central nervous system, which may show itself by anxiety, restlessness, tremors and even convulsions, which are followed by depression.
- Quinidine-like actions on the heart.

Uses

Local anaesthesia is generally used for trivial operations, when loss of consciousness is neither necessary nor desirable and also as an adjunct to major surgery to avoid high dose general anaesthesia. It can be used for major surgery, plus sedation, though many patients prefer unconsciousness. It is invaluable when the operator must also be the anaesthetist. Local anaesthetics can also be used topically for short periods to give relief from local pain or itching (but skin allergy is common).

For any but the most trivial operation premedication with a benzodiazepine is theoretically desirable to counteract the central excitant action of local anaesthetics, especially cocaine, but the doses used may in fact provide little or no protection.

Local anaesthetics may be used in several ways to provide:

- Surface anaesthesia, as solution, jelly, cream or lozenge. Chronic use is liable to cause allergy.
- Infiltration anaesthesia, to paralyse the sensory nerve endings and small cutaneous nerves.
- Regional anaesthesia.

Regional anaesthesia

Intravenous. A cuff is applied to the arm, inflated above arterial pressure after elevating the limb to drain the venous system, and the veins filled with local anaesthetic, e.g. 0.5% prilocaine, *without* adrenaline. The arm is anaesthetised in 6–8 min, and the effect lasts for up to 40 min if the cuff remains inflated. The cuff cannot safely be deflated until 20 min have passed. The technique is useful in providing anaesthesia for the treatment of injuries speedily and conveniently, and many patients can leave hospital as soon as 15 min after the cuff has been let down (during which time sensation and power return). The technique must be meticulously conducted for if the *full* dose of local anaesthetic is accidentally suddenly released into the general circulation severe toxicity and even death may result. Even if correctly performed, drug enters the general circulation through vessels in the bone that are not obstructed by the tourniquet. If toxicity occurs, convulsions and cardiac arrest may have to be treated. Patients should be fasted and someone (in addition to the surgeon) who is fully able to resuscitate should be present.

Nerve block means to anaesthetise a region, which may be small or large, by injecting the drug around, not into, the appropriate nerves, usually either a peripheral nerve or a plexus. Nerve block provides its own muscular relaxation as motor fibres are blocked as well as sensory fibres, although with care differential block can be achieved. Areas of selective sensory, but not motor, nerve block, are found at the edges of some regional nerve blocks. Even when motor fibres are intact, provided there is sensory block, muscular relaxation will occur if the patient's consciousness is blunted with a hypnotic drug. There are various specialised forms: paravertebral, paracervical, pudendal block. Sympathetic nerve blocks may be used in vascular disease to induce vasodilatation.

Extradural (epidural) anaesthesia can be used in thoracic, lumbar and sacral (caudal) regions: it is widely used in obstetrics. As the term implies, the drug is injected into the extradural space where it acts on the nerve roots. This technique avoids the potentially serious hazards of putting foreign substances into the CSF; the risk of headache and hypotension is less than with spinal anaesthesia.

Subarachnoid (intrathecal) block (spinal anaesthesia). By using a solution of appropriate specific gravity and tilting the patient the drug can be kept at an appropriate level. Hypotension due to block of the sympathetic nervous system outflow occurs. Headache due to CSF leakage may be troublesome and prolonged.

Serious local neurological complications have occurred rarely, both from the drug and from accidentally introduced bacteria.

Opioid analgesics may also be used *intrathecally* and extradurally. They diffuse into the spinal cord and are highly effective in skilled hands for intractable pain, including post-surgical pain. They are less effective in childbirth. Respiratory depression may occur. Onset of effect is in 20 min with duration of about 5 h. Adrenaline may be used to prolong effect. Morphine or other more lipid-soluble opioids may be used.

Regional anaesthesia requires considerable knowledge of anatomy and attention to detail for both success and safety.

Adverse reactions

Excessive absorption results in paraesthesiae (face and tongue) nervousness, tremors and even *convulsions*. These latter are very dangerous and are followed by respiratory depression. Diazepam or thiopentone, or even suxamethonium, may be necessary to control the convulsions as in status epilepticus. Respiratory stimulants are useless and dangerous as the patient has already passed through a phase of overstimulation. Nausea, vomiting and abdominal pain may occur, and also sudden *cardiovascular collapse* and *respiratory failure* for which there is no specific treatment other than respiratory and cardiac resuscitation. When systemic toxicity follows injection of a local anaesthetic into an extremity, a tourniquet may be used to delay entry of what remains into the general circulation, but resuscitation is the first priority. Hypertension can occur with cocaine (below).

Table 20.1 Reference data (approx) on 3 widely used local anaesthetics (amide class) (Other concentrations are used, especially in dentistry)

		Solution	Dose by vol. (adult)	Duration of effect
Lignocaine	infiltration	0.5% + adren	up to 60 ml	
	nerve block	1% + adren	up to 50 ml	
	(peripheral)	2% + adren	up to 25 ml	1.5 h
	surface anaesth.	2%	up to 20 ml	
		4%	up to 5 ml	
Bupivacaine	infiltration	0.25%	up to 60 ml	
	nerve block	0.25%	up to 60 ml	up to 8 h
	(peripheral)	0.5%	up to 30 ml	
Prilocaine	infiltration	0.5%	up to 80 ml	
	nerve block	1%	up to 40 ml	
	(peripheral)	2%	up to 20 ml	1.5–3 h
		3% + felypressin (dental use)	up to 20 ml	

Notes: 1. Time of onset of full effect is about 5 min, except bupivacaine (see text).
2. Maximum doses of local anaesthetic plus vasoconstrictor are toxic in absence of th' vasoconstrictor and so substantially less should be used. All doses are approximate only; larger amounts may be safe, but deaths have occurred with smaller amounts, so that the minimum dose that will do the job should be used.
3. Maximum dose of adrenaline is 500 micrograms (see below).
4. Concentrations of solutions and dose of drug: errors of calculation occur with sometimes fatal results. We provide these figures because experience of conducting examinations with medical students has taught us that they frequently lack the facility of calculating the dose of a drug in a given volume of known concentration.

1% means *one gram* in *100 ml* = 1000 mg in 100 ml = 10 mg per ml:
2% = 20 mg per ml, and so on.

It is traditional to express adrenaline concentrations as 1 in 200 000, or 1 in 80 000, or 1 in 1000.
1 in 1000 means 1000 mg (1.0 g) in 1000 ml = 1 mg per ml.
1 in 200 000 means 1000 mg (1.0 g) in 200 000 ml = 5 micrograms per ml.
Thus the maximum dose of adrenaline, 500 micrograms (see above), is contained in 100 ml of 1 in 200 000 solution.

Allergic reactions such as rashes, asthma and anaphylactic shock rarely occur,[11] and the subject may be allergic to more than one drug. Regular users are wise if they take care to keep them off their own skin when filling syringes.

Individual local anaesthetics (Table 20.1)

Lignocaine (Xylocaine) (lidocaine) (amide) (t_2^1 1.5 h) is a first choice drug for surface use as well as for injection, combining efficacy with comparative lack of toxicity. It is also useful in cardiac dysrhythmias (see index). Structurally, lignocaine differs from most other local anaesthetics and so is especially suitable for trial in cases of known allergy to other drugs.

Prilocaine (Citanest) (amide) (t_2^1 1.5 h) is used similarly to lignocaine, but it is less toxic. Lignocaine and prilocaine can cause *methaemoglobinaemia* (due to an aniline metabolite) at highest doses and this is only clinically important in patients in whom slight decrease of oxygen-carrying capacity is harmful, e.g. severe heart failure.

Bupivacaine (Marcain) (amide) (t_2^1 3 h) is particularly long acting and is used for nerve blocks in general, including obstetric epidural anaesthesia and for post-surgical and chronic pain relief. Whilst onset of effect is comparable to the above, peak effect occurs later (30 min).

Adverse reactions, see above.

Cocaine (alkaloid and ester) is used medicinally solely as a surface anaesthetic (for abuse toxicity, see p. 351) usually as a 4% solution, because adverse effects are both common and dangerous when it is injected. Even as a surface

---

[11] Most 'reactions' occurring in the dental chair are the result of fear, posture, dose, and not of allergy.

anaesthetic sufficient absorption may take place to cause serious adverse effects. Cocaine prevents the uptake of catecholamines (adrenaline, nor-adrenaline) into sympathetic nerve endings, thus increasing their concentration at receptor sites, so that cocaine has a built-in vasoconstrictor action, which is why it retains a declining place as a surface anaesthetic for surgery involving mucous membranes, e.g. nose. Other local anaesthetics do not have this action, indeed are vasodilator and added adrenaline is not so efficient.

There are numerous *other local anaesthetics*, e.g. procaine, amethocaine, proxymetacaine, cinchocaine, benzocaine, oxybuprocaine, butacaine, orthocaine, and their omission here is not meant to imply that good results are not obtainable with them.

Choice of local anaesthetic

The many agents available are proof that all have disadvantages and that no agent is unchallengeably the best for all occasions. This is particularly the case for *surface* anaesthesia, although a claim that lignocaine is safest and best could not easily be dismissed; prilocaine is a contender when dosage must be heavy. For *infiltration injection* by the occasional user lignocaine or prilocaine are satisfactory.

Warning. There have been many deaths due to confusion of the names, all ending in 'caine' and to the use of wrong concentrations of unfamiliar drugs.

OBSTETRIC ANALGESIA AND ANAESTHESIA

Although this soon ceased to be considered immoral on religious grounds, it has been a technically controversial topic since 1853 when it was announced that Queen Victoria had inhaled chloroform during the birth of her eighth child. The *Lancet* recorded 'intense astonishment ... throughout the profession' at this use of chloroform, 'an agent which has unquestionably caused instantaneous death in a considerable number of cases'. But the Queen took a different view, writing in her private Journal of 'that

blessed chloroform' and adding that 'the effect was soothing, quieting and delightful beyond measure'.

Pain-free labour sometimes occurs spontaneously but, rightly or wrongly, most women in Western civilisations anticipate pain and demand relief. The reason for lack of general agreement on which drugs are best is that requirements are stringent, and much depends on the skill with which they are used. *The ideal drug* must relieve pain without making the patient confused or uncooperative. It must not interfere with uterine activity nor must it influence the fetus (respiratory depression is the chief disadvantage and may occur by a direct action of the drug on the fetus, by prolonging labour or by reducing uterine blood supply). It should also be suitable for use by a midwife without supervision.

Innumerable schemes have been proposed and good results can be obtained with many, by those who take the trouble to familiarise themselves with them. Generally, strong analgesic drugs should not be started before uterine contractions are well advanced as they can arrest labour if started sooner. The following may be taken as a general guide:

- Onset of labour, up to three-quarter dilatation of cervix: non-inhalational tranquillisers and analgesics, e.g. pethidine.
- From three-quarter dilatation of cervix till birth: inhalation analgesia, e.g. nitrous oxide/oxygen (below) to avoid respiratory depression of the fetus, which occurs with effective doses of narcotic analgesics.

Pethidine is widely used. It seldom causes serious respiratory depression but has been shown to reduce respiratory minute volume in the baby. The mother may experience drowsiness and nausea. Morphine depresses fetal respiration more than pethidine. Opioids may impair infant feeding for 48 h. Naloxone administered to the mother before birth or to the child after birth will reverse opioid effect. Opioids delay gastric emptying, which can carry hazard of vomiting if general anaesthesia is then needed. The effect is not antagonised by metoclopramide.

Diazepam, as tranquilliser (it is not analgesic)

during labour and as anticonvulsant in pre-eclampsia and eclampsia, has a depressant effect on the newborn if the maternal dose exceeds 30 mg in the 15 h before delivery (apnoeic spells, failure to feed, hypothermia), and these effects can last several days.

In general the baby will be about as depressed as the mother at the time of birth, and respiratory depressant should be withheld if birth is imminent. The intervals between doses are judged on clinical progress.

Sympathomimetic amines and other vasoconstrictors may cause fetal distress by reducing placental blood supply. They do not enter the fetus. Extreme hypotension from any cause also results in fetal anoxia.

Nitrous oxide and oxygen (50% of each: Entonox) may be administered for each pain from a machine the patient works herself or supervised by a midwife (about 10 good breaths are needed for maximal analgesia). Nitrous oxide and air mixtures are obsolete because hypoxia is unavoidable at effective concentrations of nitrous oxide.

Special techniques, e.g. extradural, caudal and pudendal nerve block, are highly effective in skilled hands.

General anaesthesia during labour presents a special problem in that the safety of the fetus must also be considered, and the anaesthetist must consider the patient to have a full stomach, so that regurgitation and aspiration is a particular risk (see p. 525). All anaesthetics and analgesics in general use cross the placenta in varying amounts and, apart from respiratory depression, produce no important effects except that high doses interfere with uterine retraction and may be followed by uterine haemorrhage. Neuromuscular blocking agents can be used safely, although gallamine is best avoided as it crosses the placenta and suxamethonium stimulates the uterus; none interferes with uterine retraction.

ANAESTHESIA IN PATIENTS ALREADY TAKING DRUGS

Anaesthetists are in an unenviable position. They are expected to provide safe service to patients in any condition, taking any drugs. Sometimes there is opportunity to modify drug therapy before surgery but often there is not. Anaesthetists require a particularly complete drug history of the patient.

Drugs that affect anaesthesia

The most important groups of drugs that affect anaesthesia are adrenal steroids, tranquillisers, antidepressants and antihypertensives. There is a paucity of useful data.

Adrenal steroids: chronic corticosteroid therapy within the previous 2 years can be associated with collapse due to the failure of the hypothalamic/pituitary/cortical axis to respond to stress (see Ch. 33).

Antibiotics: aminoglycosides, e.g. neomycin, gentamicin, are themselves neuromuscular blocking agents in high dose and are additive with non-depolarising neuromuscular blocking drugs.

Anticholinesterases: can potentiate suxamethonium.

Anticoagulants: see index.

NSAIDs: interfere with blood platelet function and may cause oozing at the operation site.

Antiepilepsy drugs: continued medication is essential to avoid status epilepticus. Drugs must be given parenterally until the patient can swallow. Valproate can impair coagulation.

Antihypertensives of all kinds: hypotension may complicate anaesthesia, but it is best to continue therapy. Hypertensive patients are particularly liable to excessive rise in blood pressure and heart rate during intubation, which can be dangerous if there is ischaemic heart disease. Postoperatively, parenteral therapy may be needed for a time. Abrupt withdrawal of antihypertensive drugs can lead to rebound hypertension, especially with clonidine.

Calcium channel blocking drugs: patients taking verapamil may develop heart block with halothane.

Digoxin: cardiac dysrhythmias are more likely with general anaesthesia.

β-*adrenoceptor blocking drugs*: can prevent the homeostatic sympathetic cardiac response to cardiac depressant anaesthetics and to blood loss; bronchospasm may occur.

Diuretics: if hypokalaemia occurs, this will potentiate neuromuscular blocking agents and perhaps general anaesthetics.

Oral contraceptives containing oestrogen and postmenopausal hormone replacement therapy: predispose to thromboembolism (see p. 603).

Psychotropic drugs: neuroleptics potentiate or synergise with opioids, hypnotics and general anaesthetics. Those with antihypertensive properties, e.g. chlorpromazine, may cause severe hypotension during anaesthesia.

Antidepressants: monoamine oxidase inhibitors can potentiate opioids (especially pethidine) and sometimes general anaesthetics as well as some sympathomimetics. Tricyclics potentiate catecholamines and some other adrenergic drugs.

Lithium: may be continued unless there is serious risk of electrolyte disturbance or renal insufficiency, when it should be stopped a week before surgery.

Opioid analgesics, hypnotics and alcohol: if enough of these has been habitually taken for tolerance to result, there will be some cross-tolerance with general anaesthetics.

ANAESTHESIA IN THE DISEASED, IN OLD AGE AND CHILDHOOD

The normal response to anaesthesia may be greatly modified by disease. The possibilities are vast and only some of the more important aspects will be mentioned here.

Respiratory disease and smoking predispose the patient to postanaesthetic pulmonary complications such as collapse and pneumonia. The site of operation and the occurrence of pain are also relevant when they cause defective ventilation due to pain and fear of coughing.

Cardiac disease. The aim is to avoid the circulatory stress (with increased cardiac work which can compromise the myocardial oxygen supply), caused by struggling, coughing, laryngospasm and breath holding. Drugs given i.v. should be injected slowly to avoid hypotension, which may occur with very many substances if they are given too fast.

Patients with fixed cardiac output, e.g. mitral stenosis or constrictive pericarditis, are specially liable to a drop in cardiac output, for which they cannot compensate, with drugs that depress the myocardium and vasomotor centre. Thiopentone induction is liable to do this and inhalation induction may be preferable. Anoxia is obviously harmful. It will be seen that skilled technique rather than choice of drugs on pharmacological grounds is the important factor. If heart failure or dysrhythmias are anticipated from the condition of the patient or the nature of the operation, appropriate treatment may be begun preoperatively.

Hepatic and renal disease. Very many drugs are metabolised by the liver or excreted by the kidney so that disease of these organs is liable to lead to increased drug effects. This should be taken into account when selecting drugs and their doses. General anaesthetics can also impair hepatic function.

Malignant hyperthermia occurs in from 1:15 000 (children) to 1:40 000 of unselected subjects of general anaesthesia. It is a result of an inherited muscle disorder (autosomal dominant). The condition occurs during or within several hours of anaesthesia. It is precipitated by almost any drug, but especially by potent inhalation agents (especially halogenated), and by suxamethonium; but it is possible that it may also result from stress alone. The patient may previously have safely experienced a general anaesthetic. The mechanism involves a sudden rise in release of bound (stored) calcium of the sarcoplasm, stimulating contraction and a hypermetabolic state.

Malignant hyperthermia is a life-threatening medical emergency. Oxygen consumption increases by up to 3 times normal, and body temperature may rise as fast as 1°C every 5 min, reaching as high as 43°C. Rigidity of voluntary muscles may not be evident at the outset or in mild cases.

Administration of *dantrolene* ($t_{\frac{1}{2}}$ 9 h) i.v., 1 mg/kg, is urgently required; further doses are given if there is not a quick response (5 min); the average total effective dose is 2.5 mg/kg, but as much as 10 mg/kg may be needed. Dantrolene probably acts by preventing the release of calcium from the sarcoplasm store that ordinarily follows depolarisation of the muscle membrane.

Non-specific treatment is needed for the hyperthermia. Cardiac dysrhythmias occur (due to potassium release from contracted muscle).

Any *future anaesthesia* in patients who have experienced the syndrome can be achieved with minimal risk by using opioids, barbiturates, diazepam, neuroleptics, nitrous oxide, probably propofol or ester-class local anaesthetics; pancuronium or atracurium may be safe for neuromuscular block. Dantrolene orally may be used as prophylaxis.

It is recommended that i.v. formulation of dantrolene should be available in every surgical theatre. Where it is not available an ester-class local anaesthetic (e.g. procaine) given cautiously i.v. may be better than nothing.

The relation of malignant hyperthermia syndrome with neuroleptic malignant syndrome is uncertain.

Diabetes mellitus: see p. 579.
Thyroid disease: see p. 588.
Porphyria: see p. 122.

Muscle diseases. Patients with myasthenia gravis are very sensitive (intolerant) to competitive but not to depolarising neuromuscular blocking drugs. Those with dystrophia myotonica may recover less rapidly than normal from central respiratory depression and neuromuscular block; they may fail to relax with suxamethonium. All patients with generalised muscular weakness or disease should be treated with special attentiveness.

Sickle-cell disease: hypoxia can precipitate a crisis.

Atypical pseudocholinesterase (or deficiency) delays metabolism of suxamethonium seriously: any effect on ester class local anaesthetics is probably unimportant clinically.

Raised intracranial pressure will be made worse by inhalation agents, e.g. halothane, nitrous oxide, by hypoxia or hypercapnia and in response to intubation, it depresses the respiratory centre and these patients are liable to respiratory failure with central nervous depressants, especially opioids. Therefore, premedication may consist of atropine alone.

Old age (see p. 107). Old people are liable to become confused by cerebral depressants, especially by hyoscine, and atropine is usually substituted. Apart from this there are no special problems for anaesthesia, but mistakes and overdose are less easily retrieved in the old and frail than in the young and healthy. In general, elderly patients require smaller doses than the young. Hypotension should be especially avoided as it readily causes cerebral hypoxia.

Childhood (see p. 107). Here again the problems are more technical, physiological and psychological than pharmacological. Premedication is often by sedatives, e.g. benzodiazepine, orally or by rectum, rather than by injected morphine or papaveretum with hyoscine, although children in fact tolerate these well.

Sedation in intensive therapy units. Patients who are not too sick are likely to feel frightened. Charity requires that they be relieved (by sympathetic care and, if necessary, by drugs). Benzodiazepines are an obvious choice, e.g. midazolam; also propofol, chlormethiazole, neuroleptics.

But there are other reasons for sedation. Some patients will 'fight' the mechanical ventilator they require, and endotracheal tubes are extremely uncomfortable and even painful. Opioids are an obvious choice, e.g. phenoperidine (where short $t_{\frac{1}{2}}$, 30 min, is desired). These not only relieve pain and discomfort, but tranquillise and depress respiration so that the patient fights the ventilator less. A competitive neuromuscular blocking agent may have to be added to reduce the need for high doses of opioids, especially where there is reduced renal and hepatic function. But its use adds the risk of death due to accidental disconnection of the ventilator. Neuromuscular blockers do *not* impair consciousness and an aware and paralysed patient is in great distress, and is unable to communicate this to attendants. Everyone will wish to avoid this and it can be done by skilled use of sedatives and opioids.

GUIDE TO FURTHER READING

Editorial 1987 Pain, anaesthesia, and babies. Lancet 2: 543

Editorial 1989 Nausea and vomiting after general anaesthesia. Lancet 1: 651

Editorial 1989 Epidural morphine, hypertension and aortic surgery. Lancet 2: 598

Editorial 1990 Neuromuscular blockade. Lancet 335: 382

Editorial 1991 Postoperative pain relief and non-opioid analgesics. Lancet 337: 524

Editorial 1991 Pain relief in labour: old drugs, new route. Lancet 337: 1446

Evans C et al 1988 Improved recovery and reduced postoperative stay after therapeutic suggestion during general anaesthesia. Lancet 2: 491

Hanks G W et al 1988 Local anaesthetic creams: preparations effective on skin should increase use. British Medical Journal 297–1215

Jacobsen B et al 1990 Opiate addiction in adult offspring through possible imprinting after obstetric treatment. British Medical Journal 301: 1067

Jones J G et al 1986 Hearing and memory in anaesthetised patients. British Medical Journal 292: 1291

Jones M J T et al 1990 Cognitive and functional competence after anaesthesia in patients aged over 60: controlled trial of general and regional anaesthesia for elective hip and knee replacements. British Medical Journal 300: 1683

Kong K L et al 1989 Isoflurane compared with midazolam for sedation in the intensive care unit. British Medical Journal 298: 1277

Neil H A W et al 1987 Mortality among male anaesthetists in the United Kingdom 1957–83. British Medical Journal 295: 360

Ngai S H 1982 Effects of anaesthetics on various organs. New England Journal of Medicine 302: 564

Noble D W et al 1989 Screening for antibodies to anaesthetics. British Medical Journal 299: 2

21

Cholinergic (cholinomimetic) and antimuscarinic (anticholinergic) drugs

SYNOPSIS

Acetylcholine acts as a chemotransmitter at a wide variety of sites, mediating a wide variety of physiological effects.

Cholinergic drugs (acetylcholine agonists) mimic acetylcholine at all sites but with differences of emphasis.

Acetylcholine receptor (cholinoceptor) blocking drugs are selective for different physiological classes of receptor which have been selectively defined by use of the alkaloids nicotine (from tobacco) and muscarine (from a fungus).

Acetylcholine antagonists (blockers) that oppose the nicotine-like effects (neuromuscular blockers and autonomic ganglion blockers) are described elsewhere, see index.
Acetylcholine antagonists that block the muscarine-like effects, e.g. atropine, are often imprecisely called anticholinergics. The more precise term antimuscarinic is preferred here.

- Cholinergic drugs
  Classification
  Sites of action
  Choline esters
  Cholinergic alkaloids
  Anticholinesterases
  Myasthenia gravis
- Drugs which oppose acetylcholine
  Antimuscarinic drugs

CHOLINERGIC DRUGS

These substances act on acetylcholine receptors (*cholinoceptors*) at all the sites in the body where acetylcholine is the transmitter of the nerve impulse. They stimulate and later paralyse. In addition, like acetylcholine, they act on non-innervated dilator receptors on peripheral blood vessels.

USES OF CHOLINERGIC DRUGS

- For myasthenia gravis, both to diagnose (edrophonium) and to treat (neostigmine, pyridostigmine, distigmine).
- To stimulate the bladder and bowel after surgery (bethanecol, carbachol).
- To lower intraocular pressure in chronic simple glaucoma (pilocarpine).

CLASSIFICATION

Direct acting

- *Choline esters* (carbachol, bethanechol) which act at all sites like acetylcholine. Muscarinic effects are more prominent than nicotinic (see p. 383).
- *Alkaloids* (pilocarpine, muscarine) which act selectively on end-organs of postganglionic, cholinergic neurons.

Indirect acting

- *Cholinesterase inhibitors*, or anticholinesterases (physostigmine, neostigmine, pyridostigmine,

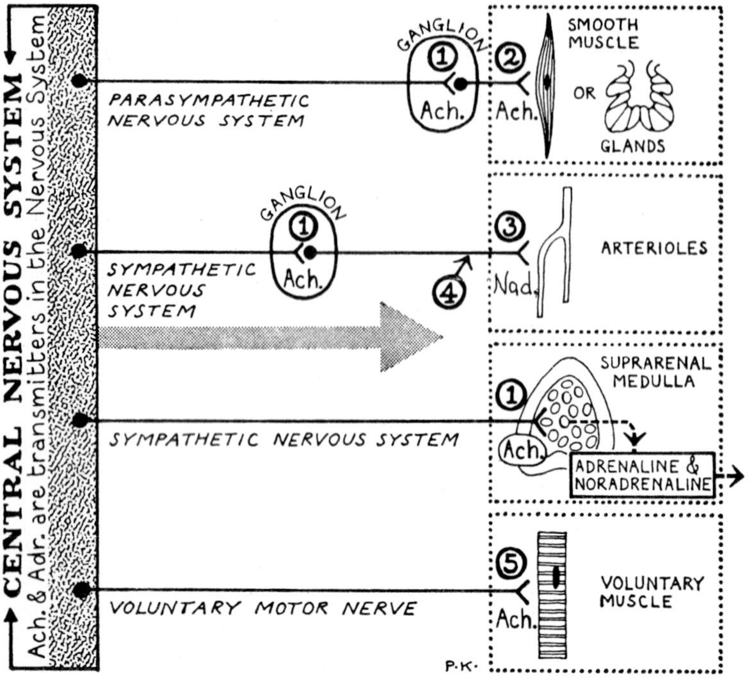

Fig. 21.1 Diagram showing sites of chemical transmitters of nerve impulse (This is the classic oversimplification that is sufficient for this account)
Ach. = acetylcholine
Nad. = noradrenaline
Site 1 is blocked by ganglion-blocking agents and stimulated by nicotine and big doses of some choline esters and anticholinesterases.
Site 2 is blocked by atropine and stimulated by some choline esters, anticholinesterases and pilocarpine.
Site 3 is blocked by adrenoceptor blocking agents and function is interfered with by drugs that deplete noradrenaline stores in nerve-endings and end-organs (reserpine).
Sympathomimetic amines stimulate here.
Site 4 is blocked by adrenergic neuron-blocking agents (guanethidine).
Site 5 is blocked by neuromuscular blocking agents and stimulated by choline esters and anticholinesterases.

distigmine), which inactivate the enzyme that destroys acetylcholine, allowing the chemical transmitter to persist and produce intensified effects.

SITES OF ACTION OF CHOLINERGIC DRUGS

1. Autonomic nervous system
a. *Parasympathetic division*
   ganglia
   postganglionic endings (all)
b. *Sympathetic division*
   ganglia
   a minority of postganglionic endings, e.g. sweat glands
2. Neuromuscular junction
3. Central nervous system
4. Non-innervated sites: blood vessels, chiefly arterioles.

Acetylcholine is the chemotransmitter of the nerve impulse at all these sites, acting on a postsynaptic receptor, except on most blood vessels in which the action of cholinergic drugs is

unrelated to cholinergic vasodilator nerves. It is also produced in tissues unrelated to nerve endings, e.g. placenta, ciliated epithelial cells, where it acts as a local hormone (autacoid) on local receptors.

A list of principal effects is given below. Not all occur with every drug and not all are noticeable at therapeutic doses. For example, central nervous system effects of cholinergic drugs are best seen in cases of anticholinesterase poisoning. Atropine antagonises all the effects of cholinergic drugs except those at *autonomic ganglia* and the *neuromuscular junction*, i.e. it does not act at receptors served by neurons arising in the central nervous system; it has antimuscarinic but not antinicotinic effects (see below).

Details of cholinergic pharmacology

1. Autonomic nervous system

Parasympathetic division. Stimulation of cholinoceptors in autonomic ganglia and at the postganglionic endings affects chiefly the following organs:

Eye: miosis and spasm of the ciliary muscle occur so that the eye is accommodated for near vision. Intraocular pressure falls due, perhaps, to dilation of vessels at the point where intraocular fluids pass into the blood.

Exocrine glands: there is increased secretion most noticeably of the salivary, lachrymal, bronchial and sweat glands. The last are cholinergic, although anatomically part of the sympathetic system; some sweat glands, e.g. axillary, may be adrenergic.

Heart: bradycardia occurs with atrioventricular block and eventually cardiac arrest.

Bronchi: bronchoconstriction occurs, also increased secretion, which effects may be clinically serious in asthmatic or other allergic subjects, in whom cholinergic drugs should be avoided as far as possible.

Alimentary tract: there is increased motor activity and exocrine secretion and colicky pain may occur. Sphincter tone is reduced and the patient may defaecate embarrassingly. Lowering of oesophageal sphincter tone creates a risk of regurgitation and inhalation, e.g. in anaesthesia.

Bladder and ureters contract and the drugs promote micturition.

Sympathetic division. *The ganglia* only are stimulated, also the cholinergic nerves to the adrenal medulla. These effects are overshadowed by effects on the parasympathetic system and are commonly evident only if atropine has been given to block the latter, when tachycardia, vasoconstriction and hypertension occur.

2. Neuromuscular (voluntary) junction

The neuromuscular junction has a cholinergic nerve ending, and so is activated, causing muscle fasciculation, followed if excess is given, by a depolarisation neuromuscular block.

3. Central nervous system

There is usually stimulation followed by depression, but variation between drugs is great, possibly due to differences in penetration into the nervous system. In overdose, mental excitement occurs, with confusion and restlessness, insomnia (with nightmares when sleep does come), tremors and dysarthria, and sometimes even convulsions and coma.

4. Blood vessels

There is stimulation of cholinergic vasodilator nerve endings in addition to the more important dilating action on arterioles and capillaries mediated through non-innervated receptors. Anticholinesterases potentiate acetylcholine which exists in the vessel walls independently of nerves.

Nicotinic and muscarinic effects

The actions of acetylcholine and substances acting like it at autonomic ganglia and the neuromuscular junction (i.e. at the end of cholinergic nerve fibres which arise in the central nervous system) are described as *nicotinic* because they are like the stimulant effects of nicotine. The actions at postganglionic cholinergic endings (parasympathetic endings plus the cholinergic sympathetic nerves to the sweat glands) and those non-innervated receptors on blood vessels are described as *muscarinic* because they resemble those of the alkaloid muscarine. The central nervous system actions are not included in this curious categorisation. The terms are useful because it is more concise to say that atropine blocks the muscarinic but not the nicotinic effects of neostigmine than it is to describe this antagonism in any other way, i.e. jargon is useful in the right place.

CHOLINE ESTERS

Acetylcholine

Since acetylcholine has such great importance in the body it is not surprising that attempts have been made to use it in therapeutics. But a substance with such a huge variety of effects and so rapidly destroyed in the body is unlikely to be useful when given systemically, as its history in psychiatry illustrates.

Acetylcholine was first injected intravenously as a therapeutic convulsant in 1939, in the justified expectation that the fits would be less liable to cause fractures than those following therapeutic leptazol convulsions. Recovery rates of up to 80% were claimed in various psychotic conditions. Enthusiasm began to wane however when it was shown that the fits were due to anoxia resulting from cardiac arrest and not to pharmacological effects on the brain.[1] The following description is illustrative:

A few seconds after the injection (which was given as rapidly as possible, to avoid total destruction in the blood) the patient sat up 'with knees drawn up to the chest, the arms flexed and the head bent forward. There were repeated violent coughs, sometimes with flushing. Forced swallowing and loud peristaltic rumblings could be heard'. Respiration was laboured and irregular. 'The coughing abated as the patient sank back in the bed. Forty seconds after the injection the radial and apical pulse were zero and the patient became comatose.' The pupils dilated, and deep reflexes were hyperactive. In 45 seconds the patient went into opisthotonos with brief apnoea. Lachrymation, sweating and borborygmi were prominent. The deep reflexes became diminished. The patient then relaxed and 'lay quietly in bed — cold moist and gray. In about 90 seconds, flushing of the face marked the return of the pulse'. The respiratory rate rose and consciousness returned in about 125 seconds. The patients sometimes micturated but did not defaecate. They 'tended to lie quietly in bed after the treatment'. 'Most of the patients were reluctant to be treated.'[2]

Other choline esters

Carbachol is a choline ester which is not destroyed by cholinesterase; its actions are most pronounced on the bladder and bowels, so that the drug is used to stimulate these organs, e.g. after surgery. Carbachol is stable in the alimentary tract; it is extremely dangerous if given i.v. but may be administered s.c.

Bethanechol is not destroyed by cholinesterase. It acts chiefly on the bowel and bladder and is preferable to carbachol because of this partial selectivity.

ALKALOIDS WITH CHOLINERGIC EFFECTS

Nicotine: see p. 328.

Pilocarpine, from an American plant (*Pilocarpus* spp.), acts directly on end-organs innervated by postganglionic nerves (parasympathetic system plus sweat glands); it also stimulates and then depresses the central nervous system. The chief clinical use of pilocarpine is to lower intraocular pressure in chronic simple glaucoma, as an adjunct to a topical β-blocker; it produces miosis, opens drainage channels in the trabecular network and improves the outflow of aqueous humour.

Arecoline is an alkaloid in the betel nut which is chewed in the East. It produces a mild dependence for, like other parasympathomimetic drugs, it stimulates the brain.

Muscarine is of no therapeutic use but it has pharmacological interest. It is present in small amounts in the fungus *Amanita muscaria* (Fly agaric), named after its capacity to kill the domestic fly (*Musca domestica*); muscarine was so named because it was thought to be the insecticidal principle, but it is relatively non-toxic to flies (orally administered). The fungus may contain other antimuscarinic substances and GABA-receptor agonists in amounts sufficient to be psychoactive in man.

Poisoning with these fungi may present with antimuscarinic, with cholinergic or with GABA-ergic effects. All have CNS actions. Happily, poisoning by *Amanita muscaria* is seldom serious. Species of *Inocybe* contain larger amounts of muscarine (see Ch. 9).

The lengths to which man is prepared to go in taking 'chemical vacations' when life is hard, are shown by the inhabitants of Eastern Siberia who used *Amanita muscaria* recreationally, for its cerebral stimulant effects. They were apparently prepared to put up with the autonomic actions to escape briefly from reality. The fungus was scarce in winter and the frugal devotees discovered that by drinking their own urine they could prolong the intoxication. Sometimes, in generous mood, the intoxicated person would offer his urine to others as a treat.

[1] Harris M et al. Arch Neurol Psychiat 1943; 50: 304.
[2] Cohen L H et al. Arch Neurol Psychiat 1944; 51: 171.

ANTICHOLINESTERASES

In the region of cholinergic nerve endings and in erythrocytes there is an enzyme that specifically destroys acetylcholine; *true* cholinesterase or acetylcholinesterase. In various tissues, especially blood plasma, there are other esterases which are not specific for acetylcholine but which also destroy other esters, e.g. suxamethonium, procaine. These are called non-specific or *pseudocholinesterases*. Chemicals which inactivate these esterases (anticholinesterases) are used in medicine, and in agriculture as pesticides. They act by allowing naturally formed acetylcholine to accumulate instead of being destroyed and their effects are almost entirely due to this accumulation in the central nervous system, at the neuromuscular junction, autonomic ganglia, postganglionic cholinergic nerve endings (which are principally in the parasympathetic nervous system) and in the walls of blood vessels, where acetylcholine is a local hormone not necessarily associated with nerve endings. Some of these effects oppose each other, e.g. the effect of anticholinesterase on the heart will be the resultant of stimulation at sympathetic ganglia and the opposing effect of stimulation at parasympathetic (vagal) ganglia and postganglionic nerve endings.

Physostigmine (eserine) is an alkaloid, obtained from the seeds of a West african plant (Physostigma), which has long been used both as a weapon and as an ordeal[3] poison. It acts for a few hours. Physostigmine is used synergistically with pilocarpine to reduce intraocular pressure. It has been shown to have some efficacy in improving cognitive function in Alzheimer type dementia.

Neostigmine (Prostigmin) is a synthetic reversible anticholinesterase ($t_{\frac{1}{2}}$ 2 h) whose actions are more prominent on the neuromuscular junction and the alimentary tract than on the cardiovascular system and eye. It is therefore principally used in myasthenia gravis, to stimulate the bowels and bladder after surgery, and as an antidote to competitive neuromuscular blocking agents. Neostigmine is effective orally (15–30 mg, 3 or 4 times a day), and by injection (usually s.c.) 0.5–2.0 mg. But higher doses may be used in myasthenia gravis, often combined with atropine to reduce the unwanted muscarinic effects.

Pyridostigmine (Mestinon) is similar to neostigmine but has a less powerful action that is slower in onset and slightly longer in duration, and perhaps fewer visceral effects. It is used in myasthenia gravis.

Distigmine (Ubretid) is a variant of pyridostigmine (2 linked molecules as the name implies).

Edrophonium (Tensilon) is structurally related to neostigmine but its action is brief and autonomic effects are minimal except at high doses. The drug is used to diagnose myasthenia gravis and to differentiate a *myasthenic* crisis (weakness due to inadequate anticholinesterase treatment or severe disease) from a *cholinergic* crisis (weakness caused by overtreatment with an anticholinesterase). Myasthenic weakness is substantially improved by edrophonium whereas cholinergic weakness is aggravated but the effect is transient; the action of 3 mg i.v. is lost in 5 minutes.

Metriphonate is used for urinary schistosomiosis.

Anticholinesterase poisoning

The anticholinesterases used in therapeutics are generally those which reversibly inactivate cholinesterase for a few hours. *Pesticides* of the carmabate type act by reversible inhibition of cholinesterase but organophosphorus compounds inhibit the enzyme almost or completely irreversibly so that recovery depends on formation of fresh enzyme. This process may take weeks although clinical recovery is usually evident in days. Cases of poisoning are usually met outside therapeutic practice, e.g. after agricultural, industrial or transport accidents. Substances of this type have also been developed and used in war (nerve 'gas'). Where there is known risk of exposure prior use of pyridostigmine, which oc-

---

[3]To demonstrate guilt or innocence according to whether the accused died or lived after the judicial dose. The practice had the advantage that the demonstration of guilt provided simultaneous punishment.

cupies cholinesterases reversibly for a few hours (the lesser evil), competitively protects them from access by the irreversible warfare agent (the greater evil); soldiers expecting attack have been provided with self-injection loaded syringes. Organophosphorus agents are absorbed through the skin, the gastrointestinal tract and by inhalation. Diagnosis depends on observing a substantial part of the list of actions below.

Typical features involve the gastrointestinal tract (salivation, vomiting, abdominal cramps, diarrhoea, involuntary defaecation), the respiratory system (bronchorrhoea, bronchoconstriction, cough, wheezing, dyspnoea), the cardiovascular system (bradycardia), the genitourinary system (involuntary micturition), the skin (sweating), the skeletal system (muscle weakness, twitching) and the nervous system (miosis, anxiety, headache, convulsions, respiratory failure). Death is due to a combination of the actions in the central nervous system, to paralysis of the respiratory muscles by peripheral depolarisation neuromuscular block, and to excessive bronchial secretions and constriction causing respiratory obstruction. At autopsy, ileal intussusceptions are commonly found.

Treatment. Since the most common circumstance of accidental poisoning is exposure to pesticide spray or spillage, contaminated clothing should be removed and the skin washed. Gastric lavage is needed if any of the substance has been ingested. Attendants should take care to ensure that they themselves do not become contaminated.

● *Atropine* is the mainstay of treatment; 2 mg is given i.m. or i.v. as soon as possible and repeated every 15–60 min until dryness of the mouth and a heart rate in excess of 70 beats per minute indicate that its effect is adequate. A poisoned patient may require 100 mg or more for a single episode. Atropine antagonises the parasympathomimetic effects of the poison, i.e. due to stimulation at postganglionic nerve endings (excessive secretion) and vasodilatation, i.e. the muscarinic actions. Neuromuscular block is not relieved, for atropine does not antagonise acetylcholine at the endings of nerve fibres which arise

in the central nervous system (nicotinic effects).

● *Mechanical ventilation* may therefore be needed to assist the respiratory muscles; special attention to the airway is vital because of bronchial constriction and excessive secretion.

● *Diazepam* may be needed for convulsions. Atropine eye-drops may relieve the headache caused by miosis.

● *Enzyme reactivation.* The organophosphorus pesticides inactivate cholinesterase by *irreversibly* phosphorylating the active centre of the enzyme. Substances that reactivate the enzyme lessen the effects of the accumulated acetylcholine, and, unlike atropine, they have both antinicotinic and antimuscarinic effects. The principal agent is *pralidoxime*, 1.0 g of which should be given 4-hourly i.m. or (diluted) by slow i.v. infusion, as indicated by the patient's condition; efficacy is best if it is administered within 12 hours of poisoning and is probably valueless after 24 hours for by then insecticide and enzyme are irreversibly bound.

Poisoning with *reversible* anticholinesterases is appropriately treated by atropine and the necessary general support; it lasts only hours.

Erythrocyte or plasma cholinesterase content should be measured if possible, both for diagnosis and to determine when a poisoned worker may return to his task in the event of his being willing to do so. This should not be allowed until the cholinesterase exceeds 70% of normal, which may take several weeks.

DISORDERS OF NEUROMUSCULAR TRANSMISSION

Myasthenia gravis

In myasthenia gravis synaptic transmission at the neuromuscular junction is impaired; most cases appear to have an autoimmune basis, for 90% of patients have a raised titre of autoantibodies to the acetylcholine receptor, but the condition is probably heterogeneous as a minority do not have antibodies.

Neostigmine was introduced in 1931 for its stimulant effects on intestinal activity. In 1934 it occurred to Dr. Mary Walker that since the paralysis of myasthenia had been (erroneously) attributed to a curare-like substance in the blood, physostigmine (eserine), an anticholinesterase drug known to antagonise curare, might be beneficial. It was, and she reported this important observation in a short letter.[4] Soon after this she used neostigmine by mouth with greater benefit.

The sudden appearance of an effective treatment for an hitherto untreatable chronic disease must always be a dramatic event for its victims. The impact of the discovery of the action of neostigmine has been described by one patient.

'My myasthenia started in 1925, when I was 18. For several months it consisted of double vision and fatigue . . . An ophthalmic surgeon . . . prescribed glasses with a prism. However, soon more alarming symptoms began.' Her limbs became weak and she 'was sent to an eminent neurologist. This was a horrible experience. He . . . could find no physical signs . . . declared me to be suffering from hysteria and asked me what was on my mind. When I answered truthfully, that nothing except anxiety over my symptoms, he replied "my dear child, I am not a perfect fool . . .", and showed me out.' She became worse and at times she was unable to turn over in bed. Eating, and even speaking were difficult. Eventually, her fiancé, a medical student, read about myasthenia gravis and she was correctly diagnosed in 1927. 'There was at that time no known treatment and therefore many things to try'. She had gold injections, thyroid, suprarenal extract, lecithin, glycine and ephedrine. The last had a slight effect. 'Then in February 1935, came the day that I shall always remember. I was living alone with a nurse . . . It was one of my better days, and I was lying on the sofa after tea . . . My fiancé came in rather late saying that he had something new for me to try. My first thought was 'Oh bother! Another injection, and another false hope.' I submitted to the injection with complete indifference and within a few minutes began to feel very strange . . . when I lifted my arms, exerting the effort to which I had become accustomed, they shot into the air, every movement I attempted was grotesquely magnified until I learnt to make less effort . . . it was strange, wonderful and at first, very frightening . . . we danced twice round the carpet. That was my first meeting with neostigmine, and we have never since been separated'.[5]

[4]Walker M B. Lancet 1934; 1: 1200.
[5]Disabilities and how to live with them. London: Lancet, 1952.

Pathogenesis. Evidence indicates that the clinical features of myasthenia gravis are caused by specific antibodies which either block or cause complement-mediated lysis of the acetylcholine receptor. In common with all body tissues, receptors are constantly being broken down and re-synthesised. Cholinoceptors exist for about 7 days in normal individuals but for only one day in myasthenic patients. The thymus gland is in some way involved in the process and three-quarters of patients have either thymitis or a thymoma.

Diagnosis is made with the anticholinesterase drug, edrophonium, which dramatically and transiently (5 min) relieves muscular weakness. A syringe is loaded with edrophonium 10 mg; 2 mg are given i.v. and if there is no improvement in weakness in 30 s the remaining 8 mg are injected. A syringe loaded with atropine should be at hand to block severe cholinergic autonomic (muscarinic) effects, e.g. bradycardia, should they occur. Acetylcholine receptor antibodies should also be measured in the plasma for an elevated titre confirms the diagnosis.

Treatment involves immunosuppression, thymectomy (unless contraindicated) and symptom relief with drugs.

● *Immunosuppressive* treatment is directed at eliminating the acetylcholine receptor antibody. *Prednisolone* induces improvement or remission in 80% of cases. The dose should be increased slowly using an alternate day regimen until the minimum effective amount is attained; an immunosuppressive improvement may take several weeks. *Azathioprine* may be used as a steroid-sparing agent. Prednisolone is effective for ocular myasthenia, which is fortunate, for this variant of the disease responds poorly to thymectomy or anticholinesterase drugs. Some acute and severe cases respond poorly to prednisolone with azathioprine and, for these, intermittent plasmapheresis (to remove circulating antibody) can provide dramatic short-term relief.

● *Thymectomy* should be offered once the clinical state allows and unless there are powerful contraindications to surgery, for most cases benefit and about 25% can discontinue drug treatment. Thymectomy should also be undertaken in all myasthenic patients who have a thymoma, but the main reason is to prevent local infiltration for the procedure is less likely to relieve the myasthenia.

• *Symptomatic* drug treatment is decreasingly used. Its aim is to increase the concentration of acetylcholine at the neuromuscular junction with anticholinesterase drugs. The mainstay is usually pyridostigmine, starting with 60 mg by mouth 6-hourly. It is preferred because its action is smoother than that of neostigmine, but the latter is more rapid in onset and can with advantage be given in the mornings to get the patient mobile. Either drug can be given parenterally if bulbar paralysis makes swallowing difficult. An antimuscarinic drug, e.g. propantheline, should be added if muscarinic effects are troublesome.

Too high a dose of anticholinesterase drugs may make the weakness worse by causing excess build-up of acetylcholine (*cholinergic crisis*) and it is important to distinguish this from an exacerbation of the disease (*myasthenic crisis*). A dose of edrophonium will make the diagnosis; a myasthenic crisis gets better and cholinergic crisis gets worse — dangerously so if the vital bulbar and respiratory muscles are involved; this test is best left to those with special experience, and mechanical ventilation facilities should be at hand.

A cholinergic crisis should be treated by withdrawing all anticholinesterase medication, mechanical respiration if required, and atropine i.v. for muscarinic effects of the overdosage. The neuromuscular block is a nicotinic effect and will be unchanged by atropine. A resistant *myasthenic crisis* may be treated by withdrawal of drugs and artificial respiration for a few days. Plasmapheresis may be beneficial by removing antibodies.

Drug-induced disorders of neuromuscular transmission

Quite apart from the neuromuscular blocking agents used in anaesthesia, a number of drugs possess actions that impair neuromuscular transmission and in appropriate circumstances, give rise to:

• postoperative respiratory depression in people whose neuromuscular transmission is otherwise normal;
• aggravation or unmasking of myasthenia gravis or,
• a drug-induced myasthenic syndrome.

These drugs include:

Antibiotics: Aminoglycosides (neomycin, streptomycin, gentamicin) and polypeptides (colistin, polymyxin B) may cause postoperative breathing difficulty if they are instilled into the peritoneal or pleural cavities. It appears that the antibiotics both interfere with the release of acetylcholine and also have a curare-like effect on the acetylcholine receptor.

Cardiovascular drugs: Those that possess local anaesthetic properties (quinidine, procainamide, lignocaine) and certain β-blockers (propranolol, oxprenolol, practolol) act by interfering with acetylcholine release and may aggravate or reveal myasthenia gravis.

Other drugs: *Penicillamine* causes some patients, especially those with rheumatoid arthritis, to form antibodies to the acetylcholine receptor and a syndrome indistinguishable from myasthenia gravis results. Spontaneous recovery occurs in about two-thirds of cases when penicillamine is withdrawn. *Phenytoin* may rarely induce or aggravate myasthenia gravis, or induce a myasthenic syndrome, possibly by depressing acetylcholine release. *Lithium* may impair presynaptic neurotransmission by substituting for sodium ions in the nerve terminal.

DRUGS WHICH OPPOSE ACETYLCHOLINE

These may be divided into:

1. Antimuscarinic drugs
These act principally at postganglionic cholinergic (parasympathetic) nerve endings, i.e. atropine-related drugs (see Fig. 21.1 site 2).

2. Antinicotinic drugs
Ganglion-blocking drugs (Fig. 21.1, site 1) (see Ch. 23)
Neuromuscular blocking drugs (Fig. 21.1, site 5) (see Ch. 20).

ANTIMUSCARINIC DRUGS

The principal effect of atropine and related drugs is to block competitively the binding of acetylcholine to receptors at the postganglionic

---

USES OF ANTIMUSCARINIC DRUGS

- For their actions in the central nervous system some (benzhexol, orphenadrine) are used against the rigidity and tremor of *parkinsonism*, in which disease doses higher than the usual therapeutic amounts are often needed and tolerated.

  They are used as *anti-emetics* (principally hyoscine, promethazine). Their *sedative* action is used in anaesthetic premedication (hyoscine).
- For their peripheral actions, atropine, homatropine and cyclopentolate are used in *ophthalmology* to dilate the pupil and to paralyse ocular accommodation. If it is desired to dilate the pupil and to spare accommodation, a sympathomimetic, e.g. phenylephrine, is useful.

  In *anaesthesia*, atropine, glycopyrronium and hyoscine block the vagus and reduce secretion.

  In the *respiratory tract* ipratropium is an effective bronchodilator.
- For their actions on the *alimentary tract* against muscle spasm and hypermotility, e.g. against colic (pain due to spasm of smooth muscle) and to prevent morphine-induced muscle spasm when that analgesic is used against colic.
- In the *urinary tract*, flavoxate, propantheline and oxybutynin are used to relieve muscle spasm accompanying infection in cystitis, and for detrusor instability.
- In disorders of the *cardiovascular system* atropine is useful in bradycardia following myocardial infarction.
- In *cholinergic poisoning*, atropine is an important antagonist of both central nervous, parasympathomimetic and vasodilator effects though it has no effect at the neuromuscular junction and will not prevent voluntary muscle paralysis. It is also used to block autonomic effects when cholinergic drugs, such as neostigmine, are used for their effect on the neuromuscular junction in myasthenia gravis.

Disadvantages of the antimuscarinics include their capacity to precipitate narrow-angle glaucoma, or urinary retention where there is prostatic hypertrophy.

---

cholinergic (parasympathetic) endings (Fig. 21.1, site 2) and at the non-innervated receptors on blood vessels, hence their description as *antimuscarinic* drugs. They also block effects of acetylcholine in the central nervous system; some have a blocking effect at autonomic ganglia also, but none blocks the neuromuscular junction at clinical doses.

The actions of atropine will first be described; other drugs will be dealt with chiefly in so far as they differ. Many antimuscarinic drugs have a variety of other actions, e.g. antihistamine, but find a place in therapeutics as antimuscarinic agents.

Atropine

Atropine is an alkaloid from the plant *Atropa belladonna*.[6]

In general, the effects of atropine are inhibitory but in large doses it stimulates the CNS (see poisoning, below). Atropine also blocks the effects of injected cholinergic drugs both peripherally and on the central nervous system. The clinically important actions of atropine are listed below; they are mostly the opposite of the activating effects on the parasympathetic system produced by cholinergic drugs.

Actions at parasympathetic postganglionic nerve endings

Exocrine glands. All secretions except milk are diminished. Dry mouth and dry eye are common. Gastric acid secretion is reduced but so also is the total volume of gastric secretion so that H^+ concentration (pH) may be little altered. *Sweating* (sympathetic nerve supply, but largely cholinergic) is inhibited. *Bronchial* secretions are reduced

---

[6] The first name commemorates its success as a homicidal poison, for it is derived from the senior of 3 legendary Fates, Atropos, who cuts with shears the web of life spun and woven by her sisters Clotho and Lachesis (there is a minor synthetic atropine-like drug called lachesine). The term belladonna refers to the once fashionable female practice of using an extract of the plant to dilate the pupils (incidentally blocking ocular accommodation) as part of the process of 'making myself attractive'.

and may become viscid, which can be a disadvantage, as removal of secretion by cough and ciliary action is rendered less effective.

Smooth muscle is relaxed. In the gastrointestinal tract there is reduction of tone and peristalsis. Muscle spasm of the intestinal tract induced by morphine is reduced, but such spasm in the biliary tract is not. Atropine relaxes bronchial muscle, an effect which is useful in some asthmatics. Micturition is slowed and urinary retention may be induced especially when there is pre-existing prostatic enlargement.

Ocular effects. Mydriasis occurs with a rise in intraocular pressure in an eye predisposed to narrow-angle glaucoma (but only rarely in chronic open-angle glaucoma). This is due to the dilated iris blocking drainage of the intraocular fluids from the angle of the anterior chamber. An attack of glaucoma may be induced. There is no significant effect on pressure in normal eyes. The ciliary muscle is paralysed and so the eye is accommodated for distant vision. After atropinisation, normal pupillary reflexes may not be regained for 2 weeks. Atropine is a cause of unequal sized and unresponsive pupils.

Cardiovascular system. Atropine reduces vagal tone thus increasing the heart rate, and enhancing conduction in the bundle of His, effects which are less marked in the elderly in whom vagal tone is low. Full atropinisation may increase rate by 30 beats/min in the young, but has little effect in the old. Transient vagal stimulation, probably in the CNS, may cause bradycardia, e.g. if atropine is given i.v. with neostigmine and the effects of the two drugs summate.

Atropine has no significant effect on peripheral blood vessels in therapeutic doses but, in poisoning, there is marked vasodilatation.

Atropine is effective against both tremor and rigidity of *parkinsonism*. It prevents or abates *motion sickness*.

Antagonism to cholinergic drugs. Atropine opposes the effects of all cholinergic drugs on the CNS, at postganglionic cholinergic nerve endings and on the peripheral blood vessels. It does not oppose cholinergic effects at the neuromuscular junction or significantly at the autonomic ganglia, i.e. atropine opposes the *muscarine-like* but not the *nicotine-like* effects of acetylcholine.

Pharmacokinetics. Atropine is readily absorbed from the alimentary tract and may also be injected by the usual routes. The occasional cases of atropine poisoning following use of eye drops are due to the solution running down the lacrimal ducts into the nose and being swallowed. Atropine is in part destroyed in the liver and in part excreted unchanged by the kidney. The $t_{\frac{1}{2}}$ is 2 h.

Dose. 0.25–2.0 mg by mouth or 0.4–1.0 mg i.v.; for chronic use it has largely been replaced by other antimuscarinic drugs.

Poisoning with atropine (and other antimuscarinic drugs) presents with the more obvious peripheral effects: dry mouth (with dysphagia), mydriasis, blurred vision, hot dry skin, and, in addition, hyperthermia (CNS action plus absence of sweating), restlessness, anxiety, excitement, hallucinations, delirium, mania and later, cerebral depression and coma or, as it has been described with characteristic American verbal felicity, 'hot as a hare, blind as a bat, dry as a bone, red as a beet and mad as a hen.'[7] It may occur in children who have eaten berries of solanaceous plants, e.g. deadly nightshade and henbane. When the diagnosis is doubtful, it is said to be worth putting a drop of the patient's urine in *one* eye of a cat. Mydriasis, if it results, confirms the diagnosis, but absence of effect proves nothing.

Treatment of atropine poisoning involves giving activated charcoal to adsorb the drug, and diazepam for excitement.

Other antimuscarinic drugs

In the following accounts of drugs, the principal peripheral atropine-like effects of the drugs may be assumed; differences from atropine are described.

Hyoscyamine is less active in the central nervous system. Atropine is racemic hyoscyamine; 'hyoscyamine' is the laevo form; the dextro form is only feebly active. Atropine is more stable chemically and so is preferred.

Hyoscine (scopolamine) is structurally related to atropine. It differs chiefly in being a central nervous system depressant, although it may

---

[7] Cohen H L et al. Arch Neurol Psychiat 1944; 51: 171.

sometimes cause excitement. The old are often confused by hyoscine and so it is avoided in their anaesthetic premedication. Mydriasis is briefer than with atropine.

Hyoscine butylbromide (Buscopan) also blocks autonomic ganglia. If injected, it is an effective relaxant of smooth muscle, including the cardia in achalasia, the pyloric antral region and the colon, which properties are utilised by radiologists and endoscopists. It may sometimes be useful for colic.

Homatropine is used for its ocular effects (1% and 2% solutions as eye drops). Its action is shorter than atropine and therefore less likely to cause serious rise of intraocular pressure; the effect wears off in a day or two. Complete cycloplegia cannot always be obtained unless repeated instillations are made every 15 min for 1–2 h. It is especially unreliable in children, in whom cyclopentolate or atropine is preferred. The pupillary dilation may be reversed by physostigmine eyedrops.

Tropicamide (Mydriacyl) and *cyclopentolate* (Mydrilate) are useful (as 0.5 or 1% solutions) for mydriasis and cycloplegia. They are quicker and shorter acting than is homatropine. The differences between the two are trivial. Mydriasis occurs in 10–20 min and cycloplegia shortly after. The duration of action is 6–12 h.

Ipratropium (Atrovent) is used by inhalation as a bronchodilator.

Flavoxate (Urispas) is used for urinary frequency, tenesmus and urgency incontinence because it increases bladder capacity and reduces unstable detrusor contractions (see Ch. 26).

Oxybutynin is also used for detrusor instability, but antimuscarinic adverse effects may limit its value.

Glycopyrronium is used in anaesthetic premedication to reduce salivary secretion; given i.v. it causes less tachycardia than does atropine.

Propantheline (Pro-Banthine) also has ganglion-blocking properties. It may be used as a smooth muscle relaxant, e.g. for irritable bowel syndrome and diagnostic procedures.

Dicyclomine (Merbentyl) is used for infantile pyloric stenosis and infantile colic.

Benzhexol and *orphenadrine*: see parkinsonism. *Promethazine*: see p. 509.

Other antimuscarinics used as antispasmodics include: ambutonium, mepenzolate, pipenzolate, poldine.

GUIDE TO FURTHER READING

Cohen H L et al 1944 Acetylcholine treatment of schizophrenia. Archives of Neurology and Psychiatry 51: 171

Fonseca V, Havard C W H 1990 The natural course of myasthenia gravis. British Medical Journal 300: 1409

Goyal R K 1989 Muscarinic receptor subtypes. New England Journal of Medicine 321: 1022

Hawkins J R et al 1956 Intravenous acetylcholine therapy in neurosis. A controlled trial (p 43), Carbon dioxide inhalation therapy in neurosis. A controlled clinical trial (p 52), The placebo response (p 60). Journal of Mental Science 102: 43

HMSO 1987 Medical manual of defence against chemical agents. JSP 312

Lambert D 1981 Personal paper; Myasthenia gravis. Lancet 1: 937

Morton H G, et al 1939 Atropine intoxication. Journal of Pediatrics 14: 755

22

Cardiovascular system I: adrenergic mechanisms, sympathomimetics, shock, hypotension

SYNOPSIS

Anyone who administers drugs acting on cardiovascular adrenergic mechanisms requires an understanding of how they act in order to use them to the best advantage and with safety.

- Adrenergic mechanisms
- Classification of sympathomimetics: by mode of action; by selectivity for adrenoceptors
- Individual sympathomimetics
- Mucosal decongestants
- Shock
- Chronic orthostatic hypotension

ADRENERGIC MECHANISMS

The discovery in 1895 of the hypertensive effect of adrenaline was initiated by Dr. Oliver, a physician in practice, who conducted a series of experiments on his young son into whom he injected an extract of bovine suprarenal. The effect was confirmed in animals and led eventually to the isolation and synthesis of adrenaline in the early 1900s. Many related compounds were examined and, in 1910, Barger and Dale invented the word *sympathomimetic*[1] and also pointed out that noradrenaline mimicked the action of the sympathetic nervous system more closely than did adrenaline.

Adrenaline, noradrenaline and dopamine are formed in the body and are used in therapeutics. The natural synthetic path is:

tyrosine → dopa → **dopamine→ noradrenaline → adrenaline.**

---

[1]'Compounds which . . . simulate the effects of sympathetic nerves not only with varying intensity but with varying precision . . . a term . . . seems needed to indicate the type of action common to these bases. We propose to call it 'sympathomimetic'. A term which indicates the relation of the action to innervation by the sympathetic system, without involving any theoretical preconception as to the meaning of that relation or the precise mechanism of the action'. (Barger G, Dale, H H. J Physiol 1910; XLI: 19–59.)

CLASSIFICATION OF SYMPATHOMIMETICS BY MODE OF ACTION

Noradrenaline is synthesised and stored in adrenergic nerve terminals and can be released from these stores by stimulating the nerve or by drugs (ephedrine, amphetamine). These noradrenaline stores may be replenished by i.v. infusion of noradrenaline, and abolished by reserpine or by cutting the sympathetic neuron.

Sympathomimetics may be classified as those that act:

1. **directly**, i.e. *adrenoceptor agonists* (adrenaline, noradrenaline, isoprenaline, methoxamine, xylometazoline, oxymetazoline, metaraminol, entirely; and dopamine and phenylephrine mainly).
2. **indirectly**, by causing a release of noradrenaline from stores at nerve endings (amphetamines, tyramine; and ephedrine, largely).
3. **by both mechanisms** (1) *and* (2), though often with a preponderance of one or other: other synthetic agents.

It is evident that *tachyphylaxis* (diminishing response to frequent or continuous administration) is particularly to be expected with drugs in group (2), and that they are less suitable for use in maintaining blood pressure than drugs of group (1). Tachyphylaxis to group (1) may be due to receptor changes.

The *interactions* of sympathomimetics with other drugs affecting the vascular system are complex. Some drugs prevent the uptake of noradrenaline from the circulation into stores (this may account for the potentiation of the pressor effect of noradrenaline by tricyclic antidepressants) and some drugs deplete or destroy the stores (reserpine) and thus block the action of sympathomimetics that act by releasing noradrenaline from stores. It is now evident that the sympathetic system is a lot more complicated than many had previously supposed, and that some drugs will act differently after acute and after chronic administration, according to whether the noradrenaline stores are depleted or

not, and receptors may change in number and activity; and there are subclasses of receptors.

Many sympathomimetics are racemic compounds and one form is commonly much more active: for instance levo-noradrenaline is at least 50 times as active as the dextro form.

Up to 1958 it was known that the peripheral motor (vasoconstriction) effects of adrenaline were preventable and that the peripheral inhibitory (vasodilatation) and the cardiac stimulant actions were not preventable by the then available antagonists (ergot alkaloids, phenoxybenzamine).

In 1948, Ahlquist introduced a hypothesis to account for this. He proposed **two different sorts of adrenoceptors** (α and β). For a further 10 years, only antagonists of α-receptor effects (α-adrenoceptor block) were known, but in 1958 the first substance selectively and competitively to prevent β-receptor effects (β-adrenoceptor block), dichloroisoprenaline, was synthesised. However, it was unsuitable for clinical use (it also had strong agonist activity, i.e. it was a partial agonist or agonist/antagonist), and it was not until 1962 that the first reasonably satisfactory β-adrenoceptor blocker (pronethalol) was introduced to medicine. Unfortunately it had a low therapeutic index and also proved to be carcinogenic in some mice (but not in rats), and was soon replaced by propranolol (Inderal).

It is evident that the site of action has an important role in selectivity, e.g. drugs that act on end-organ receptors *directly* and stereospecifically may be highly selective, whereas drugs that act *indirectly* by discharging noradrenaline indiscriminately from nerve endings, e.g. amphetamine, will have a wider range of effects.

Subclassification of adrenoceptors is shown in Table 22.1.

Consequences of activating the adrenoceptor

Catecholamines (adrenaline, noradrenaline, dopamine) act at β-adrenoceptors as *first messenger* transmitters, combining with receptors on the outside of the cell membrane of the end-organ, thus activating the enzyme adenylyl cyclase on

Table 22.1 Clinically relevant aspects of adrenoceptor functions and actions of agonists and antagonists

α_1-adrenoceptor effects[1]	β-adrenoceptor effects
Eye[2]: mydriasis	**Heart** (β_1, β_2)[3] increased *rate* (SA node) increased *automaticity* (AV node and muscle) increased *velocity* in conducting tissue increased *contractility* of myocardium increased O_2 consumption decreased *refractory period* of all tissues
Arterioles: constriction (only slight in coronary and cerebral)	**Arterioles**: dilatation (β_2) **Bronchi** (β_2): relaxation **Anti-inflammatory effect**: inhibition of release of autacoids (histamine, leukotrienes) from mast cells, e.g. asthma in type I allergy
Uterus: contraction (pregnant)	**Uterus** (β_2): relaxation (pregnant)
	Skeletal muscle: tremor (β_2)
Skin: sweat, pilomotor	
Male ejaculation	**Blood platelet**: aggregation
Metabolic effect: hyperkalaemia	**Metabolic effects**: hypokalaemia (β_2) hepatic glycogenolysis (β_2) lipolysis (β_1, β_2)
Bladder sphincter: contraction	**Bladder detrusor**: relaxation

Intestinal smooth muscle relaxation is mediated by α- and β-adrenoceptors.
α_2-**adrenoceptor effects**[1]: α_2-receptors on the nerve ending, i.e. presynaptic autoreceptors mediate negative feedback which inhibits noradrenaline release.

[1] For the role of subtypes (α_1 and α_2) see prazosin.
[2] Effects on intraocular pressure involve both α- and β-adrenoceptor as well as cholinoceptors.
[3] Cardiac β_1-receptors mediate effects of sympathetic nerve stimulation.
Cardiac β_2-receptors mediate effects of circulating catecholamines. Both receptors mediate the same biological effects.
   The use of the term *cardioselective* to mean β_1-receptor selective only, especially in the case of β-receptor blocking drugs, is no longer strictly appropriate; the drugs are *beta-selective*.

the inside of the cell membrane, which causes an increase in intracellular cyclic AMP, the *second messenger* (destroyed by intracellular phosphodiesterase[2]). This second messenger initiates a sequence (cascade) of changes that open calcium ion channels and initiate the characteristic effect of that receptor, whether this be contraction of arteriolar smooth muscle or release of glucose or potassium from liver cells. Many hormones act via cyclic AMP. Specificity is provided by the receptor, not by the messengers. Mechanisms of action at α_1- and α_2-adrenoceptors differ in detail.

The complexity of adrenergic mechanisms is shown by the following:

Drugs may mimic or impair adrenergic mechanisms

- *directly*, binding on adrenoceptors: *agonist* (adrenaline) or *antagonist* (propranolol)
- *indirectly*, by discharging noradrenaline stored in nerve endings[3] (amphetamine)
- by *preventing re-uptake* into the adrenergic nerve ending of released noradrenaline (cocaine, tricyclic antidepressants)
- by *preventing the destruction* of noradrenaline (and dopamine) in the nerve ending (monoamine oxidase inhibitors)
- by *depleting the stores* of noradrenaline in nerve endings (reserpine)
- by *preventing the release* of noradrenaline from nerve endings in response to a nerve impulse (guanethidine)
- by causing the nerve ending to synthesise a *false transmitter* instead of noradrenaline (methyldopa)
- by *blocking sympathetic autonomic ganglia* (pentolinium, trimetaphan)

All the above mechanisms operate in both the *central* and *peripheral* nervous systems. This discussion is chiefly concerned with agents that influence peripheral adrenergic mechanisms.

[2] Aminophylline (in high dose only) inhibits phosphodiesterase and so enhances cyclic AMP concentrations. In the treatment of asthma with a β-receptor agonist plus aminophylline there is thus a desired interaction on the bronchi, but an undesired interaction on the heart.
[3] Fatal hypertension can occur when this class of agent is taken by a patient treated with a monoamine oxidase inhibitor.

CLASSIFICATION OF SYMPATHOMIMETICS BY SELECTIVITY FOR ADRENOCEPTORS

The following classification of sympathomimetics and antagonists is based on selectivity for receptors and on use. But selectivity is relative, not absolute; some agents act on both α and β-receptors, some are partial agonists, and if enough is administered, many will extend their range; the same applies to selective antagonists (receptor blockers); e.g. an agonist used to arrest premature labour (β_2-receptor) will also cause tachycardia (β_1) as the dose increases; a β_1-(cardio) selective adrenoceptor blocker can cause severe exacerbation of asthma (β_2) even at low dose. It is important to remember this because patients have died in the hands of doctors who have forgotten or been ignorant of it.

Adrenoceptor agonists (Table 22.1)

α- + β-*effects, non-selective, adrenaline:* now used as vasoconstrictor (α) with local anaesthetics, as a mydriatic and in the emergency treatment of anaphylactic shock, for which condition it has the right mix of effects (bronchodilator, positive cardiac inotropic, vasoconstriction at high dose); it has been superseded for asthma by more selective (β_2) agents.

$\alpha_{1,2}$-*effects, noradrenaline* (with slight beta effect on heart): is best left to its essential role in physiology; it is selectively released where it is wanted. As a therapeutic agent it has been almost entirely superseded for hypotensive states by dopamine and dobutamine; also having predominantly α-effects are methoxamine and imidazolines (xylometazoline, oxymetazoline), metaraminol, phenylephrine, phenylpropanolamine, ephedrine, pseudoephedrine: some are used solely for topical vasoconstriction (nasal decongestants).

α_2-**effects in the central nervous system:** clonidine.

β-**effects, non-selective** (i.e. β_1 + β_2): **isoprenaline.** Its uses as bronchodilator (β_2), for positive cardiac inotropic effect and to enhance conduction in heart block (β_1, β_2) have been largely superseded by agents with a more appropriately selective profile of effects. Other agents with non-selective β-effects: ephedrine, orciprenaline are also obsolescent for asthma.

β_1-**effects, with some α-effects:** dopamine, used in vascular shock.

β_1-**effects: dobutamine,** used for cardiac inotropic effect.

β_2-**effects,** used in *asthma*, include: salbutamol, terbutaline, fenoterol, isoetharine, pirbuterol, reproterol, rimiterol; only used to relax the *uterus*: isoxsuprine, orciprenaline, ritodrine, terbutaline.

Adrenoceptor antagonists (blockers): see p. 416 and after
see p. 416 and after

Effects of a sympathomimetic

The *overall effect* of a sympathomimetic depends on the *site* of action (receptor agonist or indirect action), on *receptor specificity* and on *dose*; for instance adrenaline ordinarily dilates muscle blood vessels (β_2; mainly arterioles, but veins also) but in very large doses constricts them (α). The end results are often complex and unpredictable, partly because of the variability of homeostatic reflex responses and partly because what is observed, e.g. a change in blood pressure, is the result of many factors, e.g. vasodilatation [β] in some areas, vasoconstriction [α] in others, and cardiac stimulation [β].

To block all the effects of adrenaline and noradrenaline, antagonists for both α- and β-receptors must be used. This can be a matter of practical importance, e.g. in phaeochromocytoma.

Adverse effects may be deduced from their actions (Table 22.1, Fig. 22.1). Tissue necrosis due to intense vasoconstriction (α) around injection sites occurs as a result of leakage from i.v. infusions. The effects on the heart (β_1) include tachycardia, palpitations, cardiac dysrhythmias including ventricular tachycardia and fibrillation, and muscle tremor (β_2). Sympathomimetic drugs should be used with great caution in patients with heart disease.

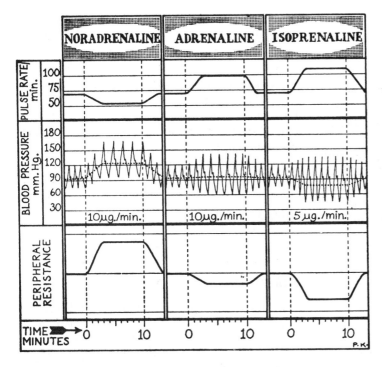

Fig. 22.1 Cardiovascular effects of noradrenaline, adrenaline and isoprenaline: pulse rate/min, blood pressure in mm Hg (dotted line is mean pressure), peripheral resistance in arbitrary units.

The differences are due to the differential α and β agonist selectivities of these agents, see text.

By permission, after Ginsburg J, Cobbold A F. In: Vane J R et al. eds. Adrenergic mechanism. London: Churchill. 1960

Sympathomimetics are particularly likely to cause cardiac dysrhythmias (β_1) in patients under halothane anaesthesia. The effect of the sympathomimetic drugs on the pregnant uterus is variable and difficult to predict, but serious fetal distress can occur, due to reduced placental blood flow as a result both of contraction of the uterine muscle (α) and arterial constriction (α). β_2-agonists are used to relax the uterus in premature labour, but unwanted cardiovascular actions can be troublesome (see Phaeochromocytoma p. 432).

Sympathomimetics and plasma potassium. Adrenergic mechanisms have a role in the physiological control of plasma potassium concentration. The biochemical pump that shifts K into cells is activated by β_2-adrenoceptor agonists (adrenaline, salbutamol, isoxsurpine) and can cause *hypo*kalaemia. The effect is blocked by β_2-adrenoceptor antagonists. The α-adrenoceptor has a suppressive effect on the pump and activation tends to cause *hyper*kalaemia.

The hypokalaemia effects of administered (β_2)

sympathomimetics may be clinically important, particularly in patients having pre-existing hypokalaemia, e.g. due to intense adrenergic activity such as occurs in myocardial infarction,[4] in fright (admission to hospital is accompanied by transient hypokalaemia), or with previous diuretic therapy, and taking digoxin. In such subjects use of a sympathomimetic infusion or of an adrenaline-containing local anaesthesic may precipitate cardiac dysrhythmia. Hypokalaemia may occur during treatment of severe asthma, particularly where the β_2-receptor agonist is combined with theophylline.

β-adrenoceptor blockers, as expected, enhance the hyperkalaemia of muscular exercise; and one of their benefits in preventing cardiac dysrhythmias after myocardial infarction may be due to block of β_2-receptor-induced hypokalaemia.

---

[4] Normal subjects, infused i.v. with adrenaline in amounts that approximate to those found in the plasma after severe myocardial infarction, show a fall in plasma K of about 0.8 mmol/l. Brown M J N Engl J Med 1983; 309: 1414.

Pharmacokinetics

Catecholamines (adrenaline, noradrenaline, dopamine, dobutamine, isoprenaline) are metabolised by two enzymes, monoamine oxidase (MAO) and catechol-O-methyltransferase (COMT). These enzymes are present in large amounts in the liver and kidney and account for most of the metabolism of injected catecholamines. MAO is also present in the intestinal mucosa (and in nerve endings, peripheral and central). Because of these enzymes catecholamines are ineffective when swallowed (though isoprenaline in enormous dose can be used by this route to treat heart block); noncatecholamines, e.g. salbutamol, amphetamine, are effective orally.

A physiological note

The termination of action of noradrenaline released at nerve endings is by (a) re-uptake into nerve endings where it is stored and also subject to MAO degradation, (b) diffusion away from the area of the nerve ending and the receptor (junctional cleft), and (c) metabolism (by MAO and COMT). These processes are slower than the extraordinarily swift destruction of acetylcholine at the neuromuscular junction by acetylcholinesterase situated outside the cells alongside the receptors. The difference reflects a different physiological requirement, the almost instantaneous (millisecond) responses required of voluntary muscle are not required (indeed might be disastrous) of arteriolar muscle.

The *plasma* $t_{\frac{1}{2}}$ of catecholamines is about 2 min.

Synthetic non-catecholamines in clinical use have $t_{\frac{1}{2}}$ of hours, e.g. salbutamol (albuterol) 4 h, because they are more resistant to enzymatic degradation and conjugation. They may be given orally. They penetrate the central nervous system and may have prominent effects, e.g. amphetamine. Substantial amounts appear in the urine.

Overdose of sympathomimetics

Overdose is treated according to rational con-sideration of mode and site of action, see adrenaline (below).

INDIVIDUAL SYMPATHOMIMETICS

The actions are summarised in Table 22.1. The classic type-substances will be described first despite their limited role in therapeutics, and then the more selective analogues that have largely replaced them.

Catecholamines

For pharmacokinetics, see above.

Adrenaline

Adrenaline (epinephrine) (both α- and β-receptor effects) is used as a vasoconstrictor with local anaesthetics (1:80 000 or weaker) to prolong their effects (about × 2); as a topical mydriatic (sparing accommodation; it also lowers intra-ocular pressure); and for allergic reactions, s.c., i.m. (or i.v.). The route must be chosen with care. Given s.c. there is intense vasoconstriction, which slows absorption and so prolongs and smooths effects. If there is circulatory collapse (as in anaphylactic shock) absorption will be too much delayed and the i.m. route is preferred; use i.v. requires dilution of the standard solution (1:1000, i.e. 1 mg/ml) and careful, frequent monitoring of heart rate and blood pressure. Intra-cardiac (or intra-airway) injection is used in cardiac arrest; even though ventricular fibrillation may be provoked, normal rhythm can be restored by electric cardioversion.

Adrenaline is used in **anaphylactic shock** (i.m.) because its mix of actions, cardiovascular and bronchial, provide the best compromise for speed and simplicity of use in an emergency; it may also stabilise mast cell membranes and reduce release of vasoactive autacoids. The dose for this indication is 0.5–1 mg (0.5–1 ml of 1:1000 solution: 1 mg/ml, i.m.): it is repeated as necessary and generally 2 mg in 5 min should be regarded as maximal. It may be exceeded, but palpitations, cardiac dysrhythmia and hypertension are likely to occur. Lower doses s.c., e.g. 200–500 µg are used for less urgent situations.

Adrenaline (topical) decreases intraocular pressure in chronic open-angle glaucoma, as does *dipivefrine*, an adrenaline ester prodrug. They are contraindicated in closed angle glaucoma because they are mydriatics.

Thyrotoxic patients are intolerant of adrenaline.

Accidental **overdose** with adrenaline occurs occasionally. It is rationally treated by propranolol to block the cardiac β-effects (cardiac dysrhythmia) *and* phentolamine or chlorpromazine to control the α-effects on the peripheral circulation that will be prominent when the β-effects are abolished; labetalol would be an alternative. β-adrenoceptor block alone is hazardous as the then unopposed α-receptor vasoconstriction causes (severe) hypertension; see phaeochromocytoma. Antihypertensives of most other kinds are irrational and some may also potentiate the adrenaline.

Noradrenaline (norepinephrine) (chiefly α-effects)

The main effect of administered noradrenaline is to raise the blood pressure by constricting the arterioles and so raising the total peripheral resistance, with *reduced blood flow* (except in coronary arteries which have few α-receptors). Though it does have slight cardiac stimulant (β$_1$) effect, the tachycardia of this is masked by the profound reflex bradycardia caused by the hypertension. Noradrenaline is given by i.v. infusion to obtain a gradual sustained response; the effect of a single i.v. injection would last only a minute or so. It is obsolete except where strong peripheral vasoconstriction is specifically desired, which is very rare. It can cause peripheral gangrene and local necrosis; tachyphylaxis occurs; withdrawal must be gradual.

Isoprenaline

Isoprenaline (isoproterenol, isopropylnoradrenaline) is a non-selective β-receptor agonist, i.e. it activates both β$_1$ and β$_2$-receptors. It relaxes smooth muscle, including that of the blood vessels, has negligible metabolic or vasoconstrictor effects, but has a vigorous stimulant effect on the heart. This latter is its main disadvantage in the treatment of bronchial asthma and virtually precludes injection except in complete heart block. It can be given as tablets, to be dissolved under the tongue or as a sustained-release preparation (Saventrine) to be swallowed. In asthma it has been superseded by selective β$_2$-agonists.

Dopamine

Dopamine is an agonist for specific *dopamine* (D$_1$) *receptors* in the CNS and the renal and other vascular beds (dilator); it also activates presynaptic autoreceptors (D$_2$) which suppress release of noradrenaline. In addition it is an agonist at β$_1$-adrenoceptors in the heart and at high doses activates α-adrenoceptors (vasoconstrictor) and also releases noradrenaline from nerve endings. It is given by continuous i.v. infusion because, like all catecholamines, its t$\frac{1}{2}$ is 2 min. An i.v. infusion (2–5 µg/kg/min) causes increased renal blood flow. As the dose rises the heart is stimulated, with tachycardia and increased cardiac output. On the peripheral circulation the combination of effects usually causes overall slight reduction in total peripheral resistance. This combination of effects renders dopamine a drug of choice in management of shock (provided any intravascular volume deficit has been corrected). But at rates exceeding 5 µg/kg/h vasoconstriction and hypertension may occur. An i.v. infusion should start at about 2 µg/kg/min and may be increased (by 5–10 µg/kg/min) at intervals of 15–30 min until the desired effect or adverse effects occur, e.g. excessive tachycardia or dysrhythmia. Increasingly close monitoring (blood pressure, urine output, etc.) should be conducted as the rate exceeds 5 µg/kg/min; it should rarely be taken above 20 µg/kg/min. The infusion should be withdrawn gradually over hours to avoid hypotension. Dopamine is stable for about 24 h in sodium chloride or dextrose; it is inactivated by alkaline solutions, e.g. sodium bicarbonate. Subcutaneous leakage causes vasoconstriction and necrosis and should be treated by local injection of an α-adrenoceptor blocking agent (phentolamine 5 mg, diluted).

It may be mixed with *dobutamine*.

For CNS aspects of dopamine, agonists and antagonists, see neuroleptics, parkinsonism.

Dobutamine is primarily a β_1-adrenoceptor agonist with greater inotropic than chronotropic effects on the heart; it has some α-agonist effect, but less than dopamine. It may be useful in shock (with dopamine) and in low output heart failure (in the absence of severe hypertension).

Dopexamine is an agonist for cardiac β_2-adrenoceptors (positive inotropic effect); it also induces pulmonary and renal vasodilation; it is used for short-term treatment of low cardiac output states, e.g. after cardiac surgery.

Non-catecholamines

Salbutamol, isoetharine, fenoterol, rimiterol, reproterol, pirbuterol, salmeterol and terbutaline are β-adrenoceptor agonists that are relatively *selective for* β_2-*receptors*, so that cardiac (β_1-receptor) effects are less prominent, though these can be serious with high dosage. They are longer acting than isoprenaline probably because they are not substrates for catechol-O-methyl-transferase, which methylates catecholamines in the blood. They are used principally in asthma.

Salbutamol

Salbutamol (Ventolin) is taken orally, 2–4 mg up to 4 times/day; it also acts quickly by inhalation and the effect can last as long as 4 h, which makes it suitable for both prevention and treatment of asthma. Of an inhaled dose (100–200 μg, i.e. 0.1–0.2 mg), about 20% is absorbed and can cause cardiovascular effects. The t_2^1 is 4 h. It can also be given by injection, e.g. in asthma, premature labour (β_2-receptor) and for cardiac inotropic (β_1) effect in heart failure (where the β_2 vasodilator action is also useful). Clinically important hypokalaemia can occur (shift of K into cells). The other drugs above are similar.

Orciprenaline (metaproterenol) is a non-selective β_1- and β_2-adrenoceptor agonist. Ritodrine and isoxsuprine have some selectivity for β_2-adrenoceptors (see uterus).

Salmeterol is a variant of salbutamol that has additional binding property to a site adjacent to the β_2-adrenoceptor, which results in slow onset of action (it is not suitable for asthma that requires quick relief), but the action persists for 12 h.

Clenbuterol is similar to salbutamol. It has found an unorthodox use as a growth promoter in cattle. Liver from treated cattle eaten by humans has caused illness compatible with its pharmacology.

Ephedrine

Ephedrine is a plant alkaloid with actions similar to adrenaline though it acts indirectly; but it has a relatively greater stimulant effect on the central nervous system in adults, producing alertness, anxiety, insomnia, tremor and nausea. Children may be sleepy when taking it. In practice central effects limit its use as a sympathomimetic in asthma.

Ephedrine is well absorbed when given by mouth and unlike most other sympathomimetics is not much destroyed by the liver: it is largely excreted unchanged by the kidney. The t_2^1 is about 4 h. It is usually given by mouth but can be injected. It differs from adrenaline principally in that its effects come on more slowly and last longer. Tachyphylaxis occurs, probably because it acts by discharging noradrenaline from stores, which it exhausts.

Ephedrine can be used as a bronchodilator, in heart block, as a mydriatic and as a mucosal vasoconstrictor, but it is being displaced by newer drugs, which are often better for these purposes. It sometimes is useful in myasthenia gravis (adrenergic agents enhance cholinergic neuromuscular transmission).

Phenylpropanolamine (norephedrine) is similar but with less CNS effect.

Amphetamine (Benzedrine) and dexamphetamine (Dexedrine) act indirectly. They are seldom used for their peripheral effects, which are similar to those of ephedrine, but usually for their effects on the central nervous system (narcolepsy, attention deficit in children). For a general account of amphetamine see p. 295.

Phenylephrine has actions qualitatively similar to noradrenaline but a longer duration of action, up to an hour or so. It can be used as a nasal decongestant (0.25–0.5% solution), but sometimes irritates. In the doses usually given, the central nervous effects are minimal, as are the direct effects on the heart. It is also used as a mydriatic and briefly lowers intraocular pressure.

Xamoterol

Xamoterol (Corwin) is a partial agonist at β_1-adrenoceptors; it acts as agonist or antagonist according to circumstances, particularly the level of sympathetic autonomic activity present. At low levels of sympathetic activity it increases heart rate and contractility (inotropic) by its agonist effect, and at high rates it reduces them by its antagonist action. It has little action on bronchial (β_2) receptors. Xamoterol may benefit *mild* chronic heart failure *only*; it may worsen moderate and severe failure because sympathetic activity increases with worsening heart failure. It has benefited some cases of hypotension caused by autonomic neuropathy. Skilled selection of patients is all-important.

MUCOSAL DECONGESTANTS

Nasal and bronchial decongestants (vasoconstrictors) are widely used in allergic rhinitis, colds, coughs and sinusitis, and to prevent otitic barotrauma, as nasal drops or as sprays to be sniffed; sprays reach a greater area of the mucous membrane. All the sympathomimetic vasoconstrictors, i.e. with α-effects, have been used for the purpose, with or without an antihistamine (H_1-receptor), and there is little to choose between them. If used more often than 3-hourly and for above 3 weeks the mucous membrane is likely to be damaged. The occurrence of rebound congestion or allergic reaction is liable to lead to overuse. The least objectionable drugs are ephedrine 0.5% and xylometazoline 0.1% (Otrivine). Naphazoline and adrenaline should

not be used, and nor should blunderbuss mixtures of vasoconstrictor, antihistamine, adrenal steroid and antibiotics. Oily drops and sprays, used frequently and long term, may enter the lungs and eventually cause lipoid pneumonia.

It may sometimes be better to give the drugs orally rather than up the nose. They interact with antihypertensives and can be a cause of unexplained failure of therapy unless enquiry into patient self-medication is made. Deaths (hypertension) have occurred when such preparations have been taken by patients treated for depression with a monoamine oxidase inhibitor.

SHOCK

Definition: Shock is a state of inadequate capillary perfusion (oxygen deficiency) of vital tissues to an extent that adversely affects cellular metabolism (capillary endothelium and organs) causing malfunction, including release of enzymes and vasoactive substances,[5] i.e. it is a *low flow* or *hypoperfusion state*.

The cardiac output and blood pressure are low in fully developed cases. But a maldistribution of blood (due to constriction, dilatation, shunting) can be sufficient to produce tissue injury even in the presence of high cardiac output and arterial blood pressure (warm shock), e.g. some cases of septic shock.

The essential element, hypoperfusion of vital organs, is present whatever the cause, whether pump failure (myocardial infarction), maldistribution of blood (septic shock) or loss of total intravascular volume (bleeding or increased permeability of vessels damaged by bacterial cell products, by burns or by anoxia). Function of vital organs, brain (consciousness, respiration) and kidney (urine formation) are clinical indicators of adequacy of perfusion of these organs.

---

[5]In fact, a medley of substances (autacoids), kinins, prostaglandins, leukotrienes, histamine, endorphins, serotonin, vasopressin, angiotensin. Prevention or reversal of shock by antagonism of these mediators is not yet practical therapeutics. Endogenous opioid mechanisms may be involved but trials of naloxone have been inconclusive.

Treatment may be summarised:

- *Treatment of the cause*: pain, wounds, bleeding, infections, adrenocortical deficiency.
- *Replacement of any fluid lost* from the circulation; but extra fluid is dangerous when the primary fault is in the heart or pulmonary circulation.
- *Maintenance of the diastolic blood pressure and perfusion of vital organs* (brain, heart, kidneys).

Blood flow (oxygen delivery) rather than blood pressure is of the greatest immediate importance for the function of vital organs. But a reasonable blood pressure is needed to ensure organ perfusion, e.g. brain and myocardium, and pressure for formation of urine. Hypotension due to *low peripheral resistance* is of little importance if the patient is horizontal or tilted head down, for venous return to the heart, and so the cardiac output, is then maintained; blood flow to brain, myocardium and kidneys remains adequate until the diastolic pressure falls below about 40 mm Hg. But *low cardiac output* is always serious even though compensatory vasoconstriction maintains the arterial pressure, for blood flow is reduced.

The decision how to treat shock depends on assessment of the pathophysiology:

- whether cardiac output, and so peripheral blood flow, is inadequate (low pulse volume, cold-constricted periphery),
- whether cardiac output is normal and peripheral blood flow is adequate (good pulse volume and warm dilated periphery), but there is maldistribution of blood;
- whether the patient is hypovolaemic or not, or needs a cardiac inotropic agent, a vasoconstrictor or a vasodilidator.

In poisoning by a cerebral depressant the principal cause of hypotension is low peripheral resistance due to sympathetic block. The cardiac output can be restored by tilting the patient head down and by increasing the venous filling pressure by cautiously raising the blood volume with a plasma expander. Use of vascular drugs is unnecessary and may be harmful.

In central circulatory failure (cardiogenic shock, e.g. myocardial infarction) the cardiac output and blood pressure are low due to loss of pumping power; myocardial perfusion is dependent on aortic pressure. Venous return (central venous pressure) is normal or high. The low blood pressure may trigger the sympathoadrenal mechanisms of peripheral circulatory failure summarised below.

Not surprisingly, the use of drugs in low output failure due to acute myocardial damage is disappointing. Vasoconstriction (by α-adrenoceptor agonist), by increasing peripheral resistance, may raise the blood pressure by increasing afterload, but this additional burden on the damaged heart can further reduce cardiac output. Cardiac stimulation with a β_1-adrenoceptor agonist may fail; it increases myocardial oxygen consumption and may cause a dysrhythmia. Dobutamine (or dopamine) offers a reasonable choice if a drug is needed.

If there is bradycardia (as there sometimes is in myocardial infarction), minute output can be increased by vagal block with atropine.

Vasodilators may be needed to treat severe cardiac *failure*.

Septic shock is caused by endotoxins from Gram-negative organisms and other cell products from Gram-positive organisms; they injure tissues and cause release of cytokines, e.g. interleukin-I, that are responsible for many of the adverse manifestation of shock. First there is a peripheral vasodilatation with eventual fall in arterial pressure. This initiates a vigorous sympathetic discharge that causes constriction of arterioles and venules; the cardiac output may be high or low according to the balance of these influences. There is a progressive peripheral anoxia of vital organs and acidosis. The veins (venules) dilate and venous pooling occurs so that blood is sequestered in the periphery and effective circulatory volume falls because of this and of fluid loss into the extravascular space.

The *immediate aim of treatment* is to restore cardiac output and vital organ perfusion by increasing venous return to the heart and to reverse the maldistribution of blood. This can be done by increasing intravascular volume (plasma transfusion), keeping a close watch on central venous pressure to avoid overloading the heart, and by tilting the patient head down. Oxygen is useful as there is often uneven pulmonary perfusion.

In addition a drug with a mix of cardiac inotropic and peripheral vascular actions may restore essential blood flow to vital organs. Dopamine provides such actions, is least likely to do harm and may even do good. Dobutamine may be added for extra cardiac inotropic effect.

Drugs that increase peripheral resistance (sympathomimetics with α-effects and *no* β_1-effect) are likely only to make matters worse by further reducing blood flow to vital organs, in the event of the resistance vessels (arterioles) retaining their reactivity and responding to them, which they may not do. Noradrenaline does have some cardiac inotropic (β_1) effect and may be used if substantial vasoconstriction is judged to be the principal requirement. Administration of a vasodilator drug to a patient with low blood volume is, of course, disastrous.

Monoclonal antibodies against bacterial endotoxins, and also antagonists to the endogenous cytokines released by tissue damage are entering use, e.g. Centoxin (HA-IA).

Adrenocortical steroids in enormous (and costly) doses, e.g. dexamethasone 2–6 mg/kg i.v., may benefit by reducing the consequences of damage to cellular membranes by toxins or anoxia and so preventing the release of biologically active damaging substances. Any effect probably has nothing to do with the ordinary actions of corticosteroids. The balance of evidence does not favour routine use and there is no doubt that secondary (opportunistic) infections are increased; these may be fatal. Ordinary replacement doses of adrenocortical steroid are irrelevant. Use of high doses in cardiogenic shock may cause cardiac dysrhythmia (hypokalaemia) and may possibly delay healing of the infarct.

Hypotension in patients with atherosclerosis (occlusive vascular disease) is more serious than in others, for they are specially dependent on pressure to provide the necessary blood flow in vital organs because the vessels are less able to dilate. Dopamine may be considered.

Choice of drug in shock

On present knowledge the best drug would be one that stimulates the myocardium as well as selectively modifying peripheral resistance to increase flow to vital organs.

Dopamine comes closest to meeting these requirements. Where high doses are used and vasoconstriction predominates it may sometimes be useful to add a vasodilator, e.g. an α-adrenoceptor blocking drug.

Dobutamine is used when cardiac inotropic effect is the primary requirement.

Noradrenaline is used when vasoconstriction is the first priority, plus some slight cardiac inotropic effect.

As well as reducing peripheral blood flow, prolonged vasoconstriction reduces blood volume due to passage of fluid into the extravascular space. Thus abrupt cessation of use may be followed by a drop in cardiac output.

Monitoring drug use

Modern monitoring by both invasive and non-invasive techniques has reached such heights of complexity that it can give more information than some doctors know how to put to good use, even if it is indeed the right information. We are liable

to measure everything at once, losing ourselves in a sea of numbers many of which are derived by arithmetical exercises from other numbers.[6]

At least the heart rate and rhythm, blood pressure and urine flow should be closely watched. No attempt should be made to raise the pressure to normal; about 80–90 mm Hg systolic pressure is enough, for the drugs are not restoring normal physiology. Prognostic indices tell us

whether the patient will live or die, but such studies do not reveal by which parameters we should 'fly' the patient, and so we end up flying the patient by the seat of our pants instead of our other end.[6]

These words, of an expert, may give some comfort when the complexities of rational management seem overwhelming.

Warning. The use of drugs in shock is secondary to accurate assessment of cardiovascular state (especially of peripheral *flow*) and to other

[6]Thompson W L Proceedings of the Royal Society of Medicine 1977; 70: 25.

essential management, treatment of infection and maintenance of intravascular volume.

Restoration of intravascular volume

Ideally the transfusion should be similar to that which has been lost: blood for haemorrhage, plasma for burns, saline for gastrointestinal loss.

In an emergency, speed of replacement is more important than its nature. Isotonic saline and saline/lactate (crystalloid) solutions are immediately effective and are cheap, but they leave the circulation quickly. Macromolecules (colloids) remain in the circulation longer. The two classes (crystalloids and colloids) may be used together. Isotonic solutions of human plasma proteins and human albumin are available (concentrated solution of albumin is used in severe hypovolaemia with oedema to move fluid into the circulation).

Colloidal isotonic solutions of macromolecules include: dextrans (glucose polymer), gelatin (hydrolysed collagen) and hetastarch (hydroxyethyl starch).

Dextran 70 or 110 (these are the molecular weights in thousands) have a plasma $t_\frac{1}{2}$ of 12 h. Dextran 40 is used to decrease blood sludging and so to improve peripheral blood flow, e.g. prophylaxis of post-surgical thrombosis.

Gelatin products (Haemaccel, Gelofusine) have a plasma $t_\frac{1}{2}$ of 5 h. **Hetastarch** has a plasma $t_\frac{1}{2}$ of 17 days.

Adverse effects include anaphylactoid reactions; dextran and hetastarch can impair haemostatic mechanisms; dextran interferes with blood group cross matching and clinical biochemical measurements.

CHRONIC ORTHOSTATIC HYPOTENSION

Chronic orthostatic hypotension occurs with age, in primary progressive autonomic failure and secondary to parkinsonism and diabetes.

Initial treatment is by expansion of blood volume using a sodium-retaining adrenocortical steroid (fludrocortisone[7]) or desmopressin plus

---

[7]Effective doses may not affect blood volume and may work by sensitising vascular adrenoceptors.

---

elastic support stocking to reduce venous pooling of blood when erect.

The possibility that vasodilator prostaglandins in excess could be a factor in some cases had led to trial of an inhibitor of prostaglandin synthesis (indomethacin) with success, particularly when combined with fludrocortisone.

Other measures include drugs having a mix of receptor actions: β_1-adrenoceptor agonist, β_2-adrenoceptor block, α-adrenoceptor agonist (on veins) and dopamine receptor block; they include pindolol, xamoterol, dihydroergotamine, metoclopramide and domperidone. These agents carry a risk of hypertension when the patient is supine and should be used to treat disabling symptoms only.

Postprandial fall in blood pressure (probably due to redistribution of blood to the splanchnic area) is characteristic of this condition; it especially occurs after breakfast (blood volume is lower in the morning). Substantial doses of caffeine (2 large cups of coffee) can mitigate this, but they need to be taken before or early in the meal. The action may be due to block of splanchnic vasodilator adenosine receptors.

The discrepant reported results of drug therapy may be due to differences in adrenergic function dependent on whether the degeneration is central, peripheral, preganglionic, postganglionic or due to changes in adrenoceptors on end-organs (age).

GUIDE TO FURTHER READING

Ahlquist R P 1948 A study of adrenotropic receptors. American Journal of Physiology 153: 586

Cryer P E 1980 Physiology and pathophysiology of the human sympathoadrenal neuroendocrine system. New England Journal of Medicine 303: 436

Editorial 1968 Gas gangrene from adrenaline. British Medical Journal 1: 721

Fowler M B et al 1982 Comparison of haemodynamic responses to dobutamine and salbutamol in cardiogenic shock after acute

myocardial infarction. British Medical
Journal 284: 73

Jack D 1991 A way of looking at agonism and
antagonism: lessons from salbutamol,
salmeterol and other β-adrenoceptor
agonists. British Journal of Clinical
Pharmacology 31: 501

Motulsky H J et al 1982 Adrenergic receptors
in man: direct identification, physiologic
regulation and clinical alterations. New
England Journal of Medicine 307: 18

Onrot J et al 1985 Haemodynamic and

humoral effects of caffeine in autonomic
failure: therapeutic implications for
postprandial hypotension. New England
Journal of Medicine 313: 549

Williams M E et al 1985 Catecholamine
modulation of rapid potassium shifts during
exercise. New England Journal of Medicine
312: 823

Wolff S M 1991 Monoclonal antibodies and
the treatment of Gram-negative
bacteraemia. New England Journal of
Medicine 324: 486

23

Cardiovascular system II: drugs used in arterial hypertension and angina pectoris

SYNOPSIS

Hypertension and angina are common diseases of great importance. Hypertension affects above 20% of the total population of the USA with its major impact on those over age 50, when above 40% are affected. Management requires attention to detail, both clinical and pharmacological.

The way drugs act in these diseases is outlined and the drugs are described according to class.

- Hypertension and angina pectoris: how drugs act
- Diuretics
- Vasodilators, especially organic nitrates, calcium channel blockers, ACE inhibitors
- Adrenoceptor blocking drugs, α and β
- Drugs acting on the peripheral sympathetic nerve terminal
- Autonomic ganglion-blocking drugs
- Drugs acting on the central nervous system
- Treatment of angina pectoris
- Treatment of arterial hypertension
- Sexual function and cardiovascular drugs
- Phaeochromocytoma

HYPERTENSION: HOW DRUGS ACT

- Dilatation of arteriolar *resistance vessels*; the heart pumps against lower resistance (afterload), with more rapid run-off of pressure.
- Dilatation of venous *capacitance vessels;* reduced venous return to the heart (preload) leads to reduced cardiac output, especially in the upright position.
- Reduction of *cardiac contractility and rate* leads to reduced output at lower pressure, especially in response to stress, e.g. upright posture, exercise.
- Depletion of *body sodium* reduces plasma volume (transiently), and reduces arteriolar response to noradrenaline.
- Inhibition of *angiotensin II formation* leads to vasodilatation.

The drugs preferred in therapy are those that lower blood pressure with minimal interference with homeostatic control, i.e. posture, exercise. Postural and exercise hypotension may be particularly limiting with antihypertensives that block the sympathetic neuron (they are more effective at high rates of impulse transmission, i.e. standing, than at low rates, i.e. lying), with α-adrenoceptor blockers, and with drugs that dilate capacitance vessels (venules).

Drugs that reduce sympathetic autonomic activity may act in the central nervous system or on peripheral nerves.

ANGINA PECTORIS: HOW DRUGS ACT

Drugs used in angina pectoris are those that reduce *cardiac work* and *myocardial oxygen need*: by unloading the heart, by dilating capacitance and resistance vessels, by dilating coronary arteries, and by blocking β-adrenoceptors.

Note: Some drugs benefit both hypertension and angina pectoris and the following account embraces drugs used in both conditions.

DRUGS USED IN HYPERTENSION AND ANGINA

DIURETICS

Diuretics, particularly the thiazides, are useful antihypertensives. They cause sodium loss with reduced volume of blood and extracellular fluid (up to 10% with chronic treatment though this may not be maintained beyond 3 months). The principal blood pressure lowering effect is probably due to reduced responsiveness of resistance vessels to noradrenaline, caused by sodium depletion. Maximum effect on blood pressure is delayed for several weeks and other drugs are best added after this time. Adverse metabolic effects characteristic of thiazides (blood lipids, glucose intolerance, hyperuricaemia) have led to suggestions that they should be replaced by newer agents not having these effects (calcium antagonists, ACE inhibitors), but it is now recognised that unnecessarily high doses of thiazides have been used in the past and that with low doses, e.g. bendrofluazide 1.25–2.5 mg/d or less (or cyclopenthiazide 125 μg), thiazides are both effective and well-tolerated. The characteristic *reduction in renal calcium excretion* induced by thiazides may, in long-term therapy, reduce the occurrence of hip fractures in older patients and benefit women with postmenopausal osteoporosis.

VASODILATORS

Organic nitrates

Organic nitrates (and nitrite: amyl nitrite) were introduced into medicine in the 19th century. Denitration in the smooth muscle cell releases nitric oxide (NO), which is, or is structurally close to, the physiological endothelium derived relaxing factor (EDRF), which activates an enzyme process via cyclic GMP (guanosine monophosphate) that alters calcium fluxes in the cell and induces relaxation. The result is a *generalised dilatation of venules* (capacitance vessels) and to a less extent of arterioles (resistance vessels), causing a fall of blood pressure that is postural at first; the larger coronary arteries especially dilate.

The venous dilatation causes a reduction in venous return, a fall in left ventricular filling pressure with reduced stroke volume, but cardiac output (per min) is sustained by the reflex tachycardia induced by the fall in blood pressure (diastolic chiefly).

Uses. Nitrates are chiefly used to relieve angina pectoris and sometimes left ventricular failure. A too-severe drop in blood pressure will reduce coronary flow as well as cause fainting due to reduced cerebral blood flow, and so it is important to ensure that an overdose is not taken. Patients with angina should be instructed on the signs of overdose: palpitations, dizziness, blurred vision, headache and flushing followed by pallor, and what to do about it (below). The optimum dose is probably just below that which causes slight tachycardia and a feeling of fullness in the head.

Transient relief of pain due to spasm of other smooth muscle (colic), can sometimes be obtained.

Pharmacokinetics. The nitrates are generally well absorbed through oral and intestinal mucosae and the skin and are used by these routes. They are subject to extensive and rapid metabolism in the liver at first pass after absorption from the gut, as is shown by the substantially larger doses required by that route over sublingual (this is why it is acceptable to swallow a sublingual tablet of glyceryl trinitrate to terminate excess effect should it be socially embarrassing to spit it out). They are first denitrated to mononitrates (and to glycerol) and then conjugated with glucuronic acid. The $t_{\frac{1}{2}}$ periods vary, see below. The *systemic* bioavailability of swallowed formulations and $t_{\frac{1}{2}}$ increase when there is hepatic insufficiency.

Tolerance to the characteristic vasodilator headache comes and goes quickly (hours). Explosives factory workers exposed to a nitrate-contaminated environment lost it over a weekend and some chose to maintain their intake by using nitrate impregnated headbands (transdermal absorption) rather than have to accept the headaches and reacquire tolerance so frequently. In therapeutics tolerance is prevented by ensuring that *steady-state plasma concentration is avoided.* This is easy with occasional use of glyceryl trinitrate, but with nitrates having longer $t_{\frac{1}{2}}$ (see below) and sustained release formulations it is necessary to plan the dosing to allow low plasma concentration for 4–8 h, e.g. at night; transdermal patches may be removed for a few hours if tolerance is suspected.

Adverse effects. Collapse due to fall in blood pressure resulting from overdose or allergy may occur. The patient should remain supine, and the legs should be raised above the head to restore venous return to the heart.

These drugs are obviously contraindicated for the pain of myocardial infarction and in angina due to anaemia.

Nitrate headache, which may be severe, is probably due to the stretching of pain-sensitive tissues around the meningeal arteries resulting from the increased pulsation that accompanies the local vasodilatation. If headache is severe the dose should be halved.

Methaemoglobinaemia occurs with heavy dosage.

Glyceryl trinitrate (see also above)

Glyceryl trinitrate (1879) (trinitrin, nitroglycerin) is an oily, non-flammable liquid that explodes on concussion with a force greater than that of gunpowder. However, physicians meet it mixed with inert substances and made into a tablet, in which form it is both innocuous and fairly stable. Tablets more than 8 weeks old or exposed to heat or air will have lost potency by evaporation and should be discarded.

Glyceryl trinitrate is the drug of choice in the treatment of an attack of angina pectoris. The tablets should be chewed and dissolved under the tongue, or placed in the buccal sulcus, where absorption is rapid and reliable. Time spent ensuring that patients understand the way to take the tablets and that the feeling of fullness in the head is harmless is time well spent. The $t_{\frac{1}{2}}$ is 3 min. The action begins in 2 min and lasts up to 30 min. The initial dose of the standard tablet is 300 or 500 µg, but the amount required for each patient must be found by trial, up to 6 mg a day total. It is taken at the onset of pain, when stopping exercise to find and take the tablet no doubt contributes to the relief, and as a prophylactic immediately before any exertion that experience has taught usually brings on the pain. Sustained release buccal tablets are available (Suscard), 1–5 mg. Absorption from the intestine is good, but there is such extensive hepatic first-pass metabolism that the sublingual or buccal route is ordinarily preferred; an oral mucosal spray (Nitrolingual Spray) is an alternative. For *prophylaxis*, glyceryl trinitrate can be given as an oral (buccal or to swallow) sustained-release formulation or via the skin as a patch (or ointment); these formulations can be useful for victims of nocturnal angina.

Venepuncture: the ointment can assist difficult venepuncture and a transdermal patch adjacent to an i.v. infusion site can prevent extravasation and phlebitis and prolong infusion survival.

An i.v. formulation is available for use in *left ventricular failure* and severe angina.

Isosorbide dinitrate (Cedocard) ($t_{\frac{1}{2}}$ 20 min) is used for prophylaxis of angina pectoris and for congestive heart failure (tabs sublingual, and to swallow).

Isosorbide mononitrate (Elantan) ($t_{\frac{1}{2}}$ 4 h) is used for prophylaxis of angina (tabs to swallow). Hepatic first-pass metabolism is much less than for the dinitrate so that systemic bioavailability is more reliable.

Pentaerythritol tetranitrate (Peritrate) ($t_{\frac{1}{2}}$ 8 h) is less efficacious than its metabolite pentaerythritol trinitrate ($t_{\frac{1}{2}}$ 11 h).

Amyl nitrite (1867) is a flammable volatile liquid. It is inhaled through the open mouth. The social disadvantage of having to break (pop) a glass capsule and the distinctive smell, with no compensatory advantage, has rendered it obsolete for angina pectoris.

'Poppers' (amyl nitrite and allies) have acquired a spurious reputation as an aphrodisiac[1] and indeed may seem so to those individuals who cannot distinguish between genital vasodilatation and true sexual pleasure. No sympathy need be expended on individuals who suffer severe hypotension by such misuse. Nor on its use to relax the anal sphincter to accommodate sexual procedures.

Calcium channel blockers

Calcium is involved in the initiation of smooth muscle and cardiac cell contraction and in the propagation of the cardiac impulse. Actions on cardiac pacemaker cells and conducting tissue are described in Chapter 24.

Vascular smooth muscle cells. Contraction of these cells requires an influx of calcium across the cell membrane. This occurs through ion channels that are largely specific for calcium and are called 'slow calcium channels' to distinguish them from 'fast' channels that allow the rapid influx and efflux of sodium.

Activation of calcium channels by an action potential allows calcium to enter the cells. There follows a sequence of events which results in activation of the contractile proteins myosin and actin, with shortening of the myofibril and contraction of smooth muscle. During relaxation calcium is released from the myofibril and, as it cannot be stored in the cell, it passes out through the channel.

The calcium channel blockers inhibit the passage of calcium through the voltage gated membrane channels of smooth muscle, reduce

available intracellular calcium and cause the muscle to relax. Members of this group therefore are vasodilators, have *negative* cardiac inotropic action and negative chronotropic effect via pacemaker cells and depress conducting tissue. These important properties give rise to the following:

Indications for use

- *Hypertension*: amlodipine, isradipine, nicardipine, nifedipine, verapamil.
- *Angina*: amlodipine, diltiazem, nicardipine, nifedipine, verapamil.
- *Raynaud's disease*: nifedipine.
- *Prevention of ischaemic neurological damage following subarachnoid haemorrhage*: nimodipine.
- *Cardiac dysrhythmia*: verapamil (see p. 437).

Pharmacokinetics. Calcium channel blockers in general are well absorbed from the gut, undergo first-pass elimination in the liver and their action is terminated by hepatic metabolism. Dose adjustments for patients with impaired renal function are therefore either minor or unnecessary.

Adverse effects. Headache, flushing, dizziness, palpitations and hypotension may occur, particularly if the dose is increased too rapidly; ankle oedema may also develop. These effects are ascribed to vasodilatation. Bradycardia and dysrhythmia may occur. Gastrointestinal effects include constipation, nausea and vomiting; palpitation and lethargy may be felt.

Interactions. As the drugs in this group in general are extensively metabolised, there is risk of decreased effect with enzyme inducers, e.g. rifampicin, and increased effect with enzyme inhibitors, e.g. cimetidine. Beta-adrenoceptor blockers may aggravate atrioventricular (AV) block and cardiac failure. Diltiazem, nicardipine and verapamil raise plasma cyclosporin concentration.

Individual drugs

Amlodipine has a $t_\frac{1}{2}$ of 40 h and is suitable for once-daily dosing (5–10 mg/d).

---

[1] From *Aphrodite*, the Greek name for Venus, 'the goddess of beauty, the mother of love, the queen of laughter ... and the patroness of courtesans' (Lemprière). An aphrodisiac would be a drug that provided a reliable, selective, dose-related increase in sexual desire and performance, lasting ideally, we suppose, a few hours; there should be a competitive antagonist. Perhaps fortunately there is no such drug. If there were, its social disadvantages might well be found to outweigh any benefits to an occasional individual.

Diltiazem ($t_{\frac{1}{2}}$ 5 h) is given × 3/d (total dose 180–480 mg/d). It causes less myocardial depression and prolongation of AV conduction than does verapamil but should not be used where there is bradycardia, second or third degree heart block or sick sinus syndrome.

Isradipine ($t_{\frac{1}{2}}$ 8 h) is given × 1–2/d (total dose usually 2.5–10 mg/d) it is similar to nifedipine.

Nicardipine ($t_{\frac{1}{2}}$ 4 h) is given × 3/d (total dose 60–120 mg/d).

Nifedipine ($t_{\frac{1}{2}}$ 2 h) selectively dilates arteries with little effect on veins; its negative myocardial inotropic and chronotropic effects are less than those of verapamil. It is given × 3/d (30–90 mg/d total), or × 2/d (20–80 mg/d total) in a sustained-release formulation. In addition to the adverse effects listed above, gum hypertrophy may occur.

Nimodipine has a moderate cerebral vasodilating action. Cerebral ischaemia after subarachnoid haemorrhage may be partly due to vasospasm; clinical trial evidence[2] indicates that nimodipine given after subarachnoid haemorrhage reduces cerebral infarction (incidence and extent).

Verapamil ($t_{\frac{1}{2}}$ 4 h) is an arterial vasodilator with some venodilator effect; it also has marked negative myocardial inotropic and chronotropic actions. It is given × 3/d as a conventional tablet (120–480 mg/d total) or × 1/d (120–480 mg/d total) as a sustained-release formulation. Because of its negative effects on myocardial conducting and contracting cells it should not be given to patients with bradycardia, second or third degree heart block, or patients with Wolff-Parkinson-White syndrome who have atrial flutter or fibrillation. Amiodarone and digoxin increase the AV block. Verapamil increases plasma quinidine concentration and this interaction may cause dangerous hypotension.

Other members include: felodipine, nisoldipine, nitrendipine.

Angiotensin converting enzyme (ACE) inhibitors

Renin is an enzyme produced by the kidney in response to a number of factors including adrenergic activity (β_1-receptor) and sodium depletion. Renin converts a circulating glycoprotein (angiotensinogen) into the biologically inert angiotensin I, which is then changed by *angiotensin converting enzyme* (ACE or kininase II) into the highly potent *vasoconstrictor* angiotensin II (ACE is located on the luminal surface of capillary endothelial cells, particularly in the lungs; and there are also renin-angiotensin systems in many organs, e.g. brain, heart, the relevance of which is uncertain). Angiotensin II also stimulates production of aldosterone (sodium-retaining hormone) by the adrenal cortex. It is evident that angiotensin II can have an important effect on blood pressure. Bradykinin (an endogenous vasodilator occurring in blood vessel walls) is also a substrate for ACE; it is uncertain whether this is important in the antihypertensive effect, but may cause cough (below).

The antihypertensive effect of ACE inhibitors results primarily from vasodilatation (reduction of peripheral resistance) with little change in cardiac output or rate; renal blood flow may increase (desirable): a fall in aldosterone production may also contribute. Claims that ACE inhibitors reverse the vascular hypertrophy of hypertension and postpone diabetic nephropathy need confirmation.

ACE inhibitors are particularly efficacious when the raised blood pressure results from excess renin production (renovascular hypertension). The effect is immediate and there may be an initial brisk, even serious, drop in blood pressure (*first dose effect*) so that therapy is best initiated at bedtime and the patient warned. Patients already taking a diuretic should omit this for a few days before the first dose. The antihypertensive effect increases progressively over weeks with continued administration (as with other antihypertensives) and the dose may be increased at intervals of 2 weeks.

ACE inhibitors can be useful vasodilators in refractory *heart failure*, given with a diuretic (great caution on initiating dual therapy).

Dose. The elderly and patients on concomitant antihypertensive therapy should be started on half the standard dose.

Captopril (Capoten) has a $t_{\frac{1}{2}}$ of 2 h and is

[2] Pickard J D et al. Br Med J 1989; 289: 636.

partly metabolised and partly excreted unchanged; in renal failure elimination is reduced and adverse effects are more common; it is given × 2/day.

Enalapril (Innovace) is a prodrug ($t_{\frac{1}{2}}$ 35 h) that is converted to the active enalaprilat ($t_{\frac{1}{2}}$ 10 h). Some enzyme inhibition is still present at 24 h and enalapril may be given once a day.

Other members include lisinopril, perindopril, ramipril, fasinopril and quinapril.

Adverse effects include persistent dry cough, angioneurotic oedema which may be severe, other rashes, loss of taste (which may recover though therapy is continued), stomatosis (like aphthous ulcers), abdominal pain, neutropenia, liver injury, raised plasma K (see effect on aldosterone above), deterioration of renal function, proteinuria and blood disorders.

Other vasodilators

Diazoxide (Eudemine) is a thiazide but without diuretic effect; indeed it causes salt and water retention. It is a potent antihypertensive by reducing *arteriolar* peripheral resistance with little effect on veins. Sympathetic homeostatic reflexes can still act so that there is generally little postural hypotension except shortly after an i.v. injection.

It is chiefly used to obtain immediate control of *severe hypertension* and heart failure: 1–3 mg/kg (max 150 mg) is given i.v. *rapidly* (<30 s) (repeat after 5–15 min); the patient must be lying down. The reason for speed was thought to be that diazoxide was so extensively bound to plasma protein that a sufficiently high free plasma concentration may not be attained if the dose was given slowly; but this is probably not so. The maximum effect occurs within 5 min and lasts for at least 4 h. It is strongly alkaline and extravasation should be avoided. The dose may be repeated according to response; i.v. use will rarely need to be prolonged beyond 24 h. The $t_{\frac{1}{2}}$ is 36 h. Alternative therapy suitable for long-term use should be instituted at the same time.

Diazoxide causes sodium retention, and concurrent use of a *non-thiazide* diuretic will be needed; blood glucose and potassium should be monitored. It also relaxes the *uterus* and may stop labour, which may be restarted with oxytocin.

Diazoxide causes hyperglycaemia by inhibiting release of *stored* (but not of newly synthesised) insulin from β-islet cells; the hyperglycaemia can be antagonised by a sulphonylurea. This action (reversible on withdrawal) renders it unsuitable for long-term oral use in hypertension. But it can be used orally in treatment of *insulinoma*.

Hydralazine has a place in combined oral therapy of hypertension and in congestive cardiac failure. It reduces peripheral resistance by directly relaxing *arterioles*, but has negligible effect on veins. For this reason postural hypotension is not generally a problem in treatment of hypertension. The compensatory baroreceptor-mediated sympathetic discharge induced by the hypotension causes tachycardia and increased cardiac output, even causing angina pectoris in predisposed subjects. This can be eliminated by a β-adrenoceptor blocker. The usual compensatory increase in blood volume that occurs with all drugs that increase the intravascular capacity, leads to loss of effect (tolerance); a diuretic can eliminate this. Therefore combination therapy is usual practice. Some of the adverse effects of hydralazine can be accounted for by the hyperkinetic circulatory changes: headache, flushing, nasal and conjunctival congestion, lacrimation, palpitations and vomiting. With prolonged use of doses above 100 mg total/day (the safe maximum oral dose) a reversible syndrome of myalgia and arthralgia proceeding to disseminated lupus erythematosus is liable to occur.

Hydralazine is metabolised by acetylation with the same genetic bimodal distribution as isoniazid. But the difference is more evident in presystemic metabolism and so affects systemic bioavailability rather than postsystemic elimination; ($t_{\frac{1}{2}}$ 1 h). Twice-daily dosing is usual.

In hypertensive emergency hydralazine 5–20 mg i.v. may be given over 20 min; the maximum effect will be seen in 10–80 min; it can be repeated according to need and the patient transferred to oral therapy within 1–2 days.

In *congestive heart failure* hydralazine is largely superseded by calcium channel blockers.

Minoxidil (Loniten) is a vasodilator selective for *arterioles* rather than for veins, similar to diazoxide and hydralazine; it is highly effective in severe hypertension, but causes increased cardiac output, tachycardia, fluid retention and hypertrichosis (see alopecia).

Sodium nitroprusside (Nipride) is a highly effective antihypertensive agent when given i.v. Its effect is almost immediate and lasts for 1–5 min. Therefore it must be given by a precisely controllable infusion. It dilates both *arterioles and veins*, which would be disastrous if the patient stood up. But no patient who needs this drug is likely to want to stand up. There is a compensatory sympathetic discharge with tachycardia and tachyphylaxis to the drug. Nitroprusside action is terminated by metabolism. It penetrates erythrocytes, where electron transfer from haemoglobin iron to nitroprusside yields methaemoglobin and an unstable nitroprusside radical. This breaks down, liberating cyanide radicals. Most of the cyanide remains in the erythrocytes and is firmly bound; it is the free cyanide that passes into the plasma that is toxic, diffusing throughout the body and inhibiting cellular respiration (cytochrome oxidase). The cyanide is converted to thiocyanate and so accumulates over days as the infusion is prolonged (3 days should generally not be exceeded).

Measurement of plasma thiocyanate may be useful in determining whether the patient is suffering from toxicity from prolonged (days) infusion. Poisoning can cause delirium and psychotic symptoms. Metabolic acidosis may occur as a result of cell metabolism becoming anaerobic. Animals and man poisoned by nitroprusside are reputed to manifest the characteristic cyanide smell.

Prolonged infusions of nitroprusside may be made safer by concurrent administration of hydroxocobalamin by i.v. infusion, to take up cyanide and become cyanocobalamin, and of sodium thiosulphate intermittently. These should not be mixed before administration (see also Cyanide poisoning). Methaemoglobinaemia may occur.

It is plain that use of this drug requires unusual knowledge and care. It is particularly dangerous in patients with renal or hepatic insufficiency.

Sodium nitroprusside is used in *hypertensive emergencies, refractory heart failure and for controlled hypotension in surgery*. An infusion[3] may be begun at 0.3–1.0 µg/kg/min and control of blood pressure is likely to be established at 0.5–6.0 µg/kg/min; close monitoring of blood pressure is mandatory; rate changes of infusion may be made every 5–10 min. Use lower doses at first if the patient is taking an antihypertensive agent and for heart failure.

Papaverine is an alkaloid present in opium, but is structurally unrelated to morphine. It inhibits phosphodiesterase and its principal effect is relaxation of smooth muscle throughout the body, especially in the vascular system. It is occasionally injected into an area where local vasodilatation is desired, especially into and around arteries and veins to relieve spasm during vascular surgery and when setting up i.v. infusions. It is also used to treat *male sexual impotence* by self-injection into the corpora cavernosa of the penis shortly before intercourse (sometimes with phentolamine).[4] (Papaver*etum* has occasionally been supplied in error, to the surprise, distress and hazard of the subject.) A physician who prescribes papaverine for this purpose must be ready to treat the occasional case of priapism (defined as erection lasting more than 4 h) (aspirate the corpora cavernosa and inject an α-adrenoceptor agonist, e.g. metaraminol).

Vasodilators in heart failure: see p. 449.

Vasodilators in peripheral vascular disease

The aim has been to produce peripheral arteriolar vasodilatation without a concurrent significant

[3] Light causes sodium nitroprusside in solution to decompose; when made, a solution should be immediately protected by an opaque cover, e.g. metal foil, and used fresh; the fresh solution has a faint brown colour; if the colour is strong it should be discarded.
[4] Brindley G S 1986 Pilot experiments on the actions of drugs injected into the human corpus cavernosum penis. Br J Pharmacol 87: 495. An account of self-experimentation with 17 drugs.

drop in blood pressure, so that an increased blood flow in the limbs will result. Drugs are naturally more useful in patients in whom the decreased flow of blood is due to *spasm* of the vessels (Raynaud's phenomenon) than where it is due to *organic obstructive* changes that may make dilatation in response to drugs impossible (arteriosclerosis, intermittent claudication, Buerger's disease).

Vasodilators such as naftidrofuryl (Praxilene) and oxpentifylline (Trental) increase blood flow to skin rather than muscle; they have also been successfully used in the treatment of *venous leg ulcers* (varicose and traumatic).

Intermittent claudication. Naftidrofuryl or oxpentifylline may be tried but should be withdrawn if there is no benefit in a few weeks. Patients should *stop smoking* and take *frequent exercise* within their capacity. *Night cramps* occur in the disease and quinine has a somewhat controversial reputation in their prevention.

Raynaud's phenomenon may be helped by nifedipine, reserpine, an α-adrenoceptor blocker (in sub-hypotensive dose) and also by topical glyceryl trinitrate; indeed any vasodilator is worth trying in resistant cases; enalapril (ACE inhibitor) seems to lack efficacy.

β-adrenoceptor blockers may exacerbate peripheral vascular disease by leaving α-receptor vasoconstriction unopposed.

Blood viscosity and blood flow. Viscosity of blood in the microcirculation depends on plasma viscosity, e.g. fibrinogen concentration, and erythrocyte deformability (the smallest vessels are half the diameter of a red cell). Oxpentifylline, a methylxanthine, is claimed usefully to increase the deformability of erythrocytes by activating cyclic AMP; it also reduces aggregation of erythrocytes and platelets and the fibrinogen content of blood; it appears to have less efficacy in peripheral vascular disease than does regular exercise.

Dextran 40 reduces blood viscosity briefly.

ADRENOCEPTOR BLOCKING DRUGS

Adrenoceptor blocking drugs occupy the adrenoceptor in competition with adrenaline and noradrenaline (and other sympathomimetic amines) whether released in the body or injected; circulating adrenaline and noradrenaline are antagonised more readily than are the effects of adrenergic nerve stimulation.

Some adrenoceptor blocking drugs have to be altered in the body before they become effective, i.e. they are prodrugs, and this explains the slow onset of action of phenoxybenzamine.

There are two principal classes of adrenoceptor, α and β: for details of *receptor effects* see Table 22.1.

α-adrenoceptor blocking drugs

There are two subtypes of α-adrenoceptor:
- the α_1- and α_2-*adrenoceptors*, on the effector organ (postsynaptic), mediate vasoconstriction;
- the α_2-*adrenoceptor* (autoreceptor) on the nerve ending (presynaptic), mediates a reduction of release of chemotransmitter (noradrenaline), i.e. it provides negative feedback control of transmitter release.

Most α-adrenoceptor blockers are non-selective, blocking both α_1- and α_2-receptors. When subjects taking such a drug rise from supine to erect posture or take exercise, the sympathetic system is physiologically activated (via baroreceptors). The normal vasoconstrictive (α_1) effect (to maintain blood pressure) is blocked by the drug and the failure of this response causes the sympathetic system to be further activated and to release more and more transmitter. This increase in transmitter would normally be reduced by negative feedback via the α_2-autoreceptors; but these are blocked too.

The β-adrenoceptors however are not blocked and the excess transmitter released at adrenergic endings is free to act on them, causing a tachycardia that may be unpleasant. It is for this reason that non-selective α-adrenoceptor blockers are not used alone in hypertension.

An α_1-adrenoceptor blocker that spared the α_2-receptor so that negative feedback inhibition of noradrenaline release was maintained, could be useful in hypertension (less tachycardia and postural and exercise hypotension); prazosin is such a drug (below).

Adverse effects of α-adrenoceptor block are postural hypotension, nasal stuffiness, red sclerae and in the male, failure of ejaculation. Effects peculiar to each drug are mentioned below.

Prazosin (Hypovase) acts as just described, i.e. it blocks postsynaptic α_1-receptors but not presynaptic α_2-autoreceptors. It has a curious transient disadvantage, the 'first-dose effect'; within 2 h of the first (rarely after another) dose there may be a brisk hypotension sufficient to cause loss of consciousness. It is prudent to initiate treatment with a low dose, with food, at home and on going to bed, since to experience this effect would not be a reassuring introduction to what is likely to be life-long therapy. Lower doses of prazosin may be used if it is combined with a diuretic or β-adrenoceptor blocker. The $t_\frac{1}{2}$ is 3 h. For use in prostatic hypertrophy, see p 627.

Doxazosin, alfuzosin and terazosin are similar.

Phentolamine (Rogitine) is a non-selective α-adrenoceptor blocker. It is given i.v. for brief effect in adrenergic hypertensive crises, e.g. phaeochromocytoma or MAOI-sympatho-mimetic interaction. It can be used to terminate dental anaesthesia when adrenaline has been used to provide vasoconstriction (for convenience or to reduce self-injury by cheek and tongue chewing as is liable to occur in mentally retarded subjects). In addition to α-receptor block it has direct vasodilator and cardiac inotropic actions. Dose for hypertensive crisis is 5–10 mg i.v. or i.m. repeated as necessary (minutes to hours). The use of phentolamine as a diagnostic test for phaeochromocytoma is only appropriate when biochemical measurements are impracticable, since it is less reliable.

Phenoxybenzamine (Dibenyline) is a powerful non-selective α-adrenoceptor blocking drug whose effects may last 2 days or longer. Accumulation may therefore occur at the beginning of treatment and the dose must be increased slowly. It is impossible to reverse the circulatory effects of an overdose by noradrenaline or other sympathomimetic drugs, because, although the amount of receptor binding at the outset is competitive, once the drug is on the receptor it binds irreversibly and is not displaced by administering increased amounts of agonist. Its effects are thus unsurmountable, which may be a useful property for treating phaeochromocytoma, and this is why its action is so prolonged. The full effect of an i.v. dose may take up to an hour to develop, since it is a prodrug.

It is wise to observe the effects of a single test dose closely before starting regular administration.

Indigestion and nausea are common with oral therapy.

Thymoxamine (Opilon) and ***indoramin*** (Baratol) are non-selective receptor blockers.

Labetalol has *both* α- and β-receptor blocking activities; see under β-adrenoceptor block, below.

Ergot alkaloids (see index). The naturally occurring alkaloids with effective α-adrenoceptor blocking actions are also powerful α-adrenoceptor agonists (i.e. they are partial agonists); the latter action obscures the vasodilatation that is characteristic of α-adrenoceptor blocking drugs.

Hydrogenation of the natural alkaloids largely eliminates α-adrenoceptor smooth muscle agonist effect but spares α-adrenoceptor block. The alkaloids are also thought to reduce sympathetic tone by a depressant action on the central nervous system. The principal preparation is *co-dergocrine* (Hydergine; a mixture of 3 dihydrogenated alkaloids). It is liable to cause malaise, nausea and vomiting at effective doses. Co-dergocrine may increase cerebral blood flow without lowering the blood pressure and its use has been associated with improvement in senile cerebral insufficiency, but the mechanism of any benefit is more likely to be enzyme changes secondary to effects on receptors than to changes in flow.

Chlorpromazine has many actions of which α-adrenoceptor block is a minor one, but sufficient to cause hypotension, and to be clinically useful in amphetamine overdose.

Yohimbine is an alkaloid from a West African tree. It is a weak α_2-adrenoceptor (autoreceptor) blocking agent, i.e. it blocks the negative feedback receptor so that sympathetic activity is enhanced. It also stimulates the central nervous system, causing a release of antidiuretic hormone. When given with a barbiturate it causes seminal ejaculation in mice, but despite this it neither affects penile diameter in healthy volunteers, nor enhances the response to visual erotic stimuli.

Uses of α-adrenoceptor blocking drugs

- Hypertension
  — essential: prazosin
  — phaeochromocytoma
- Heart failure: as vasodilator
- Peripheral vascular disease
- Miscellaneous: in *benign prostatic hypertrophy* (to relax capsular smooth muscle that may contribute to urinary obstruction), e.g. prazosin; in *chilblains*, with dubious benefit; in *causalgia* the mechanism of relief, if any, is obscure, but anything (also i.v. regional guanethidine block) is worth trying in this diabolical condition.

β-adrenoceptor blocking drugs

Pharmacodynamics

These drugs selectively block the β-receptor effects of adrenaline and will convert the characteristic adrenaline effect on blood pressure to that of noradrenaline, i.e. rise in blood pressure due to its α-receptor actions (see Fig. 22.1). They may be pure antagonists or may have some agonist activity in addition (when they are described as partial agonists).

The cardiovascular effects of β-adrenoceptor block depend on the amount of sympathetic tone present. The chief *cardiac effects* result from reduction of sympathetic drive:

- *reduced automaticity* (heart rate)
- *reduced myocardial contractility* (rate of rise of pressure in the ventricle).

With reduced rate the cardiac output/min is reduced and the overall oxygen consumption falls. These effects are more evident on the response to exercise than at rest.

With acute administration of a pure β-adrenoceptor blocker, i.e. one without any agonist effect, *peripheral vascular resistance* tends to rise, probably chiefly a reflex response to the reduced cardiac output, but also because the α-adrenoceptor (vasoconstrictor) effects are no longer partially opposed by β-adrenoceptor (dilator) effects; peripheral flow is reduced. With *chronic use* peripheral resistance returns to about pre-treatment levels or a little below, varying according to presence or absence of partial agonist activity. But peripheral blood flow remains reduced. *Hepatic blood flow* may be reduced by as much as 30% and this is enough to prolong the $t_\frac{1}{2}$ of the lipid-soluble members whose metabolism is much dependent on hepatic flow, i.e. those with extensive hepatic first-pass metabolism, including propranolol itself; also lignocaine, which is liable to be used concomitantly for cardiac dysrhythmias. The *cold extremities* that are characteristic of chronic therapy are probably due chiefly to reduced cardiac output with reduced peripheral blood flow, rather than to the blocking of peripheral ($β_2$), dilator receptors, for the effect occurs, though less commonly, with the cardiac beta-selective agents.

Effects

At first sight the *cardiac effects* might seem likely to be disadvantageous rather than advantageous, and indeed *maximum* exercise capacity is reduced, but the heart has substantial functional reserves so that use may be made of the desired properties in the diseases listed below, without inducing heart failure. But heart failure due to the drug does occur in patients with seriously diminished cardiac reserve.

With long-term use the *resting blood pressure* falls because cardiac output falls and the normal physiological reflex response (increased peripheral resistance) passes off; indeed there may be a fall in peripheral resistance (the mechanism is obscure). But in some patients the normal compensatory reflex persists, and these non-responders must be treated with other drugs.

Most of the blood pressure effect occurs quickly (hours, days) but there is often a modest decrease over several weeks.

A substantial advantage of β-block in hypertension is that physiological stresses such as *exercise, upright posture and high environmental temperature* are not accompanied by hypotension, as they are with agents that interfere with α-adrenoceptor mediated homeostatic mechanisms. With β-block these necessary adaptive α-receptor constrictor mechanisms remain intact.

Effect on *plasma potassium concentration*, see p. 397.

β-*adrenoceptor selectivity*

Some β-adrenoceptor blockers have higher affinity (selectivity) for cardiac β_1-receptors than for cardiac and peripheral β_2-receptors (see Table 23.1). See note to Table 22.1, p. 395 regarding use of the term *cardioselective*. The question is whether the differences constitute clinical advantages. Potential advantages include less likelihood of causing bronchoconstriction and of provoking or prolonging hypoglycaemia in diabetics.

Some β-blockers (antagonists) also have agonist action, i.e. they are *partial agonists*. This is sometimes described as having *intrinsic sympathomimetic activity* (ISA). These agents cause less fall in heart rate, resting and with exercise, than do the pure antagonists and may be less effective in severe angina pectoris in which reduction of heart rate is particularly important. There is also less fall in cardiac output and possibly fewer patients experience unpleasantly cold extremities, though intermittent claudication may be worsened by β-block whether or not there is partial agonist effect. Both classes of drug can precipitate heart failure and indeed no important difference is to be expected since patients with heart failure already have high sympathetic drive.

Abrupt withdrawal may be less likely to lead to a rebound effect if there is some partial agonist action, since up-regulation of receptors, such as occurs with prolonged receptor block, may not occur.

Some β-blockers have *membrane stabilising* (quinidine-like or local anaesthetic) effect, but this, with currently available drugs, is probably clinically insignificant except that agents having this effect will anaesthetise the eye (undesirable) if applied topically for glaucoma (timolol is used in the eye and does not have this action). *Blood*

platelet aggregation is reduced, especially by non-selective members.

The justification for mentioning these pharmacodynamic differences, which are not great enough to warrant firm general recommendations for drug selection, is that in individual patients they may be important.

The *ankle jerk relaxation time* is prolonged by β_2-adrenoceptor block, which may be misleading if the reflex is being relied on in diagnosis and management of hypothyroidism.

Intrinsic heart rate

If the sympathetic (β) and the parasympathetic (vagus) drives to the heart are simultaneously adequately blocked by a β-adrenoceptor blocker plus atropine, the heart will be its own master and will beat at its 'intrinsic' rate. The intrinsic rate at rest is usually about 100/min, i.e. normally there is parasympathetic vagal dominance, which decreases with age.

Pharmacokinetics

First-order kinetics applies to elimination from plasma, but receptor block follows a *zero-order* decline. The reasons for this are complex but the practical application is important, e.g. within 4 h of 20 mg propranolol i.v. the plasma concentration falls by 50%, but the receptor block (as measured by exercise tachycardia) falls by only 35%.

Most β-adrenoceptor blockers can be given orally once daily in either ordinary or sustained-release formulations because the $t_\frac{1}{2}$ of pharmacodynamic effect exceeds the elimination $t_\frac{1}{2}$ of the substance in the blood.

The solubility of β-blockers is relevant to their use

Lipid-soluble agents are extensively metabolised (hydroxylated, conjugated) to water-soluble substances (some of which are active) that can be eliminated by the kidney. In particular they are subject to extensive hepatic first-pass metabolism after oral administration, e.g. propranolol 80%.

Being lipid-soluble they readily cross cell membranes into and inside the body and so have a high apparent volume of distribution; they readily enter the central nervous system, e.g. propranolol reaches concentrations in the brain × 20 those of the water-soluble atenolol; they have shorter $t_\frac{1}{2}$ (about 4 h) than do water-soluble members (7–18 h). Plasma concentrations of drugs subject to extensive hepatic first-pass metabolism vary greatly between subjects (up to × 20) because the process is so much affected by two highly variable factors, speed of absorption and hepatic blood flow, which latter is the rate-limiting factor. When hepatic first-pass processes become saturated, as does occur, a further increase in dose results in a dramatic rise in plasma concentration. β-blockade reduces hepatic blood flow (30%) and so, with chronic use, they reduce their own metabolism, e.g. the $t_\frac{1}{2}$ of propranolol may increase × 3; but this effect is less with partial agonists with which blood flow is better maintained.

Water-soluble agents show more predictable plasma concentrations because they are less subject to liver metabolism, being excreted unchanged by the kidney; thus their half lives are much prolonged in renal failure, e.g. atenolol $t_\frac{1}{2}$ increased from 7 to 24 h. Patients with renal disease are best not given drugs (of any kind) having a long $t_\frac{1}{2}$ and whose action is terminated by renal elimination. Water-soluble agents are less widely distributed and may have a lower incidence of effects attributed to penetration of the central nervous system, e.g. nightmares.

The most lipid-soluble agents are propranolol, metoprolol, oxprenolol, labetalol.

The least lipid-soluble (water-soluble) agents are atenolol, sotalol, nadolol, practolol.

Others are intermediate.

Considerations of pharmacokinetics are of importance not only because β-adrenoceptor blockers are widely used but also because a high proportion of patients is elderly.

Classification of β-adrenoceptor blocking drugs

- *Pharmacokinetic*: lipid-soluble, water-soluble, see above.

- *Pharmacodynamic* (Table 23.1). The associated properties (partial agonist action and membrane stabilising action) have only minor clinical importance with current drugs at doses ordinarily used and may be insignificant in most cases. But it is desirable that they be known, for they can sometimes matter and they may foreshadow future developments. For example, drugs having partial β-adrenoceptor agonist effect (ISA) cause less reduction of cardiac output at rest, as is to be expected.

β-*adrenoceptor blockers*[5] not listed in Table 23.1 include:

non-selective: betaxolol, bunolol, carteolol, bufuralol, bunitrolol.

β_1-*receptor selective*: bevantolol, pafenololol, tolamolol, esmolol (ultra-short acting: minutes).

β *and* α-*receptor block*: bucindolol, carvedilol.

Partial agonists having about equal proportions of antagonist and agonist action (so-called β_1-receptor stabilisers); see xamoterol.

Agents with other combinations of actions are to be expected.

Uses

β-adrenoceptor blocking drugs are likely to be of use in any condition where reduction of adrenergic activity involving β-adrenoceptors can be beneficial, whether peripheral sympathetic autonomic, adrenal medullary secretion, or CNS adrenergic activity. Such conditions are various.

Cardiovascular

- *Angina pectoris* (β-block reduces cardiac work and oxygen consumption).
- *Hypertension* (β-block reduces cardiac output and rate): there is little interference with homoeostatic reflexes. Some concurrent prevention of sudden cardiovascular deaths may occur with metoprolol.
- *Cardiac tachydysrhythmias*: (β-block reduces drive to cardiac pacemakers: subsidiary properties, see Table 23.1, may also be relevant).
- *Myocardial infarction* and β-adrenoceptor blockers. There are two modes of use that reduce

---

[5] More than 40 are available worldwide.

Table 23.1 β-adrenoceptor blocking drugs

	Drug	Partial agonist effect (intrinsic sympathomimetic effect)	Membrane stabilising effect (quinidine-like effect)
Division I: non-selective (β₁ + β₂) block			
Group I	oxprenolol ⎫ penbutolol ⎬	+	+
Group II	propranolol	–	+
Group III	pindolol	+	–
Group IV	sotalol ⎫ timolol ⎬ nadolol ⎭	–	–
Division II: β₁('cardio')² selective block¹			
Group I	acebutolol	+	+
Group III	practolol	+	-
Group IV	atenolol ⎫ metoprolol ⎬ betaxolol ⎭	–	–
	bisoprolol	–	±
Division III: non-selective β-block + α-block			
Group II	labetalol	–	+

¹β₁ (cardio) selective drugs are 50–100 times as effective against β₁-receptors as are non-selective drugs. But as the dose (concentration at receptors) rises this selectivity is gradually lost.
² See Table 22.1, p. 395 regarding use of the term *cardioselective*.
Note. Hybrid agents having β-receptor block plus vasodilatation unrelated to adrenoceptor have been developed, e.g. carvedilol.

acute mortality and prevent recurrence: the so-called 'cardioprotective' effect.

Early use within 6 hours (or at most 12 h) of onset (i.v. for 24 h then oral for 3–4 weeks); cardiac work is reduced and dysrhythmias prevented; infarct size may be reduced by up to 25%. Maximum benefit is in the first 24–36 h but mortality remains lower for up to one year.
Contraindications to early use include bradycardia (<55/min), hypotension (systolic <90 mm Hg) and left ventricular failure.
A patient already taking a β-blocker may be given additional doses.
Late use The drug is started 4–5 days after the onset of the infarct and is continued for 3 years or even for life.
Choice of drug. The agent should be a pure antagonist, i.e. without agonist action, ISA.

- *Aortic dissection* and after *subarachnoid haemorrhage* (by reducing force and speed of systolic ejection [contractility] and blood pressure).
- *Obstruction of ventricular outflow* where sympathetic activity occurs in the presence of anatomical abnormalities, e.g. Fallot's tetralogy (cyanotic attacks): hypertrophic subaortic stenosis (angina); some cases of mitral valve disease.
- *Hepatic portal hypertension* and oesophageal variceal bleeding (reduction of portal pressure).
- *Cardiac failure.* Specialist use in some cases of congestive cardiomyopathy and hypertrophic obstructive cardiomyopathy to reduce disadvantageous catecholamine effects.

Mild congestive failure, see xamoterol.

Endocrine

- *Hyperthyroidism:* β-block reduces unpleasant symptoms of sympathetic overactivity; there may also be an effect on metabolism of thyroxine.

- *Phaeochromocytoma:* (block of β-agonist effects of circulating catecholamines in combination with α-adrenoceptor block).

Central nervous system

- *Anxiety* with somatic symptoms (see *anxiety*).
- *Migraine* prophylaxis.
- Essential *tremor,* some cases.
- *Alcohol* and *opioid* acute *withdrawal symptoms.*

Eyes

- *Glaucoma:* (timolol or carteolol eye drops) act by altering production and outflow of aqueous humour.

Adverse reactions due to β-adrenoceptor block

Bronchoconstriction (β$_2$-receptor) occurs as expected, especially *in asthmatics (in whom even eye drops can be fatal).*[6] In elderly chronic bronchitics there may be gradually increasing bronchoconstriction over weeks (even with eye drops). Plainly risk is greater with non-selective agents, but β$_1$-receptor (cardio) selective members are not totally selective and may precipitate asthma; however, non-β-receptor mechanisms may also operate.

Cardiac failure. Patients near to cardiac failure need sympathetic drive to provide adequate cardiac output/min: a drop in rate may be enough to induce cardiac failure.

Heart block may be made dangerously worse.

Incapacity for vigorous exercise due to failure of the cardiovascular system to respond to sympathetic drive.

Hypotension when the drug is given after myocardial infarction.

---

[6] A 36-year-old asthmatic collected from a pharmacy, chlorpheniramine for herself and oxprenolol for a friend. She took a tablet of oxprenolol by mistake. Wheezing began in one hour and worsened rapidly; she experienced a convulsion, respiratory arrest and ventricular fibrillation. She was treated with positive-pressure ventilation (for 11 h) and i.v. salbutamol, aminophylline and hydrocortisone. She survived (Williams I P et al Thorax 1980; 35: 160).

Hypertension may occur whenever block of β-receptors allows pre-existing α-effects to be unopposed, e.g. phaeochromocytoma.

Reduced peripheral blood flow, especially with non-selective members, leading to cold extremities, which, rarely, can be severe enough to cause necrosis; intermittent claudication may be worsened.

Reduced blood flow to liver and kidneys, reducing metabolism and elimination of drugs, is liable to be important if there is hepatic or renal disease.

Hypoglycaemia, especially with non-selective members, which block β$_2$-receptors, and especially in diabetes and after substantial exercise, due to impairment of the normal sympathetic-mediated homeostatic mechanism for maintaining the blood glucose, i.e. recovery from iatrogenic hypoglycaemia is delayed. But since α-adrenoceptors are not blocked, hypertension (which may be severe) can occur as the sympathetic system discharges in an 'attempt' to reverse the hypoglycaemia. In addition, the symptoms of hypoglyacaemia, insofar as they are mediated by the sympathetic (anxiety, palpitations), will not occur (though sweating will) and the patient may miss the warning symptoms of hypoglycaemia and slip into coma. Cardioselective (β$_1$) drugs are preferred in diabetes.

Plasma lipoproteins, high density and low density, are altered in a direction adverse for coronary heart disease (decrease of HDL/LDL ratio).

Sexual function: interference is unusual.

Adverse reactions not certainly due to β-adrenoceptor block

Effects include loss of general well-being, tired legs, fatigue, depression, sleep disturbances including insomnia, dreaming, feelings of weakness, gut upsets, rashes.

Oculomucocutaneous syndrome occurred with chronic use of practolol and even occasionally after cessation of use.[7] Other members either do not cause it, or so rarely do so that they are under suspicion only, and, properly prescribed, the benefits of their use far outweigh such a very low risk. But the mechanism of the syndrome is uncertain and, that being so, prediction from tests in animals is likely to remain elusive; it may have an immunological basis.

Abrupt cessation of therapy can be dangerous in angina pectoris and after myocardial infarction and prudence counsels that withdrawal should be gradual, e.g. reduce to a low dose and continue this for 2 weeks. The risk of exacerbation of disease appears to be less with partial agonists. Rebound hypertension is insignificant.

Overdose, including self-poisoning, causes bradycardia, heart block, hypotension and low output cardiac failure that can proceed to shock; death is more likely with agents having membrane stabilising action (see Table 23.1). Bronchoconstriction can be severe, even fatal, in patients subject to any bronchospastic disease; loss of consciousness may occur with lipid-soluble agents that penetrate the central nervous system. Receptor block will outlast the persistence of the drug in the plasma.

---

[7] *Practolol* was developed to the highest current scientific standards; it was marketed (1970) only after independent review by the UK drug regulatory body. All seemed to go well for about 4 years (though skin rashes were observed) by which time there had accumulated about 200 000 patient years of experience with the drug, and then, wrote the then Research Director of the industrial developer, 'came a bolt from the blue and we learnt that it could produce in a small proportion of patients a most bizarre syndrome, which could embrace the skin, eyes, inner ear, and the peritoneal cavity' and also the lung (oculomucocutaneous syndrome). The cause is likely to be an immunological process to which a small minority of patients are prone, 'with present knowledge we cannot say it will not happen again with another drug.'

That the drug caused this peculiar syndrome was recognised by an alert ophthalmologist who ran a special clinic for external eye diseases. In 1974 he suddenly became aware that he was seeing patients complaining of dry eyes but with unusual features. Instead of the damage (blood vessel changes with metaplasia and keratinisation of the conjunctiva) being on the front of the eye exposed by the open lids, it was initially in the areas behind and protected by the lids. He noted that these patients were all taking practolol. Quite soon the whole syndrome was defined, as above. Some patients became blind and some required surgery for the peritoneal disorder and a few died as a consequence.

The drug is now available only for brief use by injection in emergency control of disorders of heart rhythm.

The developer acknowledged moral (though not legal) liability for the harm done and paid compensation to affected patients. He was not *negligent* because current science did not provide a possibility of predicting the effect, i.e. 'state of the art defence' applied. The law did not provide for strict liability or no-fault compensation (see p. 13).

Rational treatment includes: *atropine* (1–2 mg i.v. as 1 or 2 bolus doses) to eliminate the unopposed vagal activity that contributes to bradycardia; *glucagon*, which has cardiac inotropic and chronotropic actions independent of the β-adrenoceptor (dose 5–10 mg i.v. followed by infusion of 1–10 mg/h) may be used at the outset in severe cases. If there is no response, i.v. injection or infusion of a β-adrenoceptor agonist is used, e.g. isoprenaline (4 µg/min, increasing at 1–3 min intervals until the heart rate is 50–70 beats/min); in severe poisoning the dose may need to be high and prolonged to surmount the competitive block;[8] *other sympathomimetics* may be used as judgement counsels, according to the desired receptor agonist actions (β_1, β_2, α) required by the clinical condition, e.g. dobutamine, dopamine, dopexamine, noradrenaline, adrenaline.

For bronchoconstriction salbutamol may be used; aminophylline has non-adrenergic cardiac inotropic and bronchodilator actions and should be given i.v. very slowly to avoid precipitating hypotension. Treatment may be needed for days. With prompt treatment death is unusual.

Interactions

Pharmacokinetic. Agents metabolised in the liver provide higher plasma concentrations when another drug that inhibits hepatic metabolism, e.g. cimetidine, is added. Enzyme inducers enhance the metabolism of this class of β-blockers. β-adrenoceptor blockers themselves reduce hepatic blood flow (fall in cardiac output) and reduce the metabolism of other β-blockers, of lignocaine and of chlorpromazine.

Pharmacodynamic. The effect on the blood pressure of sympathomimetics having both α- and β-receptor agonist actions is increased by block of β-receptors leaving the α-receptor vasoconstriction unopposed (adrenaline added to local anaesthetics may cause hypertension); the pressor effect of abrupt clonidine withdrawal is enhanced, probably by this action. Other cardiac

---

[8] The present published record seems to be 115 mg isoprenaline i.v. over 65 h, held by Lagerfelt J et al. Acta Med Scand 1976; 199: 517.

antidysrhythmic drugs are potentiated (hypotension, bradycardia, heart block etc). Combination with verapamil (i.v.) is hazardous in the presence of atrioventricular nodal or left ventricular dysfunction because the latter has stronger negative inotropic and chronotropic effects than do other calcium channel blockers.

Most NSAIDs attenuate the antihypertensive effect of β-blockers (but not perhaps of atenolol), presumably due to inhibition of formation of renal vasodilator prostaglandins.

β-adrenoceptor blockers potentiate the effect of other antihypertensives particularly when an increase in heart rate is part of the homeostatic response (α-adrenoceptor blockers).

Non-selective (β_1 + β_2) receptor blockers potentiate hypoglycaemia of insulin and sulphonylureas.

Pregnancy

β-adrenoceptor blocking agents are used in hypertension of pregnancy, including pre-eclampsia. Both lipid- and water-soluble members enter the fetus and may cause neonatal bradycardia and hypoglycaemia. In early pregnancy they appear not to be teratogenic.

Individual β-adrenoceptor blockers

Propranolol (Inderal) standard and sustained-release formulations. Once or twice a day oral administration of 80 mg is effective; the dose may be increased weekly; maintenance dose is likely to be 160–320 mg total/day. For *angina pectoris* the maintenance dose will be 120–240 mg total day. For *prophylaxis of myocardial infarction* 160 mg total/day. When given i.v. (1 mg/min over 1 min, repeated every 2 min up to 10 mg) for *cardiac dysrhythmia* or *thyrotoxicosis* it should be preceded by atropine (1–2 mg i.v.) to prevent excessive bradycardia; hypotension may occur. *Migraine prophylaxis*: 80–160 mg/d.

Atenolol (Tenormin) is used for angina pectoris and hypertension, 50–100 mg orally once a day.

Oxprenolol is used similarly.

Practolol is used only by injection for short-term control of cardiac dysrhythmias.

β- + α-adrenoceptor blocking drug

Labetalol (Trandate) is a racemic mixture, one isomer is a β-adrenoceptor blocker (non-selective), another blocks α-adrenoceptors; its dual effect on blood vessels minimises the vasoconstriction characteristic of nonselective β-block so that for practical purposes the outcome is similar to using a β_1-selective β-blocker. See Table 23.1.

The β-block is × 4–10 greater than the α-block, varying with dose and route of administration.

Ordinary β-adrenoceptor blockers are unsuitable for quick antihypertensive effect because a quick drop in blood pressure triggers a compensatory sympathetic discharge that increases peripheral vascular resistance (via α-adrenoceptors). Block of β-adrenoceptors alone cannot prevent this compensatory response; but the addition of α-receptor block can. It is this dual action that renders labetalol suitable for gaining quick control of blood pressure (orally or i.v.). In phaeochromocytoma the additional α-receptor block has been found sufficient to prevent the characteristic rise in blood pressure that occurs with β-receptor block alone.

Chronic use of labetalol is accompanied by normal cardiac output with reduced peripheral resistance and about normal peripheral blood flow; whereas chronic pure β-receptor block is accompanied by low cardiac output, about normal peripheral resistance, and reduced peripheral blood flow.

Postural hypotension (characteristic of α-receptor block) is liable to occur at the outset of therapy and if the dose is increased too rapidly. But with chronic therapy when the β-receptor component is largely responsible for the antihypertensive effect it is not a problem.

Labetalol (but not propranolol) reduces the hypertensive response to orgasm in women.

The $t_{\frac{1}{2}}$ is 4 h; it is extensively metabolised in the hepatic first pass.

The initial oral dose is 100 mg × 2/d (50 mg in the elderly); it may be doubled after 2 weeks. The more severe cases may need a total daily dose of up to 2400 mg/day (in 3–4 divided doses).

For emergency control of severe hypertension 50 mg i.v. may be given over 1 min with the patient supine, and repeated at 5 min intervals up to a maximum of 200 mg; atropine reverses or prevents severe bradycardia. After i.v. labetalol patients are highly responsive to posture for about 3 h.

Serotonin (5-HT) receptor + α-adrenoceptor blocking drugs

Ketanserin appears to act principally to block serotonin vasoconstrictor (subtype S_2 or 5-HT$_2$) receptors and also has some α-adrenoceptor blocking effect (its affinity ratio of serotonin block to adrenoceptor block is 1:5). It is of interest as an example of an 'hybrid' drug; it has been used in hypertension.

Serotonin (5-hydroxytryptamine, 5-HT) is (synthesised in enterochromaffin cells, largely in the gut, and also extensively taken up into blood platelets from which it is released to have vascular effect). It has complex effects on the cardiovascular system, varying with the vascular bed and its physiological state; it generally constricts arterioles and veins and induces blood platelet aggregation; it stimulates intestinal and bronchial smooth muscle. Carcinoid tumours secrete 5-HT and symptoms may be benefited by serotonin antagonists, e.g. cyproheptadine, methysergide and sometimes by octreotide (see index). It is a neurotransmitter in the brain.

DRUGS ACTING ON THE PERIPHERAL SYMPATHETIC NERVE TERMINAL

Adrenergic neuron blocking drugs

Adrenergic neuron blocking drugs are selectively taken up into adrenergic nerve endings by the active, energy-requiring, saturable amine (noradrenaline) pump mechanism. They accumulate in the noradrenaline storage vesicles from which they are released in response to nerve impulses, diminishing the release of noradrenaline and so all sympathetic function. They do not adequately control supine blood pressure and are prone to interactions with other drugs affecting adrenergic function, e.g. tricyclic antidepressants and topical nasal decongestants. They are virtually obsolete in hypertension.

Guanethidine has been used to reduce intraocular pressure in open angle glaucoma and to reduce thyrotoxic eyelid retraction for cosmetic effect. Other members of the group are debrisoquine, bethanidine, guanadrel, metaiodobenzylguanidine (p. 433).

Depletion of stored transmitter
(noradrenaline)

Reserpine (Serpasil) and *methoserpidine* are alkaloids from plants of the genus *Rauwolfia*, used in medicine since ancient times in southern Asia, particularly for insanity; reserpine was extensively used in psychiatry but is now obsolete, though it retains a minor place in combination therapy (with a diuretic) of hypertension.

Reserpine depletes adrenergic nerves of noradrenaline primarily by blocking or destroying the storage mechanism within the nerve ending, so that there is less transmitter available for release. It does not block the amine pump by which extraneuronal noradrenaline is taken up into nerve endings. Its antihypertensive action is due chiefly to peripheral action, but it enters the CNS, where it can cause severe depression which persists after withdrawal; suicide has occurred. The lowest possible dose must be used, and a history of depression contraindicates the drug.

Older domestic male turkeys are liable to fatal hypertensive dissecting aneurism of the aorta. This can cause serious economic loss. The addition of reserpine to their drinking water reduces their blood pressure and preserves their lives without noticeably moderating their natural rage,[9] as may β-adrenoceptor blockers.

---

[9] Conference on use of tranquilising agent Serpasil in animal and poultry production. College Agriculture, Rutgers State University, USA, 1959. Wild turkeys have a blood pressure of 120/60 mm Hg, but domestic turkeys are hypertensive (204/144 mm Hg). Digoxin increases the incidence of aneurysm. It seems that it is the *rate* of rise of pressure in the aorta that is important in this disease (probably in man also) and that reserpine and β-adrenoceptor blockers benefit by attenuating this.

Inhibition of synthesis of transmitter

Metirosine (α-methyltyrosine) is a competitive inhibitor of the enzyme tyrosine hydroxylase, which converts tyrosine to dopa; lack of dopa means lack of dopamine and therefore of noradrenaline and adrenaline, which are made from it by further enzyme processes. It acts also in the adrenal medulla and is used to treat phaeochromocytomas that cannot be removed surgically. Catecholamine synthesis is reduced by up to 80% over 3 days.

AUTONOMIC GANGLION-BLOCKING DRUGS

Because they are not selective and block sympathetic and parasympathetic systems alike, the ganglion-blockers are obsolete in routine therapy of hypertension; they cause severe postural hypotension.

Trimetaphan (Arfonad), a short-acting agent (given by i.v. infusion), also has direct vasodilator effect; it is used for producing hypotension to provide a blood free field during surgery, and can be used for emergency control of hypertension; pressure may be adjusted by tilting the body; it provides 'minute-to-minute' control, when the lack of selectivity is important. Pentolinium is used in a diagnostic test for phaeochromocytoma (p. 432).

DRUGS ACTING ON THE CENTRAL NERVOUS SYSTEM

α$_2$-adrenoceptor agonist

Clonidine is an agonist to α$_2$-adrenoceptors (postsynaptic) in the brain, suppressing sympathetic outflow and reducing blood pressure. At high doses it also activates peripheral α$_2$-adrenoceptors (*presynaptic* autoreceptors) on the adrenergic nerve ending; these mediate negative feedback suppression of noradrenaline release. (In overdose clonidine can stimulate peripheral α$_1$-adrenoceptors (*postsynaptic*) and thus cause hypertension), i.e. there is a therapeutic window. It is evident that, as is so often the case, receptor selectivity is not an ab-

solute property, but is relative and dose related, i.e. as with the locks on 'cheap' cars, one key, used vigorously, may open the whole range, though this is not intended by the manufacturer. Clonidine was discovered to be hypotensive, not by the pharmacologists who tested it in the laboratory but by a physician who used it on himself as nose drops for a common cold.[10]

Clonidine reduces blood pressure with little postural or exercise drop and would be a drug of first choice were it not for a *serious handicap*. Abrupt or even gradual withdrawal, e.g. forgetfulness, intercurrent illness, need for surgery, causes a rebound hypertension (in up to 50% of cases) (with high plasma catecholamine concentration) akin to the hypertensive attacks of phaeochromocytoma. The onset may be rapid (a few hours) or delayed for as long as 2 days; it subsides over 2–3 days. Treatment is either to reinstitute clonidine, i.m. if necessary (t$_{\frac{1}{2}}$ 6 h), or to treat as for phaeochromocytoma. Although it does not occur invariably on withdrawal the disadvantage is potentially serious and therefore, since there are plenty of alternative drugs for hypertension, clonidine cannot be regarded as a drug of first choice, though its use is justified in resistant cases. It should never be used with a β-adrenoceptor blocker which exacerbates withdrawal hypertension (see phaeochromocytoma). Patients taking clonidine will need to be assessed for reliability of compliance as well as given careful instructions. Common adverse effects include sedation and dry mouth. Tricyclic antidepressants antagonise the antihypertensive action and increase the rebound hypertension of abrupt withdrawal.

False transmitter

Chemotransmitters and receptors in the CNS and in the periphery are similar, and the drug in this section also has peripheral actions, as is to be expected.

Methyldopa (Aldomet) probably acts primarily in the brain stem vasomotor centres.

---

[10] Page L H N Engl J Med 1981; 304: 1371.

It is a substrate for other enzymes that synthesise noradrenaline (tyrosine → *dopa* → *dopamine* → *noradrenaline*), but it follows the path (α-*methyldopa* → α-*methyldopamine* → α-*methylnoradrenaline*). Nervous activity then releases a mixture of true transmitter (noradrenaline) and false transmitter (α-methylnoradrenaline). The false transmitter is more persistent than the true transmitter and this may enhance the agonist effect on CNS α_2-adrenoceptors that mediate inhibition of sympathetic outflow with the result that there is reduction in peripheral vascular resistance and sometimes a slight reduction in cardiac output, and blood pressure falls.

The false transmitter is also produced at peripheral adrenergic endings, but as it is there about as effective an agonist as the true transmitter, peripheral action is clinically insignificant.

The chief clinically important advantage of methyldopa is that it interferes little with homeostatic reflexes, i.e. the blood pressure is controlled equally whether the patient is supine, standing or exercising. It can be used orally or i.v.

Methyldopa is reliably absorbed from the gut and readily enters the CNS. It has a $t_{\frac{1}{2}}$ of 1.5 h.

Adverse effects are largely those expected of its mode of action, and also allergy; they include: sedation (frequent), headache, nightmares, depression, involuntary movements, nausea, flatulence, constipation, sore or black tongue, positive Coombs test with, occasionally, haemolytic anaemia, leucopenia, thrombocytopenia, hepatitis.

Gynaecomastia and lactation occur due to interference with dopaminergic suppression of prolactin secretion. Any failure of male sexual function is probably secondary to sedation. Because of its adverse effects methyldopa is no longer a drug of first choice in routine long-term management of hypertension.

TREATMENT OF ANGINA PECTORIS[11]

Cause: an attack of angina pectoris[12] occurs when the need of the myocardium for oxygen ex-

ceeds the amount delivered to it by the coronary circulation.

The principal forms relevant to choice of drug therapy are angina of exercise (more common) and its worsening form, unstable (preinfarction, crescendo) angina, which occurs at rest. Variant (Prinzmetal's) angina (less common) results from spasm of a large coronary artery.

Treatment objective is to unload the heart or to prevent/relax spasm of the coronary arteries so that oxygen need is adequately met.

Myocardial oxygen consumption is chiefly determined by:

- *preload*, i.e. the venous filling and stretching of the heart and its muscle fibres, which evokes the *contractility* (extent and velocity of fibre-shortening during systole);
- *afterload*, i.e. the peripheral arteriolar resistance against which the heart must eject blood, and including the peak systolic pressure that must be reached;
- heart *rate*, which determines the duration of diastole during which intramyocardial pressure is low enough to allow myocardial perfusion to occur via the coronary arteries.

All these determinants of oxygen consumption are influenced by the activity of the *sympathetic nervous system* and it is no surprise that continuous use of a β-*adrenoceptor blocking drug* benefits angina pectoris, reducing the frequency of attacks whether induced by exercise, anxiety or excitement.

The heart can be **unloaded**, i.e. its oxygen needs diminished, by:

- halting the *provocative exercise* (physical or emotional)
- reducing the *preload* (venous return)
- reducing the *afterload* (arteriolar resistance)
- reducing the *rate*
- *dilating* the coronary arteries (even though diseased, the larger arteries may double their diameter).

---

[11] For a personal account by a physician of his experiences of angina pectoris, coronary by-pass surgery, ventricular fibrillation and recovery, see Swyer G I M. Br Med J 1986; 292: 337. Compelling and essential reading.

[12] Angina pectoris: *angina*, a strangling; *pectoris*, of the chest.

Antiangina drugs act as follows:

● *Organic nitrates* reduce preload and afterload and dilate the main coronary arteries (rather than the arterioles).

● β-adrenoceptor blocking drugs reduce myocardial contractility and slow the heart rate. They may increase coronary artery spasm in variant angina.

● *Calcium channel blocking drugs* reduce cardiac contractility, dilate the coronary arteries (where there is evidence of spasm) and reduce afterload (dilate peripheral arterioles).

These classes of drug complement each other and can be used together.

Summary of treatment

● Any contributory *cause* is treated when possible, e.g. anaemia.
● Life style is changed so as to reduce the number of attacks. *Weight reduction* can be very helpful; stop *smoking.*
● For immediate pre-exertional prophylaxis: glyceryl trinitrate sublingually or nifedipine (bite capsule and hold liquid in mouth or swallow it).
● For an acute attack: glyceryl trinitrate (sublingual): nifedipine (bite capsule, as above).
● For long-term prophylaxis:
1. β-*adrenoceptor block*, e.g. propranolol (non-selective) or a β$_1$-selective member, given continuously (not merely when an attack is expected). Dosage is adjusted by response. Some put an arbitrary upper limit to dose, but others recommend that if complete relief is not obtained the dose should be raised to the maximum tolerated, provided the resting heart rate is not reduced below 55/min; or raise the dose to a level at which an increase causes no further inhibition of exercise tachycardia. In severe angina a pure antagonist, i.e. an agent lacking partial agonist activity, is preferred, since the latter may not slow the heart sufficiently. Warn the patient of the risk of abrupt withdrawal.

2. *calcium channel blocking drug*: nifedipine, an alternative to a β-adrenoceptor blocker, especially if coronary spasm is suspected or if the patient has myocardial insufficiency or any bronchospastic disease. It can also be used with a β-blocker, or
3. a *long-acting nitrate*: isosorbide dinitrate or mononitrate (use so as to avoid tolerance, p. 409).
● Drug therapy may be adapted to the *time of attacks*, e.g. nocturnal (percutaneous glyceryl trinitrate, or isosorbide mononitrate orally at night).
● *Antiplatelet therapy* (aspirin) reduces the incidence of fatal and of non-fatal myocardial infarction in patients with unstable angina, used alone or with low dose heparin.
● Surgery in selected cases.

TREATMENT OF ARTERIAL HYPERTENSION

Clinical evaluation of antihypertensives falls into two classes:

1. Whether long-term reduction of blood pressure benefits the patient by preventing complications and prolonging life; these studies take years, require enormous numbers of patients and cost millions (£ or $).[13] It is impracticable to conduct them for each new drug or class of drug.
2. Whether a drug is capable of effective, safe and comfortable control of blood pressure for about one year. Such studies are deemed sufficient to allow the introduction of a new drug. There is sufficient evidence

---

[13] The biggest trial ever done in hypertension was single blind for logistic, not for scientific, reasons. It was deemed to be impracticable to manage a study involving treatment adjustments in 17 354 patients and lasting 5½ years if the double blind technique was used. The study cost £4.5 million (US$5.85 million at then current values) (Medical Research Council Working Party. Br Med J 1985; 291: 97). The time from commencement to publication was 8 years. The choice of drugs as well as the dose is liable to become outdated in such trials. Calcium antagonists were introduced into medicine during the course of this study.

that reduction of blood pressure is beneficial that trials of the first kind are not demanded for all new drugs by regulatory authorities. However it is recognised that the shorter trials may not reveal the long-term consequences of some metabolic effects, e.g. on blood lipids, which may adversely affect the risk of coronary heart disease. Placebo effects are prominent in these shorter trials and must be carefully controlled in trial design.

Aim of treatment

The aim of treatment is to reduce the blood pressure as near to normal as possible in the erect posture, and to keep it there whether the patient is lying, standing or exercising and whether the environment is hot or cold. This is expecting a lot, but it often can be achieved though there may be a price to pay in well-being (quality of life). When this aim is achieved in *severe cases* there is great symptomatic improvement, retinopathy clears and vision improves; headaches are abolished. However, a variable amount of irreversible damage has often been done by the high blood pressure before treatment is started; renal failure may progress despite treatment; arterial damage leads to cardiac or cerebral catastrophes. It is obviously desirable to start treatment before irreversible changes occur, and in *mild and moderately severe* cases this often means advising treatment to symptom-free people discovered by screening.

It is also obvious that to recommend what may be life-long drug treatment to youngish people who are symptom-free and who may find they feel less well taking treatment than they did before demands exact knowledge of the natural history of the disease, and of the effects of careful long-term drug use, as well as considerable knowledge of the drugs themselves and of human nature.

Which patient to treat

There is substantial evidence that effective treatment of patients with a diastolic pressure consistently above 110 mm Hg, i.e. moderate and severe cases, reduces the risk of strokes, renal failure and heart failure; though not significantly the risk of myocardial infarction (except perhaps metoprolol).

Treatment requires as much care and attention as the use of insulin in diabetes. It will almost always be life-long.

Gender. Meta-analysis of trials shows that women are only marginally more resistant to hypertension than are men.

Patients over 65 years require special consideration. Benefits are likely to be less and therapeutic misadventures are more common. Nor do old people have the resilience (psychological or physical) to endure even the milder adverse effects, e.g. loss of energy, depression; and postural hypotension is particularly dangerous. The old may be adequately treated by very low doses very well spaced out. The *minimum* effective dose should be consciously sought and patients extra carefully monitored.

Considerations of *quality of daily life* weigh specially heavily, and therapy should be less aggressive than in younger people who have so much more to gain, e.g. a slight reduction in pressure may be acceptable in the old, rather than aiming at 'normal' levels.

Mild hypertension

Mild hypertension defined as diastolic pressure above 90 mm Hg and below 110 mm Hg presents a difficult problem of balancing potential benefit against risk, and clinicians will make a decision based on their knowledge of their patients, the disease, the drugs and the results of large therapeutic trials.

Overview of the UK Medical Research Council trial on 17 354 patients with mild hypertension (see footnote 13 p. 426):

If 850 mildly hypertensive patients are given [a diuretic or a β-adrenoceptor blocker] for one year about one stroke will be prevented. This is an *important but infrequent* benefit. Its achievement subjected a substantial percentage of the patients to chronic side effects, mostly but not all minor. Treatment did not appear to save lives or substantially alter the overall risk of coronary heart disease. More than 95% of the control patients remained free of any cardiovascular event during the trial.

Neither of the two drug regimens had any clear overall advantage over the other.

For all categories of [cardiovascular] events, and in both treated and placebo groups, rates were lower in non-smoker than in smokers.

It is obvious that adverse effects of therapy are important in that very large numbers of patients must be treated in order that very small numbers may gain; *this is a salient feature of the use of drugs to prevent disease.*

Principles of antihypertensive therapy

General measures may be sufficient to control mild cases as follows:

- **Obesity**: reduce it.
- **Alcohol**: minimise intake.
- **Smoking**: stop it.
- **Diet**: no added *salt*; avoid highly salted foods. Add *potassium* and *oily fish*. Dietary supplementation with potassium reduces blood pressure, as does a high intake of fish oil (a source of eicosapentaenoic and related acids, the high intake of which in the diet of Inuit (Eskimos) may be responsible for the rarity amongst them of severe hypertension). There is not yet a consensus on the role of these items in routine antihypertension therapy beyond ensuring adequate dietary intake (in the healthy as well as in hypertensives) and avoiding diuretic-induced potassium depletion.
- Relaxation therapy: worth considering for highly motivated patients.

Drug therapy

Blood pressure may be reduced by any one or more of the actions listed at the beginning of this chapter. But drugs are selective and when this is done with one drug alone the factors that are uninfluenced are liable to adapt (homeostatic mechanism), to oppose the useful effect and to restore the previous state. There are two principal mechanisms of such adaptation or *tolerance*:

1. *Increase in blood volume* occurs with any drug that reduces peripheral resistance (increases intravascular volume) or cardiac output (reduces glomerular flow) due to activation of the *renin-angiotensin-aldosterone* system. The result is that cardiac output and blood pressure rise. This compensatory effect can be prevented by using a diuretic in combination with the other drug, and this is commonly done.

2. *Baroreceptor reflexes.* A fall in blood pressure evokes reflex activity of the sympathetic system, causing increased peripheral resistance and cardiac activity (rate and contractility).

Therefore, whenever high blood pressure is proving difficult to control and whenever a number of hypotensive drugs are used in combination, the drugs chosen should between them act on all three main determinants of blood pressure:

blood volume, peripheral resistance and *the heart*. Such combinations will achieve three objectives:

- maximise antihypertensive efficacy by adding actions exerted at 3 different points in the cardiovascular system;
- minimise the opposing homeostatic effects by blocking the compensatory changes in blood volume, vascular tone and cardiac function;
- minimise side-effects by permitting smaller doses of each drug each acting at a different site and having different side-effects.[14]

First-dose hypotension occurs with a wide range of antihypertensives, particularly those having an action on veins. It is due to venodilatation and is especially liable to occur in severe hypertension complicated by old age, heart failure, hyponatraemia and renovascular disease. 'It should no longer take the physician by surprise':[15] see prazosin for avoidance.

A graded well-tried and conventional regimen for treating hypertension

1. Start with a single morning dose of either a β-*adrenoceptor blocker*, e.g. atenolol, or a *diuretic,*

---

[14] Chalmers J P Australian Prescriber 1977; 2: 6.
[15] Capewell S and A Br Med J 1991; 31: 213.

e.g. bendrofluazide. Efficacy will begin to be seen within 2–3 days and most of it will have developed within 14 days (dose of β-blocker can be monitored by heart rate response to standard exercise).

2. If the pressure is not controlled in 2–3 weeks, *either* change to a single drug of a different group (monodrug therapy is preferred where it is possible) *or* add the second drug, above. The dose of diuretic will be fixed, but that of the β-adrenoceptor blocker will be in the small-to-moderate range.[16]

3. If this is insufficient add a *vasodilator*, e.g. nifedipine or prazosin. At this point efficacy can sometimes be improved by increasing frequency of administration, e.g. from once to twice a day.

4. If this fails, raise the dose of the β-adrenoceptor blocker until pressure is controlled or the pulse rate on standing has fallen to 55/min, or, for a β-blocker with partial agonist activity, inhibits exercise tachycardia, *or*

5. Add a drug of another class, e.g. a calcium channel blocker (nifedipine) or an ACE inhibitor (enalapril) or methyldopa.

Whilst multidrug therapy is advantageous (see above), increasingly, drugs having different pharmacodynamic actions in the same molecule are coming into use, e.g. labetalol. These are sometimes designated *hybrid drugs*.

High-efficacy drugs with quick onset of action should be given after food to avoid high peak-plasma concentrations and consequent postural hypotension.

Treatment and severity

Mild hypertension will commonly be adequately treated by a *single drug*, stage 1 above.

Moderately severe hypertension may be treated from the start as in stage 2 above (2-drug regimen).

Severe hypertension may be treated from the start as in stages 3 to 5 above (3-drug-regimen).

In a few patients with severe hypertension, lowering the blood pressure may make the patient worse, e.g. if there is severe renal impairment (blood urea above 17 mmol/l), or advanced cerebral or coronary arteriosclerosis. In these cases blood flow to vital organs may depend upon a high perfusion pressure; but when such patients have severe hypertensive symptoms a very cautious trial of antihypertensive drugs is worthwhile.

Alternatives to the conventional regimen (described above)

It is obvious that there are numerous alternative regimens, and the fact that they are not all mentioned does not mean that good results are not obtainable; but some aspects deserve special mention.

• **Initial therapy**. Concern over the adverse metabolic effects of diuretics (diabetes, hyperuricaemia, hypokalaemia) and of β-adrenoceptor blockers (blood lipids), and their lack of demonstrable benefit in preventing coronary heart disease in large trials (except possibly in non-smoking men) (except possibly metoprolol) has led physicians to turn to more recently introduced drugs that do not have these metabolic effects as first choice treatment (especially in diabetics) despite the lack of evidence from large prolonged trials. The agents so preferred are selective α_1-adrenoceptor blockers (prazosin), calcium channel blockers (nifedipine) and angiotensin converting enzyme inhibitors (enalapril). There are indeed good reasons to think these drugs may be better, but they have not been proved so. They may be combined with a β-adrenoceptor blocker.

• **Where there is haste**, then labetalol will provide quicker control than do other β-adrenoceptor blocking drugs because of its added α-adrenoceptor blocking property; alternatively, use an adrenergic neuron blocker, which is later exchanged for less unpleasant drugs.

---

[16] Drugs having a *short steep dose-response curve* for efficacy (that quickly reach a plateau) are given in fixed dose (e.g. to increase the diuretic does not add to efficacy though it does add to toxicity). Drugs having *long sloping dose-response curves* can be titrated for efficacy as well as being used as fixed-dose components of multidrug regimens.

Monitoring

Obviously the blood pressure will be monitored by a doctor (particularly important in the old) and also sometimes by the patient.

Diuretics and potassium. The potassium losing (kaliuretic) diuretics used in hypertension deplete body potassium by 10–15%. Routine potassium chloride supplements are not required, but hypokalaemia will occasionally occur. Uncomplicated patients may not need monitoring if the lowest possible doses are used, but vulnerable patients, e.g. the elderly, should be monitored for K loss at 3 months and thereafter every 6–12 months. In general a potassium-retaining diuretic (amiloride) in a fixed-dose combination with a thiazide, e.g. Moduretic, is preferred over the use of potassium supplements. With such use, a potassium supplement then becomes dangerous.

Control of K balance is particularly important if the patient is also taking digoxin.

Fixed-dose diuretic/potassium formulations contain only a little K and provide only marginal protection.

Compliance. It is obvious that multidrug therapy will pose a substantial problem of compliance. Since treatment will be life-long it is well worthwhile taking trouble to find the most convenient regimen for each individual.

A single daily dose would be ideal and to achieve this sustained release formulations and fixed-dose combinations are used; but compliance is about as good with two doses.

Perhaps the best course is to gain control of the blood pressure with separate tablets of each drug and, when the patient is stabilised, to seek to adapt the therapy to its most convenient form.

Fixed-dose combinations are useful as above, but routine initial use is undesirable in *mild* cases as a patient may well be indefinitely condemned to taking one drug he does not need and to risk its adverse effects.

It is reasonable to employ these formulations initially in *moderately severe* cases. But in *severe* cases it is particularly important to be able to adjust doses of each drug separately and to determine the patient's need accurately, before giving priority to the convenience provided by fixed-dose formulations.

Examples include: Co-betaloc (metoprolol + hydrochlorothiazide), Inderex (propranolol + bendrofluazide), Tenoretic (atenolol + chlorthalidone) and Trasidrex (oxprenolol + cyclopenthiazide).

Accelerated (malignant) hypertension and emergency reduction of blood pressure

Usually prompt oral treatment with the objective of reducing the blood pressure over at least 12 hours will suffice, e.g. labetalol (α + β-adrenoceptor block; but see Phaeochromocytoma below). Alternatives are nifedipine, hydralazine or methyldopa.

Abrupt drops in blood pressure are dangerous because cerebral blood flow may fall so low as to cause serious ischaemia (stroke, blindness). The blood pressure should not be *acutely* reduced below 160/100 mm Hg and this level should be attained over hours. A drop of 25% in pressure is about the maximum that can be tolerated over minutes. Blood pressure should be lowered over 24 h in the elderly.

When there is *encephalopathy* (an emergency), *parenteral* therapy is essential, not only for speed but for certainty that the drug is in the blood. *Sodium nitroprusside* i.v. is a drug of first choice but its action is so fast that it needs extremely careful (1 min) monitoring. Alternatives for parenteral use are diazoxide, labetalol and glyceryl trinitrate.

Lower-than-usual doses should be used if antihypertensive drugs have recently been taken or if renal function is impaired.

● *Blood pressure monitoring* is plainly essential and doses and intervals are judged by response. It is obvious that a drug acting quickly and briefly (sodium nitroprusside) needs closer supervision than a drug with slower onset of a smoother action; availability of monitoring is a factor in choice of drug.

● *Posture* (elevate the bed head) may be made use of to potentiate the drug and (head down) to diminish the effects of inadvertent overdose.

● *Severe tachycardia* consequent on brisk

pressure reduction may be controlled by propranolol i.v.

- *Oral maintenance* treatment for severe hypertension should be started at once if possible; parenteral therapy is seldom necessary for more than 48 h.

Pregnancy hypertension

Effective treatment of pregnancy-induced hypertension improves fetal and perinatal survival. Controlled trials are difficult to do and present considerable ethical problems. Methyldopa has long been a favoured agent for oral therapy,[17] and parenteral hydralazine for emergency reduction of blood pressure (but not in early pregnancy: risk of teratogenesis). Because of possible consequence to the fetus choice of drug is conservative. But β-adrenoceptor blockers (labetalol, atenolol) are increasingly regarded as effective and safe for both mother and fetus. Severe hypotension in the mother jeopardises the fetus. But where patients enter pregnancy with mild essential hypertension, drug therapy may not benefit, and atenolol (but probably not methyldopa) may retard fetal growth.[17]

A *diuretic* should not be used in prevention or treatment of pre-eclampsia as there is no evidence of efficacy and metabolic effects may increase risk to both mother and fetus.

Aspirin, in low dose, for its action inhibiting cyclo-oxygenase in platelets and vascular endothelium, has some efficacy in preventing pre-eclampsia in at-risk patients.

Unwanted interactions with antihypertensive drugs (see also individual drugs)

Alcohol should always be considered as a cause of erratic responses or failure of effect.

Sympathomimetics, including appetite suppressants (but excluding dexfenfluramine) and tricyclic antidepressants can, even in small doses, reverse the effects of adrenergic neuron blockers.

Phenothiazine and butyrophenone *neuroleptics* interact unpredictably.

Methyldopa plus an *MAO inhibitor* may cause excitement and hallucinations.

Nonsteroidal anti-inflammatory drugs (NSAIDs), e.g. indomethacin, attenuate the antihypertensive effect of β-adrenoceptor blockers and of diuretics, perhaps by inhibiting the synthesis of vasodilator prostaglandins. This can also be important when a diuretic is used for severe left *ventricular failure.*

Cimetidine *inhibits hepatic metabolism* of lipid-soluble β-adrenoceptor blockers, increasing their effect.

Surgical anaesthesia may lead to a brisk fall in blood pressure in patients taking antihypertensives. Antihypertensive therapy should not ordinarily be altered before surgery, although it obviously can complicate care both during and after the operation.

SEXUAL FUNCTION AND CARDIOVASCULAR DRUGS

All drugs that interfere with sympathetic autonomic activity, including diuretics, can interfere with sexual function. In men they cause failure of ejaculation and difficulty with erection. Substitution of a drug having a different site of action (e.g. ACE inhibitor or calcium antagonist; or even changing the drug within a group) may solve this problem, in which pharmacological effects may be potentiated by psychology. Centrally acting drugs (methyldopa, clonidine) cause sedation as well as reducing sympathetic drive, and this is an additive factor. Also, hypertensive patients are commonly of an age when non-drug causes of decline in sexual activity are increasingly common and patients may be influenced by fear of ill-health and of the consequences of their disease in general and the likelihood that sexual activity may be hazardous, as indeed it sometimes may be.

Sexual intercourse and the cardiovascular system

Normal sexual intercourse with orgasm is accompanied by transient but brisk physiological

---

[17] Methyldopa: follow-up studies show no intellectual impairment in children up to age $7\frac{1}{2}$ years. For atenolol: see Butters L Br Med J 1990; 301: 587.

changes, e.g. tachycardia of up to 180 beats/min, with increases of 100 beats/min over less than one min, can occur. Systolic blood pressure may rise by 120 mm Hg and diastolic by 50 mm Hg. Orgasm may be accompanied by transient pressure of 230/130 mm Hg in normotensive individuals. Electrocardiographic abnormalities may occur in healthy men and women. Respiratory rate may rise to 60/min.

Such changes in the healthy may reasonably be thought to bode ill for the unhealthy (hypertension, angina pectoris, post-myocardial infarction), and

sudden deaths do occur during or shortly after sexual intercourse [ventricular fibrillation or subarachnoid haemorrhage], usually in clandestine circumstances such as the bordello or the mistress's boudoir, or when the relationship is between an older man and a younger woman — or are these the ones that make the news? In one series, 0.6% of all sudden deaths were [reportedly] attributable to sexual intercourse and in about half of these cardiac disease was present. Clearly it is undesirable that the patient with coronary heart disease should achieve the haemodynamic heights attainable in youth . . .[18]

There appears to be no record of sudden cardiovascular death in a woman.

If there is substantial concern about cardiovascular stress (hypertension, dysrhythmia) during sexual intercourse in either sex, a dose of labetalol about 2 hours before the event may well be justified (taking account of other therapy already in use). The α-receptor blocking action of labetalol added to its β-blocking action renders it more effective against the hypertension of sexual arousal than is a pure β-receptor blocker.[19] But patients taking a β-blocker long term for angina prophylaxis have shown reductions in peak heart rate during coitus from 122 to 82 beats/min. Excessive doses of these drugs may attenuate performance and satisfaction.

Patients suffering from angina pectoris will use glyceryl trinitrate or isosorbide dinitrate as usual for pre-exertional prophylaxis 10 min before intercourse.

PHAEOCHROMOCYTOMA

This tumour of the adrenal medulla secretes principally noradrenaline, but also variable amounts of adrenaline. Symptoms are related to this. Hypertension may be sustained or intermittent.

Diagnostic tests include measurement of catecholamine concentrations in blood and urine or concentrations of metabolites in urine. With modern techniques interference by drugs and diet is less troublesome than formerly.

Antihypertensive drugs may alter catecholamine concentrations (particularly those that induce a reflex increase in sympathetic activity, e.g. vasodilators).

False-positive results in tests are common and patients have undergone unnecessary operations because the tests have been regarded as more reliable than they are.[20]

A variety of *pharmacological tests* can also be used; they too can give erroneous results and must be carried out meticulously, e.g. pentolinium suppression test. Provocation tests are dangerous.

A phaeochromocytoma may also be stimulated to secrete and cause a hypertensive attack by metoclopramide and by any drug that releases histamine (opioids, curare).

Control of blood pressure and heart rate when the tumour cannot be located or removed is achieved best by a combination α- and β-adrenoceptor block (see preparation for surgery, below).

The α-block controls the blood pressure chiefly by abolishing peripheral vasoconstriction, and the β-block controls the tachycardia. A β-receptor

---

[18] Editorial Br Med J 1976; 1: 414.
[19] Riley A et al 1981 The effect of labetalol and propranolol on the pressor response to sexual arousal in women. Br J Clin Pharmacol 12: 341.

[20] On the other hand, a positive test must not be ignored. In 1954, a hospital clinical chemistry laboratory was asked to set up a biological assay for catecholamines in the urine. The head of the laboratory tested urine from the lab staff to obtain a reference range for the assay. All were negative except his own which was strongly positive. He felt well and regarded the result as showing insufficient specificity of the test. Two years later a fluorimetric assay became available. The urines of the lab staff were tested again with the same result. The head of the laboratory still felt well, but this time he decided to consult a physician colleague. A few days later, before the consultation, he was quietly reading a newspaper at home in the evening when he had a fatal cerebral infarction. Autopsy revealed a phaeochromocytoma. (Robinson R. Tumours that secrete catecholamines. Chichester: Wiley, 1980).

blocker should not be given alone, for although it blocks the cardiac stimulation, it also abolishes the peripheral vasodilator effects of adrenaline, leaving the powerful α-effects unopposed, so that there is a rise in peripheral resistance and a further *rise* of blood pressure. The combined β- and α-receptor blocker (labetalol) can be used successfully (though cases of hypertension have been reported).

For surgical removal, where the site of the phaeochromocytoma is known, the patient may be largely spared the effects of liberation of dangerous amounts of catecholamines due to anaesthesia and handling of the tumour, by preparation for 2-3 days with an α- plus a β-blocker (phenoxybenzamine[21] plus propranolol). But there may yet be breakthrough hypertension, and phentolamine (or sodium nitroprusside) should be at hand to control these.

The prolonged preparation allows the reduced blood volume (due to vasoconstriction) to be restored to normal before surgery. The patient must, of course, be kept supine if large doses of α-blocker are used.

After the adrenal veins have been clamped and postoperatively a pressor infusion may be needed to maintain the blood pressure (but it may be preferable to expand plasma volume because patients can become dependent on sympathomimetic pressor infusions which also may be ineffective in the presence of existing receptor block).

Metirosine (α-methyltrosine) has been used successfully to block catecholamine synthesis (see p. 424).

Metaiodobenzylguanidine (m[131]IBG, an analogue of guanethidine) is actively taken up by adrenergic tissue and is concentrated in phaeochromocytomas. Radioactive forms allow localisation of tumours and detection of metastases; also selective therapeutic irradiation of functioning metastases or other tumours of chromaffin tissue, e.g. carcinoid.

---

[21] Phenoxybenzamine (p. 415) may be preferred because it combines irreversibly with receptors and consequently its action is not surmountable by a sudden surge of catecholamine released from the tumour.

GUIDE TO FURTHER READING

Baver K et al 1991 Assessment of systemic effects of different ophthalmic β-blockers in healthy volunteers. Clinical Pharmacology and Therapeutics 49: 658

British Hypertension Society 1989 Treating mild hypertension: agreement from the large trials. British Medical Journal 298: 694

Bulpitt C J et al 1990 The measurement of quality of life in hypertensive patients: a practical approach. British Journal of Clinical Pharmacology 30: 353; Palmer A et al p. 365; (editorial) Callender J S p. 351

Calhoun D A et al 1990 Treatment of hypertensive crisis. New England Journal of Medicine 323: 1177 and subsequent correspondence

Cameron H A et al 1988 Drug treatment of intermittent claudication: a critical analysis of the methods and findings of published clinical trials. British Journal of Clinical Pharmacology 26: 569

Cooke E D et al 1990 Raynaud's syndrome. British Medical Journal 300: 553

Donnelly R et al 1991 The description and prediction of antihypertensive drug response: an individual approach. British Journal of Clinical Pharmacology 31: 627

Fletcher A et al 1988 Quality of life on angina therapy: a randomised controlled trial of transdermal glyceryl trinitrate against placebo. Lancet 2: 4

Hong-Hao Zhau et al 1989 Interindividual differences in β-adrenoceptor antagonists. Clinical Pharmacology and Therapeutics 45: 587

Krane R J et al 1989 Impotence. New England Journal of Medicine 321: 1148

Mills B D 1989 80,000 pills: a personal history of hypertension. British Medical Journal 298: 445

Norwegian Multicentre Study Group 1981 Timolol-induced reduction in mortality and reinfarction in patients surviving acute myocardial infarction. New England Journal of Medicine 304: 803 — a classic

Orme M 1990 Thiazides in the 1990s: the

risk: benefit ratio still favours the drug. British Medical Journal 300: 1668

Packer M 1989 Combined beta-adrenergic and calcium-entry blockade in angina pectoris. New England Journal of Medicine 320: 709

Uzan S et al 1991 Prevention of fetal growth retardation with low-dose aspirin: findings of the EPREDA (Essai Pre-eclampsie Dipyridamole Aspirine) trial. Lancet 337: 1427

Van Baak M A et al 1988 Exercise haemodynamics and maximal exercise capacity during β-adrenoceptor blockade in normotensive and hypertensive subjects. British Journal of Clinical Pharmacology 25: 169

White W B 1989 Methods of blood pressure determination to assess antihypertensive agents: Are casual measurements enough? Clinical Pharmacology and Therapeutics 45: 581

24

Cardiovascular system III: cardiac dysrhythmia and cardiac failure

SYNOPSIS

The pathophysiology of cardiac dysrhythmias is complex and the actions of drugs that are useful in stopping or controlling them may seem equally so. Nevertheless many patients with dysrhythmias respond well to therapy with drugs and a working knowledge of their effects and indications pays dividends, for irregularity of the heart-beat is at least inconvenient and at worst fatal.

- Drugs for cardiac dysrhythmias, their classification and mode of action
- Treatment of specific cardiac dysrhythmias including cardiac arrest
- Drug treatment of cardiac failure

DRUGS FOR CARDIAC DYSRHYTHMIAS

Some physiology and pathophysiology

There are broadly two types of cardiac tissue.

- *The first type* is ordinary myocardial (atrial and ventricular) *muscle,* responsible for the pumping action of the heart.
- *The second type* is specialised *conducting* tissue that initiates the cardiac electrical impulse and determines the order in which the muscle cells contract. The important property of being able to form impulses spontaneously is called *automaticity* and is a feature of certain parts of the conducting tissue, i.e. the sinoatrial (SA) and atrioventricular (AV) nodes. The SA node has the highest frequency of spontaneous discharge, 70 times per minute, and thus controls the contraction rate of the heart, making the cells more distal in the system fire more rapidly than they would do spontaneously, i.e. it is the pacemaker. If the SA node fails to function, the next fastest part takes over. This is often the AV node (45 discharges per min) or a site in the His–Purkinje system (25 discharges per min).

Altered rate of automatic discharge, or abnormality of the mechanism by which an impulse is generated from a centre in the nodes or conducting tissue, is one cause of cardiac dysrhythmia, e.g. atrial fibrillation, flutter or tachycardia.

Ionic movements into and out of cardiac cells

Nearly all cells in the body exhibit a difference in electrical voltage between their interior and exterior, the membrane potential. Some cells, including the conducting and contracting cells of the heart, are excitable; an appropriate stimulus alters the properties of the cell membrane, ions flow across it and elicit an action potential. This spreads to adjacent cells, i.e. is conducted as an electrical impulse, and when it reaches a muscle cell, causes it to contract, i.e. excitation-contraction coupling.

In the resting state the interior of the cell (conducting and contracting types) is electrically *negative* with respect to the exterior due to the disposition of ions (mainly sodium, potassium and calcium) across its membrane, i.e. it is polarised. The ionic changes of the action potential first result in a rapid redistribution of ions such that the potential alters to *positive* within the cell (depolarisation); subsequent and slower flows of ions restore the resting potential (repolarisation). These ionic movements may be separated into *phases* which are briefly described here and in Figure 24.1, for they help to explain the actions of antidysrhythmic drugs.

Phase 0 is a rapid depolarisation of the cell membrane that is associated with a fast inflow of *sodium ions* through channels that are selectively permeable to these ions.

Phase 1 is a short initial period of rapid repolarisation brought about mainly by an outflow of *potassium ions*.

Phase 2 is a period when there is a delay in repolarisation caused mainly by a slow movement of *calcium ions* from the exterior into the cell through channels that are selectively permeable to these ions.

Phase 3 is a second period of rapid repolarisation during which *potassium ions* move out of the cell.

Phase 4 is the fully repolarised state during which *potassium ions* move back into and *sodium and calcium ions* move out of the cell. During this phase, the interior of cells that discharge automatically becomes gradually less negative until a potential is reached (threshold) which allows

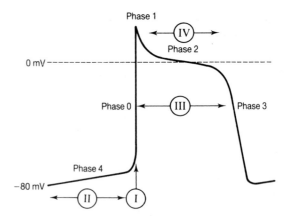

Figure 24.1 The action potential of a cardiac cell that is capable of spontaneous depolarisation (SA or AV nodal, or His–Purkinje) indicating phases 0–4; the figure illustrates the gradual increase in transmembrane potential (mV) during phase 4; cells that are not capable of spontaneous depolarisation do not exhibit increase in voltage during this phase (see text). The modes of action of antidysrhythmic drugs of classes I, II, III and IV are indicated in relation to these phases

rapid depolarisation (phase 0) to occur, and the cycle is repeated. Cells that do not discharge spontaneously rely on the arrival of an action potential from another cell to initiate depolarisation.

In phases 1 and 2 the cell is in an *absolutely refractory* state and is incapable of responding further to any stimulus, but during phase 3, the *relative refractory* period, the cell will depolarise again if a stimulus is unusually strong. The orderly transmission of an electrical impulse (action potential) throughout the conducting system may be retarded in an area of disease, e.g. ischaemia. Thus an impulse travelling down a normal Purkinje fibre may spread to an adjacent fibre which has transiently failed to transmit, and pass up it in reverse direction. If this retrograde impulse should in turn re-excite the cells which provided the original impulse, a repetitively-firing *re-entrant circuit* is established and may cause a dysrhythmia, e.g. paroxysmal supraventricular tachycardia.

In summary most cardiac dysrhythmias are probably due either to:

- *altered rate of spontaneous discharge* in conducting tissue, or

- *impaired conduction* in part of the system leading to the formation of re-entry circuits.

Classification of drugs and mode of action

Many facts about the electropharmacology of antidysrhythmic drugs are known but it is not always possible to use these satisfactorily to explain why a drug will stop one type of dysrhythmia and not another. Nevertheless in the preclinical stage of development, the anti-dysrhythmic drugs are classified according to their electropharmacological actions[1] providing a widely used system for grouping clinically useful drugs of similar properties. It is presented below together with an indication why the actions by which drugs are classified may be useful in dysrhythmias.

The system does not encompass all drugs that are used to treat dysrhythmias and others are described in a subsequent section. For routes of administration, dose, ECG effects and therapeutic plasma concentrations see Table 24.1 (p. 442).

The effects described may apply to cardiac cells in general but are taken to refer principally to cardiac conducting tissue, where most dysrhythmias are presumed to originate.

Class I: sodium channel blockade

These drugs restrict the rapid inflow of sodium during phase 0 and thus slow the maximum rate of depolarisation. Another term for this property is *membrane stabilising activity*; it may contribute to stopping dysrhythmias by limiting the *responsiveness to excitation* of cardiac cells. The drugs may be subclassified as follows:

A. *Drugs that lengthen action potential duration and refractoriness*, e.g. quinidine, procainamide, disopyramide (effective for supraventricular and ventricular dysrhythmias).
B. *Drugs that shorten action potential duration and refractoriness*, e.g. lignocaine, mexiletine,

tocainide, phenytoin (effective only for ventricular dysrhythmias).
C. *Drugs that have negligible effect on action potential duration and refractoriness*, e.g. flecainide, propafenone (effective for supraventricular and ventricular dysrhythmias).

Class II: catecholamine blockade

Propranolol and other β-adrenoceptor antagonists reduce background sympathetic tone in the heart, reduce automatic discharge (phase 4) and protect against adrenergically stimulated ectopic pacemakers.

Class III: lengthening of refractoriness (without effect on sodium inflow in phase 0)

Prolongation of cellular refractoriness (phases 1,2,3,) beyond a critical point may prevent a re-entry circuit being completed and may thereby abolish a re-entrant tachycardia (see above), e.g. amiodarone, bretylium.

Class IV: calcium channel blockade

These drugs depress the slow inward calcium current (phase 2) and prolong conduction and refractoriness particularly in the SA and AV nodes, which may explain their effectiveness in terminating paroxysmal supraventricular tachycardia, e.g. verapamil.

Although the antidysrhythmics have been entered into this classification according to a characteristic major action, most have other effects as well. For example, quinidine (class I) also has class III effects; propranolol (class II) also has class I effects, bretylium (class III) also has class II effects and sotalol (class II) also has class III effects.

INDIVIDUAL DRUGS, BY CLASS (for further data see Table 24.1)

Class I A (sodium channel blockade with lengthened refractoriness)

---

[1] Vaughan Williams E M. J Clin Pharmacol 1984; 24: 129.

Quinidine ($t_{\frac{1}{2}}$ 6 h) is the prototype class I drug, although not now the most frequently used.[2] In addition to the properties that put it in this class, quinidine depresses the contractility of the myocardium (negative intropic effect), and reduces vagus nerve activity on the heart (atropine-like or antimuscarinic effect). At therapeutic doses there is lengthening of ventricular systole and atrioventricular conduction block.

Absorption of quinidine from the gut is rapid, 75% of the drug is metabolised and the remainder is eliminated unchanged in the urine. Active metabolites may accumulate when renal function is impaired.

Quinidine can suppress and prevent supraventricular, nodal and ventricular ectopic beats and tachycardias, e.g. after myocardial infarction. It must never be used alone to treat atrial fibrillation or flutter as its antimuscarinic action enhances AV conduction and the heart rate may accelerate.

Adverse effects include diarrhoea and other gastrointestinal symptoms, cinchonism, rashes, thrombocytopenia and fever. Cardiac effects include serious ventricular tachydysrhythmias associated with electrocardiographic QT prolongation, e.g. torsade de pointes, the probable cause of 'quinidine syncope'. The negative inotropic action (above) may result in hypotension and cardiac failure. Plasma digoxin concentration is raised by quinidine (displacement from tissue binding and impairment of renal excretion) and the dose of digoxin should be decreased when the drugs are used together.

---

[2] In 1912 K F Wenckebach, a Dutch physician (who described 'Wenckebach block') was visited by a merchant who wished to get rid of an attack of atrial fibrillation (he had recurrent attacks which, although they did not unduly inconvenience him, offended his notions of good order in life's affairs). On receiving a guarded prognosis, the merchant enquired why there were heart specialists if they could not accomplish what he himself had already achieved. In the face of Wenckebach's incredulity he promised to return the next day with a regular pulse, which he did, at the same time revealing that he had done it with quinine (an optical isomer of quinidine). Examination of quinine derivatives led to the introduction of quinidine in 1918. Wenckebach K F, J Am Med Assoc 1923; 81: 472.

Procainamide ($t_{\frac{1}{2}}$ 3 h) has effects on the heart which are essentially the same as those of quinidine, but with less antimuscarinic effect. The drug is acetylated in the liver and there are genetically fast and slow acetylator phenotypes.

Procainamide is used to suppress and prevent ventricular and supraventricular dysrhythmias, especially those that follow myocardial infarction.

Adverse effects of procainamide include gastrointestinal symptoms, rashes and fever; hypotension and cardiac failure (negative inotropic effect) occur and dysrhythmias may be induced, e.g. torsade de pointes (above). In long-term use up to 80% of patients taking procainamide develop abnormal antinuclear factor titres in the blood and 30% proceed to a systemic lupus-like syndrome. The effect is dose-related, is more common in slow acetylators and usually regresses when the drug is withdrawn. Prolonged use may also cause agranulocytosis.

Disopyramide ($t_{\frac{1}{2}}$ 6 h) has significant antimuscarinic activity, in addition to the properties that place it in this group. About 50% of a dose is eliminated in the urine by glomerular filtration and the remainder is metabolised.

Disopyramide is effective in both ventricular dysrhythmias, especially after myocardial infarction and in supraventricular dysrhythmias. It may also be used for paroxysmal supraventricular tachycardias of the Wolff–Parkinson–White (WPW) syndrome.

Adverse effects: antimuscarinic activity is a significant problem and may lead to dry mouth, blurred vision, glaucoma and urinary hesitancy and retention. Gastrointestinal symptoms, rash and agranulocytosis occur. Effects on the cardiovascular system include hypotension and cardiac failure (negative inotropic effect), and tachydysrhythmia, e.g. torsade de pointes.

Class I B (sodium channel blockade with shortened refractoriness)

Lignocaine (lidocaine), (see also Local anaesthetics) can sometimes terminate a dysrhythmia when quinidine or procainamide fail, possibly because it *reduces* refractoriness. Lignocaine is used by the i.v, or occasionally by the i.m. route;

dosing by mouth is unsatisfactory because the $t_\frac{1}{2}$ (90 min) is too short to maintain a constant plasma concentration by repeated administration and because the drug undergoes extensive pre-systemic (first-pass) elimination in the liver. Lignocaine is used for ventricular dysrhythmias, especially those complicating myocardial infarction.

Adverse effects are not common unless infusion is rapid or there is significant cardiac failure; they include hypotension, dizziness, blurred sight, sleepiness, slurred speech, numbness, sweating, confusion and convulsions.

Mexiletine ($t_\frac{1}{2}$ 10 h) is similar to lignocaine but is effective by the oral route. It is used for ventricular dysrhythmias especially those complicating myocardial infarction, and those induced by cardiac glycosides.

Adverse effects are related to dose and include nausea, vomiting, hiccough, tremor, drowsiness, confusion, dysarthria, diplopia, ataxia, cardiac dysrhythmia and hypotension.

Tocainide ($t_\frac{1}{2}$ 11 h) is structurally related to lignocaine. It is effective by the oral route and eliminated partly after hepatic metabolism and partly by renal excretion. Tocainide may be used to control ventricular dysrhythmias especially following myocardial infarction, e.g. to continue treatment in place of an infusion of lignocaine, but bone marrow toxicity requires that it be reserved for patients who have not responded to lignocaine. Adverse effects include CNS symptoms similar to those with lignocaine, hypotension, bradycardia and other dysrhythmias, and aggravation of cardiac failure may occur. Marrow depression (necessitating weekly blood counts for the first 3 months), rash, fever, a lupus erythematosus-like syndrome and fibrosing alveolitis also occur.

Phenytoin is used as a cardiac antidysrhythmic as well as an antiepilepsy drug (see p. 308); it principally benefits ventricular dysrhythmias associated with digoxin overdose (i.v. by caval catheter).

Class I C (sodium channel blockade with minimal effect on refractoriness)

Flecainide slows conduction in all cardiac cells including the anomalous pathways responsible for the Wolff–Parkinson–White (WPW) syndrome. Its action is terminated by metabolism in the liver and by elimination in the urine. The $t_\frac{1}{2}$ is 14 h in healthy adults but may be over 20 h in patients with cardiac disease, in the elderly and in those with poor renal function.

Flecainide (together with encainide and moricizine) underwent clinical trials[3] to establish if suppression of asymptomatic premature beats with antidysrhythmic drugs would reduce the risk of death from dysrhythmia after myocardial infarction. The study was terminated after preliminary analysis of 1727 patients revealed that mortality in the groups treated with flecainide or encainide was 7.7% compared with 3.0% in controls. The most likely explanation for the result was the *induction* of lethal ventricular dysrhythmias by flecainide and encainide, i.e. a *prodysrhythmia* effect. In the light of these findings the *indications for use* of flecainide are restricted to treatment of:

- AV nodal tachycardia in patients with WPW syndrome or similar conditions with anomalous pathways,
- symptomatic sustained ventricular tachycardia and
- premature ventricular contractions and/or non-sustained ventricular tachycardia causing disabling symptoms where other drugs are ineffective or cannot be tolerated.

Flecainide is *contraindicated* in patients with sick sinus syndrome, with cardiac failure, and in those with a history of myocardial infarction who have asymptomatic ventricular ectopic beats or asymptomatic non-sustained ventricular tachycardia.

Adverse effects include nausea, dizziness, blurred vision, tremor, abnormal taste sensations and paraesthesiae.

Propafenone, in addition to the properties of this class, also has β-adrenoceptor blocking activity equivalent to low doses of propranolol. It is metabolised by the liver and 7% of patients

---

[3] Cardiac arrhythmia suppression trial investigators. New Engl J Med 1989; 321: 406.

are poor metabolisers (see p. 105) who thus for equivalent doses have higher plasma concentrations than the remainder of the population who are extensive metabolisers. Propafenone may be used to suppress non-sustained ventricular dysrhythmias in patients whose left ventricular function is well preserved.

Adverse effects are more common in poor metabolisers and include dizziness, taste disturbance and blurred vision. In addition, conduction block may occur, cardiac failure may worsen and ventricular dysrhythmias may be exacerbated, especially in patients with sustained ventricular tachycardia and poor left ventricular function.

Class II (catecholamine blockade)

Beta-adrenoceptor antagonists (see also Ch. 23). Beta-adrenoceptor blockers are effective probably because they counteract the dysrhythmogenic effect of catecholamines. The following actions appear to be relevant:

- The rate of automatic firing of the SA node is accelerated by β-adrenoceptor activation and this effect is abolished by β-blockers. Some ectopic pacemakers appear to be dependent on adrenergic drive.
- β-blockers prolong the refractoriness of the AV node which may prevent re-entrant tachycardia at this site.
- Many β-blocking drugs (propranolol, oxprenolol, alprenolol, acebutolol, labetalol) also possess membrane stabilising (class I) properties. Sotalol prolongs cardiac refractoriness (class III) but has no class I effects; it is often preferred when a β-blocker is indicated.

Beta-adrenoceptor antagonists are effective for a range of supraventricular dysrhythmias, in particular those associated with exercise, emotion or hyperthyroidism. They may be used in Wolff–Parkinson–White syndrome and in digoxin-induced dysrhythmias. Sotalol may be used to suppress ventricular ectopic beats and ventricular tachycardia.

For long-term use, any of the oral preparations of β-blocker is suitable. In emergencies, propranolol may be given i.v. (see Table 24.1).

Adverse cardiac effects from overdosage include heart block or even cardiac arrest. Heart failure may be precipitated when a patient is dependent on sympathetic drive to maintain output (see p. 420 for an account of other adverse effects).

Interactions: concomitant administration of calcium channel blockers that affect conduction (verapamil, diltiazem) increases the risk of bradycardia and AV block, or that depress myocardial contractility (nifedipine, verapamil) may cause hypotension or cardiac failure.

Class III (lengthening of refractoriness without sodium channel blockade)

Amiodarone prolongs the effective refractory period of myocardial cells, the AV node and of anomalous pathways. It may also block α- and β-adrenoceptors non-competitively.

Amiodarone is effective given orally; its enormous apparent distribution volume (70 1/kg) indicates that little remains in the blood. It is stored in fat and many other tissues and the $t_{\frac{1}{2}}$ of 54 d after multiple dosing signifies slow release from these sites (and slow accumulation to steady state means that a loading dose is necessary, see Table 24.1). The drug is metabolised in the liver and eliminated via the biliary and intestinal tracts.

Amiodarone is an effective agent against most cardiac dysrhythmias but, because of its adverse effects, is often reserved for cases where other drugs have failed or are contraindicated. It is effective in chronic ventricular dysrhythmias; in atrial fibrillation it slows the ventricular response and may restore sinus rhythm; it may be used to maintain sinus rhythm after cardioversion for atrial fibrillation or flutter. Amiodarone is also effective for the management of resistant re-entry supraventricular tachycardias associated with the Wolff–Parkinson–White syndrome.

Adverse cardiovascular effects include bradycardia, heart block and induction of ventricular dysrhythmia. Other effects are the development of corneal microdeposits which cause visual haloes and photophobia. These are dose-related, resolve when the drug is discontinued and are not a long-term threat to vision. Amiodarone contains iodine and both hyperthyroidism and hypothyroidism are reported; thyroid function should be monitored before and during therapy. Photosensitivity reactions are common and amiodarone may cause a bluish discolouration on exposed areas of the skin. Less commonly, pulmonary fibrosis and hepatitis occur.

Interaction with digoxin (by displacement from tissue binding sites and interference with its elimination) and with warfarin (by inhibiting its metabolism) increases the effect of both these drugs. Beta-blockers and calcium channel antagonists augment the depressant effect of amoidarone on SA and AV node function. Amiodarone raises plasma quinidine concentration.

Bretylium ($t_\frac{1}{2}$ 9 h) prevents the release of noradrenaline from sympathetic nerves. It prolongs the cardiac refractory period. It may be used for resistant ventricular tachyrhythmias, especially those complicating myocardial infarction or cardiac surgery. The main adverse effects are nausea, vomiting, hypotension and bradycardia.

Class IV (calcium channel blockade)

Calcium is involved in the contraction of cardiac and vascular smooth muscle cell, and in the automaticity of cardiac pacemaker cells. Actions of *calcium channel blockers* on vascular smooth muscle cells are described with the main account of these drugs on p. 410.

Calcium and cardiac cells

Cardiac muscle cells are normally depolarised by the fast inward flow of sodium ions, following which there is a slow inward flow of calcium ions (phase 2); the consequent rise in free intracellular calcium ions activates the contractile mechanism.

Pacemaker cells in the SA and AV nodes rely heavily on the slow inward flow of calcium ions (phase 4) for their capacity to discharge spontaneously, i.e. for their automaticity.

The calcium channel blockers inhibit the passage of calcium through the membrane channels; the result in myocardial cells is to depress contractility, and in pacemaker cells to suppress their

automatic activity. Members of the group therefore may have negative cardiac inotropic and chronotropic actions. These actions can be separated; nifedipine, at therapeutic concentrations, acts almost exclusively on non-cardiac ion channels and has no clinically useful antidysrhythmic activity whilst verapamil is a useful antidysrhythmic.

Verapamil (see also p. 411) prolongs conduction and refractoriness in the AV node and depresses the rate of discharge of the SA node. It is the drug of choice to terminate paroxysmal supraventricular tachycardia. Adverse effects include nausea, constipation, headache, fatigue, hypotension, bradycardia and heart block.

Other drugs or means used to treat cardiac dysrhythmias

Digoxin and other cardiac glycosides[4]

Crude digitalis is from the dried leaf of the foxglove plant *Digitalis purpurea*. Digitalis (purpurea or lanata) contains a number of active glycosides (digoxin, digitoxin, lanatosides) whose actions are qualitatively similar, differing principally in rapidity of onset and duration; the pure

---

[4] In 1775 Dr. William Withering was making a routine journey from Birmingham (England), his home, to see patients at the Stafford Infirmary. Whilst the carriage horses were being changed half way, he was asked to see an old dropsical woman. He thought she would die and so some weeks later, when he heard of her recovery, was interested enough to enquire into the cause. Recovery was attributed to a herb tea containing some 20 ingredients, amongst which Withering, already the author of a botanical textbook, found it 'not very difficult . . . to perceive that the active herb could be no other than the foxglove'. He began to investigate its properties, trying it on the poor of Birmingham, whom he used to see without fee each day. The results were inconclusive and his interest flagged until one day he heard that the principal of an Oxford College had been cured by foxglove after 'some of the first physicians of the age had declared that they could do no more for him'. This put a new complexion on the matter and, pursuing his investigation, Withering found that foxglove extract caused diuresis in some oedematous patients. He defined the type of patient who might benefit from it, and equally important, he standardised his foxglove leaf preparations and was able to lay down accurate dosage schedules. His advice, with little amplification, would serve today. Withering W. An account of the foxglove. London: Robinson, 1785.

Table 24.1 Drugs for cardiac dysrhythmia

Drug		Usual doses* and interval	Effect on ECG	Usually effective plasma concentration
IA:	Quinidine	p.o.: 200 mg test dose, then 200–400 mg × 6–8 h	Prolongs QRS QT and (±) PR	2–5 mg/l
	Procainamide	p.o.: 50 mg/kg/d in divided doses × 3–6 h or × 6 h (sust. release).. i.v.: see specialist literature	Prolongs QRS QT and (±) PR	4–10 mg/l (NAPA: active metabolite, 10–20 mg/l)
	Disopyramide	p.o.: 300–800 mg/d in divided doses. i.v: see specialist literature	Prolongs QRS QT and (±) PR	2–5 mg/l
IB:	Lignocaine	i.v. loading: 100 mg as a bolus over a few min. i.v. maintenance: 2–4 mg/min	No significant change	1.5–6 mg/l
	Mexiletine	p.o.: initial dose 400 mg, then after 2 h 200–250 mg × 6–8 h. i.v: see specialist literature	No significant change	0.5–2 mg/l
	Tocainide	p.o. 1.2 g/d in divided doses to 2.4 g/d max. i.v.: see specialist literature	No significant change	3–10 mg/l
	Phenytoin	i.v.: 3.5–5 mg/kg by caval catheter not exceeding 50 mg/kg with ECG and BP monitoring	No significant change	5–20 mg/l
IC:	Flecainide	p.o. and i.v.: see specialist literature	Prolongs PR and QRS	0.2–1 mg/l
	Propafenone	p.o.:see specialist literature	Prolongs PR and QRS	Active metabolite precludes establishment
II:	Propranolol	p.o.: 10–80 mg × 6 h i.v.: 1 mg over 1 min intervals to 10 mg max. (5 mg in anaesthesia)	Prolongs PR (±) No change in QRS Shortens QT Bradycardia	Not established
III:	Amiodarone	p.o. loading: 200 mg × 8 h for 1 week, then 200 mg × 12 h for 1 week; maintenance 200 mg/d	Prolongs PR, QRS and QT Sinus bradycardia	Not established
	Bretylium	i.v.: see specialist literature	No change. Sinus bradycardia	Not established
IV:	Verapamil	p.o.: 40–120 mg × 8–12 h i.v.: see specialist literature	Prolongs PR	Probably 100–300 µg/l
Other:	Digoxin	p.o. (tablets): 0.5–0.75 mg initially; additional 0.25–0.5 mg × 6–8 h maintenance: 0.125–0.5 mg/d	Prolongs PR Depresses ST segment Flattens T wave	1–2 µg/l

* Doses accord with British National Formulary recommendations. Patients with decreased hepatic or renal function may require lower doses (see text).
This table is adapted from that published in the Medical Letter on Drugs and Therapeutics (USA) 1991. We are grateful to the Chairman of the Editorial Board for allowing us to use this material.

individual glycosides are used. The following account refers to all the cardiac glycosides but *digoxin* is principally used.

Mode of action. Cardiac glycosides affect the heart both directly and indirectly in complex interactions, some of which oppose each other. The *direct* effect is to inhibit the membrane-bound adenosinetriphosphatase (ATPase) enzyme that, by hydrolysing ATP, supplies energy for the system that pumps sodium out of and transports potassium into conducting and contracting cells. The resulting rise in intracellular sodium and fall in intracellular potassium is accompanied by an influx of calcium ions. The *indirect* effect is to enhance vagal activity by complex peripheral and central mechanisms.

The clinically important consequences are:

- *On the contracting cells*: increased contractility and excitability.
- *On SA and AV nodes and conducting tissue*: decreased generation and propagation.

Pharmacokinetics. Digoxin may be administered by mouth or i.v. It is eliminated 85% unchanged by the kidney and the remainder is metabolised by the liver. The $t_\frac{1}{2}$ is 36 h. By contrast digitoxin is extensively metabolised and the $t_\frac{1}{2}$ is 150 h.

Uses of cardiac glycosides are:

1. *Atrial fibrillation*, benefiting chiefly by the vagal effect on the AV node, reducing conduction through it and thus slowing the ventricular rate.

2. *Paroxysmal supraventricular tachycardia*, benefiting chiefly by the vagal effect on the SA node, slowing its rate of discharge, and on the AV node, as in (1), above.

3. *Atrial flutter*. Cardioversion is preferred, but digoxin may be effective, chiefly by the vagus nerve action of shortening the refractory period of the atrial muscle, to convert flutter to fibrillation, in which the ventricular rate is more readily controlled.

4. *Cardiac failure*, benefiting the patient chiefly by the direct action to increase myocardial contractility. Digoxin is used in left ventricular or congestive cardiac failure due to ischaemic,

hypertensive or valvular heart disease, especially in the short term.

Dose and therapeutic plasma concentration: see Table 24.1

Reduced dose of digoxin is called for in: renal impairment (see above), the elderly (probably from decline in renal clearance with age), electrolyte disturbances (hypokalaemia accentuates the effects of digoxin, as does hypomagnesaemia), hypothyroid patients (they are intolerant of digoxin).

Adverse effects. *Abnormal cardiac rhythms* usually take the form of ectopic dysrhythmias (ventricular ectopic beats, ventricular tachy-dysrhythmias, paroxysmal supraventricular tachycardia) and heart block. *Gastrointestinal effects* include anorexia which usually precedes vomiting and is a warning that dosage is excessive. Diarrhoea may also occur. *Visual effects* include disturbances of colour vision, e.g. yellow (xanthopsia) but also red or green vision, photophobia and blurring. *Gynaecomastia* may occur in men and breast enlargement in women with long-term use (cardiac glycosides have structural resemblance to oestrogen). *Mental effects* include confusion, restlessness, agitation, nightmares and acute psychoses.

Acute digoxin poisoning causes initial nausea and vomiting and hyperkalaemia because inhibition of the sodium-potassium ATPase pump prevents intracellular accumulation of potassium. The ECG changes (see Table 24.1) of prolonged use of digoxin may be absent. There may be exaggerated sinus dysrhythmia, bradycardia and ectopic rhythms with or without heart block.

Treatment of overdose. Phenytoin 100 mg i.v. is useful in the management of digoxin-induced ventricular dysrhythmias. Atropine is effective for bradycardia. Electrical pacing may be needed, but direct current shock may lead to ventricular fibrillation. For severe digoxin poisoning infusion of the *digoxin-specific binding (Fab) fragment* (Digibind) of the antibody to digoxin, inactivates digoxin in the plasma and is an effective treatment. Because it lacks the Fc segment, this fragment is non-immunogenic and it is sufficiently small to be eliminated as the digoxin-antibody complex in the urine.

Interactions. Cardiac dysrhythmias may develop due to depletion of body *potassium* from therapy with *diuretics* or with adrenal steroids. Verapamil, nifedipine, quinidine and amiodarone raise steady-state plasma digoxin concentrations (see above) and the digoxin dose should be lowered when any of these is added. AV block caused by digoxin is increased by verapamil and by β-adrenoceptor blockers.

Adenosine

Adenosine is an endogenous purine nucleotide which slows atrioventricular conduction and dilates coronary and peripheral arteries. It is rapidly metabolised by circulating adenosine deaminase and enters cells; hence its residence in plasma is brief ($t_{\frac{1}{2}}$ several seconds) and it must be given i.v. Administered as a bolus injection, adenosine is useful for distinguishing the origin of 'broad QRS complex' tachycardias, i.e. whether ventricular, or supraventricular with aberrant conduction. If the latter is the case, AV block with adenosine allows the P waves to be seen and the diagnosis to be made; adenosine thus has the same effect as carotid massage (see below). Evidence also indicates that adenosine is effective for terminating paroxysmal supraventricular (re-entrant) tachycardias, including episodes in patients with Wolff–Parkinson–White syndrome. Adverse effects are not serious because of the brevity of its action but dyspnoea, facial flushing, chest pain and transient dysrhythmias, e.g. bradycardia, may occur.

The autonomic system

Some drugs used for dysrhythmias exert their actions through the *autonomic nervous system* by mimicking or antagonising the effects of the parasympathetic or sympathetic nerves that supply the heart.

*The **vagus nerve*** (cholinergic, parasympathetic), when stimulated, has the following effects on the heart:

1. bradycardia due to depression of the SA node

2. slowing of conduction through and increased refractoriness of the AV node
3. reduced force of contraction of atrial and ventricular muscle cells
4. shortening of the refractory period of atrial muscle cells
5. decreased myocardial excitability.

The effects 1, 2, 4 and 5 are used in the therapy of dysrhythmias.

The vagus nerve may be stimulated reflexly by various physical manoeuvres. Vagal stimulation may slow or terminate supraventricular dysrhythmias and should if possible be carried out under ECG control.

Carotid sinus massage activates stretch receptors: external pressure is applied gently to one side at a time but *never* to both sides at once. Some individuals are very sensitive to the procedure and develop severe bradycardia and hypotension. Other methods include the *Valsalva manoeuvre* (deep inspiration followed by expiration against a closed glottis, which both stimulates stretch receptors in the lung and reduces venous return to the heart); the *Muller procedure* (deep expiration followed by inspiration against a closed glottis); production of nausea and retching by inviting patients to put their *own* fingers down their throat.

The effects of vagus nerve activity are blocked by atropine (antimuscarinic action), an action that is used to accelerate the heart during episodes of sinus bradycardia as may occur after myocardial infarction. The dose is 0.6 mg i.v. and repeated as necessary to a maximum of 3 mg per day. Adverse effects are those of muscarinic blockade, namely dry mouth, blurred vision, urinary retention, confusion and hallucination.

Other antidysrhythmia drugs that have a vagal antimuscarinic action include quinidine, procainamide and disopyramide.

*The **sympathetic division*** (adrenergic component of the autonomic nervous system), when stimulated, has the following effects on the heart (receptor effects):

1. tachycardia due to increased rate of discharge of the SA node
2. increased automaticity in the AV node and His–Purkinje system

3. increase in conductivity in the His–Purkinje system
4. increased force of contraction
5. shortening of the refractory period.

(It may be noted that the effects of the two lists (parasympathetic, adrenergic) above are not all opposites).

Isoprenaline, a β-adrenoceptor agonist, may be used to accelerate the heart and to raise cardiac output when there is extreme bradycardia due to heart block, prior to the insertion of an electrical pacemaker. The dose is: i.v. 0.5–10 mg per minute; by mouth 30 mg every 8 h to a maximum of 840 mg per day. Adverse effects are those expected of β-adrenoceptor agonists and include tremor, flushing, sweating, palpitation, headache and diarrhoea.

Pro-dysrhythmic effects of antidysrhythmic drugs

Antidysrhythmic drugs can also *cause* dysrhythmia. Such pro-dysrhythmic effects are most commonly seen with drugs that prolong the QT interval or QRS complex of the ECG; hypokalaemia aggravates the danger. Quinidine may cause tachydysrhythmia in an estimated 1–4% of patients. A pro-dysrhythmic effect of flecainide and encainide resulting in a doubling of mortality was revealed by the Cardiac Arrhythmia Suppression Trial (CAST) (see p. 439).

Digoxin can induce a variety of brady- and tachydysrhythmias (above).

Recognition of this important effect requires that in general antidysrhythmic drugs be used only in patients with potentially life-threatening dysrhythmias or those that produce moderate to severe symptoms, with the least toxic drug, and with close monitoring.

The choice between drugs and electroconversion to terminate dysrhythmias

Direct current (DC) electric shock applied externally is often the best way to convert cardiac dysrhythmias to sinus rhythm. Many atrial or ventricular dysrhythmias start as a result of transiently operating factors, but once they have begun, the abnormal mechanisms are self-sustaining. When an electric shock is given, the heart is depolarised, the ectopic focus is extinguished and the SA node, the part of the heart with the highest automaticity, resumes as the dominant pacemaker.

Electrical conversion has the advantage that it is immediate, unlike drugs, which may take days or longer to act; also, the effective doses and adverse effects of drugs are largely unpredictable, and can be serious.

Uses. Electrical conversion is used in supraventricular and ventricular tachycardia, ventricular fibrillation, and in atrial fibrillation and flutter. Drugs can be useful to prevent a relapse, e.g. sotalol, amiodarone.

TREATMENT OF SPECIFIC CARDIAC DYSRHYTHMIAS

Sinus bradycardia

Sinus bradycardia requires treatment if there is hypotension or escape rhythms; extreme bradycardia may allow a ventricular focus to take over and lead to ventricular tachycardia. The foot of the bed should be raised to assist venous return and atropine should be given i.v. (as above).

Atrial ectopic beats

Reduction in the use of tea, coffee and other xanthine-containing drinks, and of tobacco, may suffice for ectopic beats not due to organic heart disease. When action is needed, a small dose of a β-adrenoceptor blocker may be effective.

Paroxysmal supraventricular (AV re-entrant) tachycardia

These manifest as recurrent attacks of abrupt onset. If vagal stimulation is unsuccessful at terminating them, verapamil i.v. is highly effective but must not be used if the patient has recently received a β-blocker; failing this a DC shock may be administered, for immediate effect. A β-adrenoceptor blocker, e.g. sotalol, may be effective at preventing attacks.

Atrial fibrillation

Atrial fibrillation (and flutter and tachycardia, below) are thought to be due to enhanced automaticity of atrial ectopic foci.

Control. The patient needs rate control to allow adequate diastolic time for the ventricle to be filled. Digoxin is the drug of choice; a rapid ventricular rate should be reduced within 2–3 hours with digoxin i.v. If digoxin does not achieve this, e.g. in hyperthyroidism, propranolol or verapamil may be added, rather than increasing the dose of digoxin. With long-standing rheumatic mitral valvular disease, it is generally better to control the heart rate with digoxin than to attempt to convert it to sinus rhythm.

Conversion to sinus rhythm. Electrical conversion has supplanted drugs. The chief indications are, uncontrollable ventricular rate, and atrial fibrillation persisting after treatment of its cause, e.g. myocardial infarction, pneumonia, hyperthyroidism. Electrical conversion should be avoided if digoxin toxicity is suspected but may proceed if the patient's dose of digoxin, serum potassium and renal function are normal. Sotalol, amiodarone or quinidine may be used to prevent relapse.

Where atrial fibrillation has been present for less than 6 months, or the left atrium is not enlarged, it is usually possible to stop it. There is a risk of arterial embolism, the result of resumed coordinated atrial contraction detaching recent, rather than old, organised, thrombus from the atrial wall. It occurs whether fibrillation is of recent onset or of long duration. *All* patients should therefore be anticoagulated for 2 weeks before conversion, and for 4 weeks after.

Atrial flutter

The atrial rate is usually 300/min. Treatment is urgent if a fast ventricular rate is causing cardiac failure or threatens extension of an area of myocardial infarction. Electrical conversion is usually preferred. Should it prove unsuccessful the heart rate may be reduced with digoxin either alone or in combination with amiodarone, or verapamil or a β-adrenoceptor blocker. Quinidine should *never* be used alone, for it may allow 1 : 1 A : V conduction both by slowing the atrial rate and by facilitating AV conduction by its antimuscarinic effect, with disastrous results, i.e. a ventricular rate of 150–200/min.

Atrial tachycardia

The atrial rate is 120–250/min, and commonly there is AV block. If the patient is taking digoxin, it should be suspected as the cause of the dysrhythmia, and stopped. If the patient is not taking digoxin, it may be used to control the ventricular rate.

Heart block

The use of artificial pacemakers is beyond the scope of this book. In an emergency, AV conduction may be improved by atropine (antimuscarinic vagal block) (0.6 mg i.v.) or by isoprenaline (β-adrenoceptor agonist) (0.5–10 μg/min, i.v.).

Pre-excitation (Wolff–Parkinson–White) syndrome

This occurs in otherwise healthy people, who possess an anomalous (accessory) artioventricular pathway; they often experience attacks of paroxysmal AV re-entrant tachycardia or atrial fibrillation. Drugs that delay conduction through the AV node are used to prevent it, i.e. a β-adrenoceptor blocker (sotalol), amiodarone or flecainide. Verapamil and digoxin may increase conduction through the anomalous pathway and should not be used. Electrical conversion may be needed to restore sinus rhythm when the ventricular rate is very rapid.

Ventricular premature beats

These are common after myocardial infarction. Their particular significance is that an ectopic beat developing during the early or peak phases of the T-wave may precipitate ventricular tachycardia or fibrillation (the R-on-T phenomenon). About 80% of patients with myocardial infarction who proceed to ventricular fibrillation have preceding ventricular premature beats.

Lignocaine is effective in suppressing ectopic ventricular beats; in the absence of clear evidence that routine prophylaxis reduces mortality, many specialists in coronary care give lignocaine if there are more than 6 ventricular ectopics per minute, if they occur near to the peak of the T-wave, if there are runs of 2 or more in succession or if they are multifocal. Propafenone, mexiletine, disopyramide or sotalol are alternatives.

Ventricular tachycardia

Ventricular tachycardia demands urgent treatment since it frequently leads to ventricular fibrillation and circulatory arrest. A powerful thump of the fist on the mid-sternum or precordium may stop a tachycardia. If the patient is in good condition i.v. treatment may begin with lignocaine or, should that fail, amiodarone i.v. For recurrent ventricular tachycardia amiodarone is often preferred but the choice is wide and includes mexiletine, tocainamide, disopyramide, procainamide, quinidine, propafenone or sotalol by mouth. The selection of a particular drug may be influenced by anticipated adverse effects, e.g. disopyramide and quinidine have antimuscarinic effects that would be undesirable in a patient with glaucoma or prostatism.

If there is rapid haemodynamic deterioration, electrical conversion is the treatment of choice. It should be followed by lignocaine as an i.v. infusion for as long as experience and wisdom counsel.

Ventricular fibrillation and cardiac arrest

Ventricular fibrillation is usually caused by myocardial infarction or ischaemia, or some other serious organic heart disease and is one of the reasons for cardiac arrest. Guidelines for the management of cardiac arrest are issued by the Resuscitation Council of the United Kingdom.[5] A protocol depicting these appears on p. 448.

---

[5] British Medical Journal 1989; 299: 446. We are grateful to the Resuscitation Council (UK) and to Laerdal Medical for permission to publish this information. DRL, PNB.

DRUG TREATMENT OF CARDIAC FAILURE

The heart may fail from disease of the myocardium itself, mainly ischaemic, or from an excessive workload imposed on it by arterial hypertension, valvular disease or an arteriovenous shunt. The management of cardiac failure requires both the relief of any treatable underlying or aggravating cause, e.g. hypertension, and therapy directed at the failure itself.

Some physiology and pathophysiology

Cardiac output (CO) depends on the heart rate (HR) and the volume of blood that is ejected with each beat, i.e. the stroke volume (SV). Their relation is expressed by the equation:

$$CO = HR \times SV$$

There are three factors that regulate the stroke volume, namely preload, afterload and contractility.

Preload is the load on the heart created by the volume of blood injected into the left ventricle by the left atrium (at the end of ventricular diastole) and that it must eject with each contraction. It can also be viewed as the amount of stretch to which the left ventricle is subject. As the preload rises so also does the degree of stretch and the length of cardiac muscle fibres. Preload is thus a *volume* load and can be excessive, e.g., when there is valvular incompetence.

Afterload refers to the load on the contracting ventricle created by the resistance to the blood injected by the ventricle into the arterial system, i.e. the total peripheral resistance. Afterload is thus a *pressure* load and is excessive, e.g., in arterial hypertension.

Contractility refers to the capacity of the myocardium to generate the force necessary to respond to preload and to overcome afterload.

When the circulation fails to meet the metabolic demands of the body various mechanisms are recruited to help sustain or increase the cardiac output:

- *The heart dilates*. The greater the length of individual cardiac fibres the greater the contrac-

CARDIOPULMONARY RESUSCITATION

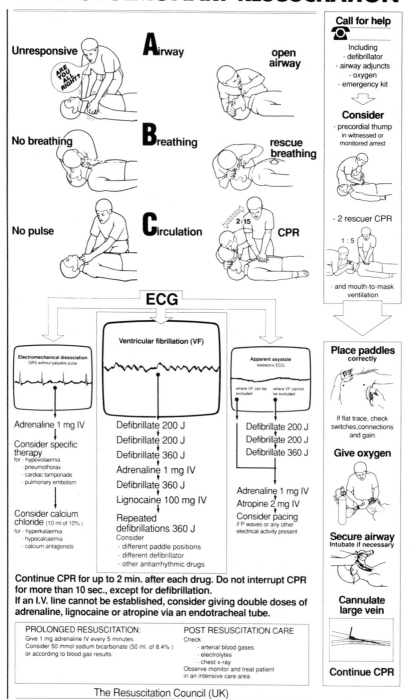

Figure 24.2 Protocol for the treatment of cardiac arrest in hospitals

tility the myocardium can develop (the Frank–Starling relation). Thus, for a time, dilatation of the heart helps to sustain cardiac output.

• *The sympathetic drive to the heart increases.* There is greater rate and force of cardiac contraction (increased *contractility*), constriction of peripheral venous capacitance vessels (increased *preload*) and arteriolar resistance vessels with raised peripheral resistance (increased *afterload*). These circulatory changes divert blood from the liver, kidneys and skin to maintain flow to the heart and brain.

• *The renin-angiotensin-aldosterone system is activated*; aldosterone causes sodium to be retained, thus enlarging blood volume (increased *preload*) and angiotensin causes peripheral vasoconstriction (increased *afterload*).

In the early stages of cardiac failure these physiological adjustments serve to maintain the blood supply to the tissues, but as failure progresses they outlive their usefulness and actually impair the effectiveness of the circulation. Elevated peripheral resistance, apart from adding directly to cardiac work (increased O_2 consumption), increases left ventricular wall tension which also raises myocardial O_2 consumption. Thus a cycle is set up which further impairs cardiac performance. Excessive retention of salt and water together with heightened venous tone, raise the ventricular filling pressure beyond the capacity of the myocardium to cope and the lungs become congested.

The distinction between the capacity of the myocardium to pump blood and the load against which the heart must work is useful in therapy. The failing myocardium is so strongly stimulated to contract by increased sympathetic drive that therapeutic efforts to induce it to function yet more vigorously are in themselves alone unlikely to be of benefit. Drugs can be used however to alleviate the load imposed on the failing heart by the physiological adjustments to cardiac failure; agents that reduce preload or afterload are very effective, especially where the left ventricular volume is raised (less predictably so for failure of the right ventricle). The main hazard of their use is a drastic fall in cardiac output in those occasional patients whose output is dependent on a high left ventricular filling pressure, e.g. those who are volume depleted by diuretic use or those with severe mitral stenosis.

Drugs used to treat cardiac failure

Drugs used may therefore be classified as producing:

Reduction of preload

Diuretics increase salt and water loss, reduce blood volume and lower excessive venous filling pressure (see Ch. 26).

Nitrates (see also Ch. 23) dilate the smooth muscle in venous capacitance vessels, increase the volume of the venous vascular bed (which normally may comprise 80% of the whole vascular system), reduce ventricular filling pressure, thus decreasing heart wall stretch, and reduce myocardial O_2 - requirements. Their arteriolar dilating action is relatively slight. Glyceryl trinitrate may be given sublingually 0.3–1 mg for acute left ventricular failure and repeated as often as necessary or by i.v. infusion, 10–200 µg/min. For chronic left ventricular failure isosorbide dinitrate 40–160 mg/d or isosorbide mononitrate 40–80 mg/d may be given by mouth in divided doses. Exercise capacity is improved but tolerance to nitrates may develop with chronic use. Headache, which tends to limit the dose of nitrate used for angina, is less of a problem in cardiac failure perhaps because the patients are more vasoconstricted.

Reduction of afterload

Hydralazine (see also Ch. 23) relaxes arterial smooth muscle and reduces peripheral vascular resistance. Reflex tachycardia, however, limits its usefulness and lupus erythematosus may be induced when the dose exceeds 100 mg per day.

Reduction of preload and afterload

Angiotensin converting enzyme (ACE) *inhibitors* (see also Ch. 23) act by:

1. reduction of afterload, by preventing the

conversion of angiotensin I to the active form angiotensin II which is a powerful artericonstrictor and is present in the plasma in high concentration in cardiac failure;

2. reduction of preload, because the formation of aldosterone, and thus retention of salt and water, is prevented by the reduction of angiotensin II.

Captopril or *enalapril* are effective. A test dose should *always* be given to patients who are in cardiac failure or who are already taking a diuretic; maintenance of blood pressure in such individuals may depend greatly on the activated renin-angiotensin-aldosterone system and a standard dose of an ACE inhibitor can cause a catastrophic fall in blood pressure. With captopril the first dose should be 6.25 mg by mouth increasing to 25 mg × 3/day if blood pressure and renal function remain satisfactory; for enalapril 2.5 or 5 mg by mouth initially increasing to 20–40 mg once daily. When therapy with an ACE inhibitor is established a diuretic may usefully be added.

Phentolamine or sodium nitroprusside (see Ch. 23) may also be used (by i.v. infusion) when cardiac failure is acute or severe, e.g. after myocardial infarction.

Stimulation of the myocardium

Digoxin improves myocardial contractility (positive inotropic effect) most effectively in the dilated, failing heart and in the longer term once an episode of cardiac failure has been brought under control. This effect occurs in patients in sinus rhythm and is separate from its (negative chronotropic) action of reducing ventricular rate and thus improving ventricular filling in atrial fibrillation.

Enoximone and *milrinone* have positive inotropic effect due to selective myocardial phosphodiesterase inhibition and may be used for short-term treatment of severe congestive cardiac failure.

Dopamine, dobutamine, dopexamine, xamoterol: see Ch. 22.

Drug management of cardiac failure

- Mild cardiac failure should be treated with a loop diuretic in low daily dose, e.g. frusemide 40 mg, to which amiloride 5 mg may be added to help conserve potassium; if necessary the frusemide may be increased.

- If failure is not adequately controlled, an ACE inhibitor may be added if hypotension is not a problem; alternatively, vasodilatation may be induced, with isosorbide mononitrate with which hydralazine may later be combined.

- Digoxin may be added if failure persists and the diuretic regimen may be intensified, e.g. by increasing the amount of loop diuretic and by replacing amiloride with spironolactone.

- Other inotropic agents should be reserved for severe congestive cardiac failure. Dobutamine produces a predictable inotropic effect and a short-term infusion may produce improvement lasting several weeks, after which the treatment can be repeated. Dopamine and dobutamine may be combined for urgent situations such as cardiogenic or septic shock. Phosphodiesterase inhibitors are not yet established in routine therapy.

- *Acute left ventricular failure* is treated by reassuring the patient, who should sit upright with the legs dependent to reduce systemic venous return. A loop diuretic, e.g. frusemide 40–80 mg i.v. is the mainstay of therapy and provides benefit both by a rapid and powerful venodilator effect reducing preload, as well as by the subsequent diuresis. Oxygen should be given, if the patient can tolerate a face mask, and diamorphine or morphine i.v. which in addition to relieving anxiety and pain, have a valuable vasodilator effect.

GUIDE TO FURTHER READING

Braunwald E 1991 ACE inhibitors — a cornerstone of the treatment of heart failure. New England Journal of Medicine 325: 351

Cohn J N 1989 Inotropic therapy for heart failure. New England Journal of Medicine 320: 729

Editorial 1989 Digoxin: new answers; new questions. Lancet 2: 79

Funck-Brentano C et al 1990 Propafenone. New England Journal of Medicine 322: 518

Garratt C et al 1989 Lessons from the cardiac arrhythmia suppression trial (CAST). British Medical Journal 299: 805.

Haddy F J 1987 Endogenous digitalis-like factor or factors. New England Journal of Medicine 3316: 621

Mason J W 1987 Amiodarone. New England Journal of Medicine 316: 455

Mehta D et al 1988 Relative efficacy of various physical manoeuvres in the termination of junctional tachycardia. Lancet 1: 1181

Quesenberry P J 1989 Cardiac asthma — a fresh look at an old wheeze. New England Journal of Medicine 320: 1346

Ruskin J N 1989 The cardiac arrhythmia suppression trial (CAST). New England Journal of Medicine 321: 386

Timmis A D 1987 Mortality in congestive heart failure: effect of vasodilator therapy. British Medical Journal 295: 1225

Timmis A D 1988 Modern treatment of heart failure. British Medical Journal 297: 83

Watt A H, Routledge P A 1986 Adenosine: an importance beyond ATP. British Medical Journal 293: 1455

25

Cardiovascular system IV: hyperlipidaemias

SYNOPSIS

Correction of blood lipid abnormalities offers scope for a major impact on cardiovascular disease. Dietary adjustment plays an important primary role in the management of hyperlipidaemias while drugs help in selected cases, and agents with a variety of modes of action are available.

- Classification of hyperlipidaemias
- Management
- Drugs used in treatment: anion-exchange resins; nicotinic-acid and derivatives; fibric acid derivatives; statins

Some physiology

Dietary triglyceride is carried in the blood stream on chylomicrons which become progressively smaller as lipolysis takes place. This is accomplished by the enzyme lipoprotein lipase attached to the capillary endothelium of certain tissues including adipose tissue and skeletal and cardiac muscle. Fatty acids released during lipolysis are taken up by the tissues and the chylomicron remnants are cleared by the liver.

Endogenous triglyceride, synthesised by the liver and carried bound to very low density lipoproteins (VLDL) is progressively removed from the circulation by the same lipolytic mechanism as above. The low density lipoproteins (LDL), which include cholesterol, are formed as a result of this process and constitute the major system for delivering cholesterol to the tissues in man. LDL are small enough to pass through the vascular endothelium, bind to specific high-affinity LDL receptors on cell membranes and enter cells by active uptake. Cholesterol within the cell is needed for membrane growth and repair, and in the liver to form bile acids.

High density lipoproteins (HDL), the other cholesterol-rich particles in the blood, appears to act as *reverse* transport mediators, accepting cholesterol from peripheral cells, e.g. in arterial walls, and taking it to the liver; they are thus protective against ischaemic heart disease (IHD).

CLASSIFICATION[1] OF HYPERLIPIDAEMIAS

Type I is very rare, characterised by high concentrations in the blood of chylomicrons and triglycerides due to genetic deficiency of lipoprotein lipase, and is associated with abdominal pain, pancreatitis and eruptive xanthomata.

Type IIa is common, characterised by high concentrations of LDL and cholesterol in the blood, and is associated with IHD in 50% of males by 50 years and females by 60 years of age. A proportion of these patients (0.2% of the general population) have heterozygous monogenic familial hypercholesterolaemia (FH) which is associated with severe premature heart disease and tendon xanthomata.

Type IIb is common, characterised by high concentrations of LDL and VLDL, cholesterol and triglycerides in the blood, and is associated with IHD.

Type III is uncommon, characterised by high concentrations of 'broad-beta' lipoprotein, cholesterol and triglyceride in the blood due to an inherited abnormal apolipoprotein, and is associated with palmar xanthomata and ischaemic heart and peripheral vascular disease.

Type IV is common, characterised by high concentrations of VLDL and triglyceride in the blood, may be associated with obesity, diabetes and high alcohol intake and gives rise to ischaemic heart and peripheral vascular disease.

Type V is uncommon, characterised by high concentrations of plasma triglyceride on chylomicrons and VLDL, in some patients in part due to excessive alcohol intake or diabetes. These patients are liable to develop pancreatitis.

MANAGEMENT OF HYPERLIPIDAEMIAS

The management of hyperlipidaemias should be viewed against the background of the following observations.

- Hyperlipidaemias are common; 66% of the adult UK population have a plasma cholesterol concentration in excess of 5.2 mmol/l (the lowest concentration associated with cardiovascular risk).

- Investigation of hyperlipidaemia must be directed initially at excluding secondary causes which include: liver and biliary disease, obesity, hypothyroidism, diabetes, diet, alcohol excess and drugs (β-adrenoceptor blockers, thiazide diuretics, oral contraceptive steroids, etretinate). Long-term decisions on management should not be initiated on the basis of a single blood lipid estimate.

- The vast majority of cases of hyperlipidaemia seen in general medical practice and perhaps half those who attend special lipid clinics can be managed by *diet* alone; all patients and their spouses, if appropriate, should have effective dietary counselling. Much of the work of lipid clinics is taken up with attending to patients' other risk factors including hypertension, diabetes, thyroid disease and smoking, as well as to the lipid abnormality.

- Lipid lowering drugs should not be considered until other measures have failed. The decision to use them is made on the basis of the overall IHD risk, e.g. evidence of existing IHD, hypertension, diabetes mellitus, positive family history. The justification is easiest in the relatively small number of patients who have major abnormalities of their lipid profiles, as correction reduces their special risk of IHD.

Management may proceed as follows:

1. *Any medical disorder* that may be causing hyperlipidaemia, e.g. diabetes, hypothyroidism, should be treated first.

2. *Dietary adjustment.* The following applies to all patients:

- Those who are overweight should reduce their total caloric intake until they have returned to the weight that is appropriate for their height; this automatically assumes reduced intake of alcohol and total (especially animal) fat. Elevated triglyceride concentrations may respond particularly well to alcohol withdrawal.

[1] Beaumont J L et al. Bull WHO 1970; 43: 891.

- Those who fail to achieve adequate weight reduction or who are already at their ideal weight should reduce their total fat intake; poly- and mono-unsaturated fats or oils may be taken partially to substitute for the reduction in animal fats. Reduction in dietary cholesterol is a much less important element of the diet, but excess egg yolks should be avoided.

3. *Specific types of hyperlipidaemia* are treated thus:

- *Types I (and some Type V)*. Reduce dietary fat to 10% of total caloric intake; this may be assisted by partial substitution of fat by medium chain triglycerides which are not carried to the systemic circulation on chylomicrons but enter the liver directly by the portal circulation.
- *Mild to moderate (or common) hypercholesteraemia (Type IIa)* usually responds to diet but those with familial hypercholesterolaemia almost always need an ion exchange resin (cholestyramine or colestipol) and often another agent, usually simvastatin.
- *Type IIb and IV* patients are usually related to overweight, to diabetes, food and alcohol, and respond to the measures indicated in (2) above; fibrates or nicotinates may be added in resistant cases.
- *Type III* patients are usually diet-sensitive, failing which fibrates are the drugs of choice and are normally very effective.
- Poorly responsive patients with familial hypercholesterolaemia (Type IIa) and those with severe (Types III, IV and V) hyperlipidaemia should preferably be advised by a specialist.

DRUGS USED IN TREATMENT

Anion-exchange resins (bile acid sequestrants)

Cholestyramine is an anion-exchange resin[2] which binds bile acids in the intestine. Bile acids are formed from cholesterol in the liver, pass into the gut in the bile and are reabsorbed at the terminal ileum. The total bile acid pool is only 3–5 g but because such enterohepatic recycling takes place 5–10 times a day, on average 20–30 g of bile acid are delivered into the intestine every 24 hours. Bile acids bound to cholestyramine are lost in the faeces and the depletion of the bile acid pool stimulates conversion of cholesterol to bile acid: the result is that plasma LDL cholesterol falls by 20–25%. In many patients there is some compensatory increase in hepatic cholesterol synthesis. Anion exchange resins (oral) are first line treatment for hypercholesteraemia but not for hypertriglyceridaemia, which may be aggravated in such patients.

About half the patients who take cholestyramine experience constipation and some complain of anorexia, abdominal fullness and occasionally of diarrhoea; these effects may limit or prevent its use. Because the drug binds anions, drugs such as warfarin, digoxin, thiazide diuretics, phenobarbitone and thyroid hormones should be taken 1 h before or 6 h after cholestyramine to avoid impairment of their absorption.

Colestipol is similar to cholestyramine.

Nicotinic acid and derivatives

Nicotinic acid ($t_{\frac{1}{2}}$ 1 h) lowers plasma triglyceride and cholesterol concentrations. It acts as an antilipolytic agent in adipose tissue, reducing the supply of non-esterified free fatty acids and hence the availability of substrate for hepatic triglyceride synthesis. Treatment of hyperlipidaemias by nicotinamide requires about × 100 the normal human nutritional needs. Flushing of the skin (preventable by low dose aspirin) and gastrointestinal upset commonly occur; the unpleasantness may be diminished by gradually building up the oral dose over 6 weeks and in time tolerance develops. Rarely there is major disturbance of liver function.

---

[2] The resins consist of aggregations of large molecules carrying a fixed positive charge which therefore bind negatively charged ions (anions).

Acipimox is better tolerated than nicotinic acid and has a longer duration of action.

Nicofuranose (tetranicotinoylfructose) (Bradilan) is a fructose ester of nicotinic acid which may be better tolerated; it may exacerbate diabetes mellitus.

Fibric acid derivatives

These drugs inhibit hepatic lipid synthesis, causing plasma cholesterol to decline by 10–15% and triglyceride by 20–30%; associated with this is a rise in the 'protective' HDL-cholesterol which may explain the reduction in non-fatal myocardial infarction with gemfibrozil in the Helsinki Heart Study.[3] Fibric acid derivatives are well absorbed from the gastrointestinal tract, are extensively bound to plasma proteins and are excreted mainly by the kidney. They are the drugs of choice for mixed hyperlipidaemia (elevated cholesterol plus triglycerides) but may be used in hypercholesterolaemia, alone or with anion exchange resins. They are contraindicated where hepatic or renal function is severely impaired (but gemfibrozil has been used in uraemic and nephrotic patients without aggravating deterioration in kidney function); all may induce a myositis-like syndrome, particularly in patients with poor renal function. Interactions may occur with oral anticoagulants and oral antidiabetic agents due to displacement of these drugs from plasma proteins, enhancing their effect.

The group includes: bezafibrate, fenofibrate, gemfibrozil and clofibrate (the latter increases the risk of gallstones and should be used only in patients who have had a cholecystectomy).

Statins

Simvastatin (Zocor) inhibits the rate-limiting enzyme in endogenous cholesterol synthesis, hydroxy-methyl-glutaryl coenzyme A (HMG CoA) reductase. This results in increased synthesis of LDL receptors (up-regulation) in the liver and clearing of LDL from the circulation;

plasma total cholesterol and LDL-cholesterol undergo a dose-related reduction (LDL-cholesterol falls by about 30% at a dose of 20 mg/d). The place of simvastatin in therapy has yet to be established but it should be considered for patients with type IIa (FH), with severe, intractable hypercholesterolaemia, especially those with established vascular disease.

It is tolerated orally, the commonest adverse effect being transient, and usually minor, abnormality of liver function tests. Elevation of muscle enzymes (creatine phosphokinase) and myositis may occur. Its long-term safety has not been established.

Pravastatin and lovastatin are similar.

Other drugs

Omega-3 marine triglycerides (Maxepa) contain the triglyceride precursors of two polyunsaturated fatty acids (eicosapentaenoic acid and docosahexaenoic acid) derived from sea fish. They have no place in treating hypercholesterolaemia. Some patients with moderate to severe hypertriglyceridaemia may respond to oral use, although LDL-cholesterol may rise. There is an associated 90 calorie per day energy load.

Probucol (Lurselle) increases the excretion of bile acids and reduces cholesterol biosynthesis; the resulting fall in plasma lipid concentration affects both LDL and the 'protective' HDL. The drug is well tolerated orally but some patients experience gastrointestinal upset and abdominal pain.

---

[3] Frick M H et al. New Engl J Med 1987; 317: 1237.

GUIDE TO FURTHER READING

Betteridge D J 1989 High density lipoprotein and coronary heart disease. British Medical Journal 298: 974

Brunzell J D, Austin M A 1989 Plasma triglyceride levels and coronary disease. New England Journal of Medicine 320: 1273

Editorial 1989 Low cholesterol and increased risk. Lancet 1: 1423

Gordon D J, Rifkind B M 1989 High density lipoprotein — the clinical implications of recent studies. New England Journal of Medicine 321: 1311

Grundy S M 1988 HMG-CoA reductase inhibitors for treatment of hypercholesterolaemia. New England Journal of Medicine 319: 24

Mansell P, Reckless J P D 1991 Garlic. British Medical Journal 303: 379

Rassouw J E et al 1990 The value of lowering cholesterol after myocardial infarction. New England Journal of Medicine 323: 1112

Shepherd J et al 1987 Strategies for reducing coronary heart disease and desirable limits of blood lipid concentrations: guidelines of the British Hyperlipidaemia Association. British Medical Journal 295: 1245

Steinberg D et al 1989 Beyond cholesterol. Modifications of low-density lipoproteins that increase its atherogenicity. New England Journal of Medicine 320: 915

26

Kidney and urinary tract

DIURETIC DRUGS

Definition: a diuretic is any substance which increases urine and solute excretion. This wide definition, however, includes substances not commonly thought of as diuretics, e.g., water. To be therapeutically useful a diuretic should increase the output of sodium as well as of water, for diuretics are normally required to remove oedema fluid which is composed of water and solutes, of which sodium is the most important.

Each day the body produces 180 l of glomerular filtrate which is modified in its passage down the renal tubules to appear as 1.5 l of urine. Thus a 1% reduction in reabsorption of tubular fluid will more than double urine output. Clearly drugs that act on the tubule have considerable scope to alter body fluid and electrolyte balance. Most clinically useful diuretics are organic anions and are transported from the blood, through the tubular cells and into tubular fluid. The following brief account of tubular function with particular reference to sodium transport will help to explain where and how diuretic drugs act; it should be read with reference to Figure 26.1.

SITES AND MODES OF ACTION

As a result of active reabsorption of sodium chloride and sodium bicarbonate from the renal tubular lumen and passive reabsorption of accompanying water, 65% of the glomerular filtrate

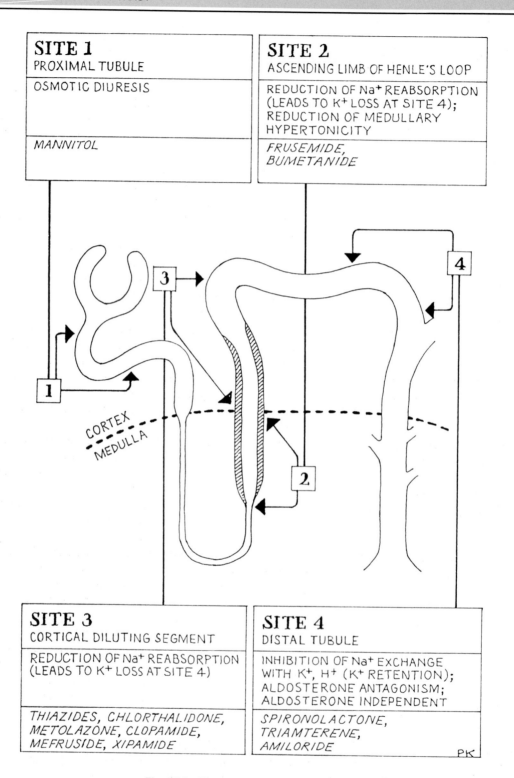

SITE 1
PROXIMAL TUBULE

OSMOTIC DIURESIS

MANNITOL

SITE 2
ASCENDING LIMB OF HENLE'S LOOP

REDUCTION OF Na$^+$ REABSORPTION
(LEADS TO K$^+$ LOSS AT SITE 4);
REDUCTION OF MEDULLARY
HYPERTONICITY

*FRUSEMIDE,
BUMETANIDE*

CORTEX
MEDULLA

SITE 3
CORTICAL DILUTING SEGMENT

REDUCTION OF Na$^+$ REABSORPTION
(LEADS TO K$^+$ LOSS AT SITE 4)

*THIAZIDES, CHLORTHALIDONE,
METOLAZONE, CLOPAMIDE,
MEFRUSIDE, XIPAMIDE*

SITE 4
DISTAL TUBULE

INHIBITION OF Na$^+$ EXCHANGE
WITH K$^+$, H$^+$ (K$^+$ RETENTION);
ALDOSTERONE ANTAGONISM;
ALDOSTERONE INDEPENDENT

*SPIRONOLACTONE,
TRIAMTERENE,
AMILORIDE*

PK

Fig. 26.1 Sites of action of diuretic drugs

is reabsorbed iso-osmotically from the proximal tubule. The epithelium of the proximal tubule is described as 'leaky' because of its free permeability to water and a number of solutes.

Osmotic diuretics such as mannitol are solutes which are not reabsorbed in the proximal tubule (site 1, Fig. 26.1) and therefore carry into the urine equivalent volumes of fluid.

The tubular fluid now passes into the loop of Henle where 25% of the filtered sodium is reabsorbed. There are two populations of nephron: those that have short loops and are confined to the cortex; and the juxtamedullary nephrons whose long loops penetrate into the inner parts of the medulla and are principally concerned with water conservation;[1] the following discussion refers to the latter. The physiological changes are best understood by considering first the ascending limb. In the thick segment (site 2, Fig. 26.1), chloride ion is transported actively from the tubular fluid into the interstitial fluid, taking with it sodium ion but not water, to which this part of the tubule is impermeable. In consequence, the tubular fluid becomes dilute, the interstitium becomes hypertonic and fluid in the descending limb, which is permeable to water, becomes more concentrated as it approaches the tip of the loop, because the hypertonic interstitial fluid sucks water out of the tubule. The 'hairpin' structure of the loop thus confers on it the property of a *countercurrent multiplier* which by active transport of ions converts a small change in osmolality into a steep osmotic gradient; the high osmotic pressure in the medullary interstitium is sustained by the vasa rectae which lie close to the loops of Henle and act as *countercurrent exchangers*, for the incoming blood receives sodium from the out-going blood.[2] Frusemide, bumetanide, piretanide and ethacrynic acid act principally at site 2 by inhibiting active chloride ion transport, which thus prevents sodium ion reabsorption and lowers the osmotic gradient between cortex and medulla; the result is that large volumes of dilute urine are formed. These drugs are called the *loop diuretics*.

As the ascending limb of the loop re-enters the renal cortex, sodium and chloride continue to be actively passed into the interstitial tissue (site 3) but are rapidly removed because cortical blood flow is high and there are no vasa rectae present; consequently the urine becomes more dilute. *Thiazides* act principally at the cortical diluting segment of the ascending limb, preventing sodium reabsorption.

In the distal tubule (site 4), sodium ions are exchanged for potassium ions and hydrogen ions. In part the mechanism of this exchange is aldosterone-dependent and may be inhibited by the selective antagonist spironolactone; an aldosterone-independent mechanism(s) also operates and is inhibited by triamterene and amiloride. Only 5% of filtered sodium is reabsorbed by the distal tubule, but by reducing sodium/potassium exchange these diuretics cause potassium *retention*. Diuretics that act proximal to this point bring about potassium *loss* because they allow more sodium to be delivered to the site at which sodium may be exchanged for potassium.

The collecting tubule then travels back down into the medulla to reach the papilla; in doing so it passes through a gradient of increasing osmotic pressure which tends to draw water out of tubular fluid. This final concentration of urine is under the influence of antidiuretic hormone (ADH) whose action is to make the collecting ducts permeable to water, and in its absence water remains in the collecting tubule; ethanol causes diuresis by inhibiting the release of ADH from the posterior pituitary gland.

Diuresis may also be achieved by extra-renal mechanisms, by raising the cardiac output and increasing renal blood flow, e.g. with dobutamine and dopamine.

---

[1] Beavers, occupying a watery habitat, have nephrons with short loops, while those of the desert rat have long loops.

[2] The most easily comprehended countercurrent exchange mechanism (in this case for heat) is that in wading birds in cold climates whereby the veins carrying cold blood from the feet pass closely alongside the arteries carrying warm blood from the body and heat exchange takes place. The result is that the feet receive blood below body temperature (which does not matter) and the blood from the feet which is often very cold, is warmed before it enters the body so that the internal temperature is more easily maintained. The principle is the same for maintaining renal medullary hypertonicity.

CLASSIFICATION

The maximum efficacy in removing salt and water that any drug can achieve is related to its site of action, and it is clinically appropriate to rank diuretics according to their natriuretic capacity, as follows:

High efficacy

Frusemide, bumetanide, piretanide and etha-crynic acid (loop diuretics) can cause 15–25% of filtered sodium to be excreted.[3] Their action impairs the powerful urine-concentrating mechanism of the loop of Henle and confers higher efficacy compared to drugs that act in the relatively hypotonic cortex (see below). Progressive increase in dose is matched by increasing diuresis, i.e they have a high 'ceiling' of effect. Indeed, they are so efficacious that overtreatment can readily dehydrate the patient. Loop diuretics remain effective at glomerular filtration rates below 10 ml/min (normal 120 ml/min).

Moderate efficacy

The *thiazide* family, bendrofluazide and the related chlorthalidone, clopamide, indapamide, mefruside, metolazone, xipamide cause 5–10% of filtered sodium load to be excreted. Increasing the dose beyond a small range produces no added diuresis, i.e. they have a low 'ceiling' of effect. Such drugs tend to be ineffective once the glomerular filtration rate has fallen below 20 ml/min (except metolazone).

Low efficacy

Potassium retaining triamterene, amiloride, spironolactone, cause 5% of filtered sodium to be excreted. They are usefully combined with more efficacious diuretics to prevent the potassium loss which other diuretics cause.

---

[3] The percentages quoted in this rank order refer to the highest fractional excretion of filtered sodium under carefully controlled conditions and should not be taken to represent the average fractional sodium loss during clinical use.

Other osmotic diuretics, e.g. mannitol, and xanthines, e.g. aminophylline, also fall into this category.

INDIVIDUAL DIURETICS

High efficacy loop diuretics: (frusemide)

Frusemide (furosemide, Lasix) acts on the thick portion of the ascending limb of the loop of Henle (site 2) to produce the effects described above. Because more sodium is delivered to site 4, exchange with potassium leads to urinary potassium loss and hypokalaemia. Magnesium and calcium loss are increased by frusemide to about the same extent as sodium; the effect on calcium is utilised in the emergency management of hypercalcaemia (see index).

Pharmacokinetics. Frusemide is well absorbed from the gastrointestinal tract and is highly bound to plasma proteins. The $t_{\frac{1}{2}}$ is 2 h, but this rises to over 10 h in renal failure.

Uses. Frusemide is highly successful for the relief of oedema. Progressive increase of dose of frusemide is matched by increase in urine production. Taken orally it acts within an hour and diuresis lasts about 6 hours. Enormous urine volumes can result and overtreatment may lead to hypovolaemia and circulatory collapse. Given i.v. it acts within 30 minutes and can relieve acute pulmonary oedema, partly by a vasodilator action which precedes the diuresis. An important feature of frusemide is its efficacy when the glomerular filtration rate is 10 ml/min or less.

The dose is 20–120 mg by mouth per day; i.m. or i.v. 20–50 mg is given initially. For use in renal failure, special high dose tablets (500 mg) are available, and a solution of 250 mg in 25 ml which should be infused i.v. at a rate not greater than 4 mg/min.

Adverse effects are uncommon, apart from excess of therapeutic effect (electrolyte disturbance, hypotension due to low plasma volume) and those mentioned in the general account for diuretics (below). They include nausea, pancreatitis and, rarely, deafness which is usually transient and associated with rapid i.v. injection in renal failure. NSAIDs, notably indomethacin, reduce frusemide-induced diuresis probably by inhibiting the formation of vasodilator prostaglandins in the kidney.

Bumetanide (Burinex), piretanide (Arelix) and ethacrynic acid are similar to frusemide. Ethacrynic acid is less widely used as it is more prone to cause adverse effects, especially nausea and deafness.

Moderate efficacy diuretics (thiazide and related diuretics)

Thiazides depress sodium reabsorption at site 3 which is just proximal to the region of sodium–potassium exchange. These drugs thus raise potassium excretion to an important extent. Thiazides lower blood pressure, chiefly due to reduction in intravascular volume but probably also to reduction of peripheral vascular resistance, for in chronic use they diminish the responsiveness of vascular smooth muscle to noradrenaline.

Thiazides are generally well absorbed from the gut and most begin to act within an hour. There are numerous derivatives and their differences lie principally in duration of action. The relatively *water soluble*, e.g. cyclopenthiazide, chlorothiazide, hydrochlorothiazide, are most rapidly eliminated, their peak effect occurring within 4–6 h and passing off by 10–12 h. They are excreted unchanged in the urine and active secretion by the proximal renal tubule contributes to their high renal clearance and $t_\frac{1}{2}$ of < 4 h. The relatively *lipid soluble* members of the group, e.g. polythiazide, methyclothiazide, hydroflumethiazide, distribute more widely into body tissues and act for over 24 h, which can be objectionable if the drug is used for diuresis, though useful for hypertension. Thiazides are not effective when renal function is severely impaired.

Adverse effects in general are discussed below. Rashes (sometimes photosensitive), thromobocytopenia and agranulocytosis occur. Long-term treatment with thiazide-type drugs causes total serum cholesterol to increase by about 7%. This must raise questions about the appropriateness of use of these drugs for mild hypertension, of which ischaemic heart disease is a common complication.

Bendrofluazide is a satisfactory member for routine use. The oral dose is 5–10 mg and diuresis usually lasts less than 12 h so that it should be given in the morning. Bendrofluazide, *used primarily for a diuresis* may be given daily for the first few days, then say, 3 days a week. Potassium supplements are best retained if not given on the same day or if on the same day, not at the same time. As an *antihypertensive* bendrofluazide 2.5 mg is given daily; in the absence of a diuresis clinically important potassium depletion is uncommon, but plasma potassium concentration should be checked in potentially vulnerable groups such as the elderly (see Ch. 23).

Cyclopenthiazide is a satisfactory alternative.

Other members of the group include: benzthiazide, chlorothiazide, hydrochlorothiazide, hydroflumethiazide, methyclothiazide, polythiazide.

Diuretics related to the thiazides. Several compounds, although strictly not thiazides, share structural similarities with them and probably act at the same site on the nephron; they therefore exhibit moderate therapeutic efficacy. Overall, these substances have a greater duration of action, are used for oedema and hypertension and their profile of adverse effects is similar to that of the thiazides. They are listed below.

Chlorthalidone acts for 48–72 h after a single oral dose.

Xipamide is structurally related to chlorthalidone and to frusemide. It induces a diuresis for about 12 h that is brisker than with thiazides, which may trouble the elderly.

Clopamide also acts for about 24 h.

Metolazone is effective when renal function is impaired. It potentiates the diuresis produced by frusemide and the combination can be effective in resistant oedema, provided the patient's fluid and electrolyte loss are carefully monitored.

Mefruside has its peak effect 6–12 h after administration and its duration may be 24 h.

Indapamide is structurally related to chlorthalidone but lowers blood pressure at sub-diuretic doses, perhaps by altering calcium flux in vascular smooth muscle. It has little apparent effect on potassium, glucose or uric acid excretion (see below).

Low efficacy diuretics
(potassium-sparing diuretics)

Spironolactone (Aldactone) is structurally similar to aldosterone and competitively inhibits its action (sodium reabsorption and potassium loss in the distal tubule); excessive secretion of aldosterone contributes to fluid retention in hepatic cirrhosis, nephrotic syndrome and congestive cardiac failure, in which conditions it is most useful as well as in primary hypersecretion (Conn's syndrome).

After oral administration, spironolactone is largely converted in the gut and liver to the active metabolite *canrenone*, which has a plasma $t_{\frac{1}{2}}$ of 9 h. Most of the diuretic effect of spironolactone is probably due to this metabolite which is available as a drug in its own right, *potassium canrenoate*. Canrenone has been shown to improve myocardial contraction, an additional action which may prove beneficial in cardiac failure.

Spironolactone is relatively ineffective when used alone, causing less than 5% of the filtered sodium load to be excreted. It may, however, be more effective when combined with a drug that reduces sodium reabsorption proximally in the tubule, e.g. a loop diuretic. Spironolactone (and also amiloride and trimaterene, below) also reduces the potassium loss that occurs with loop diuretics, but its combination with another *potassium-retaining* diuretic leads to hyperkalaemia. Dangerous potassium retention may also develop if spironolactone is given to patients with impaired renal function. Spironolactone is given orally, 50–100 mg/d total, in one or more doses. The maximum diuresis is delayed for up to 4 days but if after 5 days the response is inadequate, the dose may be increased to 200 mg/d.

Adverse effects are uncommon but include gynaecomastia, which is often painful but reverses when the drug is withdrawn, mental confusion, drowsiness, rashes, abdominal pain and menstrual irregularities including amenorrhoea. It causes negligible urate retention. Possible human metabolites are carcinogenic in rodents. Spironolactone induces hepatic microsomal enzymes.

Amiloride (Midamor) increases sodium loss and *reduces* potassium loss by a direct action on ion transport in the distal tubule, i.e. it does not antagonise the action of aldosterone and, in contrast to spironolactone, it is effective when there is no aldosterone excess. Its action is therefore complementary to that of the thiazides and, used with them, it increases sodium loss and reduces potassium loss. One such combination, co-amilozide, Moduretic (amiloride 5 mg plus hydrochlorothiazide 50 mg), is used for moderate hypertension or oedema. The maximum effect of amiloride occurs about 6 h after an oral dose and the action may last 24 h. The oral dose is 5–20 mg daily.

Trimaterene (Dytac) is a potassium-sparing diuretic which has an action and use similar to that of amiloride. The diuretic effect extends over 10 h. Gastrointestinal upsets occur. Reversible, non-oliguric renal failure may occur when triamterene is used with indomethacin (and presumably other NSAIDs).

Adverse effects characteristic of diuretics

Potassium depletion. Diuretics, which act at sites 1, 2 and 3 (Fig. 26.1), cause more sodium to reach the sodium–potassium exchange site in the distal tubule (site 4) and so increase potassium excretion. This subject warrants discussion since hypokalaemia, amongst other adverse effects, may cause cardiac dysrhythmia.

The safe lower limit for serum potassium concentration is normally quoted as 3.5 mmol/l. Whether or not diuretic therapy causes significant lowering of serum potassium depends both on the drug and on the circumstances in which it is used.

● *The loop diuretics* cause a smaller fall in serum potassium than do the thiazides, for equivalent diuretic effect, but have a greater capacity for diuresis, i.e higher efficacy especially in large dose, and so are associated with greater decline in potassium. If diuresis is brisk and continuous, potassium depletion is likely to occur.

● *Low dietary intake* of potassium predisposes to hypokalaemia; the risk is particularly notable in the elderly, many of whom ingest less than 50 mmol per day (the dietary normal is 80 mmol).

• Hypokalaemia during diuretic therapy is also more likely in *hyperaldosteronism* whether primary or more commonly secondary to severe liver disease, congestive cardiac failure or nephrotic syndrome.

• Potassium loss occurs with *diarrhoea, vomiting or small bowel fistula*, and may be aggravated by diuretic therapy.

• When a thiazide diuretic is used for *hypertension*, there is probably no case for routine prescription of a potassium supplement if no predisposing factors are present (see Ch. 23).

Potassium depletion can be minimised or corrected by:

• maintaining a good dietary potassium intake
• combining a potassium-depleting with a potassium-retaining drug
• intermittent use of potassium-losing drugs, i.e. drug holidays
• Potassium supplements: potassium chloride is preferred because chloride is the principal anion excreted along with sodium when high efficacy diuretics are used, i.e. they cause hypochloraemic alkalosis. Satisfactory formulations include: potassium chloride sustained-release tabs (Slow-K tabs) containing 8 mmol each of K and Cl and potassium chloride effervescent tabs (Sando-K tabs) containing 12 mmol of K and 8 mmol of Cl. All forms of potassium are irritant to the gastrointestinal tract. If, for example the tablet is held up in the oesophagus, ulceration may result. The elderly, in particular, should be warned never to take such tablets dry but always with a large cupful of liquid and sitting upright or standing.

Hyperkalaemia may occur, especially if a potassium conserving diuretic is given to a patient with impaired renal function. Beta-adrenoceptor blockers or angiotensin-converting enzyme inhibitors cause modest elevation of plasma potassium which may aggravate hyperkalaemia if they are also being taken.

Treatment of hyperkalaemia depends on the severity and the following measures are appropriate:

• The potassium-retaining diuretic should be discontinued.
• A cation exchange resin, e.g. polystyrene sulphonate resin (Resonium A, Calcium Resonium, see later) can be used orally (more effective than rectally) to remove body potassium via the gut.
• Potassium may be moved rapidly from plasma into cells by giving (1) sodium bicarbonate i.v. (40–160 mmol) and repeating this in a few minutes if ECG changes persist; (2) glucose 20%, 300–500 ml plus insulin 1 unit/3g glucose by i.v. infusion. If ECG changes are marked, calcium gluconate 10% solution, 10 ml i.v. and repeated if necessary in a few minutes, may be given to oppose the myocardial effect of potassium. Calcium may potentiate digoxin and should be used cautiously if at all, in a patient taking this drug. Sodium bicarbonate and calcium salt must not be mixed in a syringe or reservoir because calcium precipitates.
• Dialysis is, of course, highly effective.

Magnesium deficiency. Loop and thiazide diuretics, and in particular chlorthalidone, cause significant urinary loss of magnesium; potassium-retaining diuretics probably also cause magnesium retention. Magnesium deficiency brought about by diuretics seems rarely to be severe enough to induce the classic picture of neuromuscular irritability and tetany but cardiac dysrhythmias, mainly of ventricular origin do occur and respond to repletion of magnesium (magnesium chloride 35–50 mmol may be added to 1 litre of glucose 5% and infused over 12–24 h).

Hypovolaemia can result from overtreatment. Acute loss of excessive fluid leads to postural hypotension and dizziness. A more insidious state of *chronic hypovolaemia* can develop especially in the elderly. After initial benefit, the patient becomes sleepy and lethargic. Blood urea concentration rises but sodium and chloride concentrations are usually normal. Renal failure may result.

Urinary retention. Sudden vigorous diuresis

can cause acute retention of urine in the presence of bladder neck obstruction, e.g. due to prostatic enlargement.

Hyponatraemia may result if sodium loss occurs in patients who drink a large quantity of water. Other mechanisms are probably involved, including enhancement of antidiuretic hormone release. Such patients have reduced total body sodium and extracellular fluid and are oedema-free. Discontinuation of the diuretic and water restriction usually suffice to correct the state. The condition should be distinguished from hyponatraemia *with* oedema which develops in some patients with congestive cardiac failure, cirrhosis or nephrotic syndrome. Here salt and water intake should be restricted because extracellular fluid volume is expanded.

Urate retention with hyperuricaemia and sometimes clinical gout occurs with the high and moderate efficacy diuretics, but the effect is unimportant or negligible with the low efficacy diuretics.

Two mechanisms appear to be responsible. First, diuretics cause volume depletion, reduction in glomerular filtration and increased absorption of almost all solutes in the proximal tubule including uric acid. Second, diuretics and uric acid are organic acids and compete for the transport mechanism which carries such substances from the blood into the urine. Diuretic-induced hyperuricaemia can be prevented by allopurinol or probenecid.

Carbohydrate intolerance is caused by those diuretics which produce prolonged hypokalaemia, i.e. the loop and thiazide type. It appears that intracellular potassium is necessary for the formation of insulin, and glucose intolerance is probably due to insulin deficiency. Insulin requirements thus increase in established diabetics and the disease may become manifest in latent diabetics. The effect is generally reversible over several months.

Calcium homeostasis. Renal calcium loss is increased by the *loop diuretics*; in the short term this is not a serious disadvantage and indeed frusemide may be used in the management of hypercalcaemia after rehydration has been achieved. In the long term this effect may be harmful especially in elderly patients who tend in any case to be in negative calcium balance. Thiazides, by contrast, decrease renal excretion of calcium and this property may influence the choice of diuretic in a potentially calcium-deficient or osteoporotic individual, for thiazide use is associated with reduced risk of hip fracture in the elderly. The hypocalciuric effect of the thiazides has also been used effectively in patients with idiopathic hypercalciuria, the commonest metabolic cause of renal stones.

Interactions

Loop diuretics potentiate ototoxicity of aminoglycosides and nephrotoxicity of some cephalosporins. NSAIDs tend to cause sodium retention which counteracts the effect of diuretics; the mechanism may involve inhibition of renal prostaglandin formation. Diuretic treatment of a patient taking lithium can precipitate toxicity from this drug (see index).

Abuse of diuretics

Psychological abnormality sometimes takes the form of abuse of diuretics and/or purgatives. The subject usually desires to 'slim' to become 'attractive' or 'healthy' or may have anorexia nervosa. There can be severe depletion of sodium and potassium, with renal tubular damage due to chronic hypokalaemia.

Osmotic diuretics

Osmotic diuretics are small molecular weight substances that are filtered by the glomerulus but are not reabsorbed by the renal tubule, and thus increase the osmolarity of the tubular fluid. Their principal site of action is the proximal tubule and probably also the loop of Henle, where they prevent the reabsorption of water and also, by more complex mechanisms, of sodium. The result is that urine volume increases according to the load of osmotic diuretic.

Mannitol, a polyhydric alcohol (mol. wt. 452), is most commonly used; it is given i.v. In addition to its effect on the kidney, mannitol encourages the movement of water from inside cells to the extracellular fluid, which is thus transiently expanded. These properties define its uses, which are for rapid reduction of *intracranial* or *intraocular pressure*, and to maintain urine flow to *prevent renal tubular necrosis*. Mannitol is contraindicated in congestive cardiac failure and pulmonary oedema; where there is uncertainty that the drug will be excreted, not more that 25 g should be given.

Xanthines

The general properties of the xanthines (theophylline, caffeine) are discussed elsewhere (see p. 297). Their mild diuretic action probably depends in part on smooth muscle relaxation in the afferent arteriolar bed increasing renal blood flow, and in part on a direct inhibitory effect on salt reabsorption in the proximal tubule. Their uses in medicine depend on their other properties.

INDICATIONS FOR DIURETICS

• *Oedematous states* associated with sodium overload, e.g. cardiac, renal or hepatic disease, and also without sodium overload, e.g. acute pulmonary oedema following myocardial infarction. Note that oedema may also be localised, e.g. angioedema, or due to low plasma albumin, or immobility in the elderly, in which circumstances a diuretic is not indicated.

• *Hypertension*, by reducing intravascular volume and probably by other mechanisms too, e.g. reduction of sensitivity to noradrenergic vasoconstriction.

• *Hypercalcaemia*. Frusemide reduces calcium reabsorption in the ascending limb of the loop of Henle and this action may be utilised in the emergency reduction of elevated plasma calcium in addition to rehydration and other measures (see index).

• *Idiopathic hypercalciuria*, a common cause of renal stone disease, may be reduced by thiazide diuretics; reduction of intravascular volume favours proximal renal tubular reabsorption of calcium.

• *The syndrome of inappropriate secretion of antidiuretic hormone secretion (SIADH)* may be treated with frusemide if there is a dangerous degree of volume overload. Other measures will also be required; these include, withdrawal of a drug if it is the cause, (e.g chlorpropamide), water restriction, demeclocycline (see index) and salt replacement.

• *Nephrogenic diabetes insipidus*, paradoxically, may respond to diuretics which, by contracting vascular volume, increase salt and water reabsorption in the proximal tubule, and thus reduce urine volume.

THERAPY
Congestive cardiac failure

The main account appears in Chapter 24. It is sufficient here to note that because diuretics by mouth are easily given repeatedly, lack of supervision can result in insidious overtreatment. *Early signs of overdose* are *postural dizziness* due to reduced blood volume, and a *rising blood urea* due to falling glomerular blood flow. The simplest guide to the success or failure of diuretic regimens is to monitor *body weight*. Fluid intake and output charts are more demanding of nursing time, and often less accurate.

Acute pulmonary oedema: see
Ch. 24, p. 450.

Renal oedema

The chief therapeutic aims are to reduce dietary sodium intake and to prevent excessive sodium retention using diuretic drugs. Reduction of sodium reabsorption in the renal tubule by diuretics is most effective where glomerular filtration has not been seriously reduced by disease. Frusemide and bumetanide are effective even when the filtration rate is very low; frusemide may usefully be combined with metolazone but the resulting profound diuresis requires careful monitoring.

Secondary hyperaldosteronism complicates the *nephrotic syndrome* because albumin loss causes plasma colloid pressure to fall, and the resulting diversion of intravascular volume to the interstitium activates the renin-angiotensin-aldosterone system; then spironolactone may be added usefully to potentiate a loop diuretic and to conserve potassium, loss of which can be severe.

Hepatic ascites. Ascites and oedema are due to portal venous hypertension together with decreased plasma colloid osmotic pressure causing hyperaldosteronism as with nephrotic oedema (above). Furthermore, diversion of renal blood flow from the cortex to the medulla favours sodium retention. In addition to dietary sodium restriction, a loop diuretic plus spironolactone are used to produce a *gradual* diuresis; too vigorous depletion of sodium with added potassium loss and hypochloraemic alkalosis may cause hepatic coma. Abdominal paracentesis, usually undertaken for the sake of speed, aggravates hypoproteinaemia, and should be avoided if at all possible.

CARBONIC ANHYDRASE INHIBITORS

Carbonic anhydrase facilitates the reaction between carbon dioxide and water to form carbonic acid:

$$CO_2 + H_2O \overset{\text{carbonic anhydrase}}{\rightleftharpoons} H_2CO_3 \rightleftharpoons H^+ + HCO_3^-$$

the rate is slow in the absence of the enzyme. By making available hydrogen and bicarbonate ions, this reaction is fundamental to the production of either acid or alkaline secretions and high concentrations of carbonic anhydrase are present in the gastric mucosa, pancreas, eye and kidney. Inhibitors of carbonic anhydrase are obsolete as diuretics, but they still have uses in medicine.

Reduction of intraocular pressure. This action is due not to diuresis (thiazides actually raise intraocular pressure slightly). The formation of aqueous humour is an active process requiring a supply of bicarbonate ions, which depends on carbonic anhydrase. Inhibition of carbonic anhydrase reduces the formation of aqueous humour and lowers intraocular pressure. This is a local action and is not affected by the develop-

ment of acid-base changes elsewhere in the body, i.e. tolerance does no develop.

Prevention of high altitude mountain sickness. This condition may affect unacclimatised people at altitudes in excess of 3000 metres especially if ascent has been rapid and exertion great; symptoms range from nausea, lassitude and headache to pulmonary and cerebral oedema. The initiating cause is hypoxia: at high altitude, the normal hyperventilatory response to falling oxygen tension is inhibited because alkalosis is also induced. A carbonic anhydrase inhibitor induces metabolic acidosis, increases respiratory drive, notably at night when apnoeic attacks may occur, and thus helps to maintain arterial oxygen tension.

Acetazolamide is the most widely used carbonic anhydrase inhibitor. High doses may cause drowsiness and fever, rashes and paraesthesiae may occur, and blood disorders have been reported. Renal calculi may occur, perhaps because the urine calcium is in less soluble form owing to low citrate content of the urine.

Dichlorphenamide is similar.

CATION-EXCHANGE RESINS

Cation-exchange resins may be used to remove potassium from the intestinal contents, as a means of treating *hyperkalaemia* when urine formation is poor or has ceased, or in potential dialysis patients. The resins consist of aggregations of big insoluble molecules carrying fixed negative charges, which therefore loosely bind positively charged ions (cations); these latter readily exchange with cations in the fluid environment to an extent that depends on their affinity for the resin and their concentration. Resins loaded with sodium or calcium exchange these cations preferentially with potassium cations in the intestine (about 1 mmol of potassium per gram of resin); the freed cations are absorbed and the resin with the bound potassium is passed in the faeces. The resin does not merely prevent absorption of ingested potassium, but it also takes up the potassium normally secreted into the intestine and ordinarily reabsorbed.

In hyperkalaemia, oral administration or retention enemas of a *polystyrene sulphonate resin* may be used. A sodium phase resin (Resonium A) should obviously not be used in patients with renal or cardiac failure as sodium overload may result. A calcium phase resin (Calcium Resonium) may cause hypercalaemia and should be avoided in predisposed patients, e.g. with multiple myeloma, metastatic carcinoma, hyperparathyroidism and sarcoidosis. Enemas should ideally be retained for at least 9 h although this is usually impossible.

ALTERATION OF URINE pH

Alteration of urine pH by drugs is sometimes desirable. The most common reason is in the treatment of poisoning (a fuller account appears on p. 140). A summary of the main indications appears below.

Alkalinisation of urine

- increases the elimination of salicylate, phenobarbitone and chlorophenoxy herbicides, e.g. 2,4-D, MCPA
- reduces irritation of an inflamed urinary tract
- discourages the growth of certain organisms, e.g. *E. coli.*

The urine can be made alkaline by sodium bicarbonate i.v., or by potassium citrate by mouth. Sodium overload may exacerbate cardiac failure, and sodium or potassium excess are dangerous when renal function is impaired.

Acidification of urine

- is used as a test for renal tubular acidosis
- increases elimination of amphetamine, dexfenfluramine, quinine and phencyclidine, although it is very rarely needed.

The urine is made acid by ammonium chloride by mouth, taken with food to avoid vomiting. It should not be given to patients with impaired renal or hepatic function. Other means include arginine HCl, ascorbic acid and $CaCl_2$ by mouth.

DRUGS AND THE KIDNEY

The kidneys comprise only 0.5% of body weight, yet they receive 25% of the cardiac output. Thus, it is hardly surprising that drugs can *damage* the kidney and that disease of the kidney affects *responses to drugs.*

DRUG-INDUCED RENAL DISEASE

Drugs and other chemicals damage the kidney by:

1. Direct biochemical effect

Substances that cause direct toxicity include:

- *Heavy metals*, e.g. mercury, gold, iron, lead
- *Antimicrobials*, e.g. aminoglycosides, amphotericin, sulphonamides, cephalosporins
- *X-ray contrast media*, e.g. agents for visualising the biliary tract
- *Analgesics*, e.g. NSAID combinations
- *Solvents*, e.g. carbon tetrachloride, ethylene glycol.

2. Indirect biochemical effect

- *Cytotoxic drugs and uricosurics* may cause urate to be precipitated in the tubule.
- *Calciferol* may cause renal calcification by causing hypercalcaemia.
- *Diuretic and laxative* abuse can cause tubule damage secondary to potassium and sodium depletion.
- *Anticoagulants* may cause haemorrhage into the kidney.

3. Immunological effect

A wide range of drugs produces a wide range of injuries.

- *Drugs* include: phenytoin, gold, penicillins, sulphonamides, (especially the long-acting and extensively protein bound) hydralazine, isoniazid, rifampicin, procainamide, penicillamine, probenecid.
- *Injuries* include: arteritis, glomerulitis, interstitial nephritis, systemic lupus erythematosus.

A drug may cause damage by more than one of the above three mechanisms, e.g. sulphonamides.

The sites and pathological types of injury are as follows:

Glomerular damage. The large surface area of the glomerular capillaries renders them susceptible to damage from circulating immune complexes; glomerulonephritis, proteinuria and nephrotic syndrome may result, e.g. following treatment with penicillamine when the patient has made an immune response to the drug. The degree of renal impairment is best reflected in the *creatinine clearance* which measures the glomerular filtration rate because creatinine is eliminated entirely by this process.

Tubule damage. By concentrating 180 l of glomerular filtrate into 1.5 l of urine each day, renal tubule cells are exposed to much greater amounts of solutes and environmental toxins than are other cells in the body. The proximal tubule, through which most water is reabsorbed, experiences the greatest concentration and so suffers most drug-induced injury. Specialised transport processes concentrate acids, e.g. salicylate, cephalosporins, and bases, e.g. aminoglycosides, in renal tubular cells. Heavy metals and radiographic contrast media also cause damage at this site. Proximal tubular toxicity is best shown by leakage of *glucose, phosphate, bicarbonate* and *aminoacids* into the urine.

The counter current multiplier and exchange systems of urine concentration (see p. 461) cause some drugs to accumulate in the renal medulla. Analgesic nephropathy is often first evident at this site partly because of high tissue concentration and partly, it is believed, because of ischaemia through inhibition of locally produced vasodilator prostaglandins by NSAIDs. The distal tubule is the site of lithium-induced nephrotoxicity; damage to the medulla and distal nephron is manifested by failure to *concentrate* the urine after fluid deprivation and by failure to *acidify* urine after ingestion of ammonium chloride.

Tubule obstruction. Given certain physico-chemical conditions, crystals can deposit within the tubular lumen. Methotrexate is relatively insoluble at low pH and can precipitate in the distal nephron when the urine is acid.

Successful treatment of a leukaemia may be followed by the development of fatal urate nephropathy if breakdown of nucleic acids, released by destruction of leukaemic cells, delivers large amounts of insoluble urate to tubular fluid. This outcome can be prevented by starting the patient on allopurinol before the leukaemia is treated, for allopurinol inhibits xanthine oxidase, and the more soluble precursor, hypoxanthine, is excreted.

Other drug-induced lesions of the kidney include:

- *Vasculitis*, caused by sulphonamides, allopurinol, isoniazid.
- *Allergic interstitial nephritis*, caused by penicillins (especially), sulphonamides, thiazides, allopurinol, phenytoin.
- *Systemic lupus erythematosus*, caused by hydralazine, procainamide.

Drugs may thus induce any of the *common clinical syndromes* of renal injury, namely:

Acute renal failure, e.g. aminoglycosides, cisplatin

Nephrotic syndrome, e.g. penicillamine, gold, captopril

Chronic renal failure, e.g. NSAIDs

Functional impairment, i.e. reduced ability to dilute and concentrate urine (lithium), potassium loss in urine (loop diuretics), acid base imbalance (acetazolamide).

PRESCRIBING FOR PATIENTS WITH RENAL DISEASE

Drugs may:

- exacerbate renal disease
- be potentiated by accumulation due to failure of renal excretion
- be ineffective, e.g. thiazide diuretics in moderate or severe renal failure; uricosurics.

Problems of safety arise especially in patients with impaired renal function who must be treated with drugs that are potentially toxic and that are wholly or largely eliminated by the kidney.

A knowledge of, or at least access to, sources

Table 26.1 Drug $t_\frac{1}{2}$ (h) with normal and with severely impaired renal function

	normal	severe renal impairment*
captopril	2	25
amoxycillin	2	14
gentamicin	2.5	5
atenolol	6	100
digoxin	36	90

* glomerular filtration rate < 5 ml/min (normal is 120 ml/min)
These are examples of drugs that are excreted almost unchanged; the prolongation of their $t_\frac{1}{2}$ indicates that special care must be exercised if they are used in patients with impaired renal function.

of pharmacokinetic data is essential for safe therapy for such patients.[4] The profound influence of impaired renal function on the elimination of some drugs is illustrated in Table 26.1.

The $t_\frac{1}{2}$ of other drugs, whose activity is terminated by metabolism, is unaltered by renal impairment. Many such drugs, however, produce *pharmacologically active metabolites* which tend to be more water-soluble than the parent drug, are dependent on the kidney for their elimination, and accumulate in renal failure, e.g. acebutolol, diazepam, warfarin.

The majority of drugs fall into an intermediate class and are partly metabolised and partly eliminated unchanged by the kidney.

Administering the correct dose to a patient with renal disease must therefore take into account both the extent to which the drug normally relies on renal elimination, and the degree of renal impairment; the most convenient and useful guide to the latter is the *creatinine clearance*. These issues are now discussed.

Dose adjustment for patients with renal impairment

Adjustment of the initial dose (or where necessary the priming or loading dose, see p. 101) is

---

[4] e.g. Clinical pharmacokinetics. Drug data handbook. 1991; Auckland: Adis Press.

generally unnecessary, for the volume into which the drug has to distribute should be the same in the uraemic as in the healthy subject.

Adjustment of the maintenance dose involves either reducing each dose given or lengthening the time between doses.

Special caution is needed when the patient is hypoproteinaemic and the drug is usually extensively plasma protein bound, or in advanced renal disease when accumulated metabolic products may compete for protein binding sites; particular care is required in the early stages of dosing until response to the drug can be gauged.

General rules

1. Drugs that are wholly or largely excreted by the kidney or drugs that produce active, renally-eliminated metabolites: give a normal or, if there is special cause for caution (above), a slightly reduced initial dose, and lower the maintenance dose or lengthen the dose interval in proportion to the reduction in creatinine clearance.

2. Drugs that are wholly or largely metabolised to inactive products: give normal doses. When the special note of caution (above) applies, a modest reduction of initial dose and the maintenance dose rate are justified while drug effects are assessed.

3. Drugs that are partly eliminated by the kidney and partly metabolised: give a normal initial dose and modify the maintenance dose or dose interval in the light of what is known about the patient's renal function and the drug, its dependence on renal elimination and its inherent toxicity.

Recall that the *time to reach steady-state blood concentration* (p. 82) is dependent *only* on drug $t_\frac{1}{2}$ and a drug reaches 97% of its ultimate steady-state concentration in five $t_\frac{1}{2}$s. Thus if $t_\frac{1}{2}$ is prolonged by renal impairment, so also will be the time to reach steady state.

Schemes for modifying drug dosage for patients with renal disease do not altogether remove their increased risk of adverse effects; such patients should be observed particularly carefully throughout a course of drug therapy. Ideally, dosing should be monitored by drug plasma concentration measurements, but this service is not available to most of the world population.

NEPHROLITHIASIS

Calcareous stones result from hypercalciuria, hyperoxaluria and *hypo*citraturia. Hypercalciuria and hyperoxaluria render urine supersaturated in respect of calcium salts; citrate makes calcium oxalate more soluble and inhibits its precipitation from solution.

Non-calcareous stones occur most commonly in the presence of urea-splitting organisms which create conditions in which magnesium ammonium phosphate (struvite) stones form. Urate stones form when urine is unusually acid (*pH* <5.5).

Management. Recurrent stone-formers should maintain a urine output exceeding 2.5 l/day. Some benefit from restricting dietary calcium or reducing the intake of oxalate-rich foods (rhubarb, spinach, tea, chocolate, peanuts). *Thiazide diuretics* reduce the excretion of calcium and oxalate in the urine and reduce the rate of stone formation. *Sodium cellulose phosphate* (Calcisorb) binds calcium in the gut, reduces urinary calcium excretion and may benefit calcium stone-formers. *Allopurinol* is effective in those who have high excretion of uric acid in the urine. *Potassium citrate* which alkalinises the urine, should be given to prevent formation of pure uric acid stones.

PHARMACOLOGICAL ASPECTS OF MICTURITION

Some physiology

The detrusor, whose smooth muscle fibres comprise the body of the bladder, is innervated mainly by parasympathetic nerves which are excitatory and cause the muscle to contract. The *internal sphincter,* a concentration of smooth muscle at the bladder neck, is well developed only in the male and its principal function is to prevent retrograde flow of semen during ejaculation. It is rich in α_1-adrenoceptors, activation of which causes contraction. There is an abundant supply of oestrogen receptors in the distal two-thirds of the female urethral epithelium which degenerates after the menopause causing loss of urinary control.

When the detrusor relaxes and the sphincters close, urine is stored; this is achieved by central inhibition of parasympathetic tone accompanied by a reflex increase in α-adrenergic activity. Voiding requires contraction of the detrusor, accompanied by relaxation of the sphincters. These acts are coordinated by a micturition centre probably in the pons.

Functional abnormalities

The main abnormalities that require treatment are:

- '*Unstable bladder*' or '*detrusor instability*', characterised by uninhibited, unstable contractions of the detrusor which may be of unknown aetiology or secondary to an upper motor neuron lesion or bladder neck obstruction.
- *Decreased bladder activity* or hypotonicity due to a lower motor neuron lesion or overdistension of the bladder or to both.
- *Urethral sphincter dysfunction* which is due to various causes including weakness of the muscles and ligaments around the bladder neck, descent of the urethrovesical junction and periurethral fibrosis; the result is stress incontinence.
- *Atrophic change* affects the distal urethra in females.

Drugs may be used to alleviate abnormal micturition

Antimuscarinics block the parasympathetic supply to the bladder and are effective for incontinence due to detrusor instability. Oxybutynin or propantheline give considerable benefit to some sufferers but often at the cost of the adverse effects that accompany muscarinic blockade.

Tricyclic antidepressants. Imipramine, amitriptyline and nortriptyline are effective, especially for nocturnal but also for daytime incontinence. Their parasympathetic blocking (antimuscarinic) action is probably in part responsible but imipramine may also benefit by altering the patient's sleep profile.

Smooth muscle relaxants may benefit urinary frequency and incontinence, e.g. flavoxate which has a papaverine-like action.

Alpha-adrenoceptor antagonists. Prazosin, doxazosin and indoramin are α-adrenoceptor blockers that relax the internal sphincter, which benefits some patients, e.g. those with benign prostatic hypertrophy who are awaiting prostatectomy and are at risk of urinary retention.

Oestrogens either applied locally to the vagina or taken by mouth may benefit urinary incontinence due to atrophy of the urethral epithelium in menopausal women.

Parasympathomimetic drugs, e.g. bethanecol, carbachol and distigmine, may be used to stimulate the detrusor when the bladder is hypotonic, e.g. due to an upper motor neuron lesion. Distigmine is preferred but as its effect is not sustained, intermittent catheterisation is also needed when the hypotonia is chronic.

GUIDE TO FURTHER READING

Coburn J W, Salusky I B (editorial) 1989 Control of serum phosphorus in uremia. New England Journal of Medicine 320: 1140

Collins A J (editorial) 1987 Gold treatment for rheumatoid arthritis: reassurance on proteinuria. British Medical Journal 295: 739

Editorial 1985 Carbonic anhydrase. New England Journal of Medicine 313: 179

Editorial 1987 Acetazolamide in acute mountain sickness. British Medical Journal 295: 1161

Johnson T S, Rock P B 1988 Acute mountain sickness. New England Journal of Medicine 319: 841

LaCroix A Z et al 1990 Thiazide diuretic agents and the incidence of hip fractures. New England Journal of Medicine 322: 286

MacLennan W J (editorial) 1988 Diuretics in the elderly: how safe? British Medical Journal 296: 1551

McVeigh G et al 1988 The case for low dose diuretics in hypertension: comparison of low and conventional doses of cyclopenthiazide. British Medical Journal 297: 95

Malone–Lee J 1984 The pharmacology of urinary incontinence. In: Barbagallo–Sangiorgi G, Exton–Smith A N (eds) Aging and drug therapy. Plenum Press, New York, 419

Murphy M B et al 1982 Glucose intolerance in hypertensive patients treated with diuretics; a fourteen year follow-up. Lancet 2: 1293

Orme M L E (editorial) 1990 Thiazides in the 1990s. The risk:benefit ratio still favours the drug. British Medical Journal 300: 1668

Resnick N M, Subbaro V Y 1985 Management of urinary incontinence in the elderly. New England Journal of Medicine 313: 800

Robertson G L (editorial) 1989 Syndrome of inappropriate antidiuresis. New England Journal of Medicine 321: 538

27

Blood I: drugs and haemostasis

SYNOPSIS

Occlusive vascular disease is a major cause of morbidity and mortality. There is now a better understanding of the mechanisms by which the haemostatic system permits blood to remain liquid within vessels, yet to form a solid plug when a vessel is breached, and of the ways in which haemostasis may be altered by drugs to prevent or reverse (lyse) pathological thrombosis.

- The coagulation system: the mode of action of drugs that promote coagulation and that prevent it (anticoagulants) and their uses
- The fibrinolytic system: the mode of action of drugs that promote fibrinolysis (fibrinolytics) and their uses to lyse arterial and venous thrombi
- The platelets: the ways that drugs that inhibit platelet activity are used to treat arterial disease

The haemostatic system is complex but can be separated into the following major components:

- the formation of fibrin (coagulation)
- the degradation of fibrin (fibrinolysis)
- the platelets
- the blood vessels

Drugs that interfere with the haemostatic system are valuable in the management of pathological thrombus formation within blood vessels, or of pathological bleeding. They are classified according to which component of the system they affect.

THE COAGULATION SYSTEM

The blood coagulation system is shown in simplified form in Figure 27.1.

The *prothrombin time* monitors the *extrinsic system*. The *kaolin-cephalin clotting time* (KCCT; also known as the activated partial thromboplastin time, APTT) monitors the *intrinsic system*.

Agent that promotes coagulation

Vitamin K

Vitamin K (*Koagulation* vitamin) occurs naturally in two forms. K_1 is widely distributed in plants and K_2 is synthesised in the alimentary tract by bacteria, e.g. *E. coli*. Bile is required for the absorption of the natural vitamins K, which are fat-soluble. A synthetic analogue (K_3) of the natural vitamins also has biological activity; it is water soluble.

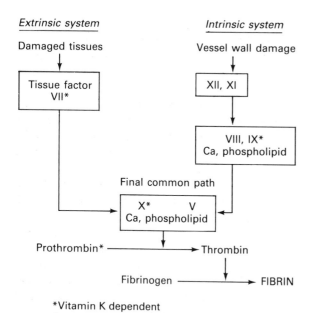

Extrinsic system

Damaged tissues

Intrinsic system

Vessel wall damage

*Vitamin K dependent

Fig. 27.1 The blood coagulation system

Vitamin K is necessary for the final stages of the synthesis of the coagulation proteins, factors II (prothrombin), VII, IX and X in the liver; when the vitamin is deficient or when its action is inhibited, functionally inert proteins result. In forming the coagulant proteins vitamin K is converted to an epoxide, an oxidation product, which is subsequently reduced again to the active vitamin K.

Vitamin K is metabolised (utilised) in the liver and is therefore less effective against hypoprothrombinaemia due to hepatic insufficiency. Indeed the response to vitamin K may be used to assess liver function, for failure of a prolonged prothrombin time to shorten after parenteral administration of vitamin K indicates considerable liver damage. A bleeding tendency due to dietary deficiency of vitamin K probably does not occur in man.

Deficiency may, however, arise from:

- bile failing to enter the intestine, e.g. obstructive jaundice or biliary fistula
- certain malabsorption syndromes, e.g. sprue, or after extensive small intestinal resections
- reduced alimentary tract flora, e.g. in

newborn infants and rarely after broad-spectrum antimicrobials.

The following preparations of vitamin K are available:

Phytomenadione (phytonadione, Konakion), the naturally occurring fat-soluble *vitamin K₁*, acts within about 12 h. The i.v. formulation is used in emergency and must be administered slowly as flushing, sweating, chest tightness and peripheral vascular collapse may occur, probably due to the castor oil it contains to make it water miscible. Otherwise phytomenadione may be given i.m., s.c. or orally.

Menadiol sodium phosphate (vitamin K₃, Synkavit), the synthetic analogue of vitamin K, being water-soluble, is preferred in malabsorption or in states in which bile flow is deficient. The main disadvantage is that it takes 24 h to act, but its effect lasts for several days. The dose is 5–40 mg daily, orally, i.v. or i.m.

Menadiol sodium phosphate in moderate doses causes haemolytic anaemia and for this reason it should not be given to neonates, especially those that are deficient in glucose-6-phosphate dehydrogenase; their immature livers are unable to cope with the heavy bilirubin load and there is danger of kernicterus.

Fat-soluble analogues of vitamin K which are available in some countries include *acetomenaphthone* and *menaphthone*.

Indications for vitamin K or its analogues

- Haemorrhage or threatened bleeding due to the coumarin or indandione anticoagulants. Phytomenadione is preferred for its more rapid action; dosage regimens vary according to the degree of urgency as described on p. 479.
- Hypoprothrombinaemia of the premature infant is treated by administration of phytomenadione to the mother (1–5 mg) 4–24 h before delivery, or, for greater reliability, to the baby (0.3 mg/kg, i.m.).
- Hypoprothrombinaemia due to intestinal malabsorption syndromes. Menadiol sodium phosphate should be used as it is water-soluble.

• Hypoprothrombinaemia due to aspirin overdose.

Drugs that prevent coagulation
(anticoagulants)

There are two types of anticoagulant:

Indirect acting: coumarin[1] and indandione drugs take about 72 h to become fully effective, act for several days, are given orally or by injection and can be antagonised (see below) by vitamin K.

Direct acting: heparin and ancrod are rapidly effective, act only for a few hours and must be given parenterally.

Indirect acting anticoagulants

Coumarins include warfarin and nicoumalone.

Indandione anticoagulants are practically obsolete because of allergic adverse reactions unrelated to coagulation but phenindione ($t_\frac{1}{2}$ 5 h) is still available.

Warfarin

Mode of action. During the formation of clotting factors II (prothrombin), VII, IX and X in the liver, vitamin K is oxidised to an epoxide and must be reduced by the enzyme epoxide reductase in order to become active again. Coumarins are structurally similar to vitamin K and competitively inhibit epoxide reductase, so limiting the availability of the active form of the vitamin to form clotting factors. The great *advantage* over heparin is that they can be given orally. Their chief *disadvantage* is the time-lag before they exert their effect, which is due to their *indirect mode of action*, i.e. although synthesis of the above clotting factors is quickly prevented, anticoagulation is delayed until the clotting factors already present in the circulation have been used up. The individual factors are eliminated at different rates and the net result is that anticoagulant protection is not effective until about 72 h after the first dose.

Pharmacokinetics. Warfarin is readily absorbed from the gastrointestinal tract and like all the oral anticoagulants it is more than 90% bound to plasma proteins. Its action is terminated by metabolism in the liver. Warfarin is a racemic mixture, i.e. it is in effect 2 drugs, namely, the enantiomorphs S(−) ($t_\frac{1}{2}$ 32 h) and R(+) ($t_\frac{1}{2}$ 54 h). S(−) warfarin is 4 times more potent than R(+) warfarin. Drugs which interact with warfarin affect these components differently.

Uses. Warfarin is the oral anticoagulant of choice, for it is reliably effective and has the lowest incidence of adverse effects. *Monitoring of therapy* is by the prothrombin time. Usually the test is carried out with a standardised thromboplastin and the result is expressed as the International Normalised Ratio (INR), which is the ratio of the prothrombin time in the patient to that in a normal, un-anticoagulated, person.

Oral anticoagulation is often undertaken in patients who are already receiving heparin. The INR reliably reflects the degree of prothrombin activity provided that the kaolin cephalin clotting time (KCCT), which is the best measure of the anticoagulant effect of heparin (see below), is within the therapeutic range (1.5–2.5 × control); this is easier to achieve when heparin is given by constant rate i.v. infusion rather than by intermittent i.v. injection.

Changeover of therapy from heparin to warfarin can then be accomplished as described below.

Dose. There is much inter-individual variation in dose requirements. A detailed scheme relating initial doses of warfarin to INR which should bring the ratio smoothly into the therapeutic range, is reproduced in Table 27.1.

Maintenance therapy should aim to keep the INR in the range 2.0–4.5. Warfarin 3–9 mg/day (taken at the same time each day) should normally achieve this. When the dose for an individual is stable the INR need be measured only every 6–8 weeks.

---

[1] Coumarins are present in many plants and are important in the perfume industry; the smell of new mown hay and grass is due to coumarins. Their discovery as anticoagulants dates from investigation of an unexplained haemorrhagic disease of cattle that had eaten mouldy sweet clover. Subsequent research culminated in the isolation of the toxic agent, dicoumarol.

Table 27.1 Loading dose schedule for warfarin administration

Day	INR	Warfarin dose (mg)
1	<1.4	10.0
2 (16 h after 1st dose)	<1.8	10.0
	1.8	1.0
	>1.8	0.5
3 (16 h after 2nd dose)	<2.0	10.0
	2.0–2.1	5.0
	2.2–2.3	4.5
	2.4–2.5	4.0
	2.6–2.7	3.5
	2.8–2.9	3.0
	3.0–3.1	2.5
	3.2–3.3	2.0
	3.4	1.5
	3.5	1.0
	3.6–4.0	0.5
	>4.0	nil
		Predicted maintenance dose
4 (16 h after 3rd dose)	<1.4	>8.0
	1.4	8.0
	1.5	7.5
	1.6–1.7	7.0
	1.8	6.5
	1.9	6.0
	2.0–2.1	5.5
	2.2–2.3	5.0
	2.4–2.6	4.5
	2.7–3.0	4.0
	3.1–3.5	3.5
	3.6–4.0	3.0
	4.1–4.5	Miss next day's dose, then give 2 mg
	>4.5	Miss next 2 days' doses, then give 1 mg

Reproduced, with permission of the authors and editor, from Fennerty A et al. Brit Med J 1984; 288: 1268.

The level of anticoagulation may be adjusted to match the perceived level of danger of thrombosis, by the following guidelines:[2]

INR 2.0–2.5   for prophylaxis of deep vein thrombosis including high risk surgery.

INR 2.0–3.0   for treatment of active deep vein thrombosis: pulmonary embolism; transient ischaemic attacks;

[2] British Society for Haematology guidelines on oral anticoagulants, 1984. Quoted by Poller L. Brit Med J 1985; 290: 1683.

prophylaxis after hip surgery and fractured femur operations.

INR 3.0–4.5   for recurrent deep vein thrombosis; recurrent pulmonary embolism; arterial disease including myocardial infarction; arterial grafts; prosthetic heart valves and grafts.

Adverse effects. Bleeding is the commonest. The incidence of major haemorrhage is 4–8% and an identifiable risk factor is often present, e.g. thrombocytopenia, liver disease or vitamin K deficiency, an endogenous disturbance of coagulation, cancer or recent surgery. Naturally, poor anticoagulant control or drug interaction with warfarin increase the risk. Haemorrhage is most likely to occur in the alimentary and renal tracts, and intracerebrally in those with cerebrovascular disease.

Cutaneous reactions, apart from purpura and bruising in those who are excessively anticoagulated, include pruritic lesions. Skin necrosis due to a mix of haemorrhage and thrombosis occurs rarely where induction of warfarin therapy is over-abrupt and/or the patient has a genetically determined or acquired deficiency of the anticoagulant protein C or its cofactor protein S; it can be very serious.

Warfarin used in early pregnancy may injure the fetus (other than by bleeding). It causes skeletal disorder (5%) (bossed forehead, sunken nose, foci of calcification in the epiphyses) and absence of the spleen. Women on long-term warfarin should be advised not to become pregnant while taking warfarin. Heparin should be substituted prior to conception and continued through the first trimester, after which warfarin should replace heparin, as continued exposure to heparin may cause osteoporosis. Warfarin being used in late pregnancy should be discontinued near term as it exacerbates neonatal hypoprothrombinaemia and its control is too imprecise for use in labour; heparin may be substituted at this stage for it can be discontinued just before labour and its anticoagulant effect passes off in about 6 h.

CNS abnormalities (microcephaly, cranial nerve palsies) are reported with warfarin used at any stage of pregnancy and are presumed to be due to intracranial haemorrhage.

Management of bleeding is guided by the clinical state and the INR:[3]

• Haemorrhage threatening life or major organs should be treated with concentrates of vitamin K-dependent clotting factors or fresh frozen plasma for immediate effect, and with phytomenadione 5 mg by slow i.v. injection, despite the thrombotic risks so created (the patient will be rendered refractory to oral anticoagulant, but not to heparin, for about 2 weeks).

• For lesser bleeding, warfarin should be withheld and phytomenadione 0.5–2 mg may be given by slow i.v. injection.

• INR > 7 but without bleeding should be corrected by withholding warfarin, and phytomenadione 0.5 mg by slow i.v. injection may be given if judged appropriate.

• INR 4.5–7.0 should be managed by withholding warfarin for 1–2 days and then reviewing the patient.

• INR 2.0–4.5 (the therapeutic range); bleeding, e.g. from the alimentary or renal tracts, should be fully investigated as a local cause frequently exists.

Withdrawal of oral anticoagulant. The balance of evidence is that abrupt, as opposed to gradual withdrawal of therapy does not, of itself, add to the risk of thromboembolism, for resynthesis of clotting factors takes several days. There is evidence that a higher incidence of thrombotic episodes occurs after withdrawal of anticoagulant therapy; the most likely explanation seems to be that this is a 'catching up' rather than a 'rebound' phenomenon, i.e. the patients now develop thromboses they would have had earlier but for anticoagulant therapy.

Interactions. Oral anticoagulant control requires to be precise both for safety and efficacy. Thus interference by other factors has only to be slight to have clinical importance. *Addition of any drug to the treatment* of a patient receiving an oral anticoagulant should be undertaken in the knowledge that *it may impair control*. If a drug which alters the action of warfarin must be used,

the INR should be monitored frequently and the dose of warfarin adjusted during the period of institution until the new stable dose of warfarin is identified; careful monitoring is also needed on withdrawal of the second drug.

The following list, although not comprehensive, identifies **medicines** which should be avoided and those which may safely be used with **warfarin**.

• *Analgesics.* Avoid if possible, all NSAIDs including aspirin because of their irritant effect on gastric mucosa and action on platelets. Paracetamol is acceptable. Dextropropoxyphene inhibits warfarin metabolism and compounds that contain it, e.g. co-proxamol, are contraindicated. Codeine, dihydrocodeine are safe.

• *Antimicrobials.* Avoid if possible: ciprofloxacin chloramphenicol, erythromycin, fluconazole, ketoconazole, metronidazole, miconazole, latamoxef and sulphonamides (including co-trimoxazole) which inhibit warfarin metabolism and potentiate anticoagulant effect. Rifampicin accelerates warfarin metabolism and reduces its effect. Penicillins, most cephalosporins and trimethoprim appear to be safe.

• *Anticonvulsants.* Carbamazepine and phenobarbitone increase warfarin metabolism; the effect of phenytoin is variable. Clonazepam and sodium valproate are safe.

• *Cardiac antidysrhythmics.* Amiodarone potentiates the effect of warfarin and dose adjustment is required, but atrophine, disopyramide and lignocaine do not interfere.

• *Antidepressants.* Avoid MAOIs which inhibit warfarin metabolism but tricyclics may be used.

• *Gastrointestinal drugs.* Avoid cimetidine which inhibits warfarin metabolism, and sucralfate which impairs its absorption; ranitidine and most antacids may be used.

• *Lipid-lowering drugs.* Bezafibrate, gemfibrate and clofibrate enhance anticoagulant effect. Cholestyramine is best avoided for it has complex effects and may impair the absorption of both warfarin and vitamin K.

• *Sex hormones.* Oestrogens increase the synthesis of some vitamin K dependent clotting factors and progestogen-only contraceptives are preferred. Tamoxifen, an oestrogen antagonist, enhances the effect of warfarin.

• *Sedatives and anxiolytics.* Benzodiazepines may be used.

---

[3] Based on recommendations of the British Society for Haematology.

Nicoumalone ($t_{\frac{1}{2}}$ 24 h) is similar to warfarin; it is eliminated in the urine mainly in the unchanged form.

Direct acting anticoagulants: heparin

Heparin was discovered by a medical student, J. McLean, working at Johns Hopkins Medical School in 1916. Seeking to devote one year to physiological research he was set to 'determine the value of the thromboplastic (clotting) substance in the body'. He found that extracts of various tissues (brain, heart, liver) accelerated clotting but that activity deteriorated during storage. To his surprise, the extract of liver which he had kept longest not only failed to accelerate but actually retarded clotting. His personal account proceeds:

After more tests and the preparation of other batches of heparophosphatide, I went one morning to the door of Dr. Howell's office, and standing there (he was seated at his desk), I said 'Dr. Howell, I have discovered antithrombin.' He was most skeptical. So I had the Deiner, John Schweinhant bleed a cat. Into a small beaker full of its blood, I stirred all of a proven batch of heparophosphatides, and I placed this on Dr. Howell's laboratory table and asked him to call me when it clotted. It never did clot. [It was heparin.][4]

Heparin is a mucopolysaccharide, occurs in mast cells and is prepared commercially from ox lung, bovine or porcine intestinal mucosa. It is the strongest organic acid in the body and in solution carries an electronegative charge.

Mode of action. Heparin depends for its action on the presence in plasma of a protein, antithrombin III, which is a naturally occurring inhibitor of several clotting factors, in particular of activated factor X (Xa) and thrombin. In the presence of small quantities of heparin antithrombin becomes vastly more active. Inhibition of factor Xa is particularly important since this factor has a role in both the intrinsic and extrinsic coagulation systems. Furthermore, inhibition of

coagulation at the factor Xa stage requires much less heparin than does inhibition at the later thrombin stage. This is the rationale for the use of low doses of subcutaneous heparin in preventing thrombus formation as opposed to the high doses which are required to treat established thrombosis (see below).

Apart from its anticoagulant properties, benefit from heparin in arterial embolus may be derived from a slight vasodilator effect which promotes collateral circulation.

Pharmacokinetics. Heparin is mainly metabolised by the liver but it is partly taken up by the reticuloendothelial system and some is excreted unchanged by the kidney. The $t_{\frac{1}{2}}$ depends on the dose given but with average doses is about 80 min, and the $t_{\frac{1}{2}}$ of its effect on the clotting time is about 100 min. Delayed elimination occurs in patients with impaired renal function. Heparin is ineffective by mouth because it is precipitated by acid; given i.v. the maximum effect is immediate.

Control of heparin therapy is by the kaolin cephalin clotting time (KCCT), the optimum therapeutic range being 1.5–2.5 times the control.

Dose

- Treatment of *established thrombosis*. The usual intravenous regimen is bolus injection of 12 500 units, follow by a constant rate infusion which delivers 10 000–20 000 units every 12 h or 5000–10 000 units by injection every 12 h. Individuals vary strikingly in their response to standard doses (apparent 'resistance' to heparin may be due to antithrombin III deficiency). The KCCT should be measured 4–6 h after starting therapy and the administration rate adjusted to keep it in the optimum therapeutic range; this usually requires daily measurements of KCCT. Alternatively 10 000–20 000 units may be given subcutaneously every 12 h but control is less even.

- *Prevention* of thrombosis. Heparin is used in lower doses for prophylaxis of venous thrombosis in high-risk cases. Postoperatively or after myocardial infarction 5000 units may be given s.c. every 8 or 12 h, or in pregnancy 10 000 units every 12 h. Monitoring is not required as

---

[4] McLean gives a fascinating account of his struggles to pay his way through medical school, as well as his discovery of heparin in: McLean J. 1959 Circulation X1X: 75.

these doses do not alter the KCCT. Subfractions prepared from crude heparin with lower molecular weights, e.g. enoxaparin and dalteparin, may be used for prophylaxis of thromboembolism after surgery. Whether their antithrombotic effect is associated with less risk of haemorrhage, remains to be established.

Adverse effects. *Bleeding* is the only serious acute complication of heparin therapy. It is uncommon, but patients with impaired hepatic or renal function, with carcinoma, and those over 60 years appear to be most at risk. A KCCT ratio > 3 is associated with an eight-fold increased chance of bleeding. *Thrombocytopenia* occurs in about 2–3% of cases, most commonly with heparin derived from bovine lung and least with that of intestinal origin; it develops after one week of use, and recurs on rechallenge. Warfarin should be substituted if the platelet count falls when a patient receives heparin. *Osteoporosis* may occur; it is dose related and may be expected with 15 000–30 000 units/day for about 6 months. Hypersensitivity reactions and skin necrosis occur but are rare. Transient alopecia has been ascribed to heparin but in fact may be due to the severity of the thromboembolic disease for which the drug was given. Skin necrosis similar to that seen with warfarin (see above) occurs rarely.

Heparin antagonism. Heparin effects wear off so rapidly that an antagonist is seldom required except after perfusion for open heart surgery. When antagonism is needed:

Protamine, a protein obtained from fish sperm, reverses the anticoagulant action of heparin. It is as strongly basic as heparin is acidic, which explains its immediate antagonism. Protamine sulphate is given by slow i.v. injection and 1 mg neutralises about 100 units of heparin derived from mucosa (mucous) or 80 units of heparin from lung; but if the heparin was given more than 15 min previously, the dose must be scaled down. Protamine itself has some anticoagulant effect and overdosage must be avoided. The maximum dose must not exceed 50 mg.

Ancrod (Arvin) is an enzyme preparation from the venom of the Malayan pit viper. It depletes fibrinogen without causing vascular occlusion and offers an alternative to heparin although it is rarely necessary.

Uses of anticoagulants

The thrombus which forms in leg *veins* characteristically has a white 'head' consisting principally of platelets adherent to the vessel wall and a red 'tail' which may be only loosely attached to the vessel wall and is comprised of a framework of fibrin in which are caught up the various cellular elements of the blood; it is the red part of the thrombus which may threaten life by breaking loose and embolising to the lungs. Thrombi that form in the chambers of the heart have a similar fibrin structure, and are also likely to embolise. *Arterial* thrombi have a different structure; the swifter flow of blood washes out many of the red cells, and the thrombus consists of fibrin and masses of platelets and leucocytes moulded to the shape of the vessel wall. It is therefore not surprising that, in general, *anticoagulant drugs* which stop formation of fibrin thrombus are more effective in venous and cardiac disease than in arterial thrombosis, and *antiplatelet drugs* (see later) are effective in arterial but not in venous thrombosis.

Anticoagulant drugs are therefore used as follows:

Venous disease

Established venous thromboembolism. An anticoagulant is used to prevent extension of an existing thrombus while its size is reduced by natural thrombolytic activity. Effective anticoagulation prevents formation of fresh thrombus, which is more likely to detach and embolise, particularly if it is in large proximal veins; it also helps to recanalise veins and to clear vein valves of thrombus and should thus prevent long-term consequences such as swelling of the leg and stasis ulceration.

Ideally the diagnosis should first be established by venography which also indicates the extent of thrombosis, and influences management. Small distal thrombi require only elevation of the limb and no anticoagulant. For a thrombus less than 10 cm long in a tibial vein heparin 5000 units s.c. × 2/d is sufficient until the patient is fully mobile. Full anticoagulation may be required for more extensive thrombosis; heparin should be used initially because of its rapid onset of effect and continued until the signs of thrombosis (heat, swelling of the limb) have settled, which may take 5–7 days. Oral anticoagulant is usually started on the third to the fifth day in the knowledge that at least 2 days must elapse before the INR is in the therapeutic range. The patient should wear a well-fitting compression stocking to increase flow in deep veins, should exercise the leg and should be encouraged to mobilise as soon as the discomfort has settled.

Thrombolytic therapy with intravenous streptokinase or urokinase may be used when thrombosis is thought to be life-threatening, and thrombectomy is recommended where the viability of the limb is threatened.

The risk of recurrence reduces with passage of time after the initial event. In cases of deep vein thrombosis uncomplicated by pulmonary embolus, 3 months of anticoagulant therapy appears adequate. Where there is evidence of pulmonary embolus it is common practice to continue therapy for 6 months.

Anticoagulant therapy may be lifesaving in *thromboembolic pulmonary hypertension*.

Prevention of venous thrombosis. Oral anticoagulant reduces the risk of thromboembolism in conditions in which there is special hazard, e.g. after surgery. Partly because of the danger of bleeding and partly because of the effort of maintaining control, oral anticoagulants have not been widely adopted and effective use has been made of mechanical methods such as intermittent calf compression during surgery. Numerous trials, however, have shown the protective effect of low doses of heparin (5000 units every 8–12 h s.c.) against deep leg vein thrombosis. The significant fact is that it takes a lot less heparin to *prevent* thrombosis than it does to treat established thrombosis, because heparin acts at an early stage in the cascade of coagulation factors which leads to fibrin formation (see before).

Apart from its use after surgery, low-dose heparin can be used to prevent venous thromboembolism in other high-risk patients, e.g. those confined to bed and immobilised with strokes, cardiac failure or malignant disease. Spontaneous bleeding has not been a problem with this form of anticoagulant treatment.

Low molecular weight *dextrans*, can reduce postoperative thromboembolism if infused i.v. at the time of operation. Dextran 70 (mol. wt. 70 000) is used; it may act by reducing platelet adhesiveness.

Cardiac disease

In general, long-term anticoagulation to prevent arterial thromboembolism should be considered for any patient who has a large left atrium, a low cardiac output and paroxysmal or established atrial fibrillation.

Arterial thrombosis

Heparin may prevent extension of a thrombus and hasten its recanalisation; it is commonly used in the acute phase following thrombosis or embolism. There is no case for treating *ischaemic peripheral vascular disease* with an oral anticoagulant. For prevention, see antiplatelet drugs.

Long-term anticoagulant prophylaxis

The decision to use warfarin long-term must take into account non-drug factors. The patient should be told of the risks of haemorrhage, including those introduced by taking other drugs, and of the signs of bleeding into the alimentary or urinary tracts. All patients should carry a card stating that they are receiving an oral anticoagulant. Such therapy should be withheld from a patient who is considered to be unlikely or unable to comply with the requirements of regular medication and blood testing. The incidence of haemorrhagic complications is directly related to the level of anticoagulation; safety and good results can only be obtained by close attention to detail.

Surgery in patients receiving anticoagulant therapy

For elective surgery warfarin may be withdrawn about 5 days before the operation and resumed about 3 days after if conditions seem appropriate; low-dose heparin may be used in the intervening period. Emergency surgery: proceed as for bleeding (p. 479). For dental extractions, omission of warfarin for 1–2 days to adjust the INR to the lower limit of the therapeutic range is adequate (INR should be tested just prior to the procedure). The usual dose of warfarin can be resumed the day after surgery.

Contraindications to anticoagulant therapy

Contraindications relate mostly to conditions in which there is a tendency to bleed, and are relative rather than absolute, the dangers being balanced against the possible benefits. They include:

- *haematological*: a pre-existing bleeding disorder
- *neurological*: stroke within 3 weeks, or surgery to the brain or eye
- *cardiovascular*: severe uncontrolled hypertension
- *alimentary*: active peptic ulcer, active inflammatory bowel disease, oesophageal varices, cirrhosis
- *renal*: if function is severely impaired
- *behavioural*: inability or unwillingness to cooperate, dependency on alcohol
- *pregnancy*: in early pregnancy the fetal warfarin syndrome is a hazard and bleeding may cause fetal death in late pregnancy.

THE FIBRINOLYTIC SYSTEM

The preservation of an intact vascular system requires not only that blood be capable of coagulating but also that there should be a mechanism for removing the products of coagulation when they have served their purpose of stopping a vascular leak. This is the function of the *fibrinolytic system* the essential features of which are show in Figure 27.2.

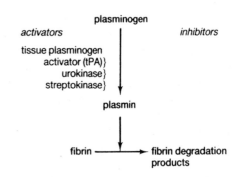

Fig. 27.2   The blood fibrinolytic system

The system depends on the formation of the fibrinolytic enzyme *plasmin* from its precursor *plasminogen* which is present in the blood. During clotting, plasminogen binds to specific sites on fibrin. Simultaneously the natural activators of plasminogen, i.e. tissue plasminogen activator (tPA) and urokinase, are released from endothelial and other tissue cells and act on plasminogen to form plasmin. The result is that plasmin formation takes place *on the fibrin surface* but not generally within the circulation. Since fibrin is the framework of a thrombus, its dissolution clears the clot away.

The therapeutic potentialities of fibrinolytic substances are obvious. *Anticoagulants* may *prevent* thrombosis, *fibrinolytics* can *remove* formed thrombi and emboli. *Inhibitors* of the fibrinolytic system (antifibrinolytics) can be of value in certain bleeding states characterised by excessive fibrinolysis.

Drugs that promote fibrinolysis

A recent and important application of fibrinolytic drugs has been to dissolve thrombi in acutely occluded coronary arteries, thereby to restore blood supply to ischaemic myocardium, to limit necrosis and to improve prognosis. The approach is to give a *plasminogen activator* intravenously by infusion or by bolus injection in order to increase the formation of the fibrinolytic plasmin. Those currently available, or being evaluated, include:

Streptokinase ($t\frac{1}{2}$ 23 min) is a protein derived from β-haemolytic streptococci: it forms a complex with plasminogen that binds loosely to fibrin where it converts plasminogen to plasmin. Too rapid administration causes abrupt fall in blood pressure.

Anistreplase (anisoylated plasminogen streptokinase activator complex, APSAC), ($t_{\frac{1}{2}}$ 90 min), is the plasminogen-streptokinase complex (above) in which the enzyme centre that converts plasminogen to plasmin, is protected from deactivation, so prolonging its action. As the full thrombolytic dose can be given by i.v. injection over 4–5 min, therapy may be initiated outside hospital; its effect persists for 6–9 h.

Urokinase ($t_{\frac{1}{2}}$ 16 min) made from human fetal kidney cells in tissue culture, is a direct activator of plasminogen.

Streptokinase, anistreplase and urokinase are not well absorbed by fibrin thrombi and are called *non-fibrin-selective*. They convert plasminogen to plasmin in the circulation, which depletes plasma fibrinogen and induces a general hypocoagulable coagulant state. This does not reduce their local thrombolytic potential but increases the risk of bleeding.

Recombinant pro-urokinase ($t_{\frac{1}{2}}$ 7 min), as the name suggests, is produced by recombinant DNA technology; on binding to fibrin it converts to urokinase.

Alteplase (rt-PA) ($t_{\frac{1}{2}}$ 5 min) is tissue type plasminogen activator produced by recombinant DNA technology.

Recombinant pro-urokinase and alteplase are termed *fibrin-selective*, for they bind strongly to fibrin, and are capable of dissolving ageing or lysis-resistant thrombi better than non-fibrin-selective agents. These drugs are less likely to produce a coagulation disturbance in the plasma i.e. they are selective for thrombi.

Apart from anistreplase (above), thrombolytic agents are normally infused i.v. over 1–3 h with most of the dose being given in the initial phase. Safe systemic administration represents a significant advance over former regimens which required direct infusion at the site of the thrombus, e.g. intracoronary.

Uses of fibrinolytic drugs

Coronary artery thrombolysis

Reduction in mortality. The idea that *thrombolysis* might improve the outcome of myocardial infarction had common-sense appeal and generated numerous clinical trials, some of which had a favourable and some an unfavourable outcome. However, an assessment by meta-analysis (see p. 51) of the combined data from 24 trials of streptokinase given 4–24 h after the onset of symptoms revealed a 24% reduction in mortality.[5] The obvious importance of this result stimulated the production and testing of newer thrombolytic agents. Evidence indicates that anistreplase and alteplase are of equivalent therapeutic efficacy to streptokinase.[6] The earlier thrombolysis is begun, the better, and reduction in mortality may approach 50% when treatment is commenced within the first hour. Follow-up for 6–12 months suggests that the benefit persists. Rethrombosis after successful coronary artery recanalisation remains a problem; anticoagulant regimens to combat this are being examined.

Aspirin, appears to add to the beneficial effect of thrombolysis. In a study of over 17 000 patients, streptokinase reduced mortality by 25% whereas with streptokinase plus aspirin 160 mg/d for one month, mortality fell by 42%.[7] The explanation may be the antiplatelet effect of aspirin, for platelets may mediate reocclusion of coronary arteries after successful thrombolysis.

Whilst the percentage reduction in mortality in these **aspirin trials** is impressive, the actual number of lives saved is small. For example, a reduction in mortality of 30% might in effect represent a fall from 10% to 7%, i.e. a saving of 3 lives from 100 treated patients.

[5] Yusuf S et al. 1985 European Heart Journal 6: 556.
[6] ISIS-3 Collaborative Group 1991, American College of Cardiology, Atlanta, USA.
[7] ISIS-2 Collaborative Group 1988 Lancet 2: 349.

Stroke may complicate myocardial infarction and is considered usually to be embolic, for its incidence correlates with the extent of myocardial infarction. Evidence[7] indicates, however, that the combination of thrombolysis plus aspirin lowers the overall risk of stroke, possibly by limiting the size of the infarct, or by reducing thromboembolic episodes, or by both. There is also an increased risk of haemorrhagic stroke with anistreplase and alteplase compared with streptokinase.[6]

Other studies show that thrombolytic agents induce in over half the cases recanalisation of the *occluded infarct-related artery*, reduction of *infarct size* and improved *left ventricular function*. Regimens involving tPA have achieved recanalisation more frequently than those using streptokinase with which they were compared but this has not resulted in lower overall mortality.

Adverse effects. *Bleeding* is the most important and usually occurs at the site of a vascular lesion, for fibrinolytic therapy does not distinguish between an undesired thrombus and a useful haemostatic plug. If the contraindications (below) are followed, the incidence of bleeding severe enough to require transfusion is <1%.

Multiple microemboli from disintegration of pre-existing thrombus anywhere in the vascular system may endanger life; these commonly originate in an enlarged left atrium, or a ventricular or aortic aneurysm.

Cardiac dysrhythmias result from reperfusion of ischaemic tissue. These vary in type and are often transient, a factor which may influence the decision whether or not to treat.

Allergy. Streptokinase and anistreplase are antigenic and anaphylactic reactions with rash, urticaria and hypotension may occur, for most people have circulating antibodies to streptococci. Antibodies persist after exposure to these drugs and their re-use should be avoided for 6 months as the recommended dose may not overcome resistance to plasminogen activation.

Evidence indicates that recombinant pro-urokinase and alteplase are not antigenic.

Contraindications to fibrinolytic drug use

- *Risk of bleeding*, where, for example the patient has had recent major surgery or trauma, or internal bleeding, or has active peptic ulcer, liver disease or portal hypertension, or coagulation defect. Relative contraindications include pregnancy, uncontrolled hypertension, diabetic proliferative retinopathy and pancreatitis.

- *Stroke* or transient ischaemic attack within the previous 6 months.
- *Thrombus* on cardiac ventricle or aneurysm wall, which may fragment and embolise.
- *Allergy* (in the case of streptokinase or anistreplase): patients with recent streptococcal infection (and high antistreptokinase titres), or who have received either drug between 5 days and 12 months previously, or who have exhibited allergy to either drug.

Conclusion. Thrombolytic agents reduce mortality in patients with myocardial infarction. Therapy should be initiated within 24 h and for best effect within 6 h of the onset of symptoms. Streptokinase is preferred because there is greater risk of haemorrhagic stroke with anistreplase or alteplase. Aspirin appears to exert an independent additive beneficial effect when given with streptokinase.

Non-coronary thrombolysis

Systemic or local thrombolysis may be considered for *arterial occlusions* distal to the popliteal artery, (thrombectomy being the usual therapeutic approach for recent occlusion proximal to this site of <24 h duration). Intravenous streptokinase will lyse 80% of occlusions if infusion begins within 12 h, and 60% if it is delayed for up to 3 days. For occlusions of longer standing, low-dose local infusion of streptokinase or urokinase is preferred, once the site of thrombosis has been defined by diagnostic arteriography. Success depends on adequate access of the fibrinolytic agent to the thrombus; obstructions in (small) digital arteries are no longer lysable after a few days, whereas thrombi in (large) iliac vessels may be cleared as long as 6 months after formation.

The criteria for selection of patients are essentially those for myocardial infarction (above).

Thrombolysis may also be considered for ocular thrombosis (urokinase), for thrombosed arteriovenous shunts (streptokinase), for life-threatening *venous thrombosis*, to reduce the risk of *persisting pulmonary hypertension* (when lung blood vessels are occluded by thromboemboli) and for *massive pulmonary embolism with shock* (to avoid embolectomy).

Drugs that prevent fibrinolysis

Antifibrinolytics are useful in a number of bleeding disorders.

Tranexamic acid occupies the sites on fibrin at which plasminogen is bound and converted to plasmin (causing dissolution of fibrin); fibrinolysis is thus retarded. The $t_{\frac{1}{2}}$ is 10 h after an i.v. bolus injection and it is excreted almost entirely in the urine.

The principal indication for tranexamic acid is to prevent the *hyperplasminaemic bleeding state* that results from damage to certain tissues rich in plasminogen activator, e.g. after prostatic surgery, tonsillectomy, uterine cervical conisation, and menorrhagia whether primary or induced by an intra-uterine contraceptive device. Tranexamic acid may also reduce bleeding after ocular trauma and in haemophiliacs after dental extraction. The drug benefits some patients with *hereditary angioedema* presumably by preventing the plasmin-induced uncontrolled activation of the complement system which characterises that condition. Tranexamic acid may be of value in thrombocytopenia (idiopathic or following cytotoxic chemotherapy) to reduce the risk of haemorrhage by inhibiting natural fibrinolytic destabilisation of small platelet plugs; the requirement for platelet transfusion is thereby reduced. It may also be used for overdose with thrombolytic agents.

Adverse effects are rare but include nausea, diarrhoea and sometimes orthostatic hypotension.

Aprotinin is a naturally occurring inhibitor of plasmin (obtained from bovine lung) which has been used for the treatment of life-threatening haemorrhage due to hyperplasminaemia complicating surgery of malignant tumours or thrombolytic therapy.

THE PLATELETS

Some physiology

Platelets do not stick to healthy endothelium but if a vessel wall is breached they react at the site by:

● *adhesion* to the exposed tissues, especially to collagen, and release of substances including adenosine diphosphate (ADP) and the prostaglandin thromboxane A_2, in response to which,

● *aggregation* of platelets on the original deposition releases further ADP and thromboxane A_2, whereupon,

● *transformation* of platelets takes place into a solid plug and simultaneously they *release* their granule contents, including proteins, enzymes, enzyme inhibitors, vasoactive and other peptides and agents that participate in the coagulation process.

The system that enables platelets to distinguish between healthy and damaged endothelium is shown in Figure 27.3. It is a continuation of, and should be studied in conjunction with, the general diagram for eicosanoids on p. 212.

1. As in so many biological systems, *cyclic AMP* plays a key role. *High* concentrations of intra-platelet cyclic AMP inhibit platelet adhesion, aggregation and the release of active substances (see above), and *low* concentrations of cyclic AMP have the opposite effect.

2. The quantity of cyclic AMP within platelets is under enzymatic control, for it is formed by the action of *adenylyl cyclase* and degraded by *phosphodiesterase*.

3. Platelet adenylyl cyclase formation in turn is stimulated by *prostacyclin* (from the endothelium) and inhibited by *thromboxane A_2* (from within platelets). Hence the action of thromboxane A_2 lowers cyclic AMP concentration and promotes platelet adhesion; prostacyclin *raises* cyclic AMP concentration and prevents platelet adhesion.

4. Prostacyclin and thromboxane A_2 are

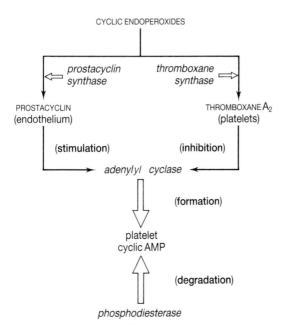

CYCLIC ENDOPEROXIDES

prostacyclin synthase ⇐   thromboxane synthase ⇒

PROSTACYCLIN (endothelium)   THROMBOXANE A₂ (platelets)

(stimulation)   (inhibition)

adenylyl cyclase

(formation)

platelet cyclic AMP

(degradation)

phosphodiesterase

Fig. 27.3 Prostacyclin, thromboxane and the formation of platelet cyclic AMP

derived from arachidonic acid which is a constituent of cell walls, both platelet and endothelial. *Cyclo-oxygenase*, an enzyme present in cells at both sites, converts arachidonic acid to cyclic endoperoxides which are further metabolised by *prostacyclin synthase* to prostacyclin in the endothelium and by *thromboxane synthase* to thromboxane A₂ in platelets. Thus prostacyclin is principally formed in the *endothelium* whereas thromboxane A₂ is formed mainly in *platelets*.

5. These differences in the prostaglandins synthesised in endothelium and platelets are important. Intact vascular endothelium does not attract platelets because of the high concentration of prostacyclin in the intima. Sub-intimal tissues contain little prostacyclin, and platelets, under the influence of thromboxane A₂, immediately adhere and aggregate to any breach in the intima. Atheromatous plaques do not generate prostacyclin which explains platelet adhesion and thrombosis at these sites.

Inhibitors or activators of platelet aggregation act directly or indirectly by altering the rate of formation or degradation of platelet cyclic AMP. Local concentrations of these substances determine whether the platelet-adhesion/aggregation process will occur.

Drugs that inhibit platelet activity

Aspirin (*acetyl*salicylic acid) acetylates and thus inactivates cyclo-oxygenase; the chemical bond is irreversible and hence lasts the 7–9 d lifetime of the platelet (the salicylate part of acetylsalicylic acid is irrelevant to this action). It follows from the diagram on p. 212 and the account above that aspirin can prevent formation of *both* thromboxane A₂ and prostacyclin. Therapeutic interest in its antithrombotic effects has centred on separating these actions and this can be achieved by using low dose. Thus 75–150 mg/d by mouth is sufficient to reduce synthesis of thromboxane A₂ without significant impairment of prostacyclin formation, i.e. amounts substantially *below* the 2.4 g/d used to control pain and inflammation.

Sulphinpyrazone ($t_{\frac{1}{2}}$ 3 h) inhibits several platelet functions possibly by competitive antagonism of platelet cyclo-oxygenase; its effects are dose-dependent and reversible. Some days must elapse before the full effect of sulphinpyrazone appears and disappears probably because active metabolites are formed. Sulphinpyrazone is a uricosuric and its primary use is in hyperuricaemia and gout.

Dipyridamole reversibly inhibits platelet phosphodiesterase (see Fig. 27.3) and in consequence cyclic AMP concentration is increased and platelet reactivity reduced; evidence also suggests that its antithrombotic effect may derive from release of prostaglandin precursors by vascular endothelium. Dipyridamole is extensively bound to plasma proteins and has a $t_{\frac{1}{2}}$ of 10 h.

Dextrans, particularly of molecular weight 70 000 (dextran 70), alter platelet function and prolong the bleeding time. Dextrans differ from the other antiplatelet drugs which tend to be used for arterial thrombosis; dextran 70 reduces the incidence of postoperative *venous* thromboembolism if it is given during or just after surgery. The dose should not exceed 10% of the estimated blood volume.

Dazoxiben, an inhibitor of thromboxane A₂

but not prostacyclin synthesis, and *ticlopidine*, an inhibitor of ADP-induced platelet aggregation are being evaluated in cardiovascular disease.

Epoprostenol (prostacyclin) (t_2^1 3 min) may be given to prevent platelet loss during renal dialysis, with or without heparin; it is infused i.v. It is a potent vasodilator.

Uses of antiplatelet drugs

• *Cerebrovascular disease.* Patients who exhibit transient ischaemic attacks (TIAs) or minor ischaemic stroke are at risk of progressing to completed stroke, the likelihood of which is reduced by about 30% by taking aspirin. Before starting treatment it is important to exclude intracerebral haemorrhage (by computed tomography), and other conditions that mimic TIAs, e.g. cardiac dysrhythmia, migraine, focal epilepsy and hypoglycaemia. The optimum dose is not known; 300 mg/d may be assumed to be effective but lower doses may be equally so, and 150 or 75 mg/d is justified where there is gastric intolerance.

• *Unstable angina.* Aspirin halves the risk of progression to myocardial infarction or death in patients with this condition, which suggests that platelet aggregates play a part in its development. It should be used with other drugs , i.e. a β-adrenoceptor antagonist, a nitrate and a calcium channel blocker as is judged appropriate.

• *Myocardial infarction.* Meta-analysis of 10 clinical trials of either aspirin, 300–1300 mg/d, alone or with dipyridamole, given long-term to survivors of myocardial infarction, i.e. *secondary prevention*, show that cardiovascular mortality fell by 13% and nonfatal reinfarction by 31%.[8]

Among 22 000 male physicians who had no history of myocardial infarction, i.e. *primary prevention*, aspirin 325 mg every other day reduced the rate of myocardial infarction by 44% in those >50 y. Put another way, in this relatively healthy population, aspirin achieved an absolute reduction of 2 myocardial infarctions per thousand subjects treated per year.[9]

Conclusion: aspirin should be given indefinitely to patients who have survived myocardial infarction; evidence indicates that 300 mg/d will protect but the optimum dose has yet to be established, and may be lower. There is as yet no case for using aspirin to prevent myocardial infarction in those without important risk factors for the disease.

• Coronary artery bypass grafts. Low-dose aspirin and dipyridamole prevent both early and late occlusion of these grafts. This combination may also be used to prevent thrombotic occlusion following percutaneous transluminal coronary angioplasty.

Haemostatics

Ethamsylate (Dicynene) is given systemically to reduce capillary bleeding, e.g. in menorrhagia.

Adrenaline may be useful in epistaxis, stopping haemorrhage by local vasoconstriction when applied by packing the nostril with ribbon gauze soaked in Adrenaline Solution.

Sclerosing agents. Chemicals may be used to cause inflammation and thrombosis in veins so as to induce permanent obliteration, e.g. Ethanolamine Oleate Injection (given i.v. for varicose veins) and Oily Phenol Injection (given submucously for haemorrhoids). Local reactions and embolus can occur.

Haemophilia

Management of the haemophilias (genetic deficiencies of the factor VIII or IX) is a matter for those with special expertise but the following points are of general interest. Bleeding can sometimes be stopped by pressure; edges of superficial wounds should be strapped, not stitched. In haemophilia A antihaemophilic globulin (factor VIII) concentrate (t_2^1 12 h) should be used for bleeding that is more than minor; and factor IX (t_2^1 18 h) for haemophilia B (Christmas disease). Desmopressin (DDAVP) administered daily for short periods, e.g. 3 days, can quadruple factor VIII activity (but not factor IX). Tranexamic acid helps stabilise thrombi, in both diseases. DDAVP may be used to prevent bleeding after dental extractions and may render transfusion unnecessary, so avoiding the risk of transmitted infection.

---

[8] Antiplatelet Trialists' Collaboration 1988 Brit Med J 296: 320.
[9] Steering Committee 1989 New Engl J Med 321: 129.

GUIDE TO FURTHER READING

Agle et al 1970 The anticoagulant malingerer. Annals of Internal Medicine 73: 67

Campbell W B, Magee T R 1989 Managing acute limb ischaemia. British Medical Journal 299: 526

Collier B S 1990 Platelets and thrombolytic therapy. New England Journal of Medicine 322: 33

de Gaetano G 1988 Primary prevention of vascular disease by aspirin. Lancet 1: 1093

Editorial 1989 Aspirin in the prevention of coronary disease. New England Journal of Medicine 321: 183

Editorial 1989 Reperfusion injury after thrombolytic therapy for acute myocardial infarction. Lancet 2: 655

Editorial 1990 Non-coronary thrombolysis. Lancet 335: 691

Fennerty A G et al 1986 Guidelines to control heparin therapy. British Medical Journal 292: 579

Hirsh J 1991 Heparin. New England Journal of Medicine 324: 1565

Hirsh J 1991 Oral anticoagulant drugs. New England Journal of Medicine 324: 1865

Loscalzo J, Braunwald E 1988 Tissue plasminogen activator. New England Journal of Medicine 319: 925

Marder V J, Sherry S 1988 Thrombolytic therapy: current status. New England Journal of Medicine 318: 1512 (first part), 1585 (second part)

Rapaport E 1989 Thrombolytic agents in acute myocardial infarction. New England Journal of Medicine 320: 861

Sandercock P (editorial) 1988 Aspirin for strokes and transient ischaemic attacks. No panacea. British Medical Journal 297: 955

Blood II: cellular disorders and anaemias

IRON

Iron, which was the metal symbolising strength in magical systems, used to be given to people suffering from weakness, and no doubt many were benefited, some psychologically (placebo reactors) and others because they had anaemia. The rational use of iron could not begin until both the presence of iron in the 'colouring matter' of the blood and the 'defective nature of the colouring matter' in anaemia were recognised.

Some facts and figures

- Total body iron is 3–5 g (male > female).
- Haemoglobin contains about two-thirds of total iron.
- Stores comprise about one-third (ferritin and an aggregate, haemosiderin) in liver, marrow, spleen and muscle.
- Diet (average Western) contains 10–15 mg iron/day.
- *Normal human* absorbs up to 10% dietary iron, i.e. 0.5–1.0 mg/day, which is adequate.
- *Anaemic human* absorbs about 30% of dietary iron.
- Iron is lost from the body mainly by desquamation.
- Menstrual loss is about 30 mg/period; menstruating women are therefore liable to be in negative balance.
- A pregnant woman absorbs 3–4 mg extra iron/day for the fetus, placenta and normal blood loss at delivery.

Iron pharmacokinetics

Iron absorption takes place chiefly in the upper part of the small intestine where the acid medium enhances solubility, but also throughout the gut, allowing sustained-release preparations to be used. Most iron in food is ferric. Ferrous iron is more readily absorbed than ferric and a reducing agent, such as ascorbic acid, increases the amount of the ferrous form; 50 mg increases iron absorption from a meal by 2 to 3 times. Food reduces iron absorption.

The *process of absorption* regulates the amount of iron entering the body according to need, i.e. the state of the iron stores. Dietary and administered iron is actively transported into the gut mucosal cell. Iron that is *not* needed by the body is bound to a protein (apoferritin) as *ferritin* and this is lost into the gut lumen when the mucosal cell is shed (2–3 days); it is eliminated at near constant rate in the faeces in healthy people (and by skin desquamation). Iron that *is* needed forms a labile pool within the cell; if this pool is excessive it stimulates more production of apoferritin to bind more iron as ferritin. Labile pool iron enters the blood bound to a transport globulin, *transferrin*, which delivers it to the sites of physiological need, principally erythrocyte precursors (80%) (where it forms haem), the rest to muscles (myoglobin), and to form iron-containing enzymes (e.g. cytochromes) in all body cells. There is a small amount of ferritin in the blood in balance with the iron stores.

Iron is *stored* as *ferritin* and its aggregate, *haemosiderin*, in the cells of the liver, bone marrow and spleen. A *measure of the state of iron stores* is provided by the amount of ferritin in the blood and by the relationship of serum iron concentration (low in iron deficiency) to the percentage saturation of transferrin (also low in iron deficiency and therefore having a high *iron binding capacity*).

Prolonged heavy excess in iron intake overwhelms the mechanism described and results in haemosiderosis.

Iron-deficient subjects absorb up to 20 times as much administered iron as those not in need.

Abnormalities of the small intestine may interfere with either the absorption of iron, as in the malabsorption syndromes and coeliac disease, or possibly with the conversion of iron into a soluble and reduced form, e.g. partial gastrectomy.

The formation of insoluble iron salts (such as phosphate and phytate) in the alkaline medium of most of the small intestine explains why much of the iron taken by mouth is not absorbed, even in severe iron deficiency.

Interactions. Iron chelates in the gut with tetracyclines, penicillamine, methyldopa, levodopa, carbidopa, and ciprofloxacin; it also forms stable complexes with thyroxine, captopril and folic acid. These interactions can be clinically important. Doses should be separated by 3 h.

Ascorbic acid increases absorption (above) but its use (200 mg/day) is not clinically important in routine therapy; *desferrioxamine* binds iron and reduces absorption (see poisoning, below); *tea* (tannins) and *bran* reduce absorption.

Iron therapy

Iron therapy is indicated only for the prevention or cure of iron deficiency; 25 mg of iron per day must be available to the bone marrow if an iron deficiency anaemia is to respond with a rise of 1% of haemoglobin (0.15 g Hb/100 ml) per day (beginning after 7 days' therapy); a reticulocyte response occurs between days 4 and 12.

Oral iron therapy. When oral therapy is used it is reasonable to assume that about 30% of the iron will be absorbed and to give 180 mg of elemental iron daily for 1–3 months according to the degree of anaemia. However calculations are necessary for **parenteral iron**. With *iron dextran i.v.* all the iron is biologically available. But with *i.m.* iron dextran about 30% of iron remains bound to muscle, and with *iron sorbitol* i.m. about 30% is lost by renal excretion. This is taken into account when calculating an i.m. course of iron. In pregnancy it is usual to add 0.5 g for the needs of placenta, fetus and blood loss at delivery.[1]

Iron stores are less easily replenished by oral

---

[1] Manufacturers provide Tables for determining the extent of iron deficiency and the size of a course of parenteral iron. These relate the Hb deficit, i.e. normal Hb minus the patient's Hb/100 ml, body weight and blood volume, with an allowance to replenish stores. Doctors unaccustomed to making such calculations will prefer the Tables.

therapy than by injection, and oral therapy (at lower dose) should be continued for 3 months after the haemoglobin concentration has returned to normal (or as long as blood loss continues).

It is illogical to give iron in the anaemia of *chronic infection* where utilisation of iron stores is impaired; but such patients may also have true iron deficiency, as in rheumatoid arthritis, due to gut bleeding from NSAIDs. Also in *haemolytic anaemias* unless there is also haemoglobinuria, for the iron from the lysed cells remains in the body, and haemosiderosis may ultimately occur.

Iron therapy is needed:

• In iron deficiency due to dietary lack or to chronic blood loss.
• In pregnancy. The extra iron required by mother and fetus totals 1000 mg, chiefly in the latter half of pregnancy. The fetus takes iron from the mother even if she is iron deficient, as she commonly is. Dietary iron is seldom adequate and iron and folic acid (50–100 mg elemental iron plus folic acid 200–500 μg/d) should be given to pregnant women from the fourth month. Opinions differ on whether all women should receive prophylaxis or whether only those who can be identified as needing it. There are numerous formulations. Parents should be particularly *warned not to let children get at the tablets*, which are often attractively coloured and sometimes sugar-coated.
• In various abnormalities of the gastrointestinal tract in which the proportion of dietary iron absorbed may be reduced, e.g. in malabsorption syndromes generally.
• In premature babies, since they are born with low iron stores, and in babies weaned late. There is very little iron in human milk and even less in cow's milk.
• In early treatment of severe pernicious anaemia with hydroxocobalamin, as the iron stores occasionally become exhausted by the sudden increase in red cell formation.

Oral iron preparations

There is an enormous variety of official and proprietary iron preparations. For each milligram of elemental iron taken by mouth, ferrous sul-phate is as effective and no more toxic than more expensive preparations. Solutions of iron salts are seldom used as they stain the teeth. It is particularly important to avoid initial overdosage with iron as the resulting symptoms may cause the patient to abandon therapy. A small dose is given at first and increased after a few days. The objective is to give 100–200 mg of elemental iron per day. *If given on a full stomach iron causes less gastrointestinal upset but less is absorbed than if it is given between meals*; however use with food is commonly preferred to improve compliance. Commonly used preparations, given in divided doses, include:

Ferrous Sulphate Tabs, 200–600 mg daily. Each 200 mg tablet contains 60–65 mg of elemental iron.

Ferrous Gluconate Tabs, 300–1200 mg daily. Each 300 mg tablet contains 35 mg of elemental iron.

Ferrous Furmarate Tabs, 200–600 mg daily. Each 200 mg tablet contains 65 mg of elemental iron.

Ferrous succinate and *ferrous glycine sulphate* are alternatives.

Choice of oral iron preparation. Oral iron is used, both for therapy and for prophylaxis (pregnancy) of anaemia in people who are feeling little, if at all, ill. Because of this, the occurrence of gastrointestinal upset is particularly important as it is liable to cause the patient to give up taking iron; in one study 30% of pregnant women were not taking the iron prescribed; in another antenatal clinic nausea, heartburn, flushes, constipation and diarrhoea were as common in patients taking dummy tablets as in those taking iron; this was attributed to gossip amongst the waiting patients.

The evidence as to which preparation provides best iron absorption with least adverse effects is conflicting. Gastrointestinal upset is minimal if the daily dose does not exceed 180 mg elemental iron.

A suggested course: Start a patient on ferrous sulphate[2] taken on a full stomach once, then

---

[2] Ferrous sulphate is the most toxic form in *acute overdose* and it may be thought best not to prescribe it to members of households where there are small children.

twice, then thrice a day. If gut intolerance occurs, stop the iron and reintroduce it with one week for each step. If this seems to cause gastro-intestinal upset, try ferrous gluconate, succinate or fumarate. If simple preparations (above) are unsuccessful, and this is unlikely, then the pharmaceutically sophisticated, and expensive *sustained-release* preparations may be tried; they release iron slowly and only after passing the pylorus, from resins, chelates (sodium iron edetate) or plastic matrices (Slow-Fe, Sytron, Feospan etc.) so that iron is released in the lower rather than the upper small intestine. It is said that the lesser incidence of symptoms is due to less iron being released and absorbed. But this is not invariably so and patients who cannot tolerate standard forms even when taken with food may get as much iron with fewer unpleasant symptoms if they use a sustained-release formulation.

Liquid formulations are available for adults who prefer them and for small children, e.g. Ferrous Sulphate Paediatric Mixture: 5 ml contains 12 mg of elemental iron. Polysaccharide-iron complex (Niferex): 5 ml contains 100 mg of elemental iron (it is diluted before use).

There are numerous other iron preparations which can give satisfactory results.

Sustained-release and *chelated* forms of iron (see above) have the advantage that poisoning is less serious if a mother's supply is consumed by young children, a real hazard.

Iron therapy blackens the faeces but does not generally interfere with tests for occult blood (commonly needed in investigation of anaemia), though it may give a false positive with some occult blood tests, e.g. guaiac test.

Failure of oral iron therapy is most commonly due to poor patient compliance persistent bleeding and, as with all drug therapy, wrong diagnosis.

Parenteral iron administration

Parenteral iron administration may be required: if iron cannot be absorbed from the intestine, if a sure response is essential in a severe iron deficiency anaemia, as in *late* pregnancy (though here a blood transfusion may be preferred); and

if, as sometimes happens for no discoverable reason, oral iron therapy fails or the patient cannot be relied on to take it or experiences intolerable gut symptoms.

The *speed of response is not quicker* than that with full doses of oral iron reliably taken and normally absorbed, for both provide as much iron as an active marrow can use. A course of injected iron is stored and utilised over months.

The approximate *total requirement* can be calculated from the haemoglobin concentration (above) or ascertained from Tables.

The ionised salts of iron used orally are powerful protein precipitants that cannot be used parenterally and un-ionised iron complexes have been developed.

Oral iron therapy should be stopped 24 h before injections begin; not only is it unnecessary, but it may promote adverse reactions to the injections by saturating the plasma protein (transferrin) binding sites so that the injection gives higher unbound iron plasma concentration than is safe. This occurs with iron sorbitol; the large molecule of iron dextran does not bind to transferrin.

Intravenous iron. *Iron Dextran* is used (see below). There is no particular reason to give intermittent i.v. injections, as it can be given by *total dose infusion* (enough iron to correct anaemia and to replenish stores on a single occasion). The technique avoids the inconvenience and unpleasantness of repeated i.m. injections and of incomplete treatment due to non-compliance. The disadvantages are that the patient must arrange to attend hospital for a day, that close supervision is necessary and that ill-effects, sometimes serious anaphylactoid (collapse and death), rarely, can occur. It should only be used where it is essential to do so. A history of any allergy is a contraindication. Resuscitation equipment should be at hand. Technique must be studied and compliance by the doctor must be meticulous.

Intramuscular iron. *Iron Sorbitol Inj* (Jectofer; 1 ml = 50 mg Fe) is an iron-sorbitol-citric-acid complex of molecular weight <5000 that is rapidly absorbed into the blood from the site of injection (unlike iron dextran). About 30%

of a dose is excreted by the kidney in 24 h and the urine may turn black transiently at the time of peak iron excretion or only on standing for some hours, (probably due to formation of iron sulphide by bacterial action).

Iron sorbitol has been found to increase the urinary leucocyte excretion rate in patients with urinary tract infections or non-infective renal disease (which can mislead diagnosis), and it should be avoided in such patients, in whom iron dextran i.m. may be preferred.

Iron sorbitol is bound to the plasma globulin, transferrin, and is stored in the marrow and liver. It is not substantially taken up in the reticulo-endothelial system. Excess unbound iron is excreted in the urine. Iron sorbitol is unsuitable for total dose i.v. infusion, probably because, after rapid saturation of transferrin, there would be very high free (toxic) iron levels in the blood (compare with iron dextran below).

Iron sorbitol is given by deep i.m. injection, which can be painful. It stains the skin (lasts up to 2 years) but this can be minimised by inserting the needle through the skin and then moving the skin and subcutaneous tissue laterally before entering the muscle so that the needle track becomes angulated when the needle is withdrawn. The dose is up to 1.5 mg/kg/day (up to 100 mg/dose) until the total amount of iron required has been given over about 10 days. The injections are usually painful and general reactions (headache, dizziness, disorientation, nausea, vomiting) occur and sometimes a metallic taste, up to 2 h after injection.

Iron Dextran Inj. (Imferon; 1 ml = 50 mg Fe) has a higher mol. wt.(>6000) than iron sorbitol and is absorbed slowly from the injection site into the lymphatics (25% remains after 3 weeks). The immediate ill-effects of both preparations i.m. are similar in kind, but are more frequent with iron sorbitol. The dose is 2–5 ml of the solution i.m. daily in active patients, or once or twice a week in inactive patients.

Iron dextran is not bound to transferrin and is stored in the reticulo-endothelial system (unlike iron sorbitol) whence utilisable iron is released over months, and this may be why the total requirements to correct anaemia and to replenish stores can be given in a single slow infusion (see above).

Folic acid deficiency may be a unmasked by effective iron therapy. Where there is a deficiency of both iron and folic acid, the deficiency of the latter may not be obvious because haemopoiesis is held back by lack of iron. If iron is supplied there will be an increased formation of red cells and the folic acid deficiency will be disclosed. This is liable to happen in pregnancy and so folic acid is commonly given to all pregnant patients with anaemia (see below); it also occurs in malabsorption syndromes.

Adverse effects

Some adverse effects of therapeutic doses have been mentioned above under oral and parenteral iron. The gastrointestinal effects of oral iron include: nausea, abdominal pain, and either constipation or diarrhoea.

Acute overdose: poisoning

High doses of iron salts by mouth (usually in small children in the home) can cause severe gastrointestinal irritation and even necrosis of the mucous membrane. Large amounts are absorbed and cardiovascular collapse occurs. Autopsy shows severe damage to brain and liver. Tablets of most iron preparations are attractive to children because they are senselessly coloured and sometimes even sugar-coated. Death may occur if an infant swallows a quantity of these 'sweets' whose danger is still not adequately recognised. Sustained-release forms (though expensive) are safer in homes where heedless parents live with small children.

Cautionary tale

. . . a girl aged 19 months was found vomiting after taking 15 or 16 ferrous sulphate tablets. She was taken to hospital and there given salt and water and she vomited again. The mother was told that there was no bed available and she was sent to another hospital. Here she was told that the tablets were not poisonous and would do the child no harm. The child was retching now but not vomiting and the mother was told to take her home and give her plenty of milk to drink. The mother was not satisfied and took the child to another doctor on the way home. He told her to give the child orange juice to drink and she would be all right. The mother then took the child home, put her in her cot, and went to make some orange juice. When she returned the child was dead . . . about four hours after the child had taken the tablets.[3]

Patients such as this can be saved by prompt chelation therapy.

The clinical course of a typical case of acute *oral* iron poisoning has four phases.[4]

- *First*, 0.5–1 h after ingestion: abdominal pain, vomiting, bloody diarrhoea, acidosis and cardiovascular collapse, with coma and death in 4–6 h in 20% of cases.
- *Second*, in 80% of cases, a period of improvement lasting 8–16 h, which may be permanent or which may pass into —
- *Third*, cardiovascular collapse, convulsions, coma and sometimes death about 24 h after ingestion.
- *Fourth*, 1–2 months later, gastrointestinal obstruction from scarring.

Treatment of acute iron poisoning is urgent and immediate efforts to chelate iron in the blood and in the intestine must be made. Raw egg and milk help to bind iron until a chelating agent is available.

The first step should be to give **desferrioxamine** 1–2 g i.m. or i.v. (see below); same dose in adults and children.

Only after this should gastric lavage or emesis (see index) be performed. If lavage is used, the water should contain 2 g desferrioxamine/litre. After emptying the stomach, 10 g desferrioxamine in 50–100 ml water should be left in the stomach; it is not absorbed.

After this, an i.v. infusion should be set up to correct abnormalities of electrolyte and water balance. Desferrioxamine may also be given i.v. in saline or dextrose infusion or i.m.

Poisoning is severe if the plasma iron concentration exceeds 90 μmol/l (500 μg/100 ml) or plasma becomes pink (vin rosé) due to the large formation of ferrioxamine (below); i.v. rather than i.m. administration of desferrioxamine is then indicated.

Where anuria occurs, exchange transfusion should be considered, for the toxicity of large amounts of the iron chelate (ferrioxamine) is unknown.

Desferrioxamine (deferoxamine) (Desferal) is an iron-chelating agent (see Chelating agents). During a systematic investigation of Actinomycete metabolites iron-containing substances (sideramines) were discovered. One of these substances was ferrioxamine. The iron in this can be removed chemically, leaving desferrioxamine.

When desferrioxamine comes into contact with ferric iron, its straight-chain molecule twines around it and forms a non-toxic complex of great stability (ferrioxamine), which is excreted in the urine giving it a reddish colour, and in the bile. It has a negligible affinity for other metals in the presence of iron excess, and serious adverse effects are rare; with chronic use cataract, retinal damage and deafness can occur.

Desferrioxamine has been shown to be effective in the therapy of acute iron poisoning and in the treatment and perhaps in the diagnosis of diseases associated with chronic iron accumulation. A topical formulation is available for ocular siderosis. It is not absorbed from the gut; injected, its $t_{\frac{1}{2}}$ is 6 h.

Chelating capacity. Desferrioxamine (5 g) chelates iron contained in about 10 tabs ferrous sulphate or gluconate (100 mg desferrioxamine chelates about 8.5 mg iron); this does not apply under the different conditions of iron overload, below.

Chronic iron overload

The body is unable to excrete any excess of iron so that, if there is uncontrolled iron intake, it accumulates in the body. Grossly excessive parenteral iron therapy or a hundred or more blood transfusions (as in treatment of thalassaemia[5]) can lead to haemosiderosis. Oral iron

---

[3] Spencer I O B Br Med J 1951; 2: 11,12.
[4] Aldrich R A In: Wallerstein R O, Metier S R, et al. Iron in clinical medicine. University of California Press, 1958.

[5] A 26-year-old subject with β-thalassaemia major had been transfused 404 units of blood over his lifetime. His iron stores were so high (estimated at above 100 g) that he triggered a metal detector at an airport security checkpoint (Jim R T S Lancet 1979; 2: 1028).

therapy over many years has also been reported to cause it.

The treatment of chronic iron overload, e.g. haemochromatosis, haemolytic anaemias and thalassaemia with transfusional iron overload: iron may be removed by repeated venesection when there is not anaemia (haemochromatosis) or by chelation (transfusional overload).

The most effective way of administration is by 12-h nocturnal s.c. infusion of desferrioxamine (on 5 nights per week). Oral ascorbic acid increases the availability of free iron for chelation. This regimen can put a patient living a life dependent on red-cell transfusions into the desired negative iron balance. The expense of doing this over a long period is currently enormous and raises serious ethical problems in economically poor countries where most of these patients live; cheap orally effective alternatives are under clinical trial.

A single venesection of 500 ml blood, *in the absence of anaemia,* removes 200 mg of iron and can be repeated weekly.

A large intake of *tea* (tannins) binds non-haem iron (as in iron-reinforced bread) and may play a modest but useful part in iron overload states.

VITAMIN B$_{12}$

Extrinsic and intrinsic factors in pernicious anaemia

In 1925, it was demonstrated that 2 factors were required to cure pernicious anaemia: one in the food (extrinsic factor) and one in gastric juice (intrinsic factor). Soon after crystalline *cyanocobalamin (vitamin B$_{12}$)* was isolated in 1948 it was generally accepted to be the *extrinsic factor.* The *intrinsic factor* (secreted by the gastric acid forming cells) is a glycoprotein. Intrinsic factor acts solely as a vehicle for carrying the important extrinsic factor into the body via receptors in the ileum, but if large doses of cobalamins are given they are absorbed (by diffusion) independently of intrinsic factor, though less reliably.

The cobalamins

The active cellular coenzymes (vitamin B$_{12}$),

methylcobalamin and deoxyadenosylcobalamin, are necessary for DNA synthesis. They are formed in the body from administered *hydroxocobalamin* and cyanocobalamin. Hydroxocobalamin is preferred for clinical use.

A deficiency of vitamin B$_{12}$ in the body leads to:

- A megaloblastic anaemia.
- Degeneration of the brain, spinal cord and peripheral nerves (subacute combined degeneration); symptoms may be psychiatric or physical.
- Abnormalities of epithelial tissue, particularly of the alimentary tract, e.g. sore tongue and malabsorption.

Requirements of cobalamins are about 3.0 µg daily. Absorption takes place mainly in the terminal ileum, and they are carried in plasma bound to proteins (transcobalamins). They are not significantly metabolised, and excretion is via the bile (there is enterohepatic circulation which can be interrupted by intestinal disease and hasten the onset of clinical deficiency), and via the kidney. Body stores amount to about 5 mg (mainly in the liver). Most animals cannot synthesise cobalamin and so are directly or indirectly dependent upon micro-organisms for it. Humans get most of their cobalamins from meat; bacteria in the human colon synthesise it but it is not absorbed from this part of the intestine, and if rabbits in the wild did not eat their own faeces they would suffer from pernicious anaemia.

Dietary deficiency is virtually confined to people who have not enough money to buy meat, and to Vegans, a sect of particularly uncompromising vegetarians.

Indications for vitamin B$_{12}$

Indications for administration are the prevention and cure of conditions due to its deficiency, which commonly presents as megaloblastic anaemia, though neurological or mental disorder (with anaemia) can occur.

In pernicious (Addisonian) anaemia the atrophic gastric mucosa is unable to produce intrinsic factor (and acid) and so vitamin B$_{12}$

deficiency occurs. Despite its name (given when no treatment was known), the prognosis of a patient with uncomplicated pernicious anaemia, properly treated with hydroxocobalamin is little different from that of the rest of the population. The neurological complications, particularly spasticity, are often permanent, although there may be considerable improvement under treatment. Total removal of the stomach or atrophy of the mucous membrane in a post-gastrectomy remnant may, after several years, lead to a similar anaemia.

Malabsorption syndromes. In *coeliac disease* and idiopathic steatorrhoea vitamin B_{12} and folic acid deficiency are common although megaloblastic anaemia occurs only relatively late.

- A variety of *drugs* can cause malabsorption including neomycin, colchicine, metformin, sustained-release KCl and antiepileptics.
- Deprivation of vitamin B_{12} by *abnormal bowel flora* occurs in tropical sprue, multiple jejunal diverticular, bowel fistulae and blind-loop syndrome. This can be remedied by a broad-spectrum antibiotic, e.g. tetracycline.

Tobacco amblyopia. It is possible there is an element of cyanide intoxication from the tobacco, and hydroxocobalamin may be given.

Diagnosis of B_{12} deficiency

The serum concentration of B_{12} is measured.

In addition the *Schilling test* of vitamin B_{12} absorption may be used. First: the patient is given a small dose of radioactive vitamin B_{12} *orally*, followed shortly by a large dose of non-radioactive vitamin B_{12} *i.m.* The large injected dose saturates binding sites in the body so that if any of the oral radioactive dose is absorbed it will not find any binding sites available and will be eliminated in the urine where it can easily be measured. In pernicious anaemia gut absorption, and therefore urinary elimination of radioactivity, is negligible. Second: the test is then repeated with intrinsic factor added to the oral dose. The radioactive vitamin B_{12} is now absorbed and is detected in the urine. Both stages of the test are needed to maximise reliability of diagnosis of pernicious anaemia.

Contraindications to vitamin B_{12}

Undiagnosed anaemia is an important contraindication. Therapy of pernicious anaemia must be both adequate and life-long, so that accurate diagnosis is essential. Even a single dose interferes with diagnosis by blood picture for weeks, although the Schilling test remains diagnostic. Inclusion of small amounts of cyanocobalamin in oral tonics is probably harmless but implies an irresponsible attitude in both promoter and prescriber. It is a bad thing that a patient's health should ever depend on not absorbing the physician's 'therapy'.

Preparations and use

Hydroxocobalamin is bound to plasma protein to a greater extent that is cyanocobalamin, with the result that there is less free to be excreted in the urine after an injection and rather lower doses at longer intervals are adequate. This is why it is preferred to cyanocobalamin, though the latter can give satisfactory results (except in tobacco amblyopia).

The initial dose in cobalamin deficiency anaemias, including uncomplicated pernicious anaemia, is hydroxocobalamin 1 mg i.m. every 2–3 days for 5 doses to induce remission and to replenish stores. Maintenance may be 1 mg 3-monthly; higher doses will not find binding sites and will be eliminated in the urine. But higher doses should probably be used in renal and hepatic disease (due to defects in conversion to the active coenzyme and excretion).

After initiation of therapy, patients feel better in 2 days, reticulocytes peak at 7 days and Hb concentration should be normal within 6 weeks.

Failure to respond implies wrong or incomplete diagnosis.

The initial stimulation of haemoglobin synthesis often depletes the *iron* and *folate* stores and supplements of these may be needed.

Hypokalaemia may occur at the height of the erythrocyte response in severe cases. It is attributed to uptake of potassium by the rapidly increasing erythrocyte mass. Oral K should be given. Acute gout occasionally occurs about the seventh day.

Inadequate response should be treated by increased frequency of injections as well as increased amount (because of urinary loss with high plasma concentrations).

Haemoglobin estimations are necessary at least every 6 months to check adequacy of therapy and for early detection of iron deficiency anaemia due to carcinoma of the stomach, which occurs in about 5% of patients with pernicious anaemia.

When injections are refused or are impracticable (rare allergy, bleeding disorder), administration as snuff or aerosol has been effective, but these routes are potentially less reliable. Large daily oral doses (1000 µg) are probably preferable; monitoring of the blood must be more frequent. *Cyanocobalamin* remains available.

Adverse effects virtually do not occur, but use of vitamin B_{12} as a 'tonic' is an abuse of a powerful remedy for it may obscure the diagnosis of pernicious anaemia, which is a matter of great importance in a disease requiring life-long therapy and prone to serious neurological complications.

In pernicious anaemia, folic acid should not be used alone. Although the anaemia improves (because vitamin B_{12} plays a role in folate metabolism), it allows progression of subacute combined degeneration of the nervous system. A patient with pernicious anaemia who has been given folic acid is thus in a dangerous situation.

'Shot-gun' haematinics

There are oral preparations containing a miscellany of substances necessary for blood formation, including iron, folic acid, cyanocobalamin and other vitamins, liver, stomach extracts, etc.

Both their indiscriminate promotion by commercial interests and their use by physicians in undiagnosed cases shows a disregard for patients' interests that is inconsiderate at best and callous at worst. Regulatory authorities are in a position to eliminate the preparations, but seem reluctant to act.

FOLIC ACID (pteroylglutamic acid)

Folic acid was so named because it was dis-covered as a bacterial growth factor present in spinach leaves (Latin: *folium*, a leaf). It is one of the B group of vitamins and was soon shown to be the same substance as that present in yeast and liver which cured a nutritional macrocytic anaemia in Indian women.

Functions

Folic acid is itself inactive; it is converted into the biologically active coenzyme tetrahydrofolic acid, which is important in the biosynthesis of amino acids and DNA, and therefore in cell division. The formyl derivative of tetrahydrofolic acid is *folinic acid* or *citrovorum factor* (leucovorin) and this can be used to bypass the block when the body fails to effect the conversion of folic acid (see folic acid antagonists).

Ascorbic acid protects the active tetrahydrofolic acid from oxidation, and the anaemia of scurvy, although usually normoblastic, may be megaloblastic due to deficiency of tetrahydrofolic acid.

Deficiency of folic acid leads to a megaloblastic anaemia probably because it is necessary for the production of the purines and pyrimidines, which are essential precursors of deoxyribonucleic acid (DNA). The megaloblastic marrow of cobalamin deficiency is due to interference with folic acid utilisation and the morphological changes of such deficiency can be reversed by folic acid. However, it is vital to realise that *folic acid does not provide adequate treatment for pernicious anaemia.* Nor does vitamin B_{12} provide adequate treatment for the megaloblastic anaemia of folate deficiency although a partial response may occur.

Folic acid antagonists are sometimes used in treatment for acute leukaemias.

Occurrence and requirements

Folic acid is widely distributed, especially in green vegetables, yeast and liver. Daily requirement of pure folic acid is about 50 µg and a diet containing 400 µg of polyglutamates will provide this. Body stores are enough for several months.

Indications

The prevention and cure of the megaloblastic anaemia due to deficiency of folic acid.

• In malabsorption syndromes, particularly steatorrhoea, gluten enteropathy and sprue, poor absorption of folic acid from the small intestine often leads to a megaloblastic anaemia.

• In pregnancy, folate requirement is increased from 400 µg to 800 µg/day and mild deficiency is common, with a minority of cases developing severe megaloblastic anaemia. For this reason folic acid is added to iron for prophylaxis of anaemia. The dose needed is about 300 µg folic acid a day, which is insufficient to alter the blood picture of pernicious anaemia and so there is no risk of masking that disease, which is also very rare in women of reproductive age and is probably incompatible with a successful pregnancy. A large number of preparations of iron with folic acid is available (see also iron therapy, p. 493). They are suitable only for prevention. Larger doses may be used in therapy of pregnancy anaemia (below); it will remit spontaneously some weeks after delivery. Vigorous iron therapy in pregnancy may unmask a folic acid deficiency.

• Prevention of fetal neural tube defect (spina bifida). Folic acid supplement taken before conception and during the early weeks of pregnancy has been shown in an 8-year trial to prevent the condition in pregnancies subsequent to an affected birth.[6] Whether all pregnancies would be protected by routine use is the subject of ongoing research.

• In chronic haemolytic states folic acid requirement is increased.

• Anticonvulsant drugs, particularly phenytoin, primidone and phenobarbitone, occasionally cause a macrocytic anaemia that responds to folic acid. This may be due to enzyme induction by the anticonvulsants increasing the need for folate to perform hydroxylations (see under epilepsy) but other factors may be involved. Some *antimalarials* e.g. pyrimethamine, may interfere with conversion, of folates to the active tetrahydrofolic acid, causing macrocytic anaemia, as may nitrofurantoin.

Contraindications: imprecisely diagnosed megaloblastic anaemia. Some cancers are folate dependent and folic acid should be used in malignant disease only where there is a specifically folic acid deficiency anaemia.

Preparations and dosage. Synthetic folic acid is taken orally; for therapy 5 mg daily is usually given for 4 months, or indefinitely if the cause of deficiency cannot be removed; 15 mg/d may be needed in malabsorption states. There is no advantage in giving *folinic acid* instead of folic acid, except in the treatment of the toxic effects of folic acid antagonists in order to bypass the site of metabolic block (see p. 629).

For prophylaxis, with iron, in pregnancy, see p. 493; for prophylaxis in haemolytic diseases and in renal dialysis: 5 mg per day or per week depending on need.

Adverse reactions: allergy occurs rarely.

HAEMOPOIETIC GROWTH FACTORS

It is now possible, once a cell growth factor has been identified, to make it by cloning and DNA technology in amounts sufficient for clinical use. Rapid developments are occurring in this area. These factors are potentially useful whenever there is deficiency of blood cell function, whether due to disease or to cytotoxic chemotherapy.

Epoietin (erythropoietin)

Epoietin is a glycoprotein hormone made in the kidney (95%) in response to anoxia. The anaemia of chronic renal failure is largely due to failure of the diseased kidney to make enough epoietin. The principal action of the hormone is to activate the proliferation and speed the development (maturation) of erythrocyte precursors.

The manufacture of enough epoietin for clinical use had to await the development of recombinant DNA technology; the human gene for epoietin is expressed in a mammalian (hamster) cell line.

Epoietin is effective in the anaemia of chronic

---

[6] MRC Vitamin Study research group. Lancet 1991; 338: 131

renal failure to an extent that significantly enhances the patients' quality of life. Patients become independent of blood transfusion, with great benefit to blood transfusion services as well as to themselves.

The hormone has also been used in severe anaemia of cancer, rheumatoid arthritis and zidovudine-treated AIDS; also to improve the quality of presurgical autologous blood collection. It is misused by sportspeople seeking advantage.

Epoietin must be given i.m. or s.c; the $t_\frac{1}{2}$ is 8 h and appears not to be affected by dialysis. Maximum reticulocyte response occurs in 4 days. Self-administration at home 3 times a week is practicable; the dose is adjusted by response.

Adverse effects include arterial hypertension which may need antihypertensive drugs; arteriovenous shunts may clot.

Iron deficiency may occur, as increased haemopoiesis outstrips available iron stores, and this can be a cause of inadequate response to the hormone; parenteral iron therapy may be needed.

Filgrastim (granulocyte colony stimulating factor: G-CSF)

Filgrastim causes immature leucocytes to differentiate into granulocytes (neutrophils). It is used in patients suffering neutropenia due to cytotoxic chemotherapy of non-myeloid malignancies; it may find use in neutropenia of other causes and in patients with increased susceptibility to infections.

Granulocyte/macrophage colony stimulating factor (GM-CSF) (sargramostim) is undergoing clinical trials.

Interleukins (of which there are many) are cell growth factors that, amongst other actions, activate lymphocytes and stimulate megakaryocytes to produce platelets. Some are already available for clinical use (see p. 628).

POLYCYTHAEMIA VERA

The principles of treatment are:
All patients: reduce packed cell volume (PCV) to normal by venesection (300–500 ml) every 2 days.

Attempt to maintain by occasional venesection to *keep* the packed cell volume normal. Iron deficiency may occur and need treatment although this may mean more frequent venesection.

If continued venesection is not acceptable or if the platelet count continues high (added risk of thrombosis) then:

Older patients: use radiophosphorus.

Younger patients: use cytotoxic chemotherapy with hydroxyurea or busulphan (see Ch. 37).

Radiophosphorus (^{32}P, sodium radiophosphate) is given i.v. Phosphorus is concentrated in bone and in cells that are dividing rapidly, so that the erythrocyte precursors in the bone marrow receive most of the β-irradiation when ^{32}P is given. The effects are similar to those of whole-body irradiation, and in polycythaemia vera ^{32}P is now a treatment of choice. The maximum effect on the blood count does not occur for 1–2 months after the dose; treatments at one year or less often give good control. Excessive depression of the bone marrow is the main adverse effect, but is seldom serious.

Secondary leukaemia occurs with both classes of therapy.

Pruritus is troublesome in polycythaemia vera; it may be helped by H_1- and H_2-histamine receptor blockers alone or together.

Hyperuricaemia occurs and is treated by allopurinol; and *iron* and *folate* deficiency by replacement doses.

Low dose aspirin (for antiplatelet action) may be used if the platelet count continues high or thrombosis occurs despite the above treatment.

APLASTIC ANAEMIA

Treatment will be chosen according to the cause (if known). Choices include bone marrow transplantation and immunosuppression, e.g. with antilymphocytic serum, corticosteroid and perhaps cyclosporin; and haemopoietic growth factors (above).

GUIDE TO FURTHER READING

Bates C J et al 1989 Vitamins, iron, and physical work. Lancet 2: 313

Beck W S 1988 Cobalamin and the nervous system. New England Journal of Medicine 318: 1753

Campbell N R C et al 1991 Iron supplements: a common cause of drug interactions. British Journal of Clinical Pharmacology 31: 251

Canadian Erythropoietin Study Group 1990 Association between recombinant human erythropoietin and quality of life and exercise capacity of patients receiving haemodialysis. British Medical Journal 300: 573

Castle W B 1966 Treatment of pernicious anaemia: historical aspects. Clinical Pharmacology and Therapeutics 7: 347

Controversies in therapeutics 1988 Iron and folate supplements during pregnancy. British Medical Journal
(i) Hibbard B M Supplementation is valuable only in selected patients. 297: 1324
(ii) Horn E Supplementing everyone treats those at risk and is cost effective. 297: 1325

Crosby W H 1977 Who needs iron? New England Journal of Medicine 297: 543

Editorial 1989 Oral iron chelators. Lancet 2: 1016

Ersley A J 1991 Erythropoietin. New England Journal of Medicine 324: 1399

Ferner R E et al 1989 Drugs in donated blood. Lancet 2: 93

Goodnough L T et al 1989 Increased preoperative collection of autologous blood with recombinant human erythropoietin therapy. New England Journal of Medicine 321: 1163

Khajwa A, Goldstone A H 1991 Haemopoietic growth factors. British Medical Journal 302: 1164

Metcalf D 1989 Haemopoietic growth factors. Lancet 1: 825, 885

MRC Vitamin study research group 1991 Prevention of neural tube defects: results of the Medical Research Council vitamin study. Lancet 338: 131, also Editorial 153 and subsequent correspondence 379

Respiratory system

COUGH

There are two sorts of cough: the useful and the useless. Cough is useful when it effectively expels secretions, exudates, transudates or extraneous material from respiratory tracts, i.e. when it is *productive*; it is useless when it is *unproductive*. Useful cough should be allowed to serve its purpose and suppressed only when it is exhausting the patient or is dangerous, e.g. after eye surgery. Useless cough should be stopped, or, if it is due to thick secretions that cannot be expelled, made useful if possible.

Clinical assessment of the frequency and intensity of cough of disease by objective recording via a microphone, allows assessment of antitussives despite the great spontaneous fluctuations. Such recording has shown patients' own reports of their cough to be too unreliable to provide valid drug comparisons. Placebo effects in cough are great.

Sites of action

Peripheral sites

On the *afferent side* of the cough reflex: by reducing input of stimuli from throat, larynx, trachea, e.g. a warm moist atmosphere, demulcents[1] in the pharynx.

---

[1] From Latin, *demulcere*: to caress soothingly.

On the *efferent side* of the cough reflex: measures to render secretions more easily removable (mucolytics, postural drainage) will reduce the amount of coughing needed, by increasing its efficiency.

The best antitussive is removal of the cause of the cough by, e.g. chemotherapy or surgery.

Central nervous system

Agents may act on the medullary paths of the cough reflex (opioids), on the cerebral cortex and on the subcortical paths (opioids and sedatives in general).

Cough is also under substantial voluntary control, as witness the increase during the louder passages of a winter orchestral concert. A good spouse with a cough may sleep better alone and free from fear of depriving an exhausted companion of sleep, whilst a child may cough less if in reassuring company in the parents' room. A cough can be induced by psychogenic factors (such as anxiety not to cough when it is socially disadvantageous to do so, e.g. during the quiet parts of a musical concert) and reduced by a placebo. Considerations such as these are relevant to practical therapeutics.

Cough suppression

Antitussives that act peripherally

The patient should stop smoking.

When the cough arises *above the larynx*, syrups and lozenges that glutinously and soothingly coat the pharynx (*demulcents*) may be used, e.g. Simple Linctus (mainly syrup; sugar). Small children are prone to swallow lozenges and so a confection on a stick may be preferred.

Linctuses are demulcent preparations that can be used alone and as vehicles of other antitussives. That their exact constitution is not critical was known and taught to medical students in 1896.

Many of you know that this (simple) linctus used to by very much thicker than it is now, and very likely the thicker linctus was more efficacious. The reason why it was made thinner was this. It was discovered

that a large number of children came to the surgery complaining of cough, and they were given the linctus, but instead of their using it as a medicine, they took it to an old woman out in Smithfield, who gave them each a penny, took their linctus, and made jam tarts with it.[2]

When cough arises *below the larynx* water aerosol inhalations and a warm environment often give relief. If it is wished to make the inhalation smell therapeutic, Compound Benzoin Tincture[3] may be added to the hot water. Benzoin inhalation may also promote secretion of dilute mucus and so help to give a protective coating to the inflamed mucous membrane. Menthol and eucalyptus provide similar therapeutic smell.

Intractable cough can be a severe problem in patients with bronchial carcinoma. Lignocaine administered by a nebuliser appears to control it effectively and delays the need to use sedative opioids such as diamorphine.

Antitussives that act on the central nervous system

In general, when it is desired to suppress cough, drugs that act on the pathways of the cough reflex in the medulla are used. Where these drugs are opioids then part of the effect may result from their actions on higher nervous centres as tranquillisers. The morphine-related antitussives are relatively non-addicting and have little depressant effect on the respiratory centre, though they may dry the mucosa and thicken the sputum. They include *codeine* and *pholcodine*.

It appears that as good results can be obtained with these as with more addicting substances, e.g. *morphine*, *diamorphine* and *methadone* which are powerful respiratory depressants. Linctuses of codeine, pholcodine and methadone are often used. Codeine needs to be given in high dose, say 60 mg, and a tablet is satisfactory. In bronchogenic carcinoma a Strong Pholcodeine

---

[2] Brunton L Lectures on the action of medicines. London: Macmillan. 1897.
[3] Friar's Balsam.

Linctus or even Diamorphine Linctus may be required to control cough. *Dextromethorphan* does not possess the CNS pharmacology of the opioids (though structurally related) and binds with high affinity and selectivity to medullary sites; it is widely used in over-the-counter antitussive preparations; overdose is antagonised by naloxone.

Sedation reduces cough. Antihistamines (H_1-receptor) with sedative and antimuscarinic actions, e.g. diphenhydramine, can also suppress cough by these (but not by antihistamine) actions; they may need to be given in doses which also cause drowsiness and thus they are usually combined with other drugs. A great many synthetic, centrally acting non-opioid antitussives have come and gone; patients will not suffer if the physician ignores these.

Mucolytics and expectorants

Normally about 100 ml of fluid is produced from the respiratory tract each day and most of it is swallowed. Respiratory mucus consists largely of water and its slimy character is due to glyco-proteins linked together by disulphide bonds to form polymers. In pathological states much more mucus may be produced, and also an exudate of plasma proteins which bond with glycoproteins and form larger polymers with the result that the mucus becomes more viscous. Patients with chest disease can have difficulty in clearing their chest of viscous sputum by cough because the bronchial cilia are rendered ineffective. They can be assisted by drugs that liquefy mucus.

Mucolytics

Acetylcysteine, carbocysteine and *methylcysteine* have free sulphydryl groups that open disulphide bonds in mucus and reduce its viscosity. They are given by inhalation (or instillation) and may be useful chiefly where particularly viscous secretion is a problem (cystic fibrosis, care of tracheostomies). Acetylcysteine may also be taken by mouth (swallowed) and achieves high concentration in the lung. Mucolytics may cause gastrointestinal irritation and allergic reaction.

Iodide stimulates the production of thin

Choice of drug therapy for cough

As always, it is necessary to have a clear idea of the underlying problem before starting to use drugs. For example, the approach to cough due to invasion of a bronchus by a neoplasm differs from that due to postnasal drip from chronic sinusitis or to that due to chronic bronchitis. The following are general recommendations.

- *For simple suppression of useless cough.* Codeine, pholcodine, dextromethorphan and methadone linctuses may be used in large, infrequent doses. In children, cough is nearly always useful and sedation at night is more effective to give rest than is codeine. Pertussis is an exception and sedation, codeine and atropine methonitrate may be tried.
- *To increase bronchial secretion slightly and to liquefy what is there.* Water aerosol with or without Menthol and Benzoin Inhalation, or Menthol and Eucalyptus Inhalation may provide comfort harmlessly.

Acetylcysteine or another mucolytic orally may be useful.

Preparations containing atropine are undesirable as muscarinic receptor block thickens bronchial secretion. Oxygen inhalation dries secretions, so rendering them even more viscous; oxygen must be bubbled through water and patients having oxygen may need measures to liquefy sputum.

- *For cough originating in the pharyngeal region.* Glutinous sweets or lozenges (demulcents), incorporating a cough suppressant or not, as appropriate, are used.

---

bronchial secretion by a direct action on secretory cells. It must generally be given to the limits of tolerance and so is not popular. Iodide has an unpleasant metallic taste and may cause painful swelling of the salivary and lachrymal glands after a few doses. With long-term treatment gastric intolerance or hypothyroidism may occur but these are largely avoided if treatment is intermittent. *Water inhalation* as an aerosol, though cheap, is not to be despised. Simply hydrating a dehydrated patient can have a beneficial effect in lowering sputum viscosity.

Expectorants

These are held to encourage productive cough by increasing the volume of bronchial secretion but may have no more than placebo value. The group includes iodide, chlorides, bicarbonates, acetates, squill, guaiphenesin, ipecacuanha, creosotes and volatile oils.

Cough mixtures

Every formulary is replete with combinations of antitussives, expectorants, mucolytics, bronchodilators and sedatives. Although choice is not critical, a knowledge of the active ingredients is useful, for some contain sedative antihistamines or ephedrine (which may antagonise antihypertensives).

RESPIRATORY STIMULANTS
(Analeptics)

The drugs used are central nervous system stimulants and the therapeutic dose is close to that which causes convulsions. Their use must therefore be carefully monitored.

Nikethamide causes an increase in the rate and depth of respiration by stimulating the medullary respiratory centres both directly and reflexly through the carotid body. It is less safe than doxapram.

Doxapram acts like nikethamide but has a larger margin between therapeutic and toxic doses. A continuous i.v. infusion of 1.5–4.0 mg/min is given according to the patient's response. Coughing and laryngospasm that develop after its use may represent a return of normal protective responses. The adverse effects include restlessness, twitching, itching, vomiting, flushing and cardiac dysrhythmias, and in addition it causes patients to experience a feeling of perineal warmth; in high doses the blood pressure is elevated.

Ethamivan is similar to nikethamide.

Aminophylline is a respiratory stimulant and may be infused slowly i.v. (500 mg in 6 h).

Acetazolamide (see also p. 468) promotes bicarbonate diuresis and metabolic acidosis which may be a useful stimulus to respiration during exacerbations of chronic obstructive lung disease or weaning from mechanical ventilation.

Uses

Respiratory stimulants have a place in some cases of acute ventilatory failure due to:

• acute exacerbations of chronic lung disease with hypercapnia, drowsiness and inability to cough or to tolerate low (24%) concentrations of inspired oxygen (air is 21% O_2). A respiratory stimulant can arouse the patient enough to allow effective physiotherapy and, by stimulating respiration, can improve ventilation-perfusion matching. As a short-term measure, this may obviate tracheal intubation and mechanical ventilation and 'buy time' for chemotherapy to control infection.

• apnoea in premature infants; aminophylline and caffeine may benefit some cases.

Avoid respiratory stimulants if possible in patients with epilepsy (risk of convulsions).

Contraindications include ischaemic heart disease, status asthmaticus, severe hypertension and thyrotoxicosis.

Irritant vapours, to be inhaled, have an analeptic effect in fainting, e.g. Aromatic Solution of Ammonia (Sal Volatile). No doubt they sometimes 'recall the exorbitant and deserting spirits to their proper stations.'[4]

PULMONARY SURFACTANT

The endogenous surfactant system produces stable low surface tension in the alveoli, preventing their collapse. Failure of production of natural surfactant occurs in respiratory distress syndrome (RDS), including that in the neonate. *Colfosceril palmitate* is a synthetic surfactant which, given endotracheally, coats the surface of

---

[4] Thomas Sydenham, 1624–89.

the alveoli and maintains their patency. Clinical trials indicate that it reduces deaths in neonatal RDS.

OXYGEN THERAPY

Oxygen used in therapy should be presented with the same care as any drug; there should be a well defined purpose and its effects should be monitored objectively.

The absolute indication to supplement inspired air is inadequate tissue oxygenation. As clinical signs may be imprecise, arterial blood gases should be measured whenever suspicion arises. Tissue hypoxia can be assumed when the PaO_2 falls below 6.7 kPa (50 mm Hg) in a previously normal acutely ill patient, e.g. with myocardial infarction, acute pulmonary disorder, drug over-dose, musculoskeletal or head trauma. Chronically hypoxic patients may maintain adequate tissue with a PaO_2 below 6.7 kPa by compensating through raised red cell mass and cerebral vasodilatation. Oxygen therapy is used as follows:

High concentration oxygen therapy is used where a low PaO_2 is associated with a normal or low $PaCO_2$, as in pulmonary embolism, pneumonia, pulmonary oedema. Here concentrations up to 60% may be used for short periods for there is little risk of inducing hypoventilation and CO_2 retention.

Low concentration oxygen therapy is reserved for patients with low PaO_2 and raised $PaCO_2$, notably those with chronic obstructive lung disease during an infective exacerbation. The normal stimulus to respiration is elevation of the $PaCO_2$ but this control is blunted in chronically hypercapnic patients whose respiratory drive comes from hypoxia. Elevating the PaO_2 in such patients by giving them high concentrations of oxygen, removes their stimulus to ventilate, exaggerates CO_2 retention and may cause fatal respiratory acidosis. The objective of therapy in such patients is to provide just enough oxygen to alleviate hypoxia without exaggerating the hypercapnia and respiratory acidosis; normally the inspired oxygen concentration should not exceed 28% and in some 24% may be sufficient.

Continuous long-term (domiciliary) oxygen therapy is given to patients with severe persistent hypoxaemia and cor pulmonale due to chronic bronchitis and emphysema. Either oxygen cylinders are delivered to the patients' homes or they are provided with an oxygen concentrator. Clinical trial evidence indicates that taking oxygen for more than 15 h per day improves survival.

HISTAMINE, ANTIHISTAMINES AND ALLERGIES

Histamine is a naturally-occurring amine that has long fascinated pharmacologists and physicians. It is found in most body tissue in an inactive bound form, often in mast cells, and pharmacologically active free histamine is released from cells in response to stimuli such as physical trauma or antigen-antibody reactions. Various chemicals can also cause release of histamine. The more powerful of these (proteolytic enzymes and snake venoms) have no place in therapeutics, but a number of useful drugs, such as tubocurarine, morphine and even some antihistamines, cause histamine release, although not usually enough to do more than transiently to lower blood pressure or cause a local reaction.

The *physiological functions* of histamine are suggested by its distribution in the body. In body epithelia (the alimentary canal, the respiratory tract and in the skin) it is released in response to invasion by foreign substances. In glands (gastric, intestinal, lachrymal, salivary) it mediates part of the normal secretory process. In most cells near blood vessels it plays a role in regulating the microcirculation.

Histamine acts as a local hormone (autacoid) similarly to serotonin or prostaglandins, i.e. it is a local chemical transmitter between the cell from which it is released and cells in the immediate vicinity. In the context of gastric secretion, for example, stimulation of receptors on the histamine-containing cell causes release of histamine which in turn acts on receptors on parietal cells which then secrete hydrogen ions (see Gastric secretion, Ch. 30).

Actions. The actions of histamine which are clinically important are those on:

Smooth muscle. In general, histamine causes smooth muscle to contract (excepting arterioles, but including the larger arteries). Stimulation of the pregnant human uterus is insignificant. A brisk attack of bronchospasm may be induced in subjects who have any allergy, particularly asthma, when it may occur even in the presence of an antihistamine.

Arterioles are dilated, with a consequent fall in blood pressure. The characteristic throbbing headache that occurs after histamine injections is due to stretching pain-sensitive structures in the dura mater by fluctuations in pressure in blood vessels and cerebrospinal fluid.

Capillaries dilate and their permeability to plasma increases, which responses comprise two parts (the flush and the wheal) of the triple response described by Thomas Lewis.[5] The third part, the flare, is arteriolar dilatation due to an axon reflex.

Skin. Histamine release in the skin can cause itch.

Gastric secretion. Histamine increases the acid and pepsin content of gastric juices. This effect is antagonised only trivially by atropine and not at all by H_1-receptor antihistamines. H_2-receptor antihistamines are highly effective.

As may be anticipated from the above actions, *anaphylactic shock,* which is largely due to histamine release, is characterised by circulatory collapse and bronchoconstriction. The most rapidly effective antidote is adrenaline (see below), and an antihistamine (H_1-receptor) may be given as well.

Metabolism and fate. Histamine is formed from the amino acid histidine and is inactivated by metabolism, largely by deamination and by methylation. In common with other local hormones, this process is extremely rapid.

Histamine antagonists

The effects of histamine can be *opposed* in three ways:

1. By using a drug with opposite effects, e.g. histamine constricts bronchi, causes vasodila-

tation and increases capillary permeability. Adrenaline opposes these effects by a mechanism unrelated to histamine. This is *physiological antagonism*.

2. By preventing histamine from reaching its site of action (receptors), e.g. *by competition*, the H_1- and H_2-receptor antagonists.

3. By preventing the release of histamine; adrenal steroids and sodium cromoglycate can suppress the effects on the tissues of antigen-antibody reactions.

Drugs that competitively block H_1-histamine receptors were the first to be introduced and are conventionally called the 'antihistamines'. They effectively inhibit the increased capillary permeability, flare and itch skin responses of histamine; they also partially prevent the vascular smooth muscle (blood pressure lowering) action but they have *no effect* on histamine-induced gastric secretion. Indeed, the standard method of testing a patient's capacity to secrete gastric acid used to be to inject histamine after first giving a large dose of a conventional (H_1-receptor) antihistamine to block the other undesired effects of the injection. Thus, if a group of drugs could block certain actions of histamine but had no effect on other actions, it was reasoned that there must be more than one kind of histamine receptor. This was the basis for the search for drugs that block histamine-induced gastric secretion (see Ch. 30) and its success established that there are at least two types of *histamine receptor*:

- H_1-*receptor*: mediates the oedema and vascular effects of histamine (see above).
- H_2-*receptor*: mediates the effect on gastric secretion.

Thus, histamine antagonists are classified:

H_1-receptor antagonists: see account below.

H_2-receptor antagonists: cimetidine, famotidine, nizatidine, ranitidine (see Ch. 30).

H_1-receptor antagonists

The term antihistamine is unsatisfactory, for the drugs have numerous other actions. This partly

---

[5] Lewis T et al. Heart 1924; 11: 209.

derives from the fact that there is a considerable similarity of structure amongst such local hormones as histamine, adrenaline, serotonin and acetylcholine. A compound which may block the action of one substance may also be capable of blocking the action of another. Thus, the H_1-antihistamines may also have antimuscarinic or sometimes α-adrenoceptor antagonist effects, and antimuscarinic drugs may exhibit some antihistaminic actions. Thus H_1-antihistamines are used as hypnotics, antitussives, expectorants, in motion sickness and in parkinsonism, all actions which are not evidently related to antihistaminic effect. These features are a disadvantage when H_1-antihistamines are used specifically to antagonise the effects of histamine, e.g. for allergies, but the introduction of drugs that are more selective H_1-antagonists and are largely free of antimuscarinic and sedative effects (see below) has been a useful advance. They can be discussed together.

Actions. H_1-antihistamines oppose, to varying degrees, the effects of liberated histamine, i.e. the oedema-producing and vascular effects. They are of negligible use in asthma, in which numerous mediators other than histamine are involved. Conventional H_1-antihistamines are *competitive*, *surmountable* inhibitors of the action of histamine except for astemizole (at therapeutic doses) and terfenadine (at very high doses) which dissociate very slowly from the receptor and exhibit unsurmountable antagonism (see p. 76). H_1-antihistamines are more effective if used *before* histamine has been liberated. Reversal of effects of histamine after it has been released is more readily achieved by *physiological* antagonism by adrenaline which should be used first in life-threatening allergic reactions.

The older H_1-antihistamines cause drowsiness and there is need to warn patients, e.g. about driving or operating machinery, and about additive effects with alcohol. Paradoxically, CNS stimulation may occur and absence epilepsy (petit mal) made worse. The newer H_1-antihistamines which penetrate the blood–brain barrier poorly are largely devoid of these effects. Antimuscarinic effects benefit parkinsonism and motion sickness.

Pharmacokinetics. H_1-antihistamines taken orally are readily absorbed. They are mainly metabolised in the liver. Enough may be excreted in the milk to cause sedation in infants. They are generally administered orally and can also be given i.m. or i.v.

Uses. The H_1-antihistamines are used for symptomatic relief of allergies such as hay fever and urticaria (see below). They are of broadly similar therapeutic efficacy.

Individual H_1-antihistamines

Non- (or less) sedative

These newer drugs are relatively selective for H_1-receptors and enter the brain less readily than do the earlier antihistamines. Differences lie principally in their duration of action.

Cetirizine ($t_{\frac{1}{2}}$ 7 h), *loratadine* ($t_{\frac{1}{2}}$ 15 h) and *terfenadine* ($t_{\frac{1}{2}}$ 20 h) are effective taken once daily and are suitable for general use. The choice may lie between cetirizine which is possibly more effective but may sedate some patients, and terfenadine which may be less effective.

Acrivastine ($t_{\frac{1}{2}}$ 2 h) must be given × 3/d and is best reserved for intermittent therapy, e.g. when breakthrough symptoms occur in a patient using topical therapy for hay fever.

Astemizole, has a slow onset of effect. Because of its long $t_{\frac{1}{2}}$ (5 days; 10 days for an active metabolite) it takes a longer time to reach steady state, and dose titration is more difficult than with short $t_{\frac{1}{2}}$ drugs.

Sedative

Mequitazine is less sedative than most members of this group.

Chlorpheniramine ($t_{\frac{1}{2}}$ 20 h) is effective when urticaria is prominent, and its sedative effect is then useful.

Diphenhydramine ($t_{\frac{1}{2}}$ 32 h) is strongly sedative and has antimuscarinic effects; it is also used in parkinsonism and motion sickness.

Promethazine ($t_{\frac{1}{2}}$ 12 h) is so strongly sedative that it is used as an hypnotic in adults and children. It may sedate the next day.

Azatadine, brompheniramine, clemastine, cyproheptadine, dimethindene, diphenylpyraline, mebhydrolin, oxatomide, phenindamine, pheniramine, trimeprazine and triprolidine are similar.

Adverse effects. Apart from sedation, these include: dizziness, fatigue, insomnia, nervousness, tremors, and antimuscarinic effects, e.g. dry mouth, blurred vision and gastrointestinal disturbance. Dermatitis and agranulocytosis can occur. Severe poisoning due to overdose results in coma and sometimes in convulsions.

Drug management of some allergic states

Histamine is released in many allergic states, but it is not the sole cause of symptoms, other chemical mediators, e.g. leukotrienes and prostaglandins, also being involved. Hence the usefulness of H_1-antihistamines in allergic states is variable, depending on the extent to which histamine, rather than other mediators, is the cause of the clinical manifestations.

Hay fever

If symptoms are limited to rhinitis, a *corticosteroid* (beclomethasone, betamethasone, budesonide or flunisolide), *ipratropium* or *sodium cromoglycate* applied topically as a spray or insufflation is often all that is required. Ocular symptoms alone respond well to sodium cromoglycate drops. When both nasal and ocular symptoms occur, or there is itching of the palate and ears as well, a systemic non-sedative H_1-antihistamine is indicated. *Sympathomimetic vasoconstrictors*, e.g. ephedrine, are immediately effective if applied topically, but rebound swelling of the nasal mucous membrane occurs when medication is stopped. Rarely, a *systemic corticosteroid*, e.g. prednisolone, is justified for a severely affected patient to provide relief for a short period, e.g. during academic examinations.

Urticaria, see p. 645.

Anaphylactic shock, see p. 125.

BRONCHIAL ASTHMA

Asthma affects 2–5% of the UK population.

Some useful pathophysiology

The bronchi become hyperreactive as a result of a persistent inflammatory process in response to a number of stimuli which include biological agents, e.g. allergens, viruses and environmental chemicals, e.g. ozone. Inflammatory mediators are liberated from mast cells, eosinophils, neutrophils, monocytes and macrophages. Some mediators such as histamine are preformed and their release causes an immediate bronchial reaction. Others are formed after activation of cells and produce more sustained bronchoconstriction; these include metabolites of arachidonic acid from both the cyclo-oxygenase, e.g. prostaglandin D_2, and lipoxygenase, i.e. leukotrienes, pathways. In addition platelet activating factor (PAF) is being increasingly recognised as an important mediator.

The relative importance of many of the mediators is not precisely defined but they interact to produce mucosal oedema, secretion of mucus which is hard to dislodge and damage to the ciliated epithelium. Breaching of the protective epithelial barrier allows hyperreactivity to be maintained by bronchoconstrictor substances or by local axon reflexes through exposed nerve fibres. Wheezing and breathlessness result. The bronchial changes also obstruct access of inhaled drug to the periphery, which is why they can fail to give full relief.

Early in an attack there is hyperventilation so that PaO_2 is maintained and $PaCO_2$ is lowered but with increasing airways obstruction the PaO_2 declines and $PaCO_2$ rises, signifying a serious asthmatic episode.

The mechanisms underlying late-onset and exercise-induced asthma are poorly understood.

Types of asthma

The following are recognised:

Asthma associated with specific allergic reactions

This *extrinsic* type is the commonest and occurs in patients who develop allergy to antigenic substances in the inspired air. In some (atopic) individuals, who have a special liability to develop allergy, the resulting reaction is of the immediate (type 1) type involving IgE antibodies; in other (non-atopic) people the reaction is delayed for some hours (type 3) and is associated with the production of precipitating antibodies. Avoidance of exposure to allergens is particularly relevant to managing this type of asthma.

Asthma not associated with known allergy

Some patients exhibit wheeze and breathlessness that is not attributable to any allergic reaction. They are considered to have *intrinsic* asthma and it follows that attempting to avoid an allergen has no place.

Exercise-induced asthma

Some patients develop wheeze that regularly follows within a few minutes of exercise; they should take a β-adrenoceptor agonist or sodium cromoglycate (see below) prior to the activity that provokes the asthma.

Asthma associated with chronic obstructive lung disease

A number of patients who have persistent airflow obstruction also exhibit considerable variation in airways resistance and are benefited by drugs used for asthma. It is important to recognise the association and to test their responses to bronchodilators or corticosteroids.

Approaches to treatment

With the foregoing discussion in mind, the following approaches to treatment are logical:

- Prevention of exposure to antigen(s)
- Reduction of the bronchial inflammation and hyperreactivity
- Dilatation of narrowed bronchi.

These objectives may be achieved as follows:

Prevention of exposure to antigen(s)

This approach is appropriate for extrinsic asthmatics. Identifying an antigen may be aided by the patient's history (wheezing in response to contact with grasses, pollens, animals), by skin prick or by intradermal injection of selected antigens or by demonstrating antibodies in the patient's serum. Avoiding an allergen may be practicable when it is related to some special situation, e.g. occupation, but is not feasible if it is widespread, as with house-dust mite. Hyposensitisation is an option for insect venoms and grass pollens but should be undertaken only where facilities for cardiopulmonary resuscitation are immediately available.

Reduction of the bronchial inflammation and hyperreactivity

As persistent inflammation is central to bronchial hyperreactivity, the use of anti-inflammatory drugs is sensible.

1. Corticosteroids bring about a gradual reduction in bronchial hyperreactivity. The exact mechanisms of this action are disputed but they probably include: inhibition of the influx of inflammatory cells into the lung that follows exposure to an allergen; inhibition of the release of mediators from macrophages and eosinophils and reduction of the microvascular leakage which these mediators cause. Some of the actions of corticosteroids may be mediated by their induction of the formation of lipocortin, a protein which inhibits phospholipase A, the enzyme that is responsible for generating arachidonic acid and which in turn gives rise to prostaglandins, leukotrienes and platelet activating factor. Corticosteroids used in asthma include *prednisolone, beclomethasone, betamethasone* and *budesonide*, see Chapter 33.

*2. **Sodium cromoglycate*** (cromolyn, Intal) impairs the immediate response to allergen and was formerly thought to act by inhibiting the release of mediators from mast cells. Evidence now suggests that the late allergic response and bronchial hyperreactivity are also inhibited, and points to effects of cromoglycate on other inflammatory cells and also on local axon reflexes.

Cromoglycate is poorly absorbed from the gastrointestinal tract but is well absorbed from the lung, which is fortunate so that it can be given by inhalation; it is eliminated unchanged in the urine and bile.

Since it does not antagonise the broncho-constrictor effect of the active substances after they have been released, cromoglycate is *not* effective at terminating an existing attack, i.e. it *prevents bronchoconstriction* as opposed to inducing bronchodilatation.

Sodium cromoglycate is chiefly of value in *extrinsic* (allergic) asthma including asthma in children, and in those whose asthma is made worse by exercise. The benefit may be delayed by several weeks. It may reduce the need to use oral adrenocortical steroid in some patients and allows a lower dose to be used (steroid sparing effect).

The drug may be inhaled as an aerosol, as a powder (using a special insufflator) or as a nebulised solution. Special formulations are used for *allergic rhinitis* (Rynacrom) and *allergic conjunctivitis* (Opticrom). Sodium cromoglycate may also be used (as Nalcrom) by mouth for food allergy, in association with avoidance of known allergens.

It is remarkably non-toxic. Apart from cough and bronchospasm induced by the powder it may rarely cause allergic reactions. Application to the eye may produce a local stinging sensation and the oral form may cause nausea.

Nedocromil sodium is structurally unrelated to cromoglycate but has a similar profile of actions.

*3. **Other drugs***. *Ketotifen* is a histamine H_1-receptor blocker which may also have some antiasthma effects but its benefit has not been conclusively demonstrated. In common with other antihistamines it causes drowsiness.

Dilatation of narrowed bronchi by physiological antagonism of bronchial muscle contraction

*1. **Beta$_2$-adrenoceptor agonists***. These are drugs of choice because the adrenoceptors in bronchi are mainly β_2 type and their stimulation causes bronchial muscle to relax. They include: salbutamol, salmeterol (slow onset, long action) terbutaline, fenoterol, pirbuterol, reproterol and rimiterol, and are discussed in Chapter 22. Less selective adrenoceptor agonists such as adrenaline, ephedrine, isoetharine, isoprenaline and orciprenaline are less safe, being more likely to cause cardiac dysrhythmias. Alpha-adrenoceptor activity contributes to bronchoconstriction but α-adrenoceptor antagonists have not proved effective.

*2. **Xanthines*** include *theophylline, aminophylline* and *choline theophyllinate*. An account of theophylline will suffice.

Theophylline relaxes bronchial muscle. Its mode of action is not understood with certainty but probably involves competitive inhibition of adenosine receptors, for theophylline is structurally similar to adenosine and blocks many of its biological actions at concentrations with the therapeutic range. Adenosine can cause bronchoconstriction in asthmatics. Formerly theophylline was thought to act by inhibiting phosphodiesterase, the enzyme that metabolises cyclic-AMP, but this effect is negligible at therapeutic concentrations. Xanthines have also been found to improve diaphragmatic contraction, which may be relevant to their role in respiratory disease.

Other actions of theophylline are to increase the rate and force of cardiac contraction, and to raise the rate of urine production.

Absorption of theophylline from the gastrointestinal tract is usually rapid and complete. It is widely distributed and 90% is metabolised by the liver; there is evidence that the process is saturable at therapeutic doses. The $t_{\frac{1}{2}}$ is 8 h, with particular variation, and it is prolonged in patients with severe cardiopulmonary disease and cirrhosis. Obesity and prematurity are associated with reduced rates of elimination, whereas smoking tobacco or cannabis enhances theophylline clearance by inducing hepatic enzymes. Attention to these factors may explain lack of responsiveness or adverse reactions to theophylline. Best therapeutic results are obtained when the plasma concentration is 10–20 mg/l (55–110 μmol/l). Theophylline is relatively insoluble and commercial preparations increase its solubility or duration of action. *Aminophylline* is a mixture of theophylline with ethylenediamine which is sufficiently soluble for i.v. use; there are numerous slow-release oral forms. Theophylline is used for both chronic asthma (by mouth) and status asthmaticus (i.v.); a suppository at night may be effective for those whose asthma is especially worse in the early morning ('morning dippers'). It is also used in the emergency treatment of left ventricular failure.

At high therapeutic doses some patients experience nausea and diarrhoea and when the plasma concentration exceeds the recommended range there is danger of cardiac dysrhythmia and epileptic seizures. The latter are prone to occur with rapid intravenous injection, which exposes the heart and brain to high concentrations before distribution is complete. It follows that i.v. injection must be slow (5 mg/kg over 20 min) and reduced i.v. dose *must* be given to any patient who is already taking a xanthine preparation (*always enquire about this before injecting*). Enzyme inhibition by erythromycin, ciprofloxacin, allopurinol or oral contraceptives increases the plasma concentration of theophylline; enzyme inducers such as carbamazepine, phenobarbitone and phenytoin reduce the concentration.

Overdose with theophylline has assumed greater importance with the advent of sustained-release preparations which prolong toxic effects, with peak plasma concentrations being reached 12–24 h after ingestion. Vomiting may be severe but the chief dangers are cardiac dysrhythmia, hypotension, hypokalaemia and seizures. After gastric lavage, activated charcoal should be given every 2–4 h until the plasma concentration is below 20 mg/l. Potassium replacement is important to prevent dysrhythmias. Diazepam is used to control convulsions.

3. Antimuscarinic bronchodilators competitively inhibit the postsynaptic receptor action of acetylcholine at vagal nerve endings to constrict bronchial smooth muscle. Atropine has been used thus but has largely been replaced for asthma by ipratropium.

Ipratropium is a synthetic analogue of atropine but, unlike the latter, is negligibly absorbed after inhalation. It acts non-selectively on the various subtypes of muscarinic receptor in the lung to inhibit cholinergic activation of airway smooth muscle and thereby to cause bronchodilation. Tolerance to its action does not appear to develop. Ipratropium is a less effective bronchodilator than are the β-adrenoceptor agonists in asthma, but it is a useful adjunct to these agents. It does, however, benefit some, notably older, patients with intrinsic asthma and chronic bronchitis. It is administered by aerosol and by nebuliser.

Inhalation of drugs for asthma

The inhalational route has been developed to advantage because the undesirable effects of systemic administration are reduced by the smaller doses that are needed. Drugs intended to be inhaled must first be converted into particulate form and the optimum *particle size* to reach and be deposited in the small bronchi is 2 μm. An *aerosol* consists of particles dispersed in a gas and may be produced as follows:

Pressurised aerosol. Drug is dissolved in a low boiling point liquid (usually one or more fluorocarbons) in a canister under pressure; when the valve is opened, a metered dose of liquid is ejected into the atmosphere, the carrier liquid evaporates instantly leaving an aerosol of the drug and is inhaled. Coordinating the act of opening the valve with that of inhalation can be difficult, especially for the young and the elderly; the problem can be overcome by interposing between the aerosol source and the patient's mouth, an extension tube (*spacer*) which prevents dispersion of the aerosol before the patient inhales.

Nebulisers convert a solution or suspension of drug into an aerosol. *Jet* nebulisers require a driving gas, usually air from a compressor unit for home use, or oxygen in hospital; the solution in the nebulising chamber is broken into droplets by the jet and the larger droplets are filtered off leaving the smaller ones to be inhaled. *Ultrasonic nebulisers* convert a solution into particles of uniform size by vibrations created by a piezo electric crystal.[6] With either method the nebulised solution is delivered to the patient by a mouthpiece or facemask, so no coordination is called for, and the dose can be altered by changing the strength of the solution. Much larger doses can be administered by nebuliser than by pressurised aerosol.

Dry powder inhalers. The drug is formulated as a micronised powder and placed in a device, e.g. a Spinhaler, from which it is inhaled. Some patients can use these when they fail with metered dose aerosols. Inhalation of powder can cause transient bronchoconstriction.

Drug treatment of asthma

This varies with the severity and type of asthma. It is a general rule that the effectiveness of changes in drug and dose should be monitored by serial measurements of the simpler respiratory function tests such as peak expiratory flow rate or forced vital capacity. Neither the patients' feelings nor ordinary physical examination are alone sufficient to determine whether there is still room for improvement. When an asthmatic attack is severe, arterial blood gases should be monitored.

Constant and intermittent asthma

A β-adrenoceptor agonist should be given by metered dose aerosol and dosing adjusted to the patients' symptoms. Salbutamol is suitable and the other $β_2$-adrenoceptor agonists referred to above; their effect is immediate. The usual dose is 1–2 puffs 4–8 hourly. The patient should be carefully instructed how to use the inhaler when treatment is begun, since failure to benefit is often due to improper use; time spent on this is never wasted. An oral β-adrenoceptor agonist can be used, e.g. salbutamol 4 mg, 3–4 times daily, but this route is more likely to give rise to tremor

---

[6] Converts electricity into mechanical vibration.

and headache. Salmeterol is slow in onset and acts for about 12 h. It is thus unsuitable for relief of acute attacks of asthma and, until its role is better defined, is best reserved to provide background bronchodilation for those patients who are already receiving high dose inhaled corticosteroid (see below).

If attacks recur, *sodium cromoglycate* or *nedocromil sodium* should be added and continued for about 4 weeks properly to assess benefit. They are most likely to prevent attacks in extrinsic asthmatics, especially children, but may be helpful in other forms.

Ipratropium by metered dose aerosol, 1–2 puffs 3–4 times daily, may benefit some asthmatics, especially elderly intrinsic asthmatics who may also have chronic bronchitis.

For the patient who fails to improve on sodium cromoglycate an inhaled *corticosteroid* by metered dose aerosol may control symptoms. Since the drug is delivered directly to the site of action, only a fraction of the oral dose is used (50–250 μg per puff). Furthermore 90% of the inhaled dose is either exhaled or is swallowed and then both poorly absorbed from the gut and rapidly metabolised in the hepatic first pass. Although reduced hypothalamic-pituitary-adrenal responsiveness has been demonstrated with inhaled steroid, it is not ordinarily a clinical problem. Dysphonia and candidiasis of the mouth and throat can develop in a minority of cases; the latter is readily treated with nystatin mouthwashes or amphotericin lozenges without interrupting asthma therapy. Washing out the mouth with water after each inhalation reduces the chance of recurrence. Beclomethasone diproprionate (50 μg/metered inhalation, 100 μg × 3 or 4/d), betamethasone valerate (100 μg/metered inhalation, 200 μg × 4/d) or budesonide (200 μg/ metered inhalation, 200μg × 2/d) are used and adjusted to the minimum effective dose. They are about as effective as prednisolone 5–10 mg by mouth.

To abort exacerbations, a β-receptor agonist aerosol, e.g. salbutamol, may be sufficient.

For more severe relapses, short courses of oral corticosteroid may be used, thus:
days 1 and 2, prednisolone 20 mg a day;

days 3 and 4, 15 mg a day;
days 5 and 6, 10 mg a day;
day 7, 5 mg.

Such use does not cause withdrawal problems (Ch. 33).

Chest infections will increase reversible airways-resistance and should be treated vigorously. The requirement of β_2-receptor agonist may increase.

Severe chronic asthma

Additions to therapy should be made sequentially with objective assessment, e.g. by peak expiratory flow rate, so than only treatments that are beneficial are continued. These are likely to include a check of the inhaler technique, a trial of sodium cromoglycate, of ipratropium and of theophylline. It is likely that higher doses of a β_2-adrenoceptor agonist will be required, possibly given by nebuliser at home.

Long-term *oral* therapy with *adrenal steroid* is used only when all else has failed in patients who relapse repeatedly into status asthmaticus or who are too disabled to lead a reasonably normal working life. This is more often the case with intrinsic asthma. Therapy may begin with prednisolone, say 40 mg/d total, reducing it as soon as feasible to a maintenance dose of 10 mg/d, which is generally well tolerated. If relapses occur, as they may, the dose may be increased to 30 mg for one day, after which it is reduced by 5 mg a day until the maintenance dose is re-established. Adrenal suppresion may be minimised by giving the corticosteroid as a single dose in the early morning when endogenous cortisol is at its peak and there is less negative feedback effect on the hypothalamic-pituitary-adrenal system. Although the $t_{\frac{1}{2}}$ of prednisolone is 3 h, once daily administration is reasonable as the *biological* effect $t_{\frac{1}{2}}$ is 18–36 h.

Patients taking long-term systemic (oral) adrenal steroid therapy should also use an inhaled steroid. The reason for this is that the inhaled steroid may allow the dose of oral (systemic) steroid to be lower than it otherwise would be, and so contribute to reducing the incidence of adverse effects of long-term systemic adrenal steroid therapy.

If systemic adrenal steroid therapy has lasted more than 6 months, great caution is required during withdrawal, because of a risk of catastrophic relapse.

Status asthmaticus

This a medical emergency requiring early vigorous treatment, for the bronchi may become refractory to β-receptor agonists (refractory to one means refractory to all) after about 36 h, perhaps the result of respiratory acidosis. In addition, drugs given by metered dose aerosol may fail to reach bronchi narrowed and blocked by mucus plugs. Proceed as follows:

• *Salbutamol* should be given by nebuliser in a dose of 2.5–5 mg over about 3 min, repeated in 15 min. Alternatively salbutamol 500 μg may be given i.m. and repeated every 4 h, or salbutamol 250 μg may be injected slowly i.v. and continued by i.v. infusion commencing at 5 μg/min and adjusted according to response. Nebulised salbutamol is usually preferred.

If this is insufficient, *ipratropium* by nebuliser may usefully be added and/or *aminophylline* i.v. Infusions of aminophylline or salbutamol may continue for 1–2 days.

• There should be no hesitation in using an adrenal steroid at the outset. *Hydrocortisone* 200 mg is given i.v. initially, and repeated 4-hourly or according to response which may not be seen for several hours. Hydrocortisone acts slightly quicker than prednisolone and the parenteral route is preferred at the outset because delayed gastric emptying may render oral administration unreliable. Once there is a response, prednisolone 15 mg 6-hourly by mouth may be used instead; this high dose may be needed for 24–48 h after which it can be reduced rapidly.

• Oxygen should be given to relieve the distress of dyspnoea (*humidified*, to help liquefy mucus). CO_2 narcosis is rare in asthma but it is generally preferable to start with O_2 28% and to check that the $PaCO_2$ has not risen before delivering O_2 35%.

Secretion of tenacious bronchial mucus adds

significantly to the respiratory obstruction; dehydration (which is usual) thickens mucus and should be remedied by i.v. fluid. Antimuscarinics reduce, but thicken, secretion. Infection should be treated with a broad-spectrum antimicrobial such as amoxycillin if suspected. Severe cases may need assisted respiration or bronchial lavage.

Warnings

Asthma may be precipitated by β-adrenoceptor block and the use of β-adrenoceptor antagonists should be avoided altogether in patients with a history of asthma; *fatal asthma has been precipitated by β-blocker eye-drops.*

Overuse of β-adrenergic agonists is dangerous. In the mid-1960s, there was an epidemic of sudden deaths in young asthmatics outside hospital. It was associated with the introduction of high-dose, metered aerosol of isoprenaline ($\beta_1 + \beta_2$ agonist); it did not occur in countries where the high concentration was not marketed.[7] The epidemic declined in Britain when the profession was warned, and the aerosols were restricted to prescription only. Though the relation between the use of β-receptor agonists and death is presumed to be causal, the actual mechanism of death is uncertain; overdose causing cardiac dysrhythmia is not the sole factor. The subsequent development of selective β_2-receptor agonists was a contribution to safety but a review in New Zealand during 1981–3 found that the use of fenoterol (β_2-selective) by metered dose inhalation was associated with increased risk of death in severe asthma[8] and the matter remains controversial.

Sedation in severe asthma. These patients are hypoxic whilst exerting maximum respiratory effort so that any diminution of respiratory drive due to depression of the respiratory centre may lead to serious underventilation. *Opioids (morphine)* are obviously contraindicated; even a small dose may stop breathing altogether.

[7] Stolley P D. Am Rev Resp Dis 1972; 105: 883.
[8] Crane J et al. Lancet 1989; 1: 917 and subsequent correspondence.

The least dangerous sedatives and hypnotics are probably diazepam, chloral derivatives, chlorpromazine and promethazine. But any sedation that will ensure sleep in a severe asthmatic may adversely effect the respiratory drive and useful cough.

GUIDE TO FURTHER READING

Avery M E, Merritt T A 1991 Surfactant-replacement therapy. New England Journal of Medicine 324: 910

Ayres J G 1990 Late onset asthma. British Medical Journal 300: 1602

Barnes P J 1989 A new approach to the treatment of asthma. New England Journal of Medicine 321: 1517

Barnes P J, Fan Chung K 1989 Difficult asthma. British Medical Journal 299: 695

British Thoracic Society (and others) 1990 Guidelines for the management of asthma in adults: 1 — chronic persistent asthma. British Medical Journal 301: 651

Cott G R, Cherniack R M 1988 Steroids and 'steroid-sparing' agents in asthma. New England Journal of Medicine 318: 634

Drazen J M, Gerard C 1989 Reversing the irreversible. New England Journal of Medicine 320: 155

Editorial 1989 PAF antagonists in asthma. Lancet 1: 592

Gross N J 1988 Ipratropium bromide. New England Journal of Medicine 319: 486

McFadden E R 1987 Exercise and asthma. New England Journal of Medicine 317: 502

Rees J 1991 Beta2 agonists and asthma. British Medical Journal 302: 1166

Shiner R J, Geddes D M 1989 Treating patients with asthma who are dependent on systemic steroids. British Medical Journal 299: 216

Stead R J, Cooke N J 1989 Adverse effects of inhaled corticosteroids. British Medical Journal 298: 403

Gastrointestinal system I: stomach and oesophagus

DRUGS FOR PEPTIC ULCER

Peptic ulcer kills few patients but troubles many. Ulcers may be transient, recurrent or chronic, and drug therapy is valuable for the relief of symptoms and to aid healing.

Some pathophysiology

The concept of a balance between the aggressive capacities of acid plus pepsin and the defensive mechanisms of the mucosa is useful. An ulcer is thought to develop when the equilibrium is disturbed either by enhanced aggressiveness or by lessened mucosal resistance.

On average, patients with duodenal ulcer produce about twice as much HCl as normal subjects, but there is much overlap and about half the patients with duodenal ulcer have acid outputs on the normal range. Patients with gastric ulcer produce normal or reduced amounts of acid.

The factors that protect the mucosa comprise: its impermeability to H^+ ion (the mucosal 'barrier' to H^+), its ability to secrete mucus and bicarbonate ion, its blood flow and its capacity rapidly to replace damaged epithelial cells; endogenous prostaglandins are probably involved in all these mechanisms.

Use of nonsteroidal anti-inflammatory drugs, cigarette smoking, the presence of *Helicobacter pylori* in the stomach and heredity (male sex, blood group O) influence the equilibrium unfavourably and are associated with increased incidence of peptic ulcer.

In general terms, duodenal ulcer is caused by an excess of the aggressive action of acid plus pepsin while defective mucosal resistance plays a more important part in gastric ulcer. Reduction of acid secretion is beneficial for both conditions.

Drugs can alter the balance towards healing and prevention of recurrence of **ulcer** in the following ways:

● Reduction of acid secretion by:
histamine H_2-receptor antagonists, e.g. ranitidine, cimetidine, famotidine and nizatidine proton pump inhibitors, e.g. omeprazole antimuscarinic drugs, e.g. pirenzepine

● Neutralisation of secreted acid by:
antacids, e.g. magnesium trisilicate, aluminium hydroxide

● Enhancement of mucosal resistance by various mechanisms:
e.g. bismuth compounds, sucralfate, prostaglandins, carbenoxolone.

The use of drugs should be seen against the background that many ulcers heal spontaneously by cessation of smoking. Medicines are justified partly because they accelerate healing with reduced risk of complications and quicker relief of symptoms, and partly because they heal some ulcers which otherwise would not heal.

REDUCTION OF ACID SECRETION
Histamine H_2-receptor antagonists

A general account of the pharmacology of histamine appears in Chapter 29. Clinically, the most important histamine H_2-receptors are those on the gastric parietal (acid secreting) cells. Numerous factors influence acid secretion by the stomach, including food, psychological conditioning and drugs. Their effects are mediated at the parietal cells by the transmitter substances histamine, gastrin, and acetylcholine which, through

a common path involving cyclic AMP and calcium ions, interact with the gastric proton pump (see p. 519) that is ultimately responsible for secreting acid into the lumen of the stomach. Histamine, however, appears to be necessary for the action of gastrin and acetylcholine, and histamine H_2-receptor antagonists inhibit acid secretion induced by these agents also; it is no surprise that histamine H_2-receptor blockade has become clinically important.

Cimetidine

Cimetidine, the first clinically important histamine H_2-receptor antagonist, is described fully and the others in so far as they differ. Cimetidine inhibits gastric secretion stimulated by injected histamine, by insulin, caffeine, protein-rich meals and (cholinergic) muscarinic drugs. All phases of gastric secretion are reduced namely, fasting and nocturnal (completely), and food-stimulated (by about 70%) by a therapeutic daily dose. Both the volume and the hydrogen ion concentration of gastric juice are reduced. Although the concentration of pepsin is not reduced, the total amount secreted falls because the volume of gastric juice is less. Parietal cells secrete intrinsic factor as well as hydrogen ions but in normal doses cimetidine does not have a sufficient effect on vitamin B_{12} turnover to lead to haematological or neurological complications. Cimetidine does not affect gastric emptying, unlike antimuscarinic drugs which delay it.

Pharmacokinetics. Cimetidine is readily absorbed from the upper small gut. The $t_{\frac{1}{2}}$ is 2 h and 60% of an oral dose is recovered as unchanged drug in the urine, the remainder appearing as metabolites. Total absorption of cimetidine is unimpaired if it is taken with food although peak blood concentrations are lower.

Uses. Cimetidine is used for conditions in which reduction of gastric secretion is beneficial. These are in the main, *duodenal ulcer, benign gastric ulcer, stomal ulcer and reflux oesophagitis.* When treating a gastric ulcer, it is desirable to confirm that it is benign by endoscopy and biopsy every 6–8 weeks until it is healed, for the symptoms of *gastric carcinoma* can be relieved by cimetidine, so that apparently successful treatment may fatally delay the correct diagnosis.

Cimetidine is also used for prophylaxis of *gastrointestinal bleeding* due to *gastric erosions* complicating the stress of such serious conditions as burns, fulminant hepatic failure, renal, failure or trauma. This success contrasts with acute bleeding in patients with peptic ulcer, oesophagitis or Mallory–Weiss syndrome (laceration of oesophagogastric junction) in which there may be erosion or trauma to larger blood vessels, and in which clinical trials have failed consistently to show benefit.

Other uses. Cimetidine is given *before anaesthesia for emergency surgery* and *before labour* to lessen the risk of aspirating gastric acid. The drug is also used to prevent peptic ulcer induced by NSAIDs in high-risk patients, e.g. elderly women and those with a previous history of ulceration, although conclusive evidence of benefit is lacking. In *chronic pancreatic insufficiency* oral enzyme supplements may fail to reach the duodenum in sufficient amount since they are destroyed by acid in the stomach; steatorrhoea and weight loss may be prevented if cimetidine is taken with the enzyme preparations.

Dose. Cimetidine 400 mg × 2/day, with breakfast and at bedtime is usually satisfactory for peptic ulcer. Alternatively, patients with duodenal ulcer who normally have a high nocturnal acid secretion, may receive 800 mg as a single dose at bedtime. Most patients become symptom-free in about 8 days but treatment should continue for 6–8 weeks, after which 85–90% of duodenal and 60% of gastric ulcers can be expected to heal; this is *about double the spontaneous healing rate*. Maintenance dose: 400 mg × 2/d or 400 mg at night. The dose should be reduced when renal or hepatic function are significantly impaired.

Adverse effects and drug interactions are few in short-term use. Minor complaints include headache, dizziness, constipation, diarrhoea, tiredness, and muscular pain. Bradycardia and cardiac conduction defects may also occur. Cimetidine is a weak antiandrogen, and may cause gynaecomastia and sexual dysfunction in males. In the elderly particularly, it may cause CNS disturbances including lethargy, confusion

and hallucinations. Cimetidine is an inhibitor of hepatic drug oxidising enzymes and raised plasma concentrations with enhanced activity of warfarin, phenytoin, lignocaine, propranolol and theophylline result when these drugs are administered with it. Indeed when cimetidine is given there is a potential for increased effect with any drug with a low therapeutic index that is inactivated by oxidation in the liver.

Ranitidine, famotidine, nizatidine

These histamine H_2-receptor antagonists have actions, uses and therapeutic efficacy that are essentially those of cimetidine. Differences from cimetidine lie chiefly in dose and profile of unwanted effects.

Pharmacokinetics. Ranitidine ($t_{\frac{1}{2}}$ 2 h) is 50%, famotidine ($t_{\frac{1}{2}}$ 3 h) is 25% and nizatidine ($t_{\frac{1}{2}}$ 1.3 h) is 10% metabolised, in each case the remainder being excreted unchanged via the kidney.

Dose. Ranitidine 150 mg × 2/day taken in the morning and in the evening will usually suffice; a single dose of 300 mg at night may be used as an alternative for duodenal ulcer. A course should last at least 4 weeks and ulcers that have not healed at this stage are normally healed by a further 4 weeks of therapy. Those with a history of recurrent ulcer may benefit from a maintenance dose of 150 mg nightly.

Adverse effects. The drugs are well tolerated but headache, dizziness, reversible confusion, constipation and diarrhoea may occur. In addition, weakness, myalgia, sleepiness, abnormal dreams, rhinitis and pruritis are reported with nizatidine. The drugs do not inhibit hepatic microsomal enzymes and drug interactions reported with cimetidine are not to be anticipated. Ranitidine and famotidine do not block androgen receptors and do not cause gynaecomastia and impotence, like cimetidine.

Proton pump inhibitors

Drugs of this class reduce gastric acid secretion not by blocking histamine-H_2 or muscarinic receptors, but by inhibiting the action of

H^+K^+-ATPase, an enzyme that occurs almost exclusively in the gastric parietal cell. The enzyme catalyses the exchange of protons (H^+) for potassium ions at the cell membrane, i.e. the final step in the acid secretory process, sometimes called the proton pump. Therefore they antagonise all stimulants of gastric secretion.

Omeprazole

Omeprazole produces a profound and long-lasting inhibition of both basal and stimulated acid secretion, a single 20 mg dose decreasing acidity by 90% over 24 h. Omeprazole must be given in enteric-coated granules for it is degraded at low pH, and it is absorbed in the small intestine. It is rapidly metabolised and indeed it is a metabolite that specifically and irreversibly inhibits the enzyme, i.e. omeprazole is a prodrug. Systemic availability increases with dose, probably because of saturation of first-pass effect; the $t_{\frac{1}{2}}$ is 1 h.

Uses. Omeprazole is highly effective for ulcerative reflux oesophagitis and is the drug of choice for Zollinger–Ellison syndrome (gastrin-producing tumour of the pancreas, causing hypersecretion of gastric acid and severe peptic ulceration). Although it heals peptic ulcers at least as well as histamine H_2-receptor antagonists, it is not first option as there are concerns about the safety of widespread and long-term use (below). Omeprazole, however, should be considered for resistant ulcers including those related to therapy with NSAIDs.

Adverse effects. Nausea, headache, diarrhoea, constipation and rash occur but are uncommon.

Concern has arisen that long-term use of highly effective antisecretory drugs may increase the risk of gastric neoplasia. Differing mechanisms have been proposed. When acid secretion is suppressed, gastrin is released as a normal homoeostatic response. Gastrin stimulates the growth of the gastric epithelium, including the enterochromaffin cells which transform into carcinoid tumours; some rats developed these tumours after prolonged and high dose exposure to omeprazole. Alternatively, prolonged hypochlorhydria favours the colonisation of the stomach by bacteria which have the potential to convert ingested nitrates into carcinogenic nitrosamines.

Surveillance studies to date have not provided evidence that this is a real hazard, and it is certainly unlikely with short-term use.

Antimuscarinic drugs

A general account appears in Chapter 21. Despite expectations, based on theoretical considerations of the importance of the parasympathetic autonomic system in gastric secretion, drugs with *general* antimuscarinic activity have not proved successful in the therapy of peptic ulcer, because of the unwanted effects of general antimuscarinic blockade, i.e. atropine-like effects.

Pirenzepine

Pirenzepine inhibits gastric secretion at doses lower than those that affect gastrointestinal motility, ocular, salivary, urinary and central nervous function. It owes this relative selectivity to its high affinity for and blockade of M_1-muscarinic receptors in autonomic ganglia; it has low affinity for the M_2-receptors of the smooth muscle of the ileum and urinary bladder. In the stomach pirenzepine appears to inhibit transmission in parasympathetic enteric ganglia.

Pirenzepine is poorly absorbed from the gastrointestinal tract and it is excreted mainly unchanged in the urine and bile. The $t_{\frac{1}{2}}$ is 11 h.

Uses. It is used for duodenal and gastric ulcer. Treatment should continue for 4–6 weeks but up to 3 months may be needed for resistant cases.

Adverse effects include dry mouth, difficulty in visual accommodation, constipation, diarrhoea and headache but it is generally well tolerated.

NEUTRALISATION OF SECRETED ACID

Antacids are basic substances that reduce gastric acidity by neutralising HCl. The *hydroxide* is the most common base but *trisilicate*, *carbonate* and *bicarbonate* ions are also used. The therapeutic efficacy and adverse effects depend also on the metallic ion with which the base is combined, and this is usually *aluminium, magnesium* or *sodium*. Calcium and bismuth have largely been abandoned for this purpose because they caused systemic toxicity.

The benefit of antacids depends on protecting the gastric mucosa from acid (by neutralisation) and from pepsin (which is inactive above pH 5, and which in addition is inactivated by aluminium and magnesium). Continuous elevation of pH by intermittent administration is limited by gastric emptying. The significant fact is that however large or small the gastric contents, if it is liquid, half will have left in about 30 minutes.

Antacids, therefore, are generally used to relieve symptoms of ulcer and non-ulcer dyspepsia and they are taken when symptoms occur, i.e. intermittently. Histamine H_2-receptor antagonists are normally preferred as ulcer-healing agents but an antacid may be taken for occasional symptomatic relief, especially during the first few days of a course of treatment with an H_2-receptor blocker.

Large amounts of a liquid magnesium-aluminium hydroxide mixture (equivalent to 1008 mmol of neutralising capacity per day) can accelerate duodenal ulcer healing with minimal adverse effects but compliance with the regimen which requires taking 30 ml × 7/day overtaxes the diligence of most patients.

Individual antacids

Magnesium oxide and hydroxide react quickly, but cause diarrhoea, as do all magnesium salts, which are also used as purgatives.

Magnesium carbonate is rather less effective.

Magnesium trisilicate reacts slowly, to form magnesium chloride which reacts with intestinal secretions to form the carbonate, the chloride being released and reabsorbed. Systemic acid–base balance is thus not significantly altered.

Aluminium hydroxide reacts with HCl to form aluminium chloride which reacts with intestinal secretions to produce insoluble salts, especially phosphate, the chloride being released and reabsorbed; thus it does not alter systemic acid–base balance. It tends to constipate. Sufficient aluminium may be absorbed from the

intestine to create a risk of encephalopathy in patients with chronic renal failure. Hypophosphataemia and hypophosphaturia may result from binding phosphate so that it is not absorbed from the gut.

Sodium bicarbonate reacts with acid and relieves pain within minutes. It is absorbed and causes alkalosis which in short-term use may not cause symptoms but can be a serious matter in patients with renal insufficiency. Sodium bicarbonate can release enough CO_2 in the stomach to cause discomfort and belching, which may have a psychotherapeutic effect or not, according to the circumstances. Excess sodium intake may cause oedema and heart failure in patients with cardiac or renal disease.

Calcium- and bismuth-containing antacids are available but should be avoided. Those that contain calcium may cause rebound acid hypersecretion and, with prolonged use, hypercalcaemia and alkalosis which may rarely be associated with renal failure (the milk-alkali syndrome). Bismuth may be absorbed and cause encephalopathy and arthropathy.

Alginic acid may be combined with an antacid to encourage adherence of the mixture to the mucosa, e.g. for reflux oesophagitis.

Dimethicone is sometimes included in antacid mixtures as an antifoaming agent to reduce flatulence. It is a silicone polymer that lowers surface tension and allows the small bubbles of froth to coalesce into large bubbles that can more easily be passed up from the stomach or down from the colon. It helps mountaineers to belch at high altitudes.

Adverse effects of antacid mixtures

Those that apply to individual antacids are described above but the following general points are also relevant.

- Some antacid mixtures contain *sodium* which may not be readily apparent from the name and for this reason may be dangerous for patients with cardiac or renal disease. For example, a 10 ml dose of Magnesium Carbonate Mixture or of Magnesium Trisilicate Mixture contains about 6 mmol of sodium.

● Aluminium- and magnesium-containing antacids may interfere with the absorption of other drugs by binding with them or by altering gastrointestinal pH or transit time. Reduced biological availability of iron, digoxin, warfarin and some NSAIDs has been ascribed to this type of interaction. It is probably advisable to avoid using antacids concurrently with drugs that are intended for systemic effect by the oral route.

Choice and use of antacids

No single antacid is satisfactory for all circumstances and mixtures are often used. They may contain sodium bicarbonate for quickest effect, supplemented by magnesium hydroxide or carbonate. Sometimes magnesium trisilicate or aluminium hydroxide is added, but these are often used alone, though they are relatively slow-acting.

Disturbed bowel habit can be corrected by altering the proportions of magnesium salts that tend to cause diarrhoea, and aluminium salts that tend to constipate, sometimes severely.

Tablets are more convenient for the patient at work but they act more slowly unless they are sucked or chewed; a liquid may be more acceptable for frequent use. An antacid taken when the stomach is empty may be effective for only 20–40 minutes because of gastric emptying but if it is taken an hour after a meal when the buffering action of food has ceased, the effect may last 2–3 hours. Patients will find their own optimal pattern of use.

ENHANCING MUCOSAL RESISTANCE

Drugs can improve mucosal resistance by different mechanisms that are described below.

Bismuth chelate (tripotassium dicitratobismuthate, bismuth subcitrate, De-Nol)

This substance was thought to act primarily by selectively chelating with protein material in the ulcer base, so forming a coating that protects it from the adverse influences of acid, pepsin and bile.

Recently, a different mechanism of action has been proposed. The organism *Helicobacter pylori* is isolated from 86% of cases of duodenal and 65% of cases of gastric ulcer.[1] *H. pylori* is specifically adapted to living in the mucus that overlies gastric epithelial cells.

Duodenal ulcer is associated with an active chronic gastritis of the antrum that extends into the duodenum where islands of ectopic gastric mucosa may occur; gastric ulcer is associated with a more severe gastritis that involves the antrum and body of the stomach. Evidence indicates that *H. pylori* plays a causative role in this gastritis. The organism is sensitive to bismuth salts but its eradication appears more effective when these are combined with another antimicrobial, e.g. amoxycillin, tinidazole or metronidazole. In addition, 60% of patients who are suspected of having a peptic ulcer on clinical grounds but who do not have an ulcer crater on endoscopy ('non-ulcer dyspepsia') have *H. pylori infection.*

Bismuth chelate is used for benign gastric and duodenal ulcer and has a therapeutic efficacy approximately equivalent to histamine H_2-receptor antagonists. Ulcer healing appears to last longer with bismuth chelate than with the histamine H_2-receptor antagonists, and this may relate to the ability of the former but not of the latter to eradicate *H. pylori*.

Bismuth chelate, particularly as the elixir, darkens the tongue, teeth and stool; the tablet is less likely to do so and is thus more acceptable. Systemic absorption of bismuth from the chelated preparation appears to be well below the levels at which encephalopathy occurs but bismuth is eliminated by the kidney and it is prudent to avoid giving the drug to patients with impaired renal function.

---

[1] These figures exclude peptic ulcers due to NSAIDs.

Sucralfate

This is a basic aluminium salt of sucrose octaphosphate. In the acid environment of the stomach, the aluminium moiety dissociates and the negatively charged sucrose octaphosphate binds electrostatically to positively charged protein molecules that transude from damaged mucosa. The result is a viscous paste that adheres selectively and protectively to the ulcer base. Its action appears also to derive from binding to and inactivating pepsin and bile acids which are ulcerogenic; it has negligible acid neutralising capacity but may prevent damaging back-diffusion of H^+ from the lumen to the mucosa.

Sucralfate is used for benign gastric and duodenal ulcer and for chronic gastritis; its therapeutic efficacy is approximately equal to that of the histamine H_2-receptor antagonists but may be better at prolonging remission after healing has occurred. Maintenance treatment is effective at preventing relapse.

Sucralfate may cause constipation but is otherwise well tolerated. It is absorbed from the gastrointestinal tract; the concentration of aluminium in the plasma may be elevated in uraemic patients, but not if renal function is normal. As the drug is effective only in acid conditions, an antacid should not be taken 30 min before or after a dose of sucralfate. The aluminium content of sucralfate may cause it to interfere with absorption of drugs (see Antacids, above).

Misoprostol

Endogenous prostaglandins are important contributors to the integrity of the gastrointestinal mucosa by a number of related mechanisms:

- stimulation of mucus and bicarbonate secretion
- maintenance of blood flow; an adequate flow not only ensures a supply of oxygen and nutrients but also helps to remove H^+ which readily diffuses from the lumen into damaged or ischaemic tissues
- prevention of luminal H^+ from diffusing into the mucosa, e.g. in response to aspirin,

ethanol and bile salts
- enhancement of the rate of cell replication in the mucosa, to hasten the repair of damaged epithelium
- reduction of gastric acid secretion.

Gastric and duodenal mucosal damage and chronic peptic ulcer associated with the use of nonsteroidal anti-inflammatory drugs may derive from interference with the above (cytoprotective) actions of prostaglandins, for NSAIDs inhibit the formation of prostaglandins.

Misoprostol is a synthetic analogue of prostaglandin E_1. It prevents the formation of gastric ulcers in patients who are taking NSAIDs, an effect which is assumed to stem from its cytoprotective action. The drug also heals chronic gastric and duodenal ulcers to an extent predictable from its inhibition of gastric acid secretion, i.e. not dependent on the cytoprotective action.

Diarrhoea and abdominal pain, transient and dose-related, are the commonest *adverse effects*. Women may experience gynaecological disturbances such as spotting and dysmenorrhoea; the drug is contraindicated in pregnancy or for women planning to become pregnant, for the products of conception may be aborted.

Liquorice derivatives

Crude liquorice contains two sources of anti-ulcer activity, one related to glycyrrhizin (a glycoside) and one that remains after glycyrrhizin is removed.

Carbenoxolone increases the amount and quality of gastric mucus, reduces diffusion of H^+ ion from the lumen into the mucosa and reduces the rate of shedding of gastric mucosal cells. It may be used to heal gastric ulcer and, to a lesser extent, duodenal ulcer. Its principal adverse effect is sodium retention which may lead to oedema, hypertension and heart failure, and which considerably limits its use especially in the old.

Deglycyrrhizinised liquorice preparations do not cause fluid retention but retain some ulcer-healing effect. Preparations include Caved-S, a mixture that includes antacids; and Rabro, which contains antacids and frangula bark (a mild bulk purgative).

OVERALL MANAGEMENT

Several drugs are now recognised as being effective for peptic ulcer and their place in the overall management of the disease may be summarised:

- *General advice* should be given to stop smoking, to avoid nonsteroidal anti-inflammatory drug use and alcohol. Both smoking and NSAIDs retard ulcer healing with histamine H_2-receptor antagonists.
- *Healing* of peptic ulcer can be accelerated by a number of types of drug. A *histamine H_2-blocker* is generally preferred because of ease of administration. Those currently available have approximately equal therapeutic efficacy and the choice in the individual case may be determined by considerations such as cost, concurrent use of drugs such as warfarin, theophylline or phenytoin with which cimetidine will interact, and experience of adverse effects. *Bismuth chelate* and *sucralfate* are alternatives that are approximately as effective as histamine H_2-receptor antagonists but the need for multiple dosing (up to ×4/d) may limit compliance. *Pirenzepine* is also satisfactory. *Antacids* as sole treatment can accelerate ulcer healing but must be taken frequently in high dose to achieve this; their use is now limited to providing supplementary symptomatic relief, e.g. in the first few days of a course of a histamine H_2-blocker and for intermittent use subsequently.
- *Most ulcers induced by NSAIDs* occur in the stomach and duodenum. The first step should be to review the necessity for using the nonsteroidal anti-inflammatory drug. *Misoprostol* may prevent peptic ulceration, in those at high risk, e.g. the elderly, and those who have previously had an ulcer. Misoprostol may also be used to treat an ulcer. A duodenal ulcer induced by NSAIDs may respond to a histamine H_2-blocker.
- *Ulcers that are difficult to heal* may respond to double the normal dose of a histamine H_2-blocker. Alternatively, *bismuth chelate plus metronidazole* and *amoxycillin* may be used with the objective of clearing *H. pylori* from the stomach. *Omeprazole* is also an option for such ulcers.
- *Prevention of relapse*, in those individuals who are prone to it, may be achieved with a *histamine H_2-blocker* taken as a single dose at night, on a long-term basis, for such drugs have a well-established safety record. Post-ulcer patients may reasonably be advised to take a histamine H_2- blocker for a few days for indigestion. Intermittent use of *bismuth chelate* (or perhaps sucralfate) is another option which may offer a lower relapse rate, but there is uncertainty about long-term effects of bismuth (and aluminium) accumulation.
- Surgery may be required for patients whose ulcers recur despite all other measures.

VOMITING

If the cause of vomiting cannot be removed, it may be desirable to attempt to prevent or to suppress it by drugs.

The pharmacology of vomiting was little studied until the world war of 1939–45, when motion sickness attained military importance as a possible handicap for landings made in the face of resistance. The British military authorities and the Medical Research Council therefore organised an investigation. Whenever there was a prospect of sufficiently rough weather, about 70 soldiers were sent to sea in small ships, again and again, after being dosed with a drug or a dummy tablet and having had their mouths inspected to detect non-compliance. The ships returned to land when up to 40% of the soldiers vomited. 'On the whole the men enjoyed their trips'; some of them, however, being soldiers, thought the tablets were given in order to make them vomit and some 'believed firmly in the efficacy of the dummy tablets.' It was concluded that, of the remedies tested, hyoscine (0.6 mg or 1.2 mg) was the most effective.[2]

Some physiology

Vomiting is a protective mechanism for eliminating irritant or harmful substances from the upper

---

[2] Holling H E et al. Lancet 1944; 1:127.

gastrointestinal tract. The act of emesis is controlled by the vomiting centre in the medulla and close to it lie other visceral centres, e.g. for respiration, salivation and vascular control which give rise to the prodromal sensations of vomiting. The *vomiting centre* does not initiate, but rather it coordinates the act of emesis on receiving stimuli from various sources, namely,

1. the chemoreceptor trigger zone (CTZ), a nearby area that is extremely sensitive to the action of drugs and other chemicals
2. the vestibular system
3. the periphery e.g. distension or irritation of the gut, myocardial infarction, biliary or renal stone
4. cortical centres.

The vomiting centre contains many muscarinic cholinergic receptors and the CTZ is rich in dopamine D_2-receptors; drugs that block these receptors are effective antiemetics. The precise role and location of 5-HT$_3$-receptors (see ondansetron, below) in relation to emesis remains to be defined but both central and peripheral mechanisms may be involved.

ANTIEMESIS AND PROKINETIC DRUGS

These may be classified as shown in Table 30.1.

Antiemetics acting on the vomiting centre have *antimuscarinic action*, e.g. hyoscine, promethazine; they alleviate vomiting from any cause. But drugs acting on the CTZ (haloperidol, odansetron) are effective only for vomiting mediated by the chemoreceptors (morphine, digoxin, cytotoxics, uraemia). The most efficacious drugs act at more than one site (see Table 30.1).

Antimuscarinic drugs (including those classed primarily as histamine H$_1$-receptor antagonists) are described elsewhere. Drugs with antimuscarinic activity probably act both centrally and in the gastrointestinal tract. Phenothiazines and butyrophenones owe their antiemetic efficacy to blockade of dopamine D_2-receptors but they readily penetrate the brain and may produce extrapyramidal effects by blocking D_2-receptors

Table 30.1 Classification of antiemesis drugs

Drug	Site of action
Dopamine D$_2$-receptor antagonists	
domperidone	CTZ and gut
metoclopramide	CTZ and gut
haloperidol	CTZ
phenothiazines, e.g.	vomiting centre
chlorpromazine	and CTZ
prochlorperazine,	
thiethylperazine,	
5-HT$_3$-receptor antagonist	
ondansetron	? CTZ and gut
granisetron	
Antimuscarinics	
hyoscine and some drugs also	Vomiting centre
classed as histamine H1-receptor	and gut
antagonists, e.g. cyclizine,	
dimenhydrinate, promethazine	
Other agents	
cisapride	CTZ and gut
corticosteroids (dexamethasone,]	
methylprednisolone]	vomiting due to
cannabinoids (nabilone)]	cytotoxics
benzodiazepines (lorazepam)]	

in the basal ganglia; many also have antimuscarinic effects.

Metoclopramide

Metoclopramide (Maxolon) acts centrally by blocking dopamine D_2-receptors in the CTZ, and peripherally by enhancing the action of acetylcholine at muscarinic nerve endings in the gut. It raises the tone of the lower oesophageal sphincter, relaxes the pyloric antrum and duodenal cap and increases peristalsis and emptying of the upper gut. The peripheral actions are utilised to empty the stomach before emergency anaesthesia and in labour (the term *prokinetic* is used for this action). If an opioid has been given, metoclopramide may fail to overcome the opioid-induced inhibition of gastric emptying and thus the risk of vomiting and inhaling gastric contents remains. The direct effects on the gut are antagonised by antimuscarinic drugs. The action of metoclopramide is terminated by metabolism in the liver; the $t_{\frac{1}{2}}$ is 4 h.

Uses. Metoclopramide is used for nausea and

vomiting associated with gastrointestinal disorders, with postsurgical conditions, and with cytotoxic drugs and radiotherapy. It is also an effective antiemetic in migraine and is used as a prokinetic agent (above).

Adverse reactions are characteristic of dopamine receptor antagonists and include extrapyramidal dystonia (torticollis, facial spasms, trismus, oculogyric crises) which occurs more commonly in children and young adults, and in those who are concurrently receiving phenothiazine drugs. The reaction is rapidly abolished by the antimuscarinic drug, benztropine, given i.v. Long-term use of metoclopramide may cause tardive dyskinesia in the elderly. Metoclopramide stimulates prolactin release and may cause gynaecomastia and lactation. Motor restlessness and diarrhoea also occur.

Cisapride (Prepulsid) is structurally related to metoclopramide but does not block dopamine receptors; rather, it appears to enhance acetylcholine release in the myenteric plexus of the gut; it increases motility throughout the gastrointestinal tract. The t_2^1 is 10 h; its action is terminated by metabolism and there is evidence of considerable first-pass inactivation by the oral route.

Cisapride is used to relieve symptoms of gastro-oesophageal reflux, for reflux oesophagitis and where gastric motility is impaired, e.g. in diabetes and systemic sclerosis.

The drug may cause abdominal cramping and diarrhoea, which are indeed extensions of its pharmacological action. It appears to have no central sedative effects.

Domperidone blocks dopamine D_2-receptors in the CTZ, and peripherally in the upper gut where it increases the tone in the lower oesophageal sphincter, enhances contractions of the gastric antrum and relaxes the pyloric sphincter. It crosses the blood–brain barrier poorly; this does not limit its therapeutic efficacy for the CTZ is functionally outwith the barrier, but there is less risk of adverse effects in the central nervous system. The t_2^1 is 7 h. Domperidone is used for nausea or vomiting associated with gastrointestinal disorders and with cytotoxic and other drug treatment. Dystonic reactions with domperidone are much fewer than with metoclopramide. It may cause gynaecomastia and galactorrhoea.

Ondansetron is a selective 5-HT₃-receptor antagonist. Drugs with this activity appear to be highly effective against nausea and vomiting induced by cytotoxic agents and radiotherapy. Evidence suggests that such anticancer treatment releases 5-HT (serotonin) from enterochromaffin cells in the gut mucosa (where resides > 80% of the 5-HT in the body) which activates specific receptors in the gut and central nervous system to cause emesis.[3] The action of ondansetron may thus be partly central and partly peripheral. Its t_2^1 is 5 h. Ondansetron may be given by i.v. injection or infusion prior to cancer chemotherapy (notably with cisplatin), followed by oral administration for up to 5 days. The drug appears to be well tolerated but constipation, headache and a feeling of flushing in the head and epigastrium may occur.

Nabilone is a synthetic cannabinoid and has properties similar to tetrahydrocannabinol (the active constituent of marijuana) which has an antiemetic action. It is used to relieve nausea or vomiting caused by cytotoxic drugs. Adverse effects include: somnolence, dry mouth, decreased appetite, dizziness, euphoria, dysphoria, postural hypotension, confusion and psychosis. These may be reduced if prochlorperazine is given concomitantly.

DRUG TREATMENT OF SOME FORMS OF VOMITING

Motion sickness

There was a young lady of Spain
Who was dreadfully sick in a train,
Not once, but again,
And again and again,
And again and again and again.[4]

Motion sickness is more easily prevented than cured. It is due chiefly to overstimulation of the

---

[3] Cubeddu L X et al. New Engl J Med 1990; 322: 810.
[4] Anonymous *limerick*, an extemporised five-line form of nonsense verse (1898).

vestibular apparatus (and does not occur if the labyrinth is destroyed). Other factors also contribute; visually, a moving horizon can be most disturbing, as can the sensations induced by the gravitational inertia of a full stomach when the body is in vertical movement. That the environment, whether close and smelly or open and vivifying, is important, is a matter of common experience amongst all who have been at sea on a rough day. Psychological factors, including observation of the fate of one's companions, are also important. Tolerance to the motion occurs, generally over a period of days.

Drugs that are used for motion sickness include: cinnarizine, cyclizine, dimenhydrinate, hyoscine and promethazine, all antimuscarinic.

For prophylaxis an antiemetic is best taken 1 h before exposure to the motion. About 70% protection may be expected by the right dose given at the right time. Once motion sickness has started, oral administration of drugs may fail, and the i.m., s.c. or rectal routes are required; alternatively, hyoscine may be administered as a dermal patch, so avoiding the enteral route. Prevention of symptoms may therefore be possible only at the expense of troublesome unwanted effects: sleepiness, dry mouth, blurred vision.

Drug-induced vomiting

If reducing the dose or withdrawing the offending drug are not options then an attempt, often unsatisfactory, may be made to oppose it by another drug. In general, chlorpromazine or another phenothiazine or metoclopramide, are best. Opioid-induced vomiting responds to one of the drugs used for motion sickness (above); cyclizine and morphine are combined as Cyclimorph.

Vomiting due to cytotoxic drugs

Prevention and alleviation of this distressing and often very severe symptom of several forms of cancer treatment may allow an optimal chemotherapeutic regimen to be used, and avoid admitting the patient to hospital. Cisplatin is notably emetic. *Dexamethasone* is effective; also

lorazepam, which gives useful amnesia although sedation and dysphoria are dose-limiting. The observation that dexamethasone and lorazepam together were more efficacious than either on its own (synergism) led to the testing of other combinations, including the addition of metoclopramide in high dose. All three drugs have been used together for the most emetogenic cytotoxic regimens.

Recognition that 5-HT (serotonin) release probably plays a key role in cytotoxic-induced vomiting stimulated the search for appropriate antagonists and has led to the introduction of *ondansetron*. 5-HT_3-receptor antagonists may become drugs of choice.

Vomiting after general anaesthesia

Postoperative vomiting is related to the duration of anaesthesia and the causation is multifactorial. Metoclopramide or a butyrophenone, e.g. haloperidol, droperidol, are preferred.

Vomiting in pregnancy

This reaches a peak at 10–11 weeks and usually resolves by 13–14 weeks of gestation. Nausea alone does not require treatment. Much can be achieved by reassurance that the problem is transient and a discussion of diet, e.g. taking food before getting up in the morning. When a decision is taken to use a drug, promethazine or thiethylperazine are preferred. Although pyridoxine deficiency has not been shown to complicate simple pregnancy vomiting, it may occur in hyperemesis gravidarum which requires i.v. fluids and multivitamin supplement.

Vertigo

A great range of drugs has been recommended to treat vertigo and labyrinthine disorders but antimuscarinics and phenothiazines are generally preferred. Cyclizine, prochlorperazine and thiethylperazine may be used to relieve an acute attack. Betahistine (a histamine analogue) is used in the hope of improving the blood circulation to the inner ear in Menière's syndrome; also cinnarizine.

GASTRO-OESOPHAGEAL REFLUX

Recurrent reflux of gastric contents into the oesophagus produces symptoms of 'heartburn' and/or oesophageal injury. This common condition may be managed as follows.

General measures include advice to avoid: 1. meals late at night or lying down after meals, 2. heavy lifting, tight clothing, bending, 3. being overweight, 4. smoking, because nicotine relaxes the lower oesophageal sphincter, 5. substances known to aggravate the condition, e.g. hot foods, or alcohol, 6. drugs which encourage reflux, i.e. those with antimuscarinic activity (e.g. tricyclic antidepressants), smooth muscle relaxants (e.g. nitrates and calcium channel blockers) and theophylline compounds. In addition elevating the head of the patient's bed by 15–20 cm will discourage nocturnal reflux.

Drugs. An antacid, either alone or combined with alginic acid, e.g. Gaviscon, Gastrocote, provides relief for milder degrees of oesophagitis. The addition of alginic acid is supposed to produce a floating viscous gel that blocks reflux and protectively coats the oesophagus. More severe oesophagitis requires acid *suppression* with a histamine H_2-receptor antagonist with a dose that is higher than that for gastric or duodenal ulcer, and given for a prolonged period. Omeprazole is also very effective but is best used in intermittent courses until issues regarding its safety during long-term use are finally resolved. Metoclopramide or cisapride may be used intermittently, especially for those patients who also complain of abdominal fullness or bloating.

MISCELLANEOUS

Therapeutic emesis: see Drug overdose, p. 136.

Diffuse oesophageal spasm may be helped by isosorbide dinitrate 5 mg sublingually or 10 mg by mouth, or by nifedipine 10 mg sublingually or swallowed.

Bitters are substances taken before meals to im-
prove appetite. They have not been scientifically investigated. They include gentian, nux vomica and quinine. Preparations can be found in the BNF and at wine merchants (Byrrh, Dubonnet, Campari).

Carminatives are substances which are used to assist in expelling gas from the stomach and intestines. Examples are: dimethicone, peppermint, dill, anise and other herbs which are commonly included in liqueurs and (in non-alcoholic solutions) for babies, and may be useful in irritable bowel syndrome. The problem is not new: the Roman Emperor Claudius (AD 10–54)

planned an edict to legitimise the breaking of wind at table, either silently or noisily, after hearing about a man who was so modest that he endangered his health by an attempt to restrain himself (Suetonius, trans R Graves).

GUIDE TO FURTHER READING

Axon A R 1991 Duodenal ulcer: the villain unmasked? Eradicating *Helicobacter pylori* will cure most patients. British Medical Journal 302: 919

Brown C, Rees W D W 1990 Dyspepsia in general practice. British Medical Journal 300: 829

Editorial 1988 Misoprostol: ulcer prophylaxis at what cost? Lancet 2: 1293

Editorial 1989 Drugs acting on 5-hydroxytryptamine receptors. Lancet 2: 717

Editorial 1989 Stress ulcer prophylaxis in critically ill patients. Lancet 2: 1255

Editorial 1990 Vomiting and chemotherapy. Lancet 335: 265

Feldman M, Burton M E 1990 Histamine H_2-receptor antagonists. Standard therapy for acid-peptic diseases. New England Journal of Medicine 323: 1672, 1749

Guslandi M 1988 Does smoking harm the duodenum? British Medical Journal 296: 311

Maton P N 1991 Omeprazole. New England Journal of Medicine 324: 965

Peterson W L 1991 *Helicobacter pylori* and pepitc ulcer disease. New England Journal of Medicine 324: 1043

Pounder R 1988 Duodenal ulcers that are difficult to heal. British Medical Journal 297:–1560

Rauws E A J, Tytgat G N J 1990 Cure of duodenal ulcer associated with eradication of Helicobacter pylori. Lancet 335: 1233

Soll A H 1990 Pathogenesis of peptic ulcer and implications for therapy. New England Journal of Medicine 322: 909

Wolfe M M, Soll A H 1988 The physiology of gastric secretion. New England Journal of Medicine 319: 1707

Gastrointestinal system II: intestines

CONSTIPATION

The terms purgative, cathartic, laxative, aperient and evacuant may be considered synonymous; they are medicines that promote defaecation largely by reducing the viscosity of the contents of the lower colon.

Purgatives may be classified as (1) bulk, (2) osmotic, (3) faecal softeners and (4) stimulant. Their properties confer some variation in the indications for use. The times that purgatives take to act are listed, for these determine whether they should be given in the morning or evening.

Bulk purgatives

These comprise indigestible vegetable fibre and hydrophilic colloids. Bulk purgatives act by increasing the volume and lowering the viscosity of intestinal contents to promote a large, soft, solid stool. The substances thus encourage *normal reflex bowel activity*, rendering it more effective and generally acting within 1–3 h. They are also helpful for anal fissure, haemorrhoids, diverticular disease and irritable bowel syndrome. All bulk purgatives must be taken with 2 l/d of fluid. If taken repeatedly with too little fluid, they can cause intestinal obstruction, especially if there is any organic obstruction or if peristalsis is weak.

Dietary fibre is essentially the cell walls of plants. It consists of a group of carbohydrate compounds including cellulose and hemicelluloses and also a non-carbohydrate component, lignin. Medicinally, fibre has two notable properties: *first*, it is not broken down by the enzymes in the human gut, so it enters the colon intact, and *second*, it has a vast capacity for retaining water; e.g. one gram of carrot fibre can hold as much as 23 grams of water.[1] It has been proposed that as humans have progressively refined the carbohydrates in their diet over the centuries, so they have deprived themselves of fibre, particularly from cereal, and that the resultant underfilling of the colon is an important cause of constipation, irritable bowel syndrome and diverticular disease. Adding fibre, e.g. bran, to the diet is thus a safe and natural way of treating constipation. *Bran* is the residue left when flour is made from cereals and contains between 25% and 50% of fibre. About 24 g per day is recommended for colonic diverticular disease but prevention should be the aim, since once the anatomical changes have occurred, they cannot be reversed and the sudden addition of a full regimen of bran to the diet of such a person may exacerbate symptoms. The fibre content of normal diet can be increased by eating wholemeal bread and bran cereals.

Ispaghula husk contains mucilage and hemicelluloses which swell rapidly in water.

Methylcellulose takes up water to swell to a colloid about 25 times its original volume. It is also used as a suspending agent in pharmacy, in lubricating jellies, in contact-lens wetting solutions and in artificial tears.

Sterculia,[2] similarly, swells when mixed with water.

Osmotic laxatives

These are but little absorbed and increase the bulk and reduce viscosity of intestinal contents to promote a fluid stool.

Some inorganic salts retain water in the intestinal lumen, or, if given as hypertonic solution, withdraw it from the body. When constipation is mild, magnesium hydroxide will suffice but mag-

nesium sulphate (Epsom[3] salt) is used when a more powerful effect is needed. Both magnesium salts act in 2–4 h. The small amount of magnesium absorbed when the sulphate is frequently used can be enough to cause magnesium poisoning in patients with renal impairment, the central nervous effects of which somewhat resemble those of uraemia. Magnesium sulphate 50% (hypertonic) is available as a single dose retention enema to reduce cerebrospinal fluid pressure in neurosurgery. Solutions of phosphates or sodium citrate may be used as enemas for constipation or when the bowel has to be cleared for a diagnostic procedure or surgery.

Lactulose is a synthetic disaccharide. Taken orally, it is unaffected by small intestinal disaccharidase, is not absorbed and thus acts as an osmotic laxative. Lactulose is also used in treatment of hepatic encephalopathy, which condition is aggravated by ammonia produced in the colon gaining access to the systemic circulation. In the colon lactulose is fermented to lactic and acetic acids which inhibit the growth of colonic ammonia-producing organisms and, by lowering pH, reduce non-ionic diffusion of ammonia from the colon into the blood. It takes 48 h to act. Apart from hepatic disease, it is useful for patients with distal ulcerative colitis who tend to have faecal stasis in the proximal colon.

Faecal softeners (emollients)

The softening properties of these agents are useful in the management of anal fissure and haemorrhoids.

Docusate sodium (dioctyl sodium sulphosuccinate) softens faeces by lowering the surface tension of fluids in the bowel which allows more water to remain in the faeces. It may also have bowel stimulant properties. Docusate sodium acts in 1–2 days but is relatively weak. *Poloxamers*, e.g. poloxalkol (poloxamer 188), act similarly and are used in combination with other agents.

Liquid paraffin is a chemically inert mineral oil

---

[1] McConnell A A, et al. 1974 J Sci Food Agric 25: 1427.
[2] Named after Sterculinus, a god of ancient Rome who presided over manuring agricultural land.

[3] Epsom, a town near London, known for its mineral spring water and for horse racing.

and is not digested. It appears to reduce water absorption in the small intestine and it may be this effect as well as the softening powers of the oil (in the colon) that promotes the passage of softer faeces. It is often presented in emulsions with magnesium hydroxide. Some paraffin is absorbed from the intestine and collects in the mesenteric lymph nodes where paraffinomas may form. Large doses may leak out of the anus causing both physical and social discomfort. Paraffin taken over long periods orally, especially at night, may cause chronic lipoid pneumonia. An unusual case resulted from successful attempts by a patient to lubricate his larynx with liquid paraffin. Because of these disadvantages, its use is declining and it should never be used long-term as a laxative.

Arachis oil is included in enemas to soften impacted faeces.

Stimulant purgatives (contact laxatives)

These increase intestinal motility by various mechanisms; they may cause abdominal cramps and should not be used where there is intestinal obstruction.

Bisacodyl stimulates sensory endings in the colon by direct action from the lumen. It is effective orally in 6–10 h, and as a suppository, acting in 1 h. In geriatric patients, bisacodyl suppositories reduce the need for regular enemas. There are no important unwanted effects.

Sodium picosulphate is similar and is also used to evacuate the bowel for investigative procedures and surgery.

Oxyphenisatin is administered as an enema to clear the colon for diagnostic procedure and surgery. It is not suitable for repeated use as this causes hepatitis.

Glycerol has a mild stimulant effect on the rectum when administered as a suppository.

The *anthraquinone group* of purgatives includes senna, danthron, cascara, rhubarb and aloes. In the small intestine soluble anthraquinone derivates are liberated and absorbed. These are excreted into the colon and act there, along with those that have escaped absorption, probably after being chemically changed by bacterial action.

Patients taking some anthraquinones may notice their urine coloured brown (if acid) or red (if alkaline). Prolonged use can cause melanosis of the colon which cognoscenti can recognise through an endoscope. Anthraquinone preparations made from crude plant extracts are to be avoided as their lack of standardisation leads to erratic results.

Danthron is available as a standardised preparation with the faecal softeners poloxamer 188 (as co-danthramer) and docusate sodium (as co-danthrusate). It acts in 6–12 h. As evidence from rodent studies indicates a possible carcinogenic risk, long-term exposure to danthron should be avoided but it may be suitable for occasional use in the elderly or the terminally ill.

Senna, available as a standardised preparation, is widely used to relieve constipation and to empty the bowel for investigative procedures and surgery. It acts in 8–12 h.

Castor oil acts as a purgative after hydrolysis in the small intestine to ricinoleic acid which stimulates peristalsis and reduces fluid absorption. The liquid contents of the small intestine pass rapidly onwards, resulting in a soft or fluid stool after 2–6 h. Its irritant action is powerful enough for it to be capable of starting pregnant women in labour. Most patients find castor oil objectionable to taste. It is also used in ointments, hair lotions and eye drops as a simple, non-irritant lubricant and vehicle.

Phenolphthalein should now be avoided as it may cause rashes and its laxative action is prolonged by enterohepatic cycling.

The drastic purgatives (jalap,[4] colocynth and podophyllum) are obsolete.

Suppositories (bisacodyl, glycerin) may be used to obtain a bowel action in about 1 hour.

For anal and rectal disease, suppositories which are astringent (hamamelis), or anti-inflammatory (adrenal steroid) or local anaesthesic (lignocaine) are used as seems necessary.

---

[4] In the 19th century 'young men proceeding to Africa' were advised to take pills named Livingstone's Rousers, consisting of rhubarb, jalap, calomel and quinine. Br Med J 1964; 2: 1583.

Enemas produce defaecation by softening faeces and distending the bowel. They are used in preparation for surgery, radiological examination and endoscopy. Preparations with sodium phosphate, which is poorly absorbed and so retains water in the gut, are generally used.

Enemas to be *retained* may be used to provide topical therapy for ulcerative colitis or Crohn's disease of the colon.

Management of constipation

Constipation may arise in the following settings:

- *Habitual constipation* is best corrected by adjusting the diet to contain more fibre, e.g. by including unpeeled fruit and vegetables, wholemeal bread, bran-based cereals, muesli[5] or simply by adding unprocessed bran. The latter may be sprinkled on the morning cereal or made up as a separate drink, the disagreeable nature of which is only partially disguised by mixing with fruit juice or milk. A faecal softener may be necessary, and if a stimulant is required, senna is perhaps the least objectionable.

Psychological factors are important. An explanation that normal bowel habit may vary between 3 motions per day and 2 per week, may be of more value to the patient than the prescription of a laxative.

- *Painful anal lesions* frequently lead to constipation because, when defaecation hurts, it is postponed for as long as possible, with the result that more water is absorbed and the faeces become harder and so hurt even more when they are eventually passed. This vicious cycle is best broken by the cure of the anal lesion, but a bulk laxative or a faecal softener, and a local anaesthetic suppository, may give relief temporarily.

- *Pregnancy.* Constipation is best treated by ensuring that there is adequate fibre in the diet and if, despite this, the bowel sluggishness persists, one of the milder stimulant laxatives, e.g. senna, should be used, as vigorous purgation can cause abortion, though this is less reliable than some women hope.

- *Acute illness* may lead to sluggish bowel habit, especially if it involves confinement to bed and is accompanied by loss of appetite. Dependence on others for assistance to the toilet or, worse, to bring a bedpan, is also a factor. If severe enough to warrant attention, this kind of constipation can usually be dealt with by a bulk laxative, a faecal softener, senna, or suppositories of glycerine or bisacodyl.

- *Elderly* patients may become constipated because their abdominal and perineal muscles lack tone and their diets are inadequate. The initial approach should be to use bran or a bulking agent, combined with improving mobility, fluid intake and establishing a regular bowel habit. Senna or bisacodyl may be used intermittently if further assistance is necessary but long-term use of a stimulant laxative may damage the myoenteric pathways. Resistant constipation may be best managed by twice-weekly phosphate enemas.

- *Drugs* may cause constipation. *Opioid* analgesics decrease propulsion in the gut. Drugs with *antimuscarinic* action reduce intestinal motility by blocking the muscarinic action of acetylcholine on gut smooth muscle; these include antispasmodics, e.g. hyoscine, antiparkinsonian drugs, e.g. orphenadrine, and tricyclic antidepressants, e.g. amitriptyline. *Aluminium-containing antacids, iron, calcium channel blockers* and *benzodiazepines*, all may constipate to varying degrees. Impaired propulsion permits water absorption from the gut contents which become more viscous. When withdrawal of the drug is not feasible, e.g. treating intractable pain with an opioid, constipation should be anticipated and a laxative prescribed with the analgesic.

MISUSE OF LAXATIVES

Dependence (abuse) may arise following laxative use during an illness or in pregnancy, or the individual may have the mistaken notion that a daily bowel motion is essential for health, or that the bowels are only incompletely opened by nature, and so indulge in regular purgation. This effectively prevents the easy return of normal

---

[5] A Swiss invention, being a delicious mixture of chopped cereals, nuts, dried fruits, honey.

habits because the more powerful stimulant purges empty the whole colon, whereas normal defaecation empties only the descending colon. Cessation of use after a few weeks is thus inevitably followed by a few days' constipation whilst sufficient material collects to restore the normal state. This may convince the patient of the continued necessity for purgatives.

To prevent purgative dependence is easier than to cure it; patients feel they understand their own bowels far better than anyone else possibly could, an opinion they seldom extend to other organs, except perhaps the liver. In Britain, there is a tradition that nurses have an intuitive understanding of the bowels that is denied to doctors.

Laxative dependence, which may be solely emotional at first, may be followed by *physical dependence*, i.e. the bowels will not open without a purgative. Excessive use of stimulant purgatives[6] may, especially in the old, lead to severe water and electrolyte depletion, even to hypokalaemic paralysis, malabsorption and protein-losing enteropathy. An atonic colon due to damage to gut nerves may result from prolonged abuse. Purgatives are dangerous if given to patients with undiagnosed abdominal pain, inflammatory intestinal disease or obstruction. Nor should they be used to get rid of hardened masses of faeces in the rectum, for they will fail and cause pain. Digital removal, generally ordered by a senior and performed by a junior doctor, is required. A faecal softener helps to prevent recurrence.

DIARRHOEA

Diarrhoea ranges from a mild and socially inconvenient illness to a major cause of death and malnutrition among children in developing countries; acute diarrhoea causes 4–5 million deaths throughout the world annually. Drugs have a place in its management but *the first priority of*

---

[6] The Roman Emperor Nero (AD 37–68) murdered his severely constipated aunt by ordering the doctors to **give** her 'a laxative of fatal strength.' He 'seized her property before she was quite dead, and tore up the will so that nothing should escape him.' (Suetonius, trans R Graves).

therapy is to preserve fluid and electrolyte balance. The condition is often assumed to be infectious, but it may be caused by anxiety, food, drugs, microbial or other toxins. Diarrhoea is measured by *volume* and *frequency* of stools.

Some physiology

Absorption and secretion of water and electrolytes occur throughout the intestine, probably as separate processes, for absorption is a function of the cells of the intestinal villi and the surface cells of the colon, while cells in the crypts between villi are responsible for secretion of water. Water follows the osmotic gradients which result from shifts of electrolytes across the intestinal epithelium, and sodium and chloride transport mechanisms are central to the causation and management of diarrhoea, especially that caused by bacteria and viruses.

Absorption of sodium into the epithelium is effected by:

- *Sodium-glucose coupled entry.* Glucose stimulates the absorption of sodium and the resulting water flow also sweeps additional sodium and chloride along with it (solvent drag). This important mechanism remains active in diarrhoea of various aetiologies and improvement of sodium and water absorption by glucose (and amino acids) is the basis of oral rehydration regimens (below).
- *Sodium-ion coupled entry.* Na^+ and Cl^- enter the epithelial cell, either as a pair, or, as seems more likely, there is a double exchange: Na^+ (extracellular) with H^+ (intracellular), and Cl^- (extracellular) with ^-OH or $^-HCO_3$ (intracellular). Oral rehydration solutions (below) contain sodium, chloride and bicarbonate.

Secretion is the opposite process to that of absorption. In response to various stimuli, crypt cells transport chloride into the gut lumen and sodium and water follow. This *stimulus-secretion coupling* is modulated by cyclic AMP and GMP, calcium, prostaglandins and leukotrienes.

Diarrhoea has numerous causes, from infections with enteric organisms (which may stimulate secretion or damage absorption), inflammation (e.g. food allergy), to nutrient malabsorption.

Motility patterns in the bowel. Segmental contractions of the smooth muscle mix the intestinal contents. Patients with diarrhoea commonly have less spontaneous activity of the sigmoid colon than do people with normal bowel habit, and patients with constipation have more. An important factor in diarrhoea may be loss of the normal segmenting contractions that delay passage of contents, so that an occasional peristaltic wave may have greater propulsive effect. Antidiarrhoeal drugs act by increasing segmentation and inhibiting peristalsis (antimotility drugs).

Therapy for diarrhoea involves *first*, the correction of fluid and electrolyte imbalance, and *second*, the use of drugs (in some cases).

Fluid and electrolyte treatment

Oral rehydration therapy (ORT) with glucose-electrolyte solution is sufficient to treat the vast majority of episodes of watery diarrhoea. As a simple, effective, cheap and readily administered therapy for a potentially lethal condition, ORT must rank as one of the major recent advances in therapy. It is effective because glucose-coupled sodium transport continues during diarrhoea and provides a means of replacing water and electrolyte losses in the stool.

The WHO/UNICEF[7] recommended **Oral Rehydration Salts** (ORS) formulation is, in 1 litre of water:

Sodium chloride	3.5 g/l
Potassium chloride	1.5 g/l
Sodium citrate	2.9 g/l
Anhydrous glucose	20.0 g/l

This provides Na^+ 90 mmol, K^+ 20 mmol, Cl^- 80 mmol, citrate 10 mmol, glucose 111 mmol.

Several other formulations[8] exist.

Rehydration therapy with commercial soft drinks alone will fail because their sodium content is too low (usually less than 6 mmol/l). The glucose may be replaced by another substrate, to give, e.g. glycine ORS, rice powder ORS. Indeed cereal-based ORS, relying on starch (to produce glucose) from many sources, e.g. rice, wheat, corn, potato, may yet prove to be a further advance. Thus almost every household in the world can find the essential components of an effective oral rehydration mixture: cereals and salt.

Most cases can be adequately treated by assiduous attention to oral intake but fluid and electrolyte depletion are especially dangerous in children for whom hospitalisation and intravenous replacement may be needed. Antimotility drugs are inappropriate for severe diarrhoea in young children; any marginal efficacy they may have is liable to be counterbalanced by hazard (see below).

Drug treatment

There are two types of drug which are often used in combination. Both types increase viscosity of faeces.

1. Drugs that increase the viscosity of gut contents directly.

Kaolin and *chalk* are adsorbent powders that are generally thought to act by providing a coating for the bowel and by adsorbing toxic substances, both unsatisfactory explanations. Their therapeutic efficacy is marginal as is shown by the fact that they are often combined with an opioid.

2. Drugs that delay passage of gut contents: *antimotility drugs.*

The action of antimotility drugs allows time for more water to be absorbed.

---

[7] World Health Organization/United Nations Children Fund (originally the words *international* and *emergency* were included).

[8] The above corresponds to Oral Rehydration Salts – Citrate (Formula C) BNF and is preferred to Formula B which contains bicarbonate and is less stable. Formula A contains sodium chloride 1.0, sodium bicarbonate 1.5, potassium chloride 1.5 and anhydrous glucose 36.4 g/l. The higher sodium content of the WHO/UNICEF formulation is based on sodium concentrations in diarrhoeal stools, but the low-sodium high-glucose Formula A may be preferred for infants, for their faecal losses of sodium are less.

Codeine activates opioid receptors on the smooth muscle of the bowel which reduce peristalsis and increase segmentation contractions so that passage of contents is delayed and more water is absorbed. Tolerance may develop if use is prolonged, as may dependence (rarely).

Diphenoxylate ($t_{\frac{1}{2}}$ 3 h) is structurally related to pethidine and affects the bowel like morphine. The drug is offered mixed with a trivial dose of atropine (to discourage abuse) as Lomotil. Nausea, vomiting, abdominal pain and depression of the central nervous system may be caused. In overdose with Lomotil, respiratory depression may be serious and can occur up to 16 h after ingestion because gastric emptying is slowed.

Loperamide ($t_{\frac{1}{2}}$ 10 h) is structurally similar to diphenoxylate. Its precise mode of action remains obscure but it impairs propulsion of gut contents by effects on intestinal circular and longitudinal muscle that are at least partly due to an action on opioid receptors. Loperamide may cause nausea, vomiting and abdominal cramps. Its potential for abuse appears to be low.

The actions of codeine, diphenoxylate and loperamide are antagonised by naloxone.

Warning*: antimotility drugs* should not be used for acute diarrhoea in children, especially babies, for there is danger of causing paralytic ileus or respiratory depression: ORT is the treatment.

Travellers' diarrhoea

So familiar is travellers' diarrhoea that it has acquired a variety of popular names: the Aztec 2-step, Montezuma's Revenge, Delhi Belly, Rangoon Runs, Tokyo Trots, Gyppy Tummy, Hong-Kong Dog, Estomac Anglais and Casablanca Crud, all indicate some of the areas deemed dangerous to visitors. The Mexican name *turista* indicates the principal sufferers.

A considerable body of medical folklore has arisen among prospective travellers fearful of the social consequences of being stricken during their coach tour of 5 European capitals in 7 days. It is now clear, however, that most cases are infective, and much of the diarrhoea that afflicts visitors to tropical and subtropical countries is associated with enterotoxigenic strains of *E. coli*; other bacterial, e.g. staphylococcal, toxins have also been implicated as have enteroviruses. Recognition that transmission is almost invariably by ingestion of contaminated food and water points to the most effective way of reducing the risk, i.e. avoiding raw, unpeeled fruit and vegetables, and unboiled water.

Acute watery diarrhoea *in adults* can ordinarily be controlled by oral rehydration salts and one of the antimotility drugs, although in mild cases the abdominal bloating produced by the latter may be less acceptable than the loose stools. If symptomatic remedies fail, then the diarrhoea is severe and the patient should consult a doctor. Choice of therapy can thereafter be based on local knowledge allied to an attempt to identify a specific organism.

Prophylactic antimicrobial therapy has been shown to reduce the incidence of attacks of diarrhoea but its routine use carries the risk of hindering the diagnosis of serious infection. A wider issue is the possible development and spread of antibiotic-resistant organisms. Thus any benefits to the *individual* must be weighed against the risk to the *community* in the future; in most instances prophylactic antimicrobials should not be used. Prophylaxis may, however, be justified for individuals who must remain well, travelling for short periods to high risk areas.

Specific infective diarrhoeas

Chemotherapy is available for certain specific organisms, e.g. amoebic dysentery, giardiasis, typhoid fever (see index).

Drug-induced diarrhoea

Antimicrobials are the commonest drugs that cause diarrhoea, probably due to alteration of bowel flora. It may range from a mild inconvenience to life-threatening enterocolitis. Magnesium-containing antacids may also produce diarrhoea, as may iron salts, NSAIDs (indomethacin, mefenamic acid, flurbiprofen) and lithium.

ABNORMAL GUT MOTILITY AND INTESTINAL SPASM

Abnormal activity of the gut (see Irritable bowel syndrome, below) may cause accelerated, retarded or retrograde (reflux) movement of its contents, with attendant symptomatology. Depending on the type of movement, patients may complain of diarrhoea, constipation, colic, and a variety of symptoms, e.g. nausea, abdominal distension and pain, generally classed as *non-ulcer dyspepsia*.[9] The symptomatic management of vomiting, constipation and diarrhoea have been discussed earlier in this and the previous chapter. In addition, certain drugs with smooth muscle relaxant properties may benefit some of these, often rather intractable, symptoms. They include:

Antimuscarinic drugs

These drugs block cholinergic transmission at parasympathetic postganglionic nerve endings, including those that innervate smooth muscle, causing it to relax. They include *atropine* and *hyoscine*, and the synthetic antimuscarinics *dicyclomine, ambutonium, mepenzolate, pipenzolate, poldine* and *propantheline*. They may be used to benefit some of the spectrum of symptoms, notably those perceived to be due to smooth muscle spasm, e.g. colic and pain. Their therapeutic efficacy is limited by the other antimuscarinic effects which include dry mouth, paralysis of visual accommodation, urinary hesitancy and constipation. Antimuscarinics should be avoided in patients with gastro-oesophageal reflux and with paralytic ileus.

Other smooth muscle relaxants

Mebeverine is a reserpine derivative which has a direct effect on colonic muscle activity, especially, it appears, on colonic hypermotility. It may be used to relieve spasm of intestinal muscle, e.g. associated with organic disease of the gut, and in irritable bowel syndrome. Not being an antimuscarinic, it does not demonstrate the troublesome side-effects of that group of drugs.

Alverine and *peppermint oil* also have direct smooth muscle relaxing activity.

Irritable bowel syndrome

This common condition is characterised by abnormal bowel activity, without obvious organic cause. Stress, psyche, lack of fibre in the diet and food allergy contribute variably to its pathogenesis. An explanation of the functional nature of the disease and avoidance of foods that obviously precipitate symptoms are important initial measures. The condition is not regularly improved by drugs but, depending on the spectrum of symptoms presented, benefit may be derived by increased dietary fibre content for constipation, by antimotility drugs (loperamide, diphenoxylate) for diarrhoea, by metoclopramide or cisapride for nausea and abdominal distension, by antimuscarinics or smooth muscle relaxants (above) for abdominal pain, by sedation with a benzodiazepine, or occasionally, by an antidepressant.

INFLAMMATORY BOWEL DISEASE

In *ulcerative colitis* and *Crohn's disease*, measures to correct anaemia, fluid and electrolyte losses and to improve the general nutritional state are important. Drugs are useful both in the termination of an acute attack and in the maintenance of remission. The following are used:

Corticosteroid (see Ch. 33). Prednisolone is effective principally for acute attacks of ulcerative colitis; it may also be used during remission in those patients who cannot be maintained on mesalazine alone. Prednisolone is also effective for Crohn's disease. The objective is to reduce the inflammatory process whilst avoiding the unwanted effects of the steroid. Thus prednisolone 21-phosphate, a water soluble salt of prednisolone, is preferred for topical use within the bowel (as suppositories or enemas), for it is less absorbed than prednisolone itself, and this preparation is also suitable for i.v. administration; prednisolone, which is absorbed, is used where systemic therapy is required.

Sulphasalazine consists of two compounds,

---

[9] Working Party 1988 Lancet 1: 576.

sulphapyridine and 5-aminosalicylic acid, joined by an azo-bond. Sulphasalazine is poorly absorbed from the small intestine and bacteria in the colon split the azo-bond to release the component parts. The therapeutically active moiety is now known to be 5-aminosalicylic acid (see below). Its precise mode of action is unknown. Sulphapyridine is well absorbed, is acetylated in the liver and excreted in the urine; it has no therapeutic action but causes adverse effects; 5-aminosalicylic acid remains largely in the colon.

Sulphasalazine is effective for maintaining remission in patients with ulcerative colitis (relapses are reduced by a factor of 3), and may also be used with a corticosteroid for treatment of the acute attack. The drug may also be given as a disease-modifying agent in rheumatoid arthritis (see index), the condition for which it was originally introduced in the 1930s.

Adverse effects include headache, malaise, anorexia, nausea and vomiting; these are related to dose and are more common in slow acetylators (of sulphonamide). Allergic reactions include rash, fever and lymphadenitis; rarely leucopenia and agranulocytosis occur. Males may become infertile due to oligospermia and reduced sperm motility; this reverses if sulphasalazine is replaced with mesalazine. Several of these adverse effects are caused by the therapeutically useless sulphapyridine moiety.

Mesalazine is 5-aminosalicylic acid (see above). When it is administered by mouth only 20% is recovered in the urine, indicating that its main action is locally in the intestine. Various sustained release preparations of, and prodrugs for, 5-amino-salicylic acid are being evaluated, the objective being to achieve high colonic concentration. Mesalazine is used to maintain remission in ulcerative colitis. Patients who are intolerant of sulphasalazine usually tolerate mesalazine. The profile of adverse effects due to mesalazine includes nausea, abdominal pain and watery diarrhoea.

Olsalazine is 2 molecules of 5-aminosalicylic acid linked by an azo-bond which is split by colonic bacteria. It is used to maintain remission in ulcerative colitis and to treat mild acute attacks of the disease. Watery diarrhoea is its main adverse effect and appears to occur more often than with mesalazine. These drugs are used as follows.

Ulcerative colitis

Mild attacks can be managed outside hospital, with a regimen of mesalazine 1.2–2.4 g/d in divided doses and prednisolone by retention enema at night. Judicious use of an antimotility drug is acceptable, e.g. for social purposes.

Moderately severe attacks should generally be managed initially in hospital with prednisolone 10 mg × 4/day and mesalazine, by mouth, and prednisolone by retention enema night and morning. The regimen should be maintained for one month, when the corticosteroid should be tailed off but the mesalazine should continue. A course of iron by mouth may be needed for anaemia.

Severe attacks must be treated in hospital for management involves correcting dehydration and electrolyte upset by i.v. fluids, parenteral nutrition and, if necessary, blood; and prednisolone 60 mg/d i.v. As the patient's condition improves, the intravenous corticosteroid may be replaced with oral prednisolone 40 mg/d in divided doses. Mesalazine should be reintroduced once improvement has been maintained, and iron supplements will usually be required. Failure to respond to this intensive regimen means that colectomy will be required.

Faecal loading (visualised on abdominal radiograph) can be a cause of spurious diarrhoea and a factor that can decrease the therapeutic efficacy of prednisolone and mesalazine; the treatment is a *laxative*, not codeine.

Idiopathic proctitis: prednisolone by enema is appropriate.

Crohn's disease

Prednisolone is best to induce remission in acutely ill patients and some benefit from continued corticosteroid therapy. Azathioprine may be useful as a steroid-sparing agent, and also in some patients who have fistula or who are resistant to corticosteroid. Metronidazole may be effective for disease of the perianal region. Mesalazine helps patients with mild or moderate disease of the colon, but is less effective than prednisolone.

GUIDE TO FURTHER READING

Bateman D N, Smith J M 1988 A policy for laxatives. British Medical Journal 297: 1420

Carpenter C C J, et al 1988 Oral rehydration therapy — the role of polymeric substrates. New England Journal of Medicine 319: 1346

Clayden G S 1989 Constipation in childhood. British Medical Journal 299: 1116

Donowitz M 1991 Magnesium-induced diarrhoea and new insights into the pathobiology of diarrhoea. New England Journal of Medicine 324: 1059

Editorial 1990 Quinolones in acute non-travellers' diarrhoea. Lancet 336: 282

Field M, et al 1989 Intestinal electrolyte transport and diarrhoeal disease. New England Journal of Medicine 321: 800, 879

Heaton K W 1990 Dietary fibre. British Medical Journal 300: 1479

Mackenzie A, Barnes G 1991 Randomised controlled trial comparing oral and intravenous rehydration therapy in children with diarrhoea. British Medical Journal 303: 393

Pfeffer M A, Pfeffer J M 1990 Diarrhoea, malnutrition, euglycaemia, and fuel for thought. New England Journal of Medicine 322: 1390

32

Gastrointestinal system III: liver, biliary tract and pancreas

DRUGS AND THE LIVER

The liver is the most important organ in which drugs are structurally altered. Some of the metabolites may be biologically inactive, some active, some toxic. Furthermore the liver is exposed to drugs at higher concentrations than are most organs, for the following reason. Most drugs are administered orally, are absorbed from the gastrointestinal tract and thus the whole dose must pass through the liver to reach the systemic circulation; subsequently, 20% of the cardiac output also passes through the liver. It is hardly surprising therefore that:

- Drugs can cause direct cellular injury to the liver or otherwise interfere with its function.
- Pharmacokinetic and pharmacodynamic changes are caused by liver disease.

These issues are now considered.

DRUG-INDUCED LIVER INJURY

Toxic effects of drugs on the liver or its function may mimic almost every naturally occurring hepatic disease. Their classification accords with that for adverse effects of drugs on the body in general (see p. 117), namely:

Type A (Augmented)

Liver injury occurs as the dose of some drugs is raised, causing:

- *Centrizonal necrosis* with *paracetamol*, in overdose; this type of injury is also caused by *carbon tetrachloride* and other non-medicinal chemicals.
- *Hepatocellular necrosis* with *salicylates*, particularly in those patients with collagen diseases, when >2 g/d are taken.
- *Fatty change in liver cells and hepatic failure* with *tetracyclines* when high doses are used; this is avoided if <2 g/day is given orally and <1 g/day i.v.
- *Hepatitis* with alcohol, especially following very heavy consumption over a short period. *Alcohol hepatitis-like* changes may be induced by amiodarone, due either to the drug or its main metabolite; the dose should be kept below 600 mg/d.
- *Interference with bilirubin metabolism and excretion* with some drugs. Jaundice is induced selectively with minimal disturbance of other liver function tests; recovery ordinarily occurs on stopping the drug. Examples are:

1. *C-17 α-substituted hormones* impair bilirubin excretion into the hepatic canaliculi; the block is biochemical not mechanical. These include some androgens and anabolic steroids (see p. 596) and oestrogens and progestogens used as oral contraceptives; but jaundice is rare with the low dose formulations now preferred.

2. *Rifampicin* impairs hepatic uptake and excretion of bilirubin; plasma unconjugated and conjugated bilirubin may be elevated during the first 2–3 weeks of dosing.

3. *Fusidic acid* interferes with hepatic bilirubin excretion to cause conjugated hyperbilirubinaemia.

4. *Cholecystographic media* compete with bilirubin for uptake into the hepatic cell, and serum bilirubin may be transiently raised after an oral cholecystogram.

Type B (Bizarre)

Many drugs can cause hepatic damage at therapeutic doses, although the incidence with any single agent is low (if it were not the drug would not be used). The injury is due to unusual properties of the patient interacting with the drug and is unrelated to dose. The reaction may or may not be associated with features of generalised allergy (fever, arthralgia, skin rash, lymphadenopathy). Patterns include:

- *Acute hepatocellular necrosis.* This reaction varies from a transient disturbance of liver function tests to acute hepatitis. It can be induced by several drugs including general anaesthetics (halothane, methoxyflurane), anticonvulsants (carbamazepine, phenytoin, sodium valproate, phenobarbitone), antidepressants (MAO inhibitors), anti-inflammatory drugs (indomethacin, ibuprofen), antimicrobials (PAS, sulphonamides, nitrofurantoin) and cardiovascular drugs (methyldopa, hydralazine).
- *Cholestatic hepatitis.* The picture is of obstructive jaundice though the block is biochemical rather than mechanical. This type is particularly associated with the phenothiazine neuroleptics, especially chlorpromazine. The jaundice generally occurs within the first month of therapy, its onset may be insidious or acute with abdominal pain, and can be accompanied by features suggesting allergy (fever, rash eosinophilia). Recovery is usual. It is also caused by antidiabetic drugs (chlorpropamide, tolbutamide, glibenclamide), carbimazole, erythromycin and gold.

Type C (Continued use)

- *Chronic active hepatitis* may develop with prolonged use of methyldopa, isoniazid, dantrolene and nitrofurantoin.
- *Hepatic fibrosis or cirrhosis* may be caused by prolonged abuse of *alcohol*, and therapeutic use of *methotrexate*, e.g. for psoriasis; the risk is lessened by giving a large dose weekly rather than a smaller dose daily and by monitoring progress by liver biopsy after every 1.5–2 g of methotrexate.

Type D (Delayed effects)

Benign liver tumours may develop when synthetic androgens, e.g. anabolic steroids usually in high dose, and oral contraceptives are used for more than 5 years; there is also increased risk of developing hepatocellular carcinoma, although the absolute risk of either complication is very low. Malignant liver tumours associated with the contraceptive pill are highly vascular and may cause recurrent or acute abdominal pain if they rupture and bleed.

In summary, **drugs** may cause any of the common, and some of the uncommon, forms of **liver disease**. Always think of the possibility of drug-induced injury when:

- plasma transaminases of hepatic origin are raised
- jaundice is unexplained
- acute hepatitis, chronic active hepatitis or cirrhosis are diagnosed
- primary hepatic tumour is present
- there is liver disease of obscure cause.

PHARMACOKINETIC AND PHARMACODYNAMIC CHANGES CAUSED BY LIVER DISEASE

Pharmacokinetic changes occur because:

- drug metabolising capacity is reduced since liver cells are either sick or, if functioning normally, are reduced in number
- liver cells that metabolise drugs are bypassed when portal-systemic shunts develop in cirrhosis
- when liver disease causes hypoproteinaemia and drug binding capacity is reduced, more unbound and pharmacologically active drug may circulate.

The following discussion refers to stable liver disease such as cirrhosis or chronic active hepatitis; there is less information about altered pharmacokinetics in acute liver disease, e.g. viral hepatitis or toxic liver necrosis. The pattern of change that is induced by disease depends on the manner in which a drug is treated by the healthy liver and there are two general classes:

1. Drugs that are rapidly metabolised and highly extracted in a single pass through the liver.

Such drugs are said to undergo *presystemic elimination* after oral administration, i.e. to exhibit the hepatic first-pass effect (see index). Poor liver cell function means that less drug is extracted from the blood as it passes through the liver and portal-systemic shunts allow a proportion of blood to bypass the liver altogether. Therefore the predominant change in the kinetics of drugs that are given orally is *increased systemic availability,* i.e. the amount that reaches the systemic circulation is larger than normal, and its effect is correspondingly greater. Accordingly the initial doses of a drug should be smaller than usual, at least until some assessment of its effect has been obtained. The normally low systemic availability of, e.g. labetalol, propranolol, pentazocine, pethidine and chlormethiazole is much increased in cirrhotic patients. When liver function is severely impaired the $t_{\frac{1}{2}}$ of drugs in this class may also be lengthened.

2. Drugs that are slowly metabolised and are poorly extracted in a single pass through the liver.

These drugs do not exhibit significant first-pass effect after oral administration. The major change caused by liver disease is *prolongation of $t_{\frac{1}{2}}$.* Consequently the interval between doses of such drugs may need to be lengthened and the time to reach steady-state concentration in the plasma $(5 \times t_{\frac{1}{2}})$ is increased, e.g. diazepam, lorazepam, phenobarbitone, theophylline and clindamycin have materially increased $t_{\frac{1}{2}}$ in patients with chronic liver disease.

Pharmacodynamic changes occur because:

- Cellular responses to drugs may alter. CNS sensitivity to opioids, sedatives and antiepilepsy drugs is increased; effect of oral anticoagulants is increased because synthesis of clotting factors is impaired.
- Fluid and electrolyte balance are altered. Sodium retention may be more readily induced by NSAIDs or corticosteroids; ascites and oedema may be more resistant to diuretics.

These issues are now discussed, as they affect the use of drugs.

PRESCRIBING FOR PATIENTS WITH LIVER DISEASE

It is especially important that drugs should be prescribed only if there is real need. Patients at greatest risk are those with ascites, jaundice or evidence of encephalopathy. The following examples provide a general guide.

Central nervous system. The brain receives concentrations of toxic substances (ammonia, amines) to which it is normally not exposed, as a result of failure of liver cells to metabolise naturally-occurring substances and also of shunting of blood from the portal to the systemic circulation. CNS function becomes impaired (hepatic encephalopathy) and response to drugs is *qualitatively* abnormal.

Opioids should be avoided as coma may occur, but if an opioid is essential, pethidine is probably less dangerous than morphine. Lorazepam and oxazepam are preferred as anxiolytics and temazepam as an hypnotic. In patients with acute alcoholic liver disease who are withdrawing from alcohol, use of chlormethiazole should be particularly closely monitored. Antiepilepsy drugs should be used in the lowest effective dose; phenobarbitone may induce coma. A tricyclic may be used when antidepressant therapy is deemed necessary but MAO inhibitors are hazardous.

Cardiovascular system. Beta-adrenoceptor blockers that are metabolised, e.g. propranolol, labetalol, should be given in reduced initial oral dose, as should calcium channel antagonists, e.g. nicardipine, nifedipine, verapamil. Hypokalaemia may precipitate coma so plasma electrolytes should be monitored carefully during diuretic therapy and a potassium-sparing drug should be included in the regimen.

Gastrointestinal system. Antacids that contain much sodium may cause fluid retention and those that contain aluminium and calcium may constipate, which predisposes to encephalopathy as there is greater opportunity for absorption of toxic substances from the gut.

Infection. Many antimicrobials are eliminated by the kidney, so ordinary doses of these are safe. Avoid, or use in reduced dose, those drugs that have known risk of hepatotoxicity, e.g. isoniazid, erythromycin, rifampicin, tetracyclines. Ketoconazole is contraindicated unless there is no alternative. The sodium content of some penicillins may be hazardously high.

Endocrine system. Avoid C-17 α-substituted androgens and anabolic steroids for they are hepatotoxic (see above). Avoid combined oral contraceptives especially in cholestatic liver disease. Metformin is normally inactivated by the liver and should be avoided as it may cause lactic acidosis; chlorpropamide and tolbutamide are more likely to induce hypoglycaemia.

Respiratory system. Reduce the dose of theophylline.

ASPECTS OF THERAPY FOR LIVER DISEASE

Ascites. Standard therapy consists of dietary sodium restriction and diuretics, the aim being slowly, rather than rapidly, to remove excess salt and water. Abrupt diuresis, e.g. with too large doses of a loop diuretic, may precipitate electrolyte imbalance, renal dysfunction and hepatic encephalopathy.

Oesophageal varices and portal hypertension. Bleeding from rupture of varices is serious, the mortality from an initial event being 36–70%, depending on the patient's hepatic reserve.

• Acute variceal bleeding. Vasopressin or terlipressin (which has a weaker action) are given by i.v. infusion or injection and the varices are sclerosed immediately. The vasopressin constricts splanchnic vessels, thus reducing flow to and pressure in the liver and the collateral (oesophageal) channels. Coronary vasoconstriction may be induced also and cause angina. Balloon tamponade, followed by obliteration of the varices by sclerotherapy is another option.

• Prophylactic therapy. β-adrenoceptor block reduces variceal bleeding in cirrhotic patients. It probably does so by lowering cardiac output, causing a fall in hepatic blood flow, and with it portal pressure; other more complex mechanisms may be involved. Propranolol seems most effective and safe in mild (compensated) cases and less so in those with severe (decompensated) disease, in whom, also, the reduction in liver blood flow may precipitate encephalopathy. Systemic availability of propranolol is greatly increased in severe hepatic disease. Prophylactic propranolol may be combined with endoscopic sclerosing injection of varices where practicable.

BILE SALTS AND GALLSTONES

Gallstone disease affects about 15% of females and 6% of males of middle age in the UK, and the prevalence increases with age. Cholesterol is the commonest constituent of stones in countries where gallstone disease is common; some stones consist almost exclusively of cholesterol while others also contain bile pigments, calcium and protein. Stones that are rich in cholesterol are amenable to medical treatment.

Some pathophysiology

Bile acids are synthesised from cholesterol in the liver, secreted into the duodenum and reabsorbed at the terminal ileum; in any one day the acids may go round this *enterohepatic cycle* 5–10 times.

Human bile has a capacity for maintaining more cholesterol in solution than, say, an equivalent volume of water. The explanation is that bile contains bile acids (mainly cholic, deoxycholic and chenodeoxycholic) and phospholipids (mainly lecithin) which together form molecular aggregates called *mixed micelles* that are capable of keeping cholesterol dissolved within them. It follows that bile can become saturated and cholesterol can precipitate (forming gallstones) if: 1. the concentration of bile acids is too low or, 2. the concentration of cholesterol in the bile is too high.

Enhancing the cholesterol holding capacity of bile is the basis of medical treatment for cholesterol gallstone and it is achieved either by increasing the bile acid content or by reducing the cholesterol content of bile.

Ursodeoxycholic acid (UDCA) is a bile acid which occurs in small amounts in the human (but in large amounts in the bile of the bear family,

Ursidae). It is effective at dissolving gallstones. The mechanism of action of UDCA is not clear but may involve reduction of cholesterol absorption from the gut, inhibition of cholesterol synthesis by the liver and, to a lesser extent, expansion of the bile acid pool. The result is that bile contains less cholesterol and more bile acid; saturated bile is converted into unsaturated bile which can redissolve cholesterol that has precipitated as gallstones. An oral cholecystogram after 6 months will show whether therapy is proving effective. Treatment should continue for up to 24 months depending on the size of the stone(s) and should be maintained for 3 months after dissolution. Unlike chenodeoxycholic acid (below), UDCA rarely causes diarrhoea and does not elevate transaminases; it is therefore usually preferred.

Chenodeoxycholic acid (CDCA) comprises about 40% of the naturally-occurring bile acids, and when it is taken as a medicine to treat gallstones the proportion rises to 70%. It is effective for gallstone dissolution but causes diarrhoea in about 40% of patients and elevates plasma aspartate transaminase concentrations. Chenodeoxycholic acid should not be given to patients at risk of pregnancy or to patients with chronic liver disease or inflammatory bowel disease.

A *terpene* mixture (Rowachol) also increases cholesterol solubility in bile but less effectively than CDCA or UDCA. It may be used in addition to CDCA and UDCA for stones in the common bile duct.

Dehydrocholic acid stimulates the formation of thin, watery bile; it is used after surgery to flush small calculi out of the bile ducts, and in radiology to help visualisation of the gallbladder.

Use of drugs to dissolve gallstones

Only about 30% of patients are suitable for treatment for the following reasons:

● The *gallstone(s)* must be completely radiolucent, for even a thin covering of calcium salts usually prevents dissolution. Pigment stones are also radiolucent but are usually associated with haemolytic disorders. Small stones (5–10 mm diameter) respond better because the surface area for dissolution is relatively large.

- The *gallbladder* must be shown by cholecystography to be functioning; in many patients with recurrent cholecystitis the gallbladder is shrunken and cannot concentrate bile.
- The *patients* for whom the treatment is most appropriate are mainly those in whom surgery is inadvisable, i.e. the elderly, the obese, the unfit. Symptoms should be infrequent, for treatment may take 1–2 years. Patients who have asymptomatic gallbladder stones need not be treated for such stones tend to remain silent.

The major concern with medical dissolution of gallstones is the recurrence of 30–50% stones in 3–5 years; low-dose UDCA may be effective prophylaxis in younger patients but the issue of what drug to use and in whom remains unresolved.

Other non-surgical treatments for gallstones

Direct contact dissolution by injecting a volatile organic solvent, methyl tert-butyl ether (MTBE), by percutaneous transhepatic cannulation of the gallbladder, can dissolve gallstones in 7 h–3 d. The role of this and other solvents is being evaluated.

Conditions caused by bile acids

Excess bile acids in the colon cause diarrhoea, e.g. after resection of the ileum, their normal site of reabsorption. In biliary obstruction pruritus is due to accumulation of bile acids. Both conditions may be helped by cholestyramine.

Cholestyramine is an anion exchange resin that is used principally to treat hyperlipidaemias (see p. 455). Taken orally, it binds bile acids in the bowel, preventing their absorption, and is thus effective for diarrhoea due to bile acids in the colon; excess effect may cause steatorrhoea. Provided biliary obstruction is partial, i.e. that there is some escape of bile acids into the intestine where they can be bound, cholestyramine will reduce the accumulation of bile acids and help pruritus.

THE PANCREAS
Digestive enzymes

In pancreatic exocrine insufficiency, the aim of therapy is to prevent weight loss and diarrhoea and to maintain adequate growth in children. The problem of getting enough enzyme to the duodenum concurrently with food is not as simple as it might appear. Gastric emptying varies with the composition of meals, e.g. high fat, calories or protein causes delay, and the pancreatic enzymes taken by mouth are destroyed by gastric juice. On the other hand, only one-tenth of the normal pancreatic output is sufficient to prevent excess fat (steatorrhoea) or excess nitrogen (azotorrhoea) loss, and it is not essential to eliminate these totally.

Preparations are of animal origin and of variable potency. Pancreatin BNF, Cotazym and Nutrizym appear to be satisfactory. A reasonable course is to start the patient on the recommended dose of a reliable formulation and to vary this according to the individual's needs, and the size and composition of meals. Some extract may be taken before, during and after food to limit destruction by gastric acid, and antacids, cimetidine or ranitidine taken 30–45 min before pancreatin may improve its efficacy. Enteric-coated formulations (Pancreatin Granules, Tablets) are available.

Acute pancreatitis

Many drugs have been tested for specific effect, and none has shown convincing benefit. The main requirements of therapy are:

- to provide adequate analgesia. Opioids are generally satisfactory; their potential disadvantage of contracting the sphincter of Oddi appears to be outweighed by their analgesic efficacy; buprenorphine has less of this effect and may therefore be preferred.
- to correct hypovolaemia due to the exudation of large amounts of fluid around the inflamed pancreas. Plasma may be required, or blood if the haematocrit falls; in addition large volumes of electrolyte solution may be needed to maintain urine flow.

Drugs and the pancreas

The strongest association with acute pancreatitis is alcohol drinking. High plasma calcium, including that caused by hypervitaminosis D and parenteral nutrition also increase the risk. Corticosteroids, diuretics, including thiazides and frusemide, and paracetamol, in overdose, have also been causally related.

GUIDE TO FURTHER READING

Bateson M C 1986 Acute pancreatitis. British Medical Journal 292: 848

Editorial 1988 Diuresis or paracentesis for ascites? Lancet 2: 775

Editorial 1989 Gallstones, bile acids, and the liver. Lancet 2: 249

Lieber C S 1988 Biochemical and molecular basis of alcohol-induced injury to the liver and other tissues. New England Journal of Medicine 319: 1693

Panos M, et al 1988 Treating the ascites of cirrhosis. British Medical Journal 297: 698

Poynard T et al 1991 Beta-adrenergic-antagonist drugs in the prevention of gastrointestinal bleeding in patients with cirrhosis and oesophageal varices. New England Journal of Medicine 324: 1532

Salen G, Tint G S 1989 Nonsurgical treatment of gallstones. New England Journal of Medicine 320: 665

Sherlock S 1986 The spectrum of hepatotoxicity to drugs. Lancet 2: 440

Terblanche J, et al 1989 Controversies in the management of bleeding esophageal varices. New England Journal of Medicine 320: 1393, 1469

33

Endocrinology I: adrenal corticosteroids, antagonists, corticotrophin

In 1855, Dr. Thomas Addison, assisted in his observations by three colleagues, published his famous monograph 'On the constitutional and local effects of disease of the suprarenal capsules' (Addison's disease). It was not until the 1920s that the vital importance of the adrenal cortex was appreciated and the distinction between the hormones secreted by the cortex and medulla.

By 1936, numerous steroids were being crystallised from cortical extracts, but not enough could be obtained to provide supplies for clinical trial.

In 1948 *cortisone* was made from bile acids in quantity sufficient for clinical trial, and the dramatic demonstration of its power to induce remission of rheumatoid arthritis was published in the following year. In 1950 it was realised that cortisone is biologically inert and that the active natural hormone is hydrocortisone (cortisol). Since then an embarrassingly large number of synthetic steroids has been made and offered to the clinician. They are made by a complicated process from natural substances (chiefly plant sterols), the constitutions of which approach most nearly to that of the steroids themselves. A principal aim in research is to produce steroids with more selective action than hydrocortisone, which induces a greater variety of effects than desired in any patient who is not suffering from adrenal insufficiency.

About the same time as cortisone was introduced, *corticotrophin* became available for clinical use.

ADRENAL STEROIDS AND THEIR SYNTHETIC ANALOGUES

Hormones normally produced by the adrenal cortex include hydrocortisone (cortisol), corticosterone, aldosterone and some androgens and oestrogens, but *not* cortisone. Cortisone is a prodrug, i.e. it is biologically inert and must be converted (largely in the liver) to hydrocortisone for biological activity; its use is obsolete for this reason.

Numerous analogues have been made in which the major actions have been separated.

When the adrenal cortex fails (Addison's disease) adrenocortical steroids are available for *replacement therapy*, but their chief use in medicine is for *their anti-inflammatory and immuno-suppressive effects (pharmacotherapy)*. These are only obtained when the drugs are given in doses far above those needed for *physiological replacement*. Various metabolic effects, which are of the greatest importance to the normal functioning of the body, then become adverse or side-effects. Much successful effort has gone into separating *glucocorticoid* from *mineralocorticoid* effects[1] and some steroids, e.g. dexamethasone, have virtually no mineralocorticoid activity. But it has not yet proved possible to separate the glucocorticoid effects from each other, so that if a steroid is used for its anti-inflammatory action the risks of osteoporosis, diabetes, etc., remain.

In the account that follows, the effects of hydrocortisone will be described and then other steroids insofar as they differ. In the context of this chapter 'adrenal steroid' means a substance with hydrocortisone-like activity. Androgens are described in Chapter 36.

Mechanism of action

Adrenocortical steroids enter cells where they combine with steroid receptors in the cytoplasm. The combination then enters the nucleus where it controls the synthesis of protein, including enzymes that regulate vital cell activities over a wide range of metabolic functions including all aspects of inflammation. There is formation of protein that inhibits the enzyme phospholipase A_2, which is needed to allow the supply of arachidonic acid from which mediators of inflammation are formed; these mediators cause increased vascular permeability and subsequent changes including oedema, leucocyte migration, fibrin deposition. Corticosteroids also act on cell membranes, altering ion permeability, and they modify the production of neurohormones.

The actions of hydrocortisone

Naturally there is a distinction between *replacement therapy (physiological effects)* and the higher doses of *pharmacotherapy*.

On inorganic metabolism (mineralocorticoid effects): increased retention of sodium by the renal tubule, and increased potassium excretion in the urine.

On organic metabolism (glucocorticoid effects):

- *Carbohydrate metabolism*: gluconeogenesis is increased and peripheral glucose utilisation (transport across cell membranes) may be decreased (insulin antagonism) so that hyperglycaemia and sometimes glycosuria result. Latent diabetes becomes overt, and this effect has been used as a test for the prediabetic state.

- *Protein metabolism*: anabolism (conversion of amino acids to protein) is decreased but *catabolism* continues unabated or even faster, so that there is a negative nitrogen balance with muscle wasting. Osteoporosis (reduction of bone protein matrix) occurs, growth slows in children, the skin atrophies and this, with increased capillary fragility, causes bruising and striae. Healing of peptic ulcers or of wounds, is delayed as is fibrosis.

- *Fat deposition*: this is increased on shoulders, face and abdomen.

- *Inflammatory response* is depressed, regardless of its cause, so that as well as being of great benefit in 'useless' or excessive inflammation, steroids can be a source of danger in infections

---

[1] The mere introduction of a double bond transforms hydrocortisone to prednisolone, a big biological change: see Table 33.1 for relative potencies 1.0:1.0 to 4:0.8.

by limiting useful protective inflammation. Neutrophil and macrophage function is depressed, including the release of chemical mediators and the effects of these on capillaries.

- *Allergic responses* are suppressed. The antigen-antibody interaction is unaffected, but its injurious inflammatory consequences do not follow.
- *Antibody production* is reduced by heavy doses.
- *Lymphoid tissue* is reduced (including leukaemic lymphocytes).
- *Renal excretion of uric acid* is increased.
- *Blood eosinophils* are reduced in number.
- *Euphoria or psychotic* states may occur, perhaps due to CNS electrolyte changes.
- *Anti-vitamin D action*, see calciferol.
- *Reduction of hypercalcaemia* chiefly where this is due to excessive absorption of Ca from the gut (sarcoidosis, vitamin D intoxication).
- *Urinary calcium excretion* is increased and renal stones may form.
- *Growth reduction* where new cells are being *added* (growth in children), but not where they are *replacing* cells as in adult tissues.
- *Suppression of hypothalamic/pituitary/ adrenocortical system* (with delayed recovery)

occurs with chronic use (see p. 554), so that abrupt withdrawal leaves the patient in a state of adrenocortical insufficiency.

The *normal daily secretion* of hydrocortisone is 10–30 mg. The exogenous daily dose that completely suppresses the cortex is hydrocortisone 40–80 mg, or prednisolone 10–20 mg, or its equivalent of other agents. Recovery of function is quick after a few days' use; but when used over months recovery takes months. A steroid-suppressed adrenal continues to secrete aldosterone.

Individual adrenal steroids

The relative potencies for glucocorticoid and mineralocorticoid effects which are shown in Table 33.1 are central to the choice of agent in relation to clinical indication.

All drugs in Table 33.1 except aldosterone are active when swallowed, being protected from hepatic first-pass metabolism by high binding to plasma proteins. Some details of preparations and equivalent doses are given in the Table. Injectable and topical forms are available (creams, suppositories, eye drops).

Table 33.1 Relative potencies of adrenal steroids

| Compound (tablet strength, mg) | Approximate relative potency | | Equivalent[1] dosage (for anti-inflammatory effect, mg)[2] |
	Anti-inflammatory (glucocorticoid) effect	Sodium-retaining (mineralocorticoid) effect	
Cortisone (25)	0.8	1.0	25
Hydrocortisone (20)	1.0	1.0	20
Prednisolone (5)	4	0.8	5
Methylprednisolone (4)	5	minimal	4
Triamcinolone (4)	5	none	4
Dexamethasone (0.5)	30	minimal	0.75
Betamethasone (0.5)	30	negligible	0.75
Fludrocortisone (0.1)	15	150	irrelevant
Aldosterone —	none	500[3]	—

[1] Note that these equivalents are in approximate inverse accord with the tablet strengths.
[2] The doses in the final column are in the lower range of those that may cause suppression of the hypothalamic/pituitary/adrenocortical axis when given daily continuously. Much higher doses, e.g. 40 mg prednisolone, can be given on alternate days or daily for up to 5 days without causing clinically significant suppression.
[3] Injected.

Hydrocortisone (cortisol) is the principal naturally occurring steroid; it is taken orally; a soluble salt can be given i.v. (as Hydrocortisone Sodium Succinate Inj.) for rapid effect in emergency (whether due to deficiency, allergy or inflammatory disease). A suspension (Hydrocortisone Acetate Inj.) can be given intra-articularly.

Cortisone is obsolete (see above).

Choice of parenteral preparation for systemic effect: the soluble Hydrocortisone Sodium Succinate Inj. is used for quick (1–2 h) effect; for continuous effect about 8-hourly administration is appropriate. Prednisolone Acetate Inj. i.m. is an alternative, once or twice a week.

Oral tablet strengths, see Table 33.1.

Prednisolone is predominantly anti-inflammatory (glucocorticoid), is biologically active and has little sodium-retaining activity; it is the standard choice for anti-inflammatory pharmacotherapy, orally or i.m.

Prednisone is a prodrug i.e. it is biologically inert and converted into prednisolone in the liver. Since there is 20% less on conversion there seems no point in using it.

Methylprednisolone is similar to prednisolone; it is used i.v. for megadose pulse therapy (see below).

Fluorinated corticosteroids: triamcinolone has virtually no sodium-retaining effect but has the disadvantage that muscle wasting may occasionally be severe and anorexia and mental depression may be more common at high doses; **dexamethasone** and **betamethasone** are similar, powerful, predominantly anti-inflammatory steroids. They are longer acting than prednisolone and are used for therapeutic adrenocortical suppression.

Fludrocortisone has a very great sodium-retaining effect in relation to its anti-inflammatory action, and only as high doses need the non-electrolyte effects be considered. It is used to replace aldosterone where the adrenal cortex is destroyed (Addison's disease).

Aldosterone ($t_{\frac{1}{2}}$ 20 min), the principal natural salt-retaining hormone, has been used i.m. in acute adrenal insufficiency. After oral administration it is rapidly inactivated in the first pass through the liver and it has no place in routine therapeutics, as fludrocortisone is as effective and is active orally.

Spironolactone is a competitive aldosterone antagonist which also blocks the mineralocorticoid effect of other steroids; it is used in treatment of *primary hyperaldosteronism* and as a diuretic.

Beclomethasone and **budesonide** are used by inhalation for asthma (see p. 514). About 90% of an inhalation dose is swallowed and these steroids are inactivated by hepatic first-pass metabolism; the rest, absorbed from mouth and lungs, gives very low systemic plasma concentration. The risk of suppression of the hypothalamic/pituitary/adrenal axis is thus minimal (but it can happen). This property of extensive hepatic first-pass metabolism with low systemic availability is an advantage in the topical treatment of inflammatory bowel disease with minimal risk of systemic adverse effects.

Pharmacokinetics of corticosteroids

Absorption of the synthetic steroids given *orally* is rapid. The $t_{\frac{1}{2}}$ of most in plasma is 1–3 h but the *maximum* biological effect occurs after 2–8 h. They are usually given 2 or 3 times a day. They are metabolised principally in the liver and are excreted by the kidney. The $t_{\frac{1}{2}}$ is prolonged in hepatic and renal disease and is shortened by hepatic enzyme induction to an extent that can be clinically important. For hepatic first-pass metabolism see immediately above.

Topical application (skin, lung, joints) allows absorption which can be enough to cause systemic effects.

In the blood, adrenal steroids are carried in the free (biologically active) form (5%) and also bound (95% in the case of hydrocortisone) to *transcortin* (a globulin with high affinity, but low binding capacity) and, when this is saturated, to albumin (80% in the case of hydrocortisone). The concentration of the transcortin is increased by oestrogens, e.g. pregnancy, oral contraception, other oestrogen therapy, so that if plasma hydrocortisone concentration is measured the *total* will be found raised, but the amount of *free* hydrocortisone may be normal, being controlled by the normal feedback mechanism. Patients may be wrongly suspected of Cushing's syndrome if the fact that they are taking oestrogen is unrecognised and only the *total* concentration is measured (as is usual).

In patients with very low serum albumin, steroid doses should be lower than usual owing to the reduced binding capacity. In addition, low albumin concentration may be caused by *liver disease*, which also potentiates steroids by delaying metabolism (t_2^1 of prednisolone may be doubled).

Dosage schedules

Various spaced-out dosage schedules have been used in the hope of reducing hypothalamic/pituitary/adrenal suppression by allowing the plasma steroid concentration to fall enough between doses to provide time for pituitary recovery, e.g. prednisolone 40 mg on alternate days does not cause appreciable pituitary suppression. But none has been both successful in wholly avoiding suppression at the same time as it was successful in controlling symptoms. Where a single daily dose is practicable it should be given in the early morning. *Alternate day schedules* are worth trying, especially where immunosuppression is the objective (organ transplants) rather than anti-inflammatory effect (rheumatoid arthritis); asthmatics taking a systemic steroid may or may not be manageable on such intermittent dosage. *Short courses* (a few days) may be practicable for some without significant suppression.

Another variant is to give *enormous doses* (grams, not mg), orally or i.v., e.g. methylprednisolone 1.0 g i.v. on 3 successive days, at intervals of weeks or months (*megadose pulses*). The technique is used particularly in collagen diseases. Definitive evaluation of efficacy and side-effects is awaited.

Choice of adrenal steroid: summary

• *For oral replacement therapy* in adrenocortical insufficiency, *hydrocortisone* should be used to supply mineralocorticoid and some glucocorticoid activity. In Addison's disease a small dose of a hormone with only mineralocorticoid effect (fludrocortisone) is normally needed in addition. Prednisolone on its own is not effective replacement therapy.

• *For anti-inflammatory and anti-allergic (immunosuppressive) effect, prednisolone,* triamcinolone or dexamethasone. It is not possible to rank these in firm order of merit. One or other may suit an individual patient best, especially as regards incidence of side-effects such as muscle wasting. By *inhalation,* beclomethasone or budesonide.

• *For hypothalamic/pituitary/adrenocortical suppression,* e.g. in adrenal hyperplasia, prednisolone or dexamethasone.

Adverse effects of systemic adrenal steroid pharmacotherapy

These consist of *too intense production of the physiological or pharmacological actions* listed under actions of hydrocortisone. Some are confined to systemic use and for this reason local therapy, e.g. inhalation, intra-articular injection, is preferred where practicable.

Unwanted effects virtually do not occur with 1 or 2 doses though some occur with a few days' use, e.g. spread of infection. They follow prolonged administration and are sufficiently frequent and dangerous to warrant serious consideration by the physician whether 'the disease which he is attempting to suppress is more dangerous to the patient than the Cushing's syndrome which he might induce'.[2] The undesired effects recounted below should never be experienced in replacement therapy, but are sometimes unavoidable when the steroid is used as pharmacotherapy. Naturally, the nature of unwanted effects depends on the choice of steroid. Fludrocortisone in ordinary doses does not cause osteoporosis and prednisolone does not normally cause oedema.

In general, *serious unwanted effects* are unlikely if the daily dose is below the equivalent of hydrocortisone 50 mg or prednisolone 10 mg.

---

[2] Liddle G W. Clin Pharmacol Ther 1961; 2: 615.

The principal evil effects of chronic administration are:

Iatrogenic Cushing's syndrome: moon face, characteristic deposition of fat on the body, oedema, hypertension, striae, bruising, acne, hirsutism, muscle wasting and *osteoporosis* of the spine (with fractures of vertebrae, ribs, femora and feet). Addition of a small dose of anabolic steroid in the hope of preventing osteoporosis and muscle wasting has been tried, but is ineffective. When these occur, change to corticortrophin may help, as may calcium supplement to diet and *small* doses of vitamin D to reduce progress of osteoporosis (which is largely irreversible).

Avascular necrosis of bone (femoral heads) is another serious complication (at higher doses); it appears to be due to restriction of blood flow through bone capillaries. Pain and restriction of movement may occur months in advance of radiographic changes. *Diabetes mellitus* may appear. *Growth* in children is impaired.

Depression and psychosis can occur, sometimes with suicide, especially in those with a history of mental disorder; *insomnia* is common.

Peptic ulceration. Patients taking continuous oral therapy probably have an excess incidence of peptic ulcer and haemorrhage of about 1–2%. It is plainly unreasonable to seek to protect all such patients by routinely giving prophylactic antiulcer therapy, i.e. to treat 98 patients unnecessarily in order to help 2. But such therapy (histamine H_2-receptor blocker, sucralfate) may be used when ulcer is particularly likely, e.g. a patient with rheumatoid arthritis taking a NSAID, or when ulcer develops whilst taking the steroid. In patients with a history of peptic ulcer disease physicians will exercise their critical judgement.

Ulcer may occur with treatment as brief as 30 days.

Other effects include: posterior subcapsular lens cataract (risk if dose exceeds 10 mg prednisolone/day or equivalent for above a year), glaucoma (with prolonged use of eye drops), raised intracranial pressure and convulsions, blood hypercoagulability, menstrual disorders and fever. Delayed tissue healing following surgery is seldom important, but it can disagreeably complicate deep radiotherapy. Major skin damage can result from minor injury of any kind.

Suppression of the inflammatory response to infection and immunosuppression causes some patients to present with atypical symptoms and signs and quickly to deteriorate. The incidence of infection is increased with high dose therapy, and any infection can be more severe when it occurs. Previously dormant tuberculosis may become active insidiously. Intra-articular injections demand the strictest asepsis.

The incidence of unwanted effects of one kind or another depends on drug used, dosage and duration of therapy but can be as high as 50% of cases.

Hypothalamic/pituitary/adrenal (HPA) suppression is dependent on the steroid used, its dose, duration and the time of administration. A single morning dose of less than 20 mg of prednisolone is usually not followed by suppression, whereas a dose of 5 mg given late in the evening is suppressive of the essential early morning activation of the HPA axis (circadian rhythm). *Substantial suppression of the HPA axis can occur within a week* (but see Withdrawal of steroid therapy, below).

Adrenal steroids and pregnancy

Adrenal steroids are teratogenic in animals. Although a relationship between steroid pharmacotherapy and cleft palate and other fetal abnormalities has been suspected in man, there is no doubt that many women taking a steroid throughout have both conceived and borne normal babies. Adrenal insufficiency due to hypothalamic/pituitary suppression in the newborn only occurs with high doses to the mother. Dosage during pregnancy should be kept as low as practicable and fluorinated steroids are best avoided as they are more teratogenic in animals (dexa- and betamethasone, triamcinolone and various topical steroids, e.g. fluocinolone). Hypoadrenal women who become pregnant may require an increase in hydrocortisone replacement therapy by about 10 mg per day to compensate for the increased binding by plasma proteins that occurs in pregnancy.

Labour should be managed as described for major surgery (below).

Precautions during chronic adrenal steroid therapy

The most important precaution during replacement and pharmacotherapy is to see the patient regularly with an awareness of the possibilities of adverse effects including fluid retention (weight gain), hypertension, glycosuria, hypokalaemia (potassium supplement may be necessary), and back pain (osteoporosis).

Mild withdrawal symptoms (iatrogenic cortical insufficiency) include conjunctivitis, rhinitis, weight loss, arthralgia and itchy skin nodules.

Patients must always carry a card giving details of therapy and simple instructions and they *must* be impressed with the importance of compliance; also, on what to do if they develop an intercurrent illness or other severe stress — to double their next dose and to tell their doctor. If a patient omits a dose then it should be made up as soon as possible so that the total daily intake is maintained, because every patient should be taking the *minimum* dose necessary to control the disease.

Treatment of intercurrent illness

The normal adrenal cortex responds to severe *stress* by secreting more than 300 mg cortisol/day. Intercurrent illness is stress and treatment is urgent, particularly of *infections*; the dose of corticosteroid should be doubled during the illness and gradually reduced as the patient improves. Effective chemotherapy of bacterial infections is specially important.

Viral infections contracted during steroid therapy can be overwhelming because the immune response of the body may be largely suppressed; continuous use of equivalent of 20 mg prednisolone/day or more is immunosuppressive. But a steroid may sometimes be useful in therapy after the disease has begun

(thyroiditis, encephalitis) and there has been time for the immune response to occur. It then acts by suppressing unwanted effects of immune responses and excessive inflammatory reaction.

Vomiting may require parenteral administration.

In the event of the misfortune of *surgery* being added to that of adrenal steroid therapy the patient should receive hydrocortisone 100–200 mg i.m. with premedication. If there is any sign suggestive that the patient may collapse, e.g. hypotension, during the operation, i.v. hydrocortisone (50–100 mg) should be infused at once. Otherwise, if there are no complications, the dose is repeated 6-hourly for 24–72 h and then reduced by half every 24 h until normal dose level is reached.

Minor operations, e.g. dental extraction, may be covered by hydrocortisone 100 mg orally 2–4 h before operation and the same dose afterwards.

In all these situations an i.v. infusion should be available for immediate use in case the above is not enough. These precautions should be used in patients who have received substantial treatment with corticosteroid within the past year, because their hypothalamic/pituitary/adrenal system, though sufficient for ordinary life, may fail to respond adequately to severe stress. If steroid therapy has been very prolonged, these precautions should be taken for as long as 2 years after stopping it. This will mean that some unnecessary treatment is given, but collapse due to acute adrenal insufficiency can be fatal and the ill-effects of short-lived increased dosage of steroid are less grave, being confined to possible increased incidence and severity of infection.

Dosage and routes of administration

Dosage depends very much on the purpose for which the steroid is being used and on individual response. It is impossible to suggest a single schedule that will suit every case.

The following *systemic commencing doses* can be used:

For a *serious disease* such as systemic lupus, dermatomyositis: prednisolone up to 30 mg/day orally in divided doses; if *life-threatening*, up to 70 mg, or its equivalent of another steroid. The dose is then increased if necessary until the disease is controlled or adverse effects occur; as much as prednisolone 300 mg a day can be needed.

Alternatively megadose pulses (methylprednisolone 1.0 g i.v. daily for 3 days); followed by oral maintenance.

For *less dangerous disease*, such as rheumatoid arthritis: prednisolone 7.5–10.0 mg daily, adjusted later according to the response.

In some special cases, including *replacement* of adrenal insufficiency, dosage is mentioned in the account of the treatment of the disease.

For continuous therapy the minimum amount to produce the desired effect must be used. Sometimes imperfect control must be accepted by the patient because full control, e.g. of rheumatoid arthritis, though obtainable, involves use of doses that must lead to long-term toxicity, e.g. osteoporosis, if continued for years. The decision to embark on such therapy is a serious matter for the patient.

Topical applications (creams, intranasal, inhalations, enemas) are used in attempts, often successful, to obtain local, whilst avoiding systemic, effects; suspensions or solutions are also injected into joints, soft tissues and subconjunctivally. However, all these can, with heavy dose, be sufficiently absorbed to suppress the hypothalamus and cause other unwanted effects. Individual preparations are mentioned in the text where appropriate.

The relatively high selectivity of *inhaled beclomethasone* in asthma is due to a combination of route of administration, high potency and rapid conversion to inactive metabolites by the liver of any drug that is absorbed (see asthma, skin); but yet hypothalamic/pituitary suppression and systemic toxicity occasionally occur.

Contraindications to the use of adrenal steroids for suppressing inflammation are all relative, depending on the advantage to be expected. They should only be used for serious reasons in patients with diabetes, a history of mental disorder or peptic ulcer, epilepsy,

tuberculosis, hypertension or heart failure. The presence of any infection demands that effective chemotherapy be begun before the steroid, but there are exceptions (some viral infections, see above). *Topical corticosteroid applied to an inflamed eye (with the very best of intention) can be disastrous if the inflammation is due to herpes virus.*

Steroids containing fluorine (see above) intensify diabetes more than others and so should be avoided in that disease.

Long-term use of adrenal steroids in children presents essentially the same problems as in adults except that growth is retarded approximately in proportion to the dose. This is unlikely to be important unless therapy exceeds 6 months; there is a spurt of growth after withdrawal. Intermittent dosage schedules (alternate day) may reduce the risk (rarely, corticotrophin may be preferred p. 562).

Some other problems loom larger in children than in adults. Common childhood viral infections may be more severe, and if a non-immune child taking an adrenal steroid is exposed to one, it is wise to try to prevent the disease with the appropriate specific immunoglobulin (if available).

Live virus vaccination is unsafe in immunosuppressed subjects, e.g. systemic prednisolone >2 mg/kg per day for >1 week in the preceding 3 months, as it may cause the disease, but active immunisation with killed vaccines or toxoids will give normal response unless the dose of steroid is high, when the response may be suppressed.

Raised intracranial pressure may occur more readily in children than in adults.

Fixed-dose combinations of adrenal steroids with other drugs in one tablet should *never* be used as they abrogate the principles for the use of such formulations (p. 102).

Indications for use of adrenal steroids

- Replacement of hormone deficiency
- Inflammation suppression
- Immunosuppression
- Suppression of excess hormone secretion

Nabarro[3] summarised *the place of adrenal steroids in therapeutics*, and this account of 1960 remains valid:

The use of physiological amounts of hydrocortisone has greatly improved the replacement therapy available for patients with Addison's disease or hypopituitarism. Larger or pharmacological amounts of steroids have been used in the treatment of diseases unrelated to the adrenal gland. Adrenocortical steroids inhibit the inflammatory reaction, but in many instances the inflammatory reaction is part of the body's defence mechanism and is to be encouraged rather than inhibited. It has, however, become apparent that there are diseases which are really due to the body's reaction being quite disproportionate to the noxious stimulus. The manifestations of the disease are, in fact, those of an exaggerated or inappropriate inflammatory response, and if steroid therapy can inhibit this inappropriate response the manifestations of the patient's disease will be suppressed. The underlying condition is not cured, though it may ultimately burn itself out.

The anti-inflammatory action of steroids is used for this purpose in allergic conditions and diseases like rheumatoid arthritis, rheumatic carditis, disseminated lupus erythematosus, and polyarteritis nodosa. Large doses of steroid will also inhibit antibody production and help in the management of auto-immune conditions like some of the haemolytic anaemias and thrombocytopenic purpuras. Steroid therapy may also be used to suppress the patient's adrenal glands; the doses required, however, are nearer the physiological levels. This may be needed in cases of adrenal dysfunction where abnormal androgenic steroids are being made, or in cases of disseminated breast cancer to inhibit adrenal secretion of oestrogens, the so-called medical adrenalectomy.

When large doses of steroids are given for their pharmacological action, the result will be to produce an iatrogenic Cushing's syndrome. There is a tendency to forget that Cushing's syndrome is a serious illness with a grave prognosis — so serious, in fact, that one has no hesitation in advising total adrenalectomy for its treatment. Admittedly, treatment with high doses of steroid may in some situations be life-saving, or produce a temporary remission in an incurable disease. There has been a tendency to overlook the dangers of treatment with adrenocortical steroids and to use them in cases where the treatment may prove more dangerous or disabling than the original disease.

[3] Nabarro J D N. Br Med J 1960; 2: 553.

Uses of adrenocortical steroids

Replacement therapy

Acute adrenocortical insufficiency
(Addisonian crisis)

This is an emergency and hydrocortisone sodium succinate 100 mg should be given i.v. immediately it is *suspected*, or the patient may die. An i.v. infusion of sodium chloride solution (0.9%) is set up immediately and a second 100 mg of hydrocortisone is added to the first litre, which may be given over 2 h (several litres of fluid may be needed in the first 24 h). The patient should then receive hydrocortisone 50–100 mg i.v. or i.m. 6–8 hourly for 24 h; then 12-hourly, initiating oral use when appropriate; then a total of 50–75 mg a day orally in 2 or 3 doses. Other treatment to restore electrolyte balance will depend on the circumstances. The cause of the crisis should be sought and treated; it is often an infection. When the dose of hydrocortisone falls below 60 mg a day, supplementary mineralo-corticoid (fludrocortisone) may be needed (see below).

The *hyper*kalaemia of Addison's disease will respond to the above regimen and must not be treated with insulin because of the risk of severe hypoglycaemia.

Chronic primary adrenocortical insufficiency (Addison's disease)

Hydrocortisone orally is used (20–40 mg total daily) in the lowest dose that maintains well-being and body weight, with two-thirds of the total dose in the morning and one-third in the evening to mimic the natural *diurnal rhythm* of secretion.[4] Plainly corticotrophin is useless.

[4] But this can be associated with an unphysiologically low plasma concentration of hydrocortisone in the late afternoon (with loss of well-being). Such patients may be best managed on 3 equal doses per day. *Air travellers* on long flights across longitude east to west (> 12 h, i.e. longer day): take an extra dose near the end of the flight. For west to east flights (> 8 h, i.e. shorter day): the normal evening dose may be taken sooner and the usual dose taken on the 'new' morning. *Night workers* may adjust their dosage to their work pattern (Drug Therap Bull 1990: 28: 71).

Some patients do well on hydrocortisone alone, with or without added salt, but most patients require a small amount of mineralocorticoid as well (fludrocortisone, 0.1–0.2 mg once a day, orally). If the dose of fludrocortisone should exceed 0.5 mg a day, an unlikely event, then its glucocorticoid effect must be taken into account.

The dosage of the hormones is determined in the individual by following general clinical progress and particularly by observing weight, blood pressure, appearance of oedema, serum sodium and potassium concentrations and haematocrit. If any complicating disease arises, such as infection, a need for surgery or other stress, the hydrocortisone dosage should immediately be doubled, see above. *If there is vomiting*, the replacement hormone must be given parenterally without delay.

There are no contraindications to replacement therapy. The risk lies in withholding rather than in giving it.

Some patients (particularly those with hypopituitarism), when first treated, cannot tolerate full doses of hydrocortisone because they become euphoric or otherwise mentally upset; 10 mg a day may be all they can take. The dose can usually soon be increased if it is done slowly. If diabetes is present the full dose is used and the diabetes controlled with insulin.

Chronic secondary adrenocortical insufficiency

This occurs in *hypopituitarism*. In theory the best treatment is corticotrophin, but the disadvantages of frequent injection are such that hydrocortisone is preferred. Usually less hydrocortisone is needed than in primary insufficiency. Special sodium-retaining hormone is seldom required, for the pituitary has little control over aldosterone production which responds principally to plasma K concentration and to the renin–angiotensin system. Thyroxine is given in appropriate dosage and sometimes sex hormones. The general conduct of therapy does not differ significantly from that in primary adrenal insufficiency.

Iatrogenic adrenocortical insufficiency

This occurs in patients who have recently received prolonged pharmacotherapy with a corticosteroid which inhibits hypothalamic production of the corticotrophin releasing hormone and so results in *secondary* adrenal failure. It is treated by reinstituting therapy or as for acute insufficiency, as appropriate. To avoid an acute crisis on stopping, steroid therapy *must* be withdrawn gradually to allow the hypothalamus, the pituitary and the adrenal to regain normal function. Also, when patients taking steroids have an infection or surgical operation (major stress) they should be treated as for primary insufficiency.

After the use of large doses of hormone to suppress inflammation or allergy, sudden withdrawal may not only lead to an adrenal insufficiency crisis but to relapse of the disease, which has only been suppressed, not cured. Such relapse can be extremely severe, sometimes life-threatening.

Pharmacotherapy

Suppression of adrenocortical function

In adrenogenital syndrome and adrenal virilism, an attempt may be made to suppress excess adrenal androgen secretion by inhibiting pituitary corticotrophin production by means of prednisolone or dexamethasone. Suppression of androgen production is effective if there is adrenal hyperplasia, but not if an adrenal tumour is present. Hairiness, which women especially dislike in themselves, is often unaffected even though good suppression is achieved, and menstruation recommences.

Use in inflammation and for immunosuppression

Adrenal steroids have been used in virtually every hitherto untreatable or obscure disease, e.g. immune complex diseases, nephrotic syndrome, sarcoidosis, with very variable results. Only a brief survey can be given here.

Drugs with primarily *glucocorticoid effects*, e.g. prednisolone, are chosen, so that dosage is not limited by the mineralocorticoid effects that are inevitable with hydrocortisone. But it remains essential to *use only the minimum dose that will achieve the desired effect*. Sometimes therapeutic effect must be partly sacrificed to avoid adverse effects, for it has not yet proved possible to separate the glucocorticoid effects from each other; indeed it is not known if it is possible to eliminate catabolic effects and at the same time retain anti-inflammatory action. In any case, in some conditions, e.g. nephrotic syndrome, the clinician cannot specify exactly what action he wants the drug developer to provide.

Diseases in which adrenal steroids may be useful

The decision to give a corticosteroid commonly depends on knowledge of the likelihood and amount of benefit (bearing in mind that very prolonged high dose *inevitably* brings serious complications such as osteoporosis) on the severity of the disease and on whether the patient has failed to respond usefully to other treatment. It often requires expertise that can only be imparted by those with wide experience of the disease concerned.

Adrenal steroids are used in *all* or *nearly all* cases of:

- *Exfoliative dermatitis and pemphigus*, if severe
- *Collagen diseases*, if severe, e.g. lupus erythematosus (systemic), polyarteritis nodosa, polymyalgia rheumatica and cranial giant cell arteritis (urgent therapy to save sight), dermatomyositis
- *Status asthmaticus*
- *Acute lymphatic leukaemia* (see Ch. 37)
- *Acquired haemolytic anaemia*
- *Severe allergic reactions* of all kinds, e.g. serum sickness, angioneurotic oedema, trichiniasis. They will not control acute manifestations of anaphylactic shock as they do not act quickly enough.
- *Organ transplant rejection*

- *Acute spinal cord injury*: early, brief, and high dose
- *Active chronic hepatitis*: a corticosteroid improves well being, liver function and histology and patient survival in the short term, but there is considerable uncertainty about the classes of patient that will benefit long term. Prednisone should not be used because it is a prodrug and the liver may fail to transform it into the active prednisolone.

Adrenal steroids are used in *some* cases of:

- *Rheumatic fever*
- *Rheumatoid arthritis*
- *Ankylosing spondylitis*
- *Ulcerative colitis and proctitis*
- *Regional ileitis*
- *Bronchial asthma and hay-fever (allergic rhinitis)*: also some bronchitics with marked airways obstruction.
- *Sarcoidosis.* If there is hypercalcaemia or threat to a major organ, e.g. eye, steroid administration is urgent. Pulmonary fibrosis may be delayed and central nervous system manifestations may improve.
- *Severe infections.* In any severe infection where the need for control of the adverse effects of the inflammatory process outweighs the risk of suppression of protective responses, e.g. severe meningitis in children (fewer CNS complications). Effective chemotherapy is essential, though this may not exist in viral diseases.
- *Acute mountain/altitude sickness*
- Prevention of *adverse reaction* to *radiocontrast media* in patients who have had a previous severe reaction.
- *Blood diseases due to circulating antibodies*, e.g. thrombocytopenic purpura (there may also be a decrease in capillary fragility with lessening of purpura even though thrombocytes remain few); agranulocytosis.
- *Eye diseases.* Allergic diseases and nongranulomatous inflammation of the uveal tract. But bacterial and virus infections may be made worse and use of steroids to suppress inflammation of infection is generally undesirable, is

best left to ophthalmologists and must be accompanied by effective chemotherapy; this is of the greatest importance in herpesvirus infection. Corneal integrity should be checked before use (by instilling a drop of fluorescein). Prolonged used of corticosteroid eye drops causes glaucoma in 1 in 20 of the population (a genetic trait). Application is generally as hydrocortisone, prednisolone or fluorometholone drops, or subconjunctival injection.

● *Nephrotic syndrome*. Patients with *minimal change disease* respond well to daily or alternate day therapy. With 60 mg/day total of prednisolone 90% of those who will lose their proteinuria will have done so within 4–6 weeks; the dose is tapered off over 3–4 months. Longer courses only induce adverse effects. Relapses are common (50%) and it is then necessary to find a minimum dose of steroid that will keep the patient well. If a steroid is for any reason undesirable, cyclophosphamide or chlorambucil, may be substituted. *Membranous nephropathy* may respond to high dose corticosteroid with or without chlorambucil. The prognosis of other forms of glomerulonephritis is not improved by drugs, indeed for some patients the disease may even made worse.

● *A variety of skin diseases*, such as eczema. Severe cases may be treated by occlusive dressings if a systemic effect is not wanted — though absorption can be substantial (see Ch. 38).

● *Acute gout* resistant to other drugs (see p. 227).

● *Hypercalcaemia* of multiple myeloma and other malignant diseases, of sarcoidosis and of vitamin D intoxication responds to prednisolone 30 mg daily (or its equivalent of other steroid) for 10 days. Hyperparathyroid hypercalcaemia does not respond.

● *Raised intracranial pressure due to cerebral oedema*, e.g. in cerebral tumour or encephalitis, probably an anti-inflammatory effect which reduces vascular permeability and acts in 12–24 h: give dexamethasone 10 mg i.m. or i.v. (or equivalent) initially and then 4 mg 6-hourly by the appropriate route, reducing dose after 2–4 days and withdrawing over 5–7 days; but much

higher doses may be used in palliation of inoperable cerebral tumour.

● *Pre-term labour*: (to mother) to enhance fetal lung maturation.

● *Vascular shock*: see p. 403.

● *Mendelsohn's syndrome* (aspiration of gastric acid).

● *Myasthenia gravis*: see p. 387.

Miscellaneous diseases. In these other lines of treatment may be tried first, where they exist: steatorrhoea, severe nasal allergy (topical application), 'aphthous' mouth ulcers (suck a 2.5 mg hydrocortisone tablet (Corlan) 4 times daily), Bell's palsy, acute polyneuritis, toxic and virus encephalitis, post-irradiation fibrosis, Hunner's ulcer of the bladder, myotonia.

Use in diagnosis: dexamethasone suppression test. Dexamethasone acts on the hypothalamus (like hydrocortisone), to reduce output of corticotrophin releasing hormone (CRH), but it does not interfere with measurement of corticosteroids in blood or urine. Normal suppression of cortisol production after administering dexamethasone indicates that the hypothalamic/pituitary/adrenal axis is intact. Failure of suppression implies pathological hypersecretion of ACTH by the pituitary or of cortisol by the adrenal. Dexamethasone is used because its action is prolonged (24 h). There is a number of ways of carrying out the test.

Withdrawal of corticosteriod pharmacotherapy

The longer the duration of therapy the slower must be the withdrawal. For use of less than 1 week (e.g. in severe asthma), although there is some hypothalamic suppression, withdrawal can be safely accomplished in a few steps. After use for 2 weeks, if rapid withdrawal is desired, a 50% reduction in dose may be made each day; but if the patient has been treated for a longer period, reduction in dose is accompanied by the dual risk of a flare up of the disease and of iatrogenic hypoadrenalism; then withdrawal should be done very slowly, e.g. 2.5–5 mg prednisolone or equivalent at intervals of 3–7 days.

An alternative scheme is to try halving the dose weekly until 25 mg prednisolone or equivalent is reached, after which it may be reduced by about 1 mg every third to seventh day. Paediatric tablets (1 mg) can be useful during withdrawal.

But these schemes may yet be found too fast (occurrence of fatigue, 'dish-rag' syndrome, or relapse of disease) and the rate may need to be even as slow as 1 mg prednisolone or equivalent per month, particularly as the dose approaches the level of physiological requirement (equivalent of 5–7 mg prednisolone daily).

The long tetracosactrin test or measurements of plasma corticotrophin concentration may be used to assess recovery of adrenal responsiveness, but a positive result should not be taken to indicate full recovery of the patient's ability to respond to stressful situations — the latter is best shown by an adequate response to insulin-induced hypoglycaemia (which tests the hypothalamic/pituitary capacity to respond).

Corticotrophin should not be used to hasten recovery of the cortex since its effects cause further suppression of the hypothalamic/pituitary axis, on the recovery of which the patient's future depends. Complete recovery of normal hypothalamic/pituitary/adrenal function sufficient to cope with severe intercurrent illnesses or surgery is generally complete in 2 months but may take as long as 2 years.

There have been many reports of collapse, even coma, occurring within a few hours of omission of steroid therapy, e.g. due to patients' ignorance of the risk to which their physicians are exposing them or failing to have their tablets with them and other trivial causes; but it is not invariable. Patients *must* be instructed on the hazards of omitting therapy and, during intercurrent disease, i.m. preparations should be freely used. Anaesthesia and surgery in adrenocortical insufficiency is discussed on p. 555.

INHIBITION OF SYNTHESIS OF ADRENAL STEROIDS

These agents have use in diagnosis of adrenal disease and in controlling excessive production of corticosteroids, e.g. by corticotrophin-producing tumours of the pituitary (Cushing's syndrome) or by adrenocortical adenoma or carcinoma where the cause cannot be removed. They must be used with special care since they can precipitate acute adrenal insufficiency.

Metyrapone (Metopirone) inhibits the enzyme, steroid 11β-hydroxylase, that converts 11-deoxy precursors into hydrocortisone, corticosterone and aldosterone. It affects synthesis of aldosterone less than that of glucocorticoids.

Trilostane (Modrenal) blocks the synthetic path earlier (3β-hydroxysteroid dehydrogenase) and thus also inhibits aldosterone synthesis.

Aminoglutethimide (Orimeten) blocks even earlier, preventing the conversion of cholesterol to pregnenolone. It therefore blocks synthesis of all steroids, hydrocortisone, aldosterone and sex hormones (including the conversion of androgens to oestrogens); it has a use in breast cancer.

Ketoconazole (Nizoral) is an effective antifungal agent by virtue of its capacity to block sterol/steroid synthesis (ergosterol in the case of fungi). In man it inhibits steroid synthesis in gonads and adrenal cortex and it has been used in Cushing's syndrome and prostatic cancer.

Competitive antagonism of adrenal steroids

Spironolactone (Aldactone; see index) antagonises the sodium-retaining effect of aldosterone and other mineralocorticoids. It is used to treat primary and secondary hyperaldosteronism (p. 552). There are no competitive antagonists to glucocorticoid effects in clinical use.

ADRENOCORTICOTROPHIC HORMONE (ACTH) (CORTICOTROPHIN)

Natural corticotrophin is a 39-amino-acid polypeptide secreted by the anterior pituitary gland; it is obtained from animal pituitaries.

The physiological activity resides in the first 24 amino acids (which are common to many species) and most immunological activity resides in the remaining 15 amino acids.

The pituitary output of corticotrophin responds rapidly to physiological requirements by the familiar negative-feedback homeostatic mechanism. Since the $t_{\frac{1}{2}}$ of corticotrophin is 10 min and the adrenal cortex responds rapidly (within 2 min) it is plain that adjustments of steroid output can be quickly made.

Synthetic corticotrophins have the advantage that they are shorter amino acid chains (devoid of amino acids 25–39) and so are less likely to cause serious allergy, though this can happen. In addition they are not contaminated by animal proteins which are potent allergens.

Tetracosactrin consists of the biologically active first 24 amino acids of natural corticotrophin (from man or animals) and so it has similar properties, e.g. $t_{\frac{1}{2}}$ 10 min.

Actions

Corticotrophin stimulates the synthesis of corticosteroids (of which the most important is *hydrocortisone*) and to a lesser extent of *androgens*, by the cells of the adrenal cortex. It has only a minor (transient) effect on aldosterone production, which can proceed independently; in the absence of corticotrophin the cells of the inner cortex atrophy.

The release of natural corticotrophin by the pituitary gland is controlled by the hypothalamus via *corticotrophin releasing hormone* (CRH or corticoliberin), production of which is influenced by environmental stresses as well as by the level of circulating hydrocortisone. High plasma concentration of any steroid with glucocorticoid effect prevents release of corticotrophin releasing hormone and so of corticotrophin, lack of which in turn results in adrenocortical hypofunction. This is the reason why catastrophe may follow sudden withdrawal of steroid therapy in the chronically treated patient who has an atrophied cortex.

The effects of corticotrophin are those of the steroids (*hydrocortisone, androgens*) liberated by its action on the adrenal cortex. Prolonged heavy dosage causes the clinical picture of Cushing's syndrome.

Uses

Corticotrophin is used principally in diagnosis and rarely in treatment. It is inactive if taken orally and has to be injected like other peptide hormones.

Diagnostic use: as a test of the capacity of the adrenal cortex to produce cortisol; the plasma cortisol (hydrocortisone) concentration is measured after an i.m. injection of tetracosactrin (Synacthen); variants of the test in cases of difficulty involve use of the depot (sustained-release) formulation i.m.

Therapeutic use is seldom appropriate because the peptide hormone has to be injected; selective glucocorticoid action (without mineralocorticoid effect) cannot be obtained, and clinical results are irregular. However, because androgens are secreted, corticotrophin is less liable to suppress growth in children, e.g. in severe chronic rheumatic disease it does not retard growth in children and adolescents and may occasionally be preferred for long-term therapy for this reason, despite the disadvantage of daily i.m. injection.

Corticotrophin is not useful during withdrawal of a steroid after prolonged therapy (it does not restore suppressed hypothalamic/pituitary function), but it can be used if these patients have an infection or other severe accidental stress during the succeeding 1–2 years when pituitary responsiveness may still be inadequate; though hydrocortisone is ordinarily preferred.

Preparations

Tetracosactrin Injection is a powder dissolved in water immediately before injection i.v. i.m. or s.c.

Tetracosactrin Zinc Injection (Synacthen Depot) in which the hormone is adsorbed on to zinc phosphate from which it is slowly released. This is the form used in therapy, for it can be given i.m. twice a week (0.5 –1.0 mg) and the doses then spaced according to response.

Corticotrophin preparations from animals (mixed with carboxymethylcellulose or gelatin for prolonged effect) remain available, but pure synthetic preparations are always preferable to inevitably impure biological preparations.

GUIDE TO FURTHER READING

Baylink D J 1983 Glucorticoid-induced osteoporosis. New England Journal of Medicine 309: 306

Bone R C et al 1987 A controlled clinical trial of high-dose methylprednisolone in the treatment of severe sepsis and septic shock. New England Journal of Medicine 317: 653

Byyny R 1976 Withdrawal from glucocorticoid therapy. New England Journal of Medicine 295: 30

Downie W W et al 1977 Steroid cards: patient compliance. British Medical Journal 2: 428

Editorial 1983 Prednisolone pulses in collagen disease: grammes or milligrammes? Lancet 1: 280

English J et al 1983 Diurnal variation in prednisolone kinetics. Clinical Pharmacology and Therapeutics 33: 381

Freidy J F 1988 Reactions to contrast media and steroid pretreatment. British Medical Journal 296: 809

Hench P S et al 1949 The effect of a hormone of the adrenal cortex (17-hydroxy-11-dehydrocorticosterone: Compound E) and of pituitary adrenocorticotrophic hormone on rheumatoid arthritis. Proceedings of the Staff Meetings of the Mayo Clinic 24: 181, 277 (acute rheumatism). The classic studies of the first clinical use of an adrenocortical steroid in inflammatory disease. See also p. 298 for an account by E C Kendall of the biochemical and pharmaceutical background to the clinical studies. Kendall writes of his collaboration with Hench, 'ne can now say "17-hydroxy-11-dehydrocorticosterone" and in turn I can say "the arthritis of lupus erythematosus". In sophisticated circles, however, I prefer to say, "the arthritis of L.E."'

Lavin M J et al 1986 Use of steroid eye drops in general practice. British Medical Journal 292: 1448

Newrick P G et al 1990 Self-management of adrenal insufficiency by rectal hydrocortisone. Lancet 335: 212

Newton R W et al 1978 Adrenocortical suppression in workers manufacturing synthetic glucocorticoids. British Medical Journal 1: 73

Odio C M 1991 The beneficial effects of early dexamethasone administration in infants and children with bacterial meningitis. New England Journal of Medicine 324: 1525

Swinburne C R et al 1988 Evidence of prednisolone induced mood change ('steroid euphoria') in patients with chronic obstructive airways disease. British Journal of Clinical Pharmacology 26: 709

Wolthers O D et al 1991 Growth of asthmatic children during treatment with budesonide: a double blind trial. British Medical Journal 303: 163

34

Endocrinology II: diabetes mellitus, insulin, oral antidiabetic agents

SYNOPSIS

Diabetes mellitus affects 1–2% of many populations. Its successful management requires close collaboration between the patient and the doctor.

- Diabetes mellitus and insulin
- Insulin (including sources, actions, choice, formulations, adverse effects, hypoglycaemia, insulin resistance)
- Oral antidiabetes drugs
- Treatment of diabetes mellitus
- Diabetic ketoacidosis
- Surgery in diabetic patients

DIABETES MELLITUS AND INSULIN

History

Insulin (as pancreatic islet cell extract) was first administered to a 14-year-old insulin-deficient patient on 11 January 1922 in Toronto, Canada. A sufferer from diabetes who developed the disease in 1920 and who, because of insulin, lived until 1968, has told[1] how

Many doctors, after they have developed a disease, take up the speciality in it ... But that was not so with me. I was studying for surgery when diabetes took me up. The great book of Joslin said that by starving you might live four years with luck. [He went to Italy and, whilst his health was declining there, he received a letter form a biochemist friend which said] there was something called 'insulin' appearing with a good name in Canada, what about going there and getting it. I said 'No thank you; I've tried too many quackeries for diabetes; I'll wait and see.' Then I got peripheral neuritis. ... So when [the friend] cabled me and said, 'I've got insulin — it works — come back quick', [I] responded, arrived at King's College Hospital, London, and went to the laboratory as soon as it opened. . ... It was all experimental for [neither of us] knew a thing about it ... So we decided to have 20 units — a nice round figure. I had a nice breakfast. I had bacon and eggs and toast made on the Bunsen. I hadn't eaten bread for months and months ... by 3 o'clock in the afternoon my urine was quite sugar free. That hadn't happened for

---

[1] Abbreviated from Lawrence R D King's College Hospital Gazette 1961; 40: 220. Transcript from a recorded after-dinner talk to students' Historical Society.

many months. So we gave a cheer for Banting and Best.[2]

But at 4 pm I had a terrible shaky feeling and a terrible sweat and hunger pain. That was my first experience of hypoglycaemia. We remembered that Banting and Best had described an overdose of insulin in dogs. So I had some sugar and a biscuit and soon got quite well, thank you.

Diabetes mellitus is classified broadly as:

Type I (insulin dependent diabetes mellitus, IDDM) which typically occurs in younger people who cannot secrete insulin;

Type II (non-insulin dependent diabetes mellitus, NIDDM), which typically occurs in older, often obese people who retain capacity to secrete insulin but who are resistant to its action.

These terms and abbreviations are used in this chapter.

INSULIN

Sources

Insulin is synthesised and stored (bound to zinc) in granules in the β-islet cells of the pancreas. Daily secretion amounts to 30–40 units, which is about 25% of total pancreatic insulin content. The principal factor that evokes insulin secretion is a high blood glucose concentration.

Insulin is a polypeptide with 2 peptide chains (A chain, 21 amino acids and B chain, 30) linked by 2 disulphide bridges. The basic structure having metabolic activity is common to all mammalian species but there are minor species differences, which result in the development of antibodies in all patients treated with animal insulins, as well as to unavoidable impurities in the preparations, minimal though these now are.

Bovine insulin differs from human insulin by 3 amino acids and is *more antigenic* to man than is *porcine* insulin, which differs from human by only 1 amino acid.

---

[2] F G Banting and C H Best, of Toronto, Canada. See also J Lab Clin Med 1922; 7: 251.

Human insulin (1980) is available as 4 forms: e.g., *e*nzyme *m*odified *p*orcine (*emp*); *c*hain, *r*ecombinant DNA, *b*acterial (*crb*) insulin, for which the gene for insulin synthesis has been artificially introduced into *E. coli*; and other insulins designated *prb* and *pyr*. All preparations contain small amounts of contaminants (animal, microbial), which can cause allergy; and human insulin itself can cause antibody formation.

Note. The chief reason for using human insulin is not difference in biological insulin activity, but reduced immunogenicity.

Insulin receptors

Insulin is bound to receptors on the surface of the target cell (mostly liver, muscle, fat) and the insulin/receptor complex enters the cell. Receptors vary in number inversely with the insulin concentration to which they are exposed, i.e. with high insulin concentration the number of receptors declines (*down-regulation*) and responsiveness to insulin also declines (insulin resistance); with low insulin concentration the number of receptors increases (*up-regulation*) and responsiveness to insulin increases. Thus obese Type II (NIDDM) patients having hypersecretion due to overeating, with insulin resistance, may recover insulin responsiveness as a result of dieting so that the insulin secretion diminishes, cellular receptors increase and insulin sensitivity is restored. Changes in *affinity* of receptors, as well as in numbers, also contribute to insulin resistance, e.g. as more insulin receptors are occupied, the affinity for insulin of those remaining unoccupied diminishes (a negative feedback control mechanism).

Actions of insulin

Cellular mechanism of action of insulin after combination with the receptor is still uncertain; the complex activates 'second messenger' processes which in turn mediate the characteristic metabolic effects. Insulin also has an immediate membrane effect increasing glucose transport as well as its utilisation, especially by muscle and adipose tissue. Its effects include:

- *Reduction in blood glucose* due to *increased glucose uptake* in the peripheral tissues (which convert it into glycogen or fat), and *reduction of hepatic output of glucose* (diminished breakdown of glycogen and diminished gluconeogenesis). When the blood-glucose concentration falls below the renal threshold (10 mmol/l or 180 mg/100 ml) glycosuria ceases, as does the osmotic diuresis of water and electrolytes. Polyuria with dehydration and excessive thirst are thus alleviated. If the blood glucose falls much below normal levels appetite is stimulated.
- *Other metabolic effects.* In addition to enabling glucose to pass across cell membranes, the transit of amino acids and potassium into the cell is enhanced. Insulin regulates carbohydrate utilisation and energy production. It *enhances protein synthesis. It inhibits breakdown of fats* (lipolysis). *An insulin-deficient diabetic* (Type I) becomes dehydrated due to osmotic diuresis, and is *ketotic* because fats break down faster than the ketoacid metabolites can be metabolised.

Uses

The main indication is **diabetes mellitus**. Insulin promotes the passage of potassium simultaneously with glucose into cells, and this effect is utilised in *hyperkalaemia* (see p. 465).

Insulin hypoglycaemia can also be used as a test of *anterior pituitary function* (growth hormone and corticotrophin are released) and to test the *completeness of surgical vagotomy* in reducing gastric secretion.

Pharmacokinetics

Insulin *naturally secreted* by the pancreas enters the portal vein and passes straight to the liver which takes up half of it. The rest enters the systemic circulation where its concentration is only about 15% (in fasting subjects) of that entering the liver. When insulin is injected s.c. it enters the systemic circulation and both liver and other peripheral organs receive the same concentration.

This difference may have clinical importance and this is why some continuous infusion pumps (see below) deliver insulin intraperitoneally rather than subcutaneously.

In conventional use, insulin is injected (s.c., i.m. or i.v.) as it is digested if swallowed.[3] It is absorbed into the blood[4] and is inactivated in the liver and kidney; about 10% appears in the urine. The $t_\frac{1}{2}$ is about 5 min. This is convenient for an accurately controlled continuously functioning biofeedback system, but poses difficulties for routine replacement in insulin deficiency. Therefore *sustained-release (depot) formulations* have been developed to provided a nearer approach to natural function compatible with the convenience of daily living. An even closer approach is provided by the development of (at present inevitably expensive) miniaturised infusion pumps which can be used by *reliable* patients.

Engineers have developed pump systems, which have been dignified with the name 'artificial pancreas'. They deliver insulin by continuous variable s.c. infusion from an electronically controlled pump (s.c. infusion can be managed by the patient) carried in a belt or harness, or even miniaturised and implanted s.c. In one, a glucose sensor monitors the blood glucose concentration and automatically changes the infused dose accordingly (closed-loop system), and in the other, less complex technically, the infusion is programmed (with varying degrees of manual control) independently of the blood glucose concentration, providing pre- and postprandial doses appropriate to the patient's habits (open-loop system). The kinetics of s.c. infusion differ from those of intermittent injection. Infusion s.c. (continuous or pulsed) provides slower absorption that does not allow rapid changes in blood concentration in relation to meals; with changed rate of infusion a steady state is reached in 6–8 h.

---

[3] Orally active formulations which protect the insulin from digestion are under development.
[4] Peak-plasma insulin (s.c.) concentration 60–90 min. Absorption is slower if there is peripheral vascular disease or smoking, and faster if the patient takes a hot bath or uses an ultraviolet light sunbed (which has induced a hypoglycaemic fit) or exercises. The effects are due to changes in peripheral blood flow.

Delivery of insulin intraperitoneally is feasible and is closer to the natural arrangements (see above).

Differences between human and animal insulins

Human insulin is absorbed from subcutaneous tissue slightly more rapidly than animal insulins and it has a slightly shorter duration of action.

Human insulin is less immunogenic than are animal insulins. When changing from *beef* to human insulin patients taking <100 units of beef insulin are likely to require 10% less human insulin, and if taking >100 units beef insulin, 25% less human insulin. The probable explanation of this is the presence of antibodies to beef insulin. With pork insulin, dose reduction is not usually necessary.

There has been concern that patients taking human insulin may experience more frequent and more severe *hypoglycaemic attacks*, especially when transferring from animal insulins. Such occurrences are likely to be due to management problems rather than to pharmacological differences.

However there is some evidence of a lessened *awareness* of hypoglycaemia with human insulin, i.e. the counter-regulatory physiological responses to animal and human insulin may differ. It is claimed that with human insulin patients experience less *adrenergic* symptoms (sweating, tremor, palpitations), which are such a useful warning, although the *neurological* (neuroglycopenic) symptoms (dizziness, headache, inability to concentrate) are unchanged. But one careful clinical study has found no difference (see Guide to Further Reading).

Preparations of insulin

There are three major factors:

- *Strength* (concentration)
- *Source* (human, porcine, bovine)
- *Formulation*
  a. *short-acting* solution of insulin for use s.c., i.m., i.v.

b. *intermediate and longer acting* (sustained-release) preparations in which the insulin has been modified by combination with other proteins or zinc or by modification of its crystalline form to give a poorly soluble product; this is given s.c. and slowly dissociates to release insulin in its soluble form (given i.m., which is not advised, the time course of release would be different).

Dosage is measured in international units (IU) now standardised by immunoassay.

Diabetes mellitus may be managed from a choice of four insulin preparations having:

1. **Short duration** of action (and rapid onset): Soluble Insulin (neutral insulin, regular insulin).
2. **Intermediate duration** of action (and slower onset): Insulin Zinc Suspension (Amorphous), Semilente.
3. **Long duration** of action: Insulin Zinc Suspension (Crystalline), Ultralente.
4. **A mixture**: Biphasic Insulin Inj. (25% is in neutral form (1, above) and 75% zinc suspension, crystalline) or other mixtures to suit the individual (see below and Table 34.1). The other insulins (see Table 34.1) will also serve. The important thing is for the doctor to get to know well a range that will serve most patients.

For insulin regimens and injection techniques, see p. 576.

Notes for prescribing insulin

- *Purity.* Earlier insulins (beef, pork) have contained substantial impurities derived from the insulin molecule and from other animal pancreatic proteins. These impurities cause allergy, but happily advances in technology have now allowed production of a range of *Highly Purified (mixed) Insulins* and *Monocomponent Insulins*, chiefly pork, which are less allergenic than the earlier forms and replace them. They often go under the same names as the earlier insulins, but with identification that they belong to the Highly

Table 34.1 Some (approximate) data on some insulins

Preparation (source)	pH	Action (h) given s.c.		
		Onset	Peak	Duration
Short duration				
Acid Insulin Inj. (b,p)	3	0.5	2–5	6–8
Neutral Insulin Inj. (h, p, b) soluble, regular)	7	0.5	2–5	6–8
Intermediate duration				
Insulin Zinc Susp (IZS) (Amorphous) (Semilente) (h, p, b) Isophane Insulin Inj. (h, p, b) (a protamine Zn suspension)	7	1–2	4–12	20–24
Intermediate duration mixed with short duration				
Biphasic Insulin Inj. and Biphasic Isophane Insulin Inj. (h, p, b) a range of mixtures of neutral and isophane in proportions (%): 10/90, 20/80, 30/70, 40/60, 50/50	7	0.5–1	3–8	24
Intermediate duration mixed with long duration				
Insulin Zinc Susp (IZS) (Mixed) (amorphous crystalline) (Lente) (h, p, b)	7	2.5	4–16	24
Long duration				
Insulin Zinc Susp (IZS) (crystalline) (Ultralente, Ultratard) (h,b)	7	3	10–20	30–40

Note. There is enormous individual variation in response to insulins. Abbreviations for species: h = human; p = porcine; b = bovine. There is a great complexity of proprietary names for insulins. Though strictly it is imprecise the term 'soluble' insulin is now taken to refer to Neutral Insulin Inj.

Purified Group (HP, MC) until such time as the less pure forms cease to be made. Human insulins are of high purity and are replacing others.

● There is no need to change a stabilised diabetic to human insulin or to a purer form if there are no clinical problems (local or general adverse reactions), or unexplained requirement of above 100 units/day (likely to be due to presence of antibodies) in which latter case the transfer should be made in hospital as the requirement of highly purified or human insulin is unpredictable.

● *Allergy* occurs to impurities, to additives (protamine) and to insulin itself. It may take the form of local reactions (inflammatory or fat atrophy) or of insulin resistance. Though less common with the highly purified preparations and human insulin it still does occur. Allergy to the preservative, e.g. phenol, cresol, may occur.

● *New cases* of diabetes needing insulin should start on human insulin or on highly purified pork insulin (beef insulin is more immunogenic).

● *Antibodies to insulin*, provided they are moderate in amount, may be actually advantageous. They act as a carrier or store, binding insulin after injection and releasing it slowly as the free insulin in the plasma declines. In this way they smooth and prolong insulin action. But too high concentrations cause insulin resistance.

● *Compatibility.* Neutral Insulin may be mixed in the syringe with Insulin Zinc Suspensions (amorphous, crystalline) and with Isophane and Biphasic Insulin, and used at once: but there are insulins in which *protamine* is used as a carrier, and spare protamine will bind some of the short-acting neutral insulin, thus blunting its effects.

Preparations of widely differing pH, (see Table 34.1) should not be mixed.

● *Intravenous insulin*: only Neutral Insulin Inj. or Acid Insulin Inj. should be used.

● The standard strength of insulin preparations is *100 IU* per ml in a large and growing number of countries. Even very low doses can be accurately measured with modern special syringes. Solutions of 40 IU remain available in many countries.

Choice of insulin preparation

That insulin preparations should be both precise and of uniform strength all over the world is vital to the health and safety of millions of diabetics. Advances in technology now allow biological standardisation in animal to be replaced by physicochemical methods (high performance liquid chromatography: HPLC).

Neutral Insulin Inj. (soluble, regular insulin) is an aqueous solution of insulin. It is simple to use, being given s.c. 2–3 times a day, 30–40 min before meals. There is little risk of serious hypoglycaemic reaction if it is used sensibly. If it is known that a meal must be delayed, then the insulin injection can be postponed. The dose can easily be adjusted according to self-performed blood or urine glucose measurements.[5] For these reasons it is often used initially to balance diabetics needing insulin and always for the treatment of diabetic ketosis. The biggest disadvantages of soluble insulin for long-term use are the need for frequent injections, and the occurrence of high blood glucose before breakfast.

There are two principal forms of neutral (soluble) insulin:

- Acid Insulin Inj., at pH 3 (which can cause discomfort at the injection site)
- Neutral Insulin Inj., at pH 7 (see Table 34.1).
- The latter is preferred.

Intravenous neutral (soluble) insulin is used in diabetic ketoacidosis. It may be given intermittently (i.v. or i.m.) but continuous infusion is preferred. If the insulin is *infused* by *drip* in physiological saline (40 units/l) as much as 60–80% can be lost due to binding to the fluid container and tubing. It is necessary to take this into account in dosing. Polygeline (Haemaccel) may be added to bind the insulin in competition with the apparatus and so carry it into the body. Use of a slow-infusion pump with a more concentrated solution (insulin 1.0 IU/ml) is preferred. Insulin loss is much less and control of dosage is more accurate when more con-centrated solutions are infused by pump, and at 1000 units/l (1 unit/ml) such as is convenient for infusion by pump, losses are not of practical importance. For i.v. doses see diabetic keto-acidosis, below. Long-acting (sustained-release) preparations *must not* be given i.v.

The *time-course of soluble insulin given i.v.* is shorter than when given s.c. (as in Table 34.1), namely: onset 0.25 h; peak 0.5–1 h; duration 2 h.

Insulin Zinc Suspensions including iso-phane insulin (see Table 34.1) have been developed following the observation that the pancreatic islet cells store insulin in association with zinc. They are sustained-release formulations in which rate of release is controlled by modifying particle size. Neutral pH, soluble insulin can be mixed with them without altering the time-course of effect of either and these formulations can be a great convenience.

Duration of action. Patients live by a 24-hour cycle and plainly insulins having a duration of action exceeding 24 hours can cause problems, especially early morning hypoglycaemia.

Dose of insulin

The total daily output of endogenous insulin from pancreatic islet cells is 30–40 units (determined by the needs of completely pancreatectomised patients), and most insulin-deficient diabetics will need 30–50 unit/day of insulin (two-thirds in the morning and one-third in the evening).

Initial treatment for a Type I (IDDM) patient with *soluble (neutral) insulin* may be thus:

- blood glucose >16.5 mmol/l (300 mg/100 ml): 20 units;
- blood glucose[6] 11–16.5 mmol/l (200–300 mg/100 ml): 10 units.

The dose is then adjusted according to the usual monitoring of blood and/or urine glucose. Daily (total) dose increments should be 4 units. When stabilised, two-thirds of the total daily dose is

---

[5] An adverse effect of easy self-monitoring is that a minority of obsessional patients, told of the desirability of blood glucose concentrations being kept in the normal range to prevent diabetic complications, become obsessed with monitoring, and experience great anxiety when they find what are, in fact, normal fluctuations. They then anxiously change their insulin doses daily and as a result induce frequent hypoglycaemia, e.g. one patient had 33 episodes in 44 days, many with loss of consciousness (Beer S F et al. Br Med J 1989; 298: 362).

[6] The normal (fasting) blood glucose range is 3.9–5.8 mmol/l (70–105 mg/100 ml).

generally given 30–40 min before breakfast and one-third before the evening meal.

If it is decided to give the patient only one injection per day, then 10–14 units of an intermediate-duration insulin zinc suspension may be given. Dose increments (4 units) may be given on alternate days.

Soluble insulin (neutral) may be added, or special mixed (biphasic) insulins used, according to the patient's response. Excessive dose of insulin leads to overeating and obesity; it also leads to hypoglycaemia (especially nocturnal), that may be followed by rebound morning hyperglycaemia that is mistakenly treated by increased insulin, thus establishing a vicious cycle (Somogyi effect).

Muscular activity increases carbohydrate utilisation, so that hypoglycaemia is likely if a well-stabilised patient changes suddenly from an inactive hospital existence to a vigorous life outside. If this is likely to happen the diet may be increased by 250–500 calories[7] or the dose of insulin reduced by up to one-third and then readjusted according to need. This is less marked in patients on oral agents.

See also Choice of regimen and Ketoacidosis, below.

Adverse effects of insulin

Adverse effects are mainly those of overdose.[8] Because the brain relies on glucose as its source of energy, an adequate blood/glucose concentration is just as essential as an adequate supply of oxygen, and hypoglycaemia may lead to coma, convulsions and even death (in 4% of diabetics under 50 years of age).

It is usually easier to differentiate **hypoglycaemia** from severe diabetic ketosis than from other causes of coma, which are as likely in a diabetic as in anyone else. If there is doubt as to the aetiology in a comatose patient it is reasonable to give glucose i.v., but only after taking blood for a glucose estimation. If

hypoglycaemia of short duration is responsible, then a rapid improvement is usual; in any case a dose of glucose generally (but not always, see below) does no harm. Hypoglycaemia may manifest itself as disturbed sleep and morning headache. For details of treatment see below.

Other adverse reactions to insulin are **lipodystrophy** (atrophy or hypertrophy) at the injection sites (rare with purified pork and human insulin), after they have been used repeatedly. These are unsightly, but otherwise harmless. The site should not be used further, for absorption can be erratic, but the patient may be tempted to continue if local anaesthesia has developed, as it sometimes does. Lipoatrophy is probably allergic and lipohypertrophy is due to a local metabolic action of insulin. Local allergy also is manifested as itching or painful red lumps. *Generalised allergic* reactions are very rare, but may occur to any insulin (including human) and to any constituent of the formulation. Change of brand of insulin, especially to highly purified preparations, (or to one with a different mode of manufacture) may rectify allergic problems. But zinc occurs in all insulins (through very little in soluble insulin) and can be the allergen.

Low pH insulins may cause local discomfort at the injection site.

Treatment of a hypoglycaemic attack

Prevention depends very largely upon patient education. In particular, they should never miss meals and must know the early symptoms of an attack.[9] Treatment is always to give sugar, either by mouth if the patient can still swallow or glucose (dextrose) i.v. (20–50 ml of 50% solution, i.e. 10–25 g; this concentration is thrombotic so do *not* withdraw the needle and compress the vein immediately after completion of injection). The response is usually dramatic. The patient should be given a meal to avoid relapse. But if the patient does not respond within 30 min, it may be because of cerebral

---

[7] 1.0 calorie ≈ 4.2 joules.
[8] Suicidal overdose (in diabetics) is well recorded. Surgical excision of the skin and subcutaneous tissue at the injection site of an enormous dose of long-acting insulin has been used.

[9] It can be useful training to allow a patient to experience hypoglycaemia once by delaying a meal.

oedema, which will require treatment with i.v. dexamethasone and perhaps mannitol. If the patient has been severely hypoglycaemic for hours or if very large amounts of insulin or sulphonylurea have been taken, then large amounts of glucose may have to be given by i.v. infusion for several days. Very severe attacks sometimes damage the central nervous system permanently. See also glucagon below.

After recovery from a severe attack and elucidation of the cause, the patient should be carefully restabilised on insulin or an oral agent.

Some advocate (see above) giving i.v. glucose to a comatose diabetic on the basis that it will revive him if he is hypoglycaemic and do no harm if he is hyperglycaemic. The latter assumption is unsound since a minority of comatose insulin-dependent diabetics have hyperkalaemia and added glucose can cause a brisk and potentially hazardous rise in serum potassium (mechanism uncertain), in contrast to non-diabetics in whom glucose causes a fall in serum potassium.

Hypoglycaemia due to other causes, e.g. alcohol, is treated similarly.

Insulin resistance and hormones that increases blood glucose

Insulin resistance may be due to a decline in *number* and/or *affinity* of receptors (see above) or to defects in *post-receptor mechanisms*.

A diabetic requiring more than 200 units/day is regarded as insulin resistant (some patients have needed as much as 5000 units/day). This is due to *antibodies* binding insulin in a biologically inactive complex (though it can dissociate as with protein binding of drugs).

As beef insulin is more antigenic than pork, change to a highly purified pork or human insulin may be successful in reducing resistance. Addition of a sulphonylurea to release endogenous insulin (non-antigenic) may also be useful when pancreatic function is not entirely lost (Type II diabetics). Responsiveness to insulin may sometimes be restored by immunosuppression, e.g. an adrenocortical steroid (prednisolone 20–40 mg/day) over weeks or months, to suppress antibody

production. Obviously, if this is successful, insulin dosage will have to be reduced in accordance with the unpredictable reduction in antibodies. Patients need to be carefully monitored to avoid severe hypoglycaemia. *Ketoacidosis* also reduces the effect of insulin.

Glucagon ($t_{\frac{1}{2}}$ 4 min) is a polypeptide hormone (29 amino acids) from the α-islet cells of the pancreas. It is released in response to hypoglycaemia and is a physiological regulator of insulin effect. It releases liver glycogen as glucose. It has been used to treat insulin hypoglycaemia, but in about 45 min from onset of *coma* the hepatic glycogen will anyway be exhausted and glucagon will be useless. Its chief advantage would seem to be that, as it can be given s.c. or i.m. (1.0 mg), it can be used in severe hypoglycaemic attack by somebody, e.g. a member of the patient's family, who is unable to given an i.v. injection of glucose. If a comatose patient does not recover sufficiently in 20 min to allow oral therapy, i.v. glucose is essential. Glucagon is ineffective in marked, e.g. alcoholic, hepatic insufficiency.

Glucagon has a positive cardiac inotropic effect; it appears to have value in acute overdose of β-adrenoceptor blockers (see index).

Adrenaline raises the blood sugar by mobilising liver and muscle glycogen; it does not antagonise the peripheral actions of insulin. Glycosuria and diabetic symptoms may occur in patients with phaeochromocytoma.

Adrenal steroids, either endogenous or exogenous, antagonise the actions of insulin, although this effect is only slight with the primarily mineralocorticoid group; the glucocorticoid hormones *increase* gluconeogenesis and reduce glucose uptake and utilisation by the tissues. Patients with Cushing's syndrome thus develop diabetes very readily and may be resistant to insulin. Patients with Addison's disease, hypothyroidism and hypopituitarism are abnormally sensitive to insulin action.

Oral contraceptives can impair carbohydrate tolerance.

Growth hormone antagonises the actions of insulin in the tissues. Acromegalic patients may develop insulin-resistant diabetes.

Thyroid hormone increases the requirements for insulin.

ORAL ANTIDIABETES DRUGS

Oral antidiabetes drugs are of two kinds, sulphonamide derivatives (*sulphonylureas*) and guanidine derivatives (*biguanides*). They are used by 30% of all diabetics. Unlike insulin they are not essential for life.

Following the observation in 1918 that guanidine had hypoglycaemic effect, guanides were tried in diabetes in 1926, but were abandoned a few years later for fear of hepatic toxicity.

In 1930 it was noted that sulphonamides could cause hypoglycaemia, and in 1942 severe hypoglycaemia was found in patients with typhoid fever during a therapeutic trial of a sulphonamide. In the 1950s a similar observation was made during a chemotherapeutic trial in urinary infections. This was followed up and effective drugs soon resulted.

Mode of action

Sulphonylureas activate receptors on the β-islet cells of the pancreas to release more stored insulin in response to glucose. They do not increase insulin formation. Insulin receptors increase in number. They are ineffective in totally insulin-deficient patients and for successful therapy probably require about 30% of normal β-cell function to be present. They cause hypoglycaemia in normal subjects as well as in diabetics.

Gain in weight is liable to occur. Because of the mode of action, *secondary failure* (after months or a few years) occurs due to declining β-cell function and to increasing insulin resistance.

Biguanides. The cellular mode of action is uncertain but the most important effect seems to be to reduce the production of glucose in the liver, i.e. gluconeogenesis. Other effects include enhancement of peripheral insulin effect (they do not act in the absence of insulin) and to increase glucose uptake in peripheral tissues. They do not (used alone) cause clinical hypoglycaemia in normal subjects nor in diabetics, but they do cause lactic acidosis. Secondary failure is not a problem.

Both groups of drugs are effective only in the presence of insulin.

Drugs of the two groups may be used together.

Individual drugs

Absorption from the alimentary tract is good for all the oral agents. If a patient fails to respond to one drug response to another of the same group may yet occur.

Sulphonylureas (see also Table 34.2)

Tolbutamide ($t_{\frac{1}{2}}$ 8 h) is rapidly metabolised by oxidation in the liver so that patients with hepatic disease should be treated with special caution, as always. It is the preferred sulphonylurea in the presence of impaired renal function. Adverse effects are unlikely to occur in more than 3% of patients. They usually consist of mild gastrointestinal upsets, which may be mitigated by taking the drug after food or by antacids, and of rashes. Alcohol intolerance (inhibition of metabolism) and alcohol-enhanced hypoglycaemia occur occasionally with all sulphonylureas. Other ill-effects are rare, but include blood disorders. The question of *increased cardiovascular mortality with long-term use* has been raised and continues to be controversial.

Sulphonamides, as expected, potentiate sulphonylureas by direct action and by plasma protein displacement.

Chlorpropamide is partly metabolised and largely excreted unchanged by the kidney. It is dangerous in patients with poor renal function because of its long $t_{\frac{1}{2}}$ (36 h) which is even longer in the elderly for whom the drug is unsuitable. Adverse effects are about twice as frequent as with tolbutamide: gastrointestinal upsets, rashes, vertigo, muscle weakness, headache, unpleasant taste, alcohol intolerance, jaundice and blood disorders; but the latter are rare and seldom serious.

Glibenclamide ($t_{\frac{1}{2}}$ 10 h) is shorter-acting than chlorpropamide but is yet suitable for use in single daily dose; its action is terminated by metabolism.

Table 34.2 The principal oral antidiabetes drugs

Drug $t_\frac{1}{2}$ h	Total daily dose	Remarks
Sulphonylureas Tolbutamide (Rastinon) ($t_\frac{1}{2}$ 8)	1–3 g in 2–3 daily doses	Very safe. Frequent administration. Less effective than chlorpropamide. Dose may be altered daily. Tolerance (resistance) occurs
Chlorpropamide (Diabinese) ($t_\frac{1}{2}$ 36)	100–500 mg in 1 dose at breakfast	Less safe than tolbutamide: long $t_\frac{1}{2}$. May succeed where tolbutamide fails. Taken only once daily and dose increment weekly
Glibenclamide (Daonil) ($t_\frac{1}{2}$ 10)	5–15 mg in 1 dose at breakfast	Its $t_\frac{1}{2}$ allows once daily dose with less risk of accumulation than with chlorpropamide. Dose increment weekly
Biguanide Metformin (Glucophage) ($t_\frac{1}{2}$ 5)	1.5–2.0 g in 1–3 doses with meals	Capable of controlling some patients when used alone. Chief use in supplementing a sulphonylurea (different mode of action) or insulin

Other sulphonylureas include gliclazide, gliquidone, glipizide, glibornuride, tolazamide.

Biguanide (diguanide) (see also Table 34.2)

Metformin ($t_\frac{1}{2}$ 5 h) is taken with meals. Minor adverse gut reactions are common, including diarrhoea, and a metallic taste in the mouth. It is not metabolised and is excreted by the kidney and should not be used in the presence of renal impairment. Heavy prolonged use can cause vitamin B_{12} deficiency due to malabsorption. Its chief *use* is in combination with a sulphonylurea when the latter alone has failed. It is particularly used in obese patients to get their weight down and so to mitigate their (maturity-onset) diabetic state.

With a biguanide ketonuria may occur in the presence of normal blood sugar. This is not generally severe and may be treated by reducing the dose; but persistence in overdose may lead to severe lactic acidosis. Indeed the frequency and severity (death) of lactic acidosis with phenformin caused the drug to be abandoned. Lactic acidosis is treated with large doses of sodium bicarbonate (i.v.).

Precautions with oral agents

Hypoglycaemia occurs with sulphonylureas, but is less common than with insulin therapy. However, it can be severe, prolonged for days, and may be fatal, especially in the elderly and in patients with heart failure.

Renal and hepatic disease. A biguanide should not be used in patients with either; the risk of lactic acidosis is too great.

Sulphonylureas are potentiated in these diseases and a drug with a short $t_\frac{1}{2}$ (*not* chlorpropamide) should be used in low doses.

Age and cardiac disease add to the hazard of oral agents.

Dietary fibre and diabetes

The addition of gel-forming (soluble) but unabsorbable fibre (*guar gum*, a hydrocolloidal polysaccharide of galactose and mannose from seeds of the 'cluster bean') to the diet of diabetics reduces carbohydrate absorption and flattens the postprandial blood glucose curve. Reduced need for insulin and oral agents has been reported, but adequate amounts are unpleasant (flatulence) and patient compliance is therefore poor.

α-glucosidase inhibitor

Acarbose inhibits this enzyme in the gut, reducing breakdown and absorption of carbohydrate; the agents are popularly known as 'starch blockers'; their role in diabetes is unestablished.

TREATMENT OF DIABETES MELLITUS

Both doctor and patient are faced with a lifetime of collaboration. Compliance is not a one-sided process, and the patients need all the consideration and support they can get. They should learn about their disease and its management, including home monitoring of blood glucose.

Good control of diabetes always involves diet and most patients need insulin or oral anti-diabetes drugs in addition.

The *aim* of treatment is:

- to keep the fasting blood glucose <7 mmol/l and the 2-hour postprandial concentration <8 mmol/l;
- to avoid ketosis and infections;
- by this regimen to avoid the long-term complications.

Each patient must be assessed individually; only an outline of the general principles involved can be given here.

Diet. Patients should be allowed to follow their own preferences as far as is practicable, and drugs should be adjusted to suit the patient rather than the other way round. Some carbohydrate restriction is necessary, but the amount varies from patient to patient according to their total caloric requirements and whether weight increase or reduction is desired. The way in which carbohydrate is distributed through the day should correspond with the type of insulin taken.

Weight. Older fat diabetics (70% of NIDDM) form a group whose blood often contains much insulin but who are resistant to its action; they seldom develop ketosis. Glycosuria may cease when their weight is reduced. Biguanide particularly helps weight reduction. Weight loss is associated with an increase in numbers of insulin receptors and so an increase in responsiveness to insulin.

Young patients with IDDM are often under-weight and need insulin to restore normal weight. The blood of these young diabetics contains negligible insulin (they are sensitive to its action), and they readily become ketotic.

Selection of therapy for diabetes

Patients are treated with:

- Diet alone.
- Diet plus oral agent.
- Diet plus insulin (± oral agent).
- For ketoacidosis: soluble insulin urgently.

Diabetics   under 30 years: almost all need insulin;
over 30 years: approximately one-third need insulin, one-third oral agents and one-third diet only.

Type I (IDDM): human insulin is preferred for new patients. For regimen see below.
Type II (NIDDM): oral antidiabetics should only be used initially when there is no significant ketonuria.

Oral drugs are useless if no insulin is present and are most useful in NIDDM. Careful trial is the only sure way of deciding who can be maintained on oral therapy rather than on insulin.

When diet alone has failed to control NIDDM it is necessary to add an oral agent, the choice should fall first on a **sulphonylurea** (except in overweight), for a biguanide, though capable of controlling some patients when used alone, carries too high an incidence of adverse effects, especially on the alimentary tract, and serious lactic acidosis.

A **biguanide** is used: *as a supplement to a sulphonylurea* when this is insufficient to give control; *in overweight diabetics*, especially those who find diet difficult; patients tend to lose their appetite and therefore to lose weight with a biguanide.

Of the principal sulphonylureas, *tolbutamide* is the safest (short $t_{\frac{1}{2}}$), especially in the elderly, but has to given up to 4 times a day. *Chlorpropamide* is prone to accumulate, but can succeed where tolbutamide fails and need only be given once a day. They thus have their advantages and disadvantages and the choice in any patient is a matter of opinion and of trial. *Glibenclamide* is popular largely because its kinetics are intermediate.

To start a patient on a sulphonylurea, glibenclamide 5 mg is given orally (or 2.5 mg in the aged) with breakfast. The dose is adjusted, according to response, at weekly intervals by increments of 2.5 or 5 mg, to a maximum of 15 mg. If control is incomplete, metformin may be added.

Failure of oral agents. If the postprandial blood sugar does not fall below 14–16 mmol/l (250–300 mg/100 ml) after 4 weeks (primary failure), then insulin is needed, for not only is this state unsatisfactory but, on the same treatment, control may worsen over succeeding weeks. For secondary failure see p. 573.

Withdrawal of oral agents, gradually, may be attempted after the patient has been controlled and stable for 3–6 months. About 30% of patients will be found not to need the drug any longer.

Monitoring of patients taking oral agents should be as close as of those on insulin and probably closer. The patient must be disabused of any notion that substitution of tablets to swallow for the tiresome routine of self-injection carries any implication that the condition is less serious, or that diet can be relaxed.

Choice of insulin regimen

The range of insulin formulations available allows flexible adjustment of the regimen to the patient's way of life. There is no need to coerce patients into a regimen favoured by the physician. There is no single regimen that suits all patients.

One of the following regimens can suit most patients:

- Three doses of Neutral (soluble) Insulin (before the main meals) plus an intermediate-acting insulin at bedtime
- A Biphasic Insulin (e.g. 30/70 see Table 34.1) twice a day before morning and evening meals
- A Biphasic Insulin before breakfast and Neutral (soluble) Insulin before the evening meal
- A single morning dose of a Biphasic Insulin before breakfast may suffice for some patients.

Injection technique has pharmacokinetic consequences according to whether the insulin is delivered into the subcutaneous tissue or muscle. Patients have been traditionally taught to pinch up a skin fold and inject obliquely, thus ensuring true subcutaneous injection. But, with the introduction of short needles and pen-shaped injectors, patients are often encouraged to inject perpendicularly to the skin, it being assumed that this will provide subcutaneous delivery. But the thickness of subcutaneous tissue is very variable between individuals and between different parts of the body and this technique may lead to superficial (and intermittent) i.m. injection, which may be unrecognised as i.m. injection is not necessarily more painful. The absorption of insulin is as much as 50% more rapid from shallow i.m. injection.

Plainly patients should standardise their technique to ensure injection is s.c. Inadvertent i.m. injection of an overnight dose of an extended duration insulin can lead to inadequate early morning control of blood glucose. Sites of injection should be rotated to avoid local complications (lipodystrophy). Absorption is faster from arm and abdomen than it is from the thigh and buttock.

Diabetic complications. A well-controlled diabetic is less liable to ketosis, infections, neuropathy and cataract. And it seems certain that good control of glycaemia at least mitigates the serious microvascular retinal and renal complication. Overzealous control of glycaemia can result in increase in hypoglycaemia attacks.

Some factors affecting control of diabetes

Intercurrent illnesses cause fluctuations in the patient's metabolic needs. If these are severe, e.g. myocardial infarction, it is prudent to substitute soluble insulin for oral agents. Infections cause an increase in insulin need (about 20%), which may drop briskly on recovery.

Surgery, see later.

Menstruation and oral contraception: insulin needs may rise slightly.

In pregnancy close control of diabetes is of the first importance to avoid fetal loss at all stages, and in the *first trimester* to reduce fetal malformations. *Insulin* requirements increase steadily after the third month.

During labour soluble insulin should be given 4-hourly (or by continuous infusion at about 1 unit/h with plenty of glucose orally or i.v. infusion of 10% glucose 1.0 l in 8 h). Substantially *less*, e.g. 25%, insulin is likely to be needed immediately after delivery, when timing and dose of insulin injections should be carefully reconsidered lest hypoglycaemia occur. Insulin need remains lower during the first 6 weeks of *lactation*.

Blood glucose estimations are necessary during the latter part of pregnancy, for glycosuria is not then a reliable guide because the renal threshold for glucose (also of lactose) falls, so that glycosuria and lactosuria may occur in the presence of a normal blood glucose.

Maternal hyperglycaemia leads to fetal hyperglycaemia with consequent fetal islet cell hyperplasia, high birth-weight babies, and postnatal hypoglycaemia.

Premature labour: use of β_2-adrenoceptor agonists, and of dexamethasone (to prevent respiratory distress syndrome in the prematurely newborn) causes hyperglycaemia and increased insulin (and potassium) need.

Oral antidiabetes agents and pregnancy: the continued use of these during pregnancy is associated with fetal loss and insulin should be given.

Interactions with non-diabetes drugs

The subject is ill-documented, but whenever a diabetic under treatment takes other drugs it is prudent to be on the watch for disturbance of control.

Adrenocorticosteroids antagonise insulin.

β-*adrenoceptor blocking drugs* impair the sympathetic mediated (β_2-receptor) release of glucose from the liver in response to hypoglycaemia and also reduce the symptoms of hypoglycaemia (except sweating). Insulin hypoglycaemia is thus both more profound and less noticeable. A diabetic needing a β-adrenoceptor blocker should be given a β_1-*cardio*selective member, e.g. atenolol. Adrenergic neuron blocking drugs potentiate insulin similarly. Since *thiazides* cause diabetes it is plain the choice of drugs for treating hypertension in diabetics requires care.

The action of sulphonylureas is intensified by heavy *sulphonamide* dosage and some sulphonamides increase free tolbutamide concentrations, probably by competing for plasma protein binding sites.

Monoamine oxidase inhibitors potentiate oral agents and perhaps also insulin. They can also reduce appetite and so upset control.

Interaction may occur with *alcohol* (hypoglycaemia with any antidiabetes drug, flushing with chlorpropamide). *Combined contraceptive pill* reduces hypoglycaemic effect.

Hepatic enzyme inducers may enhance the metabolism of sulphonylureas that are metabolised in the liver (tolbutamide). Cimetidine, an inhibitor of drug metabolising enzymes, increases metformin plasma concentration.

These examples suffice to show that the possibility of interactions of practical clinical importance is a real one.

Drug-induced diabetes

After the introduction of *thiazide diuretics*, it was soon found that their prolonged use increased hyperglycaemia in diabetics, and, later, that they impaired glucose tolerance in some non-diabetics.

Research for better antihypertensive thiazides resulted in the discovery of a non-diuretic derivative with antihypertensive effect **diazoxide**, but it proved unsatisfactory for long-term use as it often caused diabetes, though it is effective short-term (see p. 412). It is useful in treating hypoglycaemia due to islet-cell tumour (insulinoma).

An antibiotic (*streptozotocin*) is selectively toxic to malignant β-islet cell tumours. It has been used to treat functioning metastases. After a short course remission may occur in 3 weeks and last a year or longer.

Adrenocortical steroids and *oral contraceptives* are also diabetogenic.

Diuretics for diabetics. In general a non-thiazide should be chosen (see Ch. 26). Frusemide and ethacrynic acid are less prone to precipitate diabetes.

Potassium-conserving diuretics are liable to cause hyperkalaemia in patients with nephropathy and should be avoided.

DIABETIC KETOACIDOSIS

The condition is discussed in detail in medical texts and only the more pharmacological aspects will be dealt with here.

In severe ketoacidosis the patient urgently needs insulin to stop ketogenesis, i.v. fluid and electrolytes, and treatment of any precipitating factor, e.g. infection.

The objective is to supply as continuously as possible, a moderate amount of insulin.

Soluble insulin, preferably from the same species the patient has been using (never a sustained-release form), should be given by continuous i.v. infusion (rather than by intermittent, bolus, injection) ideally by a pump (which allows independent control of insulin and electrolyte administration more readily than an i.v. drip) in a concentration of 0.1 unit/ml in isotonic sodium chloride, at a dose of 0.1 unit/kg/h, i.e. 7 units/h in a 70 kg adult. The dose is raised or lowered in the light of blood glucose concentrations. If an i.v. drip is used instead of a pump the concentration should be lower (40 units/l); stringent precautions against septicaemia are necessary in these patients. It has been shown that continuous infusion i.m. (not s.c.) can be equally effective, provided the patient is not in shock, and provided there is not an important degree of peripheral vascular disease.

Intermittent doses i.v. or i.m. may be used when circumstances require it. If the i.m. route is used, a priming dose of 15–20 units should be given at the outset and then 5–10 units hourly.

Progress. When the blood glucose has fallen to 10 mmol/l the infusion rate may be reduced to, say, 0.02 unit/kg per hour until the patient can eat and drink and s.c. insulin is restarted. Similar progression is used if the insulin is given i.m., e.g. lower doses 2-hourly. Doses are always tailored to the clinical situation which requires *close* monitoring.

Less severe cases of ketosis can be treated with half the above doses (3 units/h) at the outset.

It has been shown that the rate of fall of blood glucose/hour is proportional to the rate of infusion of insulin over the range of 1–10 units/h. A reasonable rate of fall during treatment is 4–5.5 mmol/l (75–100 mg/100 ml) per hour.

Intravenous fluid and electrolytes.[10] Patients are often more deficient in water than in saline and although initial replacement is by *isotonic (0.9%) sodium chloride* solution, occurrence of hypernatraemia is an indication for half isotonic (0.45%) solution. A patient with diabetic ketoacidosis may have a fluid deficit of above 5 litres and may be given 500 ml in the first 20 min, followed by 2 litres in 90 min, then 1 litre in 90 min, and 1 litre in 120 min, watching the patient for signs of fluid overload. Fluid replacement causes a fall in blood glucose by dilution.

Glucose should only be given when its concentration in blood falls below the renal threshold (8.5–10 mmol/l: i.e. 150–180 mg/100 ml). If it is used at concentrations above the renal threshold it merely increases the diabetic osmotic diuresis causing further dehydration, and potassium and magnesium loss (but see Hypoglycaemia, above).

Potassium. Even if plasma potassium is normal or high, patients have a substantial total body deficit, and the plasma potassium will fall briskly with i.v. saline (dilution) and insulin which draws potassium into cells within minutes. Infusion of KCl may begin at about 15 mmol/h and is adjusted according to monitoring.

Bicarbonate should be used only if plasma pH is <7.0 and peripheral circulation is good; insulin corrects acidosis.

Success in treatment of diabetic ketoacidosis and its complications (hypokalaemia, aspiration

---

[10] In this situation glucose solution does not provide water replacement since the normal capacity to metabolise glucose is fully taken up.

of stomach contents, infection, shock) *attends on close, constant, informed supervision.*

Mild diabetic ketosis. If the patient is fully conscious and there has been no nausea or vomiting for at least 12 h, intravenous therapy is unnecessary. It is reasonable to give small doses of insulin s.c. 3–6 hourly and fluids by mouth.

Hyperosmolar diabetic coma occurs chiefly in non-insulin-dependent diabetics who fail to compensate for their continuing osmotic glucose diuresis. It is characterised by *severe* dehydration, a very high blood sugar (>33 mmol/l: 600 mg/100 ml) and lack of ketosis and acidosis. Treatment is with isotonic or hypotonic fluids (not glucose) with less potassium than in severe ketoacidosis and small doses of insulin. Patients are liable to thrombosis and heparin is used.

SURGERY IN DIABETIC PATIENTS

Principles:

- Surgery constitutes a major stress
- Insulin needs increase with surgery
- Avoid ketosis
- Avoid hypoglycaemia
- High blood glucose concentration matters little over short periods.

The programme for control should be agreed between anaesthetist and physician *whenever diabetics must undergo general anaesthesia* or *modify their diets.* There are many different techniques that can give satisfactory results.

Type I diabetes (IDDM)

Elective major surgery

- Admit to hospital 2 days before surgery
- Substitute soluble or biphasic for long-acting insulin
- Arrange operation for morning
- Evening before surgery: reduce insulin dose by 25%
- Day of operation: omit morning s.c. dose; set up i.v. infusion (glucose 500 ml 10% + insulin 15 IU + KCl 10 mmol) and infuse at 100 ml/h

- Modify regimen during and after surgery according to monitoring
- Stop i.v. infusion one hour after first postsurgical s.c. insulin
- Insulin requirements may be even as high as 20 units/h in cases of serious infection, corticosteroid use, obesity, liver disease.

Minor surgery

For example, simple dental extractions (for multiple extractions or when there is infection the patient should be admitted to hospital). A suitable postoperative diet of appropriate calorie and carbohydrate content must be arranged. Plan the operation for between 12 noon and 5 p.m. Omit the usual dose of long-acting insulin on the morning of the operation and substitute soluble insulin, one-quarter of the usual total daily dose, before a light breakfast 6 h preceding the operation. Take a light evening meal after the operation and soluble insulin, 10–30 units s.c., according to the blood tests. Return to the normal routine the next day.

Emergency surgery

When a surgical emergency is complicated by diabetic ketosis, an attempt should be made to control the ketosis before the operation. Management during the operation will be similar to that for major surgery except that more insulin may be needed.

In other cases small doses of soluble insulin are given 2–4 hourly, keeping the blood glucose between 8.5 and 10 mmol/l (150 and 300 mg/100 ml).

Type II diabetes (NIDDM)

Elective and emergency surgery: use the same regimen as for IDDM.

Minor surgery: continue as usual with close monitoring perioperatively. If the surgery is more than trivial, omit the oral agent on the day of operation and consider using soluble insulin s.c. If vomiting is likely, use insulin.

MISCELLANEOUS

Aldose reductase inhibition. Sorbitol accumulates in some tissues in diabetes mellitus. It is formed from glucose by the enzyme aldose reductase. There is some evidence that use of an aldose reductase inhibitor (tolrestat) can benefit diabetic nephropathy.

GUIDE TO FURTHER READING

Bogardus C et al 1990 Where all the glucose doesn't go in non-insulin dependent diabetes mellitus. New England Journal of Medicine 322: 262

Coustan D R 1988 Pregnancy in diabetic women. New England Journal of Medicine 319: 1663

Editorial 1989 Transferring diabetic patients to human insulin Lancet 1: 762

Gerich J E 1989 Oral hypoglycaemic agents. New England Journal of Medicine 321: 1231

Heine R J et al 1989 Responses to human and porcine insulin in healthy subjects. Lancet 2: 946

McCance D R et al 1989 Long-term glycaemic control and diabetic retinopathy. Lancet 2: 824

MacPherson J N et al 1990 Insulin. British Medical Journal 300: 731

Patrick A W et al 1991 Human insulin and awareness of acute hypoglycaemic symptoms in insulin-dependent diabetes. Lancet 338: 528

Saudek C D et al 1989 A preliminary trial of the programmable implantable medication system for insulin delivery. New England Journal of Medicine 321: 574

Shah S C et al 1989 A randomised trial of intensive insulin therapy in newly diagnosed insulin-dependent diabetes mellitus. New England Journal of Medicine 320: 550

Stevens A B et al 1989 Motor vehicle driving amongst diabetics taking insulin and non-diabetics. British Medical Journal 299: 591

Thow J et al 1990 Insulin injection technique. British Medical Journal 301: 3

Zinman B 1989 The physiologic replacement of insulin. New England Journal of Medicine 321: 363

35

Endocrinology III: thyroid hormones, antithyroid drugs

THYROID HORMONES

L-thyroxine (T_4 or tetraiodo-L-thyronine) and **liothyronine** (T_3 or triiodo-L-thyronine) are the natural hormones of the thyroid gland. T_4 is a less active precursor of T_3, which is the major mediator of physiological effect.

For convenience, the term *thyroid hormone* is used to comprise T_4 plus T_3. Both forms are available for oral use as therapy.
Calcitonin: see p. 656.

Physiology and pharmacokinetics

Thyroid hormone is formed from dietary iodine by iodination of tyrosine to *mono-* and *di*iodotyrosine; 2 molecules of diiodotyrosine combine to form *tetra*iodotyrosine, T_4 or *thyroxine*.

Thyroid hormone is stored in the gland as thyroglobulin from which enzymatic hydrolysis releases T_4 and a little T_3 into the circulation. About 80% of the released T_4 is deiodinated in the peripheral tissues to the biologically active T_3 (30–35%) and biologically inactive *reverse* T_3 (45–50%); thus most circulating T_3 is derived from T_4. Further deiodination, largely in the liver, leads to loss of activity.

In the blood both T_4 and T_3 are extensively (99.9%) bound to plasma proteins (thyroxine-binding globulin, TBG, and thyroxine-binding prealbumin, TBPA). *The concentration of TBG is raised* by oestrogens (including doses used in oral contraceptives), clofibrate, and prolonged use of neuroleptics, and in pregnancy. *The concentration of TBG is lowered* by adrenocortical and androgen (including anabolic steroid) therapy and by urinary protein loss in nephrotic syndrome. Phenytoin and salicylates compete with thyroid hormone for TBG binding sites. Effects such as these obviously can interfere with the assessment of the clinical significance of measurements of *total* thyroid hormone concentration. But measurement of *free* thyroid hormone by ingenious techniques (free thyroxine index) largely avoids these complicating factors.

T_4 and T_3 are well absorbed from the gut except in *severe* hypothyroidism, when initial parenteral therapy is used.

T_4 (*thyroxine*): a single dose reaches its maximum effect in about 10 days (its binding to plasma proteins is strong) and passes off in 2–3 weeks ($t_\frac{1}{2}$ 7 days in euthyroid subjects; 14 d in hypothyroid; 3 d in hyperthyroid).

T_3 (*liothyronine*) is about 5 times as biologically potent as T_4; a single dose reaches its maximum effect in about 24 h (its binding to plasma proteins is weak) and passes off in one week ($t_\frac{1}{2}$ 2 days in euthyroid subjects: see T_4 above).

Pharmacodynamics

Thyroid hormone passes into the cells to target organs, combines with specific receptors there and induces characteristic metabolic changes:

- *protein synthesis* during growth;
- increased *metabolic rate* with raised oxygen consumption;
- increased *sensitivity to catecholamines* with proliferation of β-adrenoceptors (particularly important in the cardiovascular system).

USE OF THYROID HORMONE FOR HYPOTHYROIDISM

The main indication for thyroid hormone is treatment of *deficiency* (cretinism, hypothyroidism, myxoedema) from any cause. The adult requirement of hormone is remarkably constant, and dosage does not have to be altered once the optimum is found. Children naturally need more as they grow.

Early treatment of cretinous babies is important if permanent mental defect is to be avoided. It must be life-long.

Hypothyroidism due to *panhypopituitarism* requires replacement with adrenocortical as well as with thyroid hormones. Use of thyroxine alone can cause acute adrenal insufficiency.

Small doses of thyroxine in normal subjects merely depress TSH production and consequently reduce the output of thyroid hormone by an equivalent amount.

When *thyroid enlargement* is associated with excess TSH (puberty goitre, endemic iodine deficiency, Hashimoto's autoimmune thyroiditis), thyroxine administration can be effective in suppressing TSH secretion (by the usual feedback mechanism) with reduction in size of goitre.

Thyroxine should not be used to treat simple obesity (see obesity).

A curious by-way of human nature that can cause diagnostic difficulty is secret thyroxine 'addiction'.[1] It is associated with overt psychiatric disease and/or emotional immaturity, and aggressive dependence on mothers or mother substitutes. The condition is uncommon, and afflicts women particularly.

Treatment of hypothyroidism

Thyroxine Tabs contain pure L-thyroxine sodium and should be used (preparations of dried animal glands are obsolete because they are unreliable and moulds grow on them).

The initial oral dose may be 50–100 μg daily; but in the old and patients with heart disease or hypertension, this should be achieved gradually (to minimise cardiovascular risk due to a too-sudden increase in metabolic demand), starting with 25 μg daily for the first 2–4 weeks, and then increasing by 25–50 μg every fortnight until symptoms are relieved, usually at 100–200 μg as a single daily dose. This is usually sufficient to reduce plasma TSH to normal concentrations which is the *best indicator* of adequate treatment. Patients who appear to need more are probably not taking their tablets consistently. The maxi-

---

[1] Harvey R F. Br Med J 1973; 2: 35.

mum effect of a dose is not reached for about 10 days and passes off over about 2–3 weeks. Absorption is more complete and less variable if thyroxine is taken well apart from food.

Tablets containing supposedly physiological mixtures of *thyroxine and liothyronine* offer no advantage.

Hypothyroid patients tend to be intolerant of drugs due to delayed metabolism.

Liothyronine Tabs. Liothyronine is the most rapidly effective thyroid hormone, a single dose giving maximum effect within 24 h and passing off over about a week. Its main uses are in *hypothyroid coma and psychosis*, both rare conditions. It is not used in routine treatment of hypothyroidism because the fast action can induce heart failure, but in the above conditions, particularly in coma where death is inevitable in the absence of treatment, the risk may be justified.

Hypothyroid coma follows prolonged total hormone deficiency and constitutes an emergency. An untreated patient dies of hypothyroidism and a too-vigorously treated patient dies from cardiovascular collapse due to a precipitate rise in metabolism. Thus the physician must steer between the Scylla[2] of undertreatment and the Charybdis[3] of overtreatment, both fatal. This may be done by giving thyroxine (T_4) i.v., if available. The biologically weaker T_4 is gradually converted into the highly active T_3. A single dose of 500 μg of thyroxine raises the plasma T_4 to about half the normal concentration and suffices for a week, after which routine oral maintenance dose may be used. Oral T_4 is too slow in the emergency.

Alternatively (or sometimes, judiciously, in addition in low dose) the quick-acting T_3 may be given by stomach tube, 5–10 μg 8–12 hourly (or

i.v.). Maximum dose in the first 24 h should probably not exceed 50 μg since 100 μg is the full replacement dose. The dose may be raised after 3 days and the patient transferred to thyroxine after recovery.

Hydrocortisone i.v. is also needed, as prolonged hypothyroidism is associated with hypoadrenalism, and hydrocortisone is needed to cope with the increasing metabolism.

Adverse effects of thyroid hormone parallel the increase in metabolic rate. The symptoms and signs are those of hyperthyroidism, minus exophthalmos. Angina pectoris or heart failure are liable to be provoked by too vigorous therapy or in patients having serious ischaemic heart disease who may even be unable to tolerate optimal therapy. Should they occur thyroxine must be discontinued for at least a week and begun again at lower dosage. Only slight overdose is needed to precipitate atrial fibrillation in patients over 60 years.

In pregnancy a hypothyroid patient should be carefully assessed; a small increase in dose of thyroxine may be required; breast feeding is not contraindicated though the baby's thyroid status should be watched.

ANTITHYROID DRUGS AND HYPERTHYROIDISM

Drugs used for the treatment of *hyper*thyroidism include:

- **Thionamides** which block the synthesis of thyroid hormone.
- **Iodine**: radioiodine which destroys the cells making thyroid hormone; iodide, an *excess* of which reduces the production of thyroid hormone *temporarily* by an unknown mechanism (it is also necessary for the formation of hormone, and both excess and deficiency can cause goitre).

Thionamides (thiourea derivatives)

Mode of action

The major action of thionamides is to *reduce the formation of thyroid* hormone by inhibiting the

---

[2] In classical mythology *Scylla* was a rival in love to Circe who, using her pharmacological expertise, changed Scylla into a monster having 12 feet, 6 heads and 3 rows of teeth. Terrified by this Scylla threw herself into the sea and was transformed into rocks.

[3] *Charybdis* stole the oxen of Hercules, was struck by thunder, and became a whirlpool.

Ships passing between Sicily and Italy were liable to fall victim to one or other of these hazards. The words *Incidit in Scyllam qui vult vitare Charybdim* have become a proverb to show that, *in our eagerness to avoid one evil, we often fall into a greater* (Lemprière).

organification (incorporation into organic form) of iodine (iodotyrosines), and by inhibiting the coupling of iodotyrosines to form T_4 and T_3. Maximum effect is delayed until existing hormone stores are exhausted (weeks, see below). With high dosage the reduction in hormone synthesis may be sufficient to induce the pituitary to produce more TSH, which in turn causes thyroid enlargement (hyperplasia and increase in vascularity).

Carbimazole and **methimazole** (the chief metabolite of carbimazole) ($t_\frac{1}{2}$ 4 h) and **propylthiouracil** ($t_\frac{1}{2}$ 2 h) are commonly used. Half-lives are shorter in hyperthyroid subjects and lengthen if the patient becomes hypothyroid, but $t_\frac{1}{2}$ matters little since the drugs accumulate in the thyroid and act there for 30–40 h; thus a single daily dose suffices.

Propylthiouracil differs from other members of the group in that it also inhibits peripheral conversion of T_4 to T_3 (but this is not quick enough immediately to arrest a thyroid storm, see below).

Doses

Carbimazole, initial, orally, 30–60 mg total/day until euthyroid: maintenance 5–15 mg total/day. *Propylthiouracil* orally, 300–450 mg total/day until euthyroid: maintenance 50–150 mg total/day. Higher doses are sometimes needed (even 3 times the above).

Use

It is probable that no patient is wholly refractory to these drugs. Failure to respond is likely to be due to the patient not taking the tablets or to wrong diagnosis.

The drugs are used in hyperthyroidism as *principal therapy*, and as *adjuvant to radioiodine* to control the disease until the radiation achieves its effect,[4] and to *prepare patients for surgery.*

---

[4] Use of a thionamide during the week before and after radioiodine therapy *may* impair the response to radiation (Velkeniers B et al. Lancet 1988; 1: 1127), see Mode of action of thionamides, above.

Clinical improvement is noticeable in about a week, and the patient should be euthyroid after about 6 weeks. The dose is then progressively reduced and adjusted according to the clinical picture. The best guides to therapy are the patients' feelings, their weight and pulse rate, though measurements of the latter can be misleadingly high in a well-controlled patient if they are only taken in a clinic. Measurement of the *ankle reflex time* (long in *hypo* and short in *hyper*thyroidism) is a useful guide to therapy (rather than to diagnosis) in both hyper- and hypothyroidism. Simple machines to record this are available.

Symptoms and signs are, of course, less valuable as guides if the patient is also taking a β-adrenoceptor blocker, and reliance is then put on tests, but β-blockers also prolong the ankle reflex time.

With optimal treatment the gland decreases in size, but *overtreatment* leading to low hormone concentrations in the blood activates the feedback system, inducing TSH secretion and goitre.

All three drugs give similar results.

Adverse reactions

These drugs are all liable to cause allergic effects including rashes, lymphadenopathy and most serious of all, leucopenia sometimes proceeding to agranulocytosis ($<1:10\ 000$) or aplastic anaemia (which may be due to idiosyncrasy rather than to allergy). Blood disorders are most common in the first 2 months of treatment. Repeated leucocyte counts are often advocated but agranulocytosis may be so acute that the counts give no warning; a leucocyte count should be done if the patient develops an infection (usually a sore throat, but infected haemorrhoids have heralded agranulocytosis). Patients should be warned to report this, and any suggestion of anaemia should be investigated. Cross allergy between the drugs occurs sometimes.

Pregnancy. If a pregnant woman has hyperthyroidism (2/1000 pregnancies) she should be treated with the *smallest possible* amount of these drugs because they cross the placenta; with overtreatment fetal goitre occurs. Surgery in the second trimester may be preferred to continued drug therapy.

So little of propylthiouracil passes into breast milk that it may safely be used during breast-feeding.

Goitre (fetal) may occur due to increased TSH secretion by the pituitary in response to decreased thyroxine production.

Control of antithyroid drug therapy

The aim of drug therapy is to control the hyperthyroidism until a natural remission takes place. Unfortunately, though usual, remission is not invariable and there is no way of predicting which patients will not remit and who should therefore be offered radiation or surgery at the outset.

Clinically, it is not possible to decide reliably when remission has occurred, although disappearance of bruit and reduction in gland size suggest it. Treatment should not be stopped whilst a bruit persists.

If there has never been a bruit, treatment may be stopped after the patient has been judged euthyroid for 4–6 months on the minimum dose of the drug. Lid retraction is the only eye sign that improves. But the duration of therapy that minimises the relapse rate is controversial, and 12–18 months total therapy before withdrawal as a routine is commonly advised. Plasma concentrations of T_3 and T_4 (at withdrawal and 4 weeks later) can be used to determine if remission has occurred, along with clinical monitoring.

Relapse occurs in a few months or years in as many as 50–70% of cases, and this is the major disadvantage of thionamides; a second course of treatment may be successful. The *use of thyroxine concurrently with an antithyroid drug* suppresses TSH production and decreases the production of antibodies to TSH (which are the cause of the hyperthyroid state). It may reduce the frequency of relapse.

Both successful drug treatment and follow-up require a compliant patient; but radioiodine may be preferred.

Control of hyperthyroid symptoms with drugs that block sympathetic autonomic activity

There is evidence that there is increased tissue sensitivity to catecholamines with increased number of β-adrenoceptors in hyperthyroidism and that this is a cause of some of the unpleasant symptoms.

Quick relief can be obtained with a β-adrenoceptor blocking drug (judge dose by heart rate) though these do not block all the metabolic effects of the hormone, e.g. on the myocardium, and the basal metabolic rate is unchanged. For this reason they should not be used as sole therapy; they do not alter the course of the disease, nor biochemical tests of thyroid function. Any effect on thyroid hormonal action on peripheral tissues is clinically unimportant. Plainly it is desirable to choose a drug that lacks partial agonist effect (intrinsic sympathomimetic activity).

β-adrenoceptor block is specially useful during the long wait (months) for the effect of radio-iodine, though it may be used for any patient who feels uncomfortable.

Eye signs may respond to eye drops of a β-adrenoceptor blocker (timolol) or of an adrenergic neuron blocker (guanethidine, but this can cause conjunctival fibrosis in prolonged use).

A hyperthyroid patient with urgent intercurrent disease, e.g. need for surgery, should at once be treated with a β-adrenoceptor blocker.

In thyrotoxic heart failure patients may need their sympathetic cardiac drive and may be made worse by β-adrenoceptor block.

Iodine (iodide and radioactive iodine)

Iodide

Iodide is well absorbed from the intestine, is distributed like chloride in the body and is rapidly excreted by the kidney. It is selectively taken up and concentrated (about ×25) by the thyroid gland, but more in hyperthyroidism and less in hypothyroidism. A *deficiency of iodide* reduces the amount of thyroid hormone produced, which stimulates the pituitary to secrete TSH. The result is hyperplasia and increased vascularity of the gland, with eventual goitre formation.

Effects

Iodide effects are complex and related to dose and to thyroid status of the subject.

In *hyperthyroid* subjects a *moderate* excess of iodide may enhance hormone production by providing 'fuel' for hormone synthesis. But a *substantial excess* inhibits hormone release and promotes storage of hormone and involution of the gland, making it firmer and less vascular so that surgery is easier. The effect is *transient* and its mechanism uncertain.

In *euthyroid* subjects with normal glands an excess of iodide from any source can cause goitre (with or without hyperthyroidism), e.g. use of iodide-containing cough medicines, iodine-containing radiocontrast media, amiodarone, seaweed eaters.

A euthyroid subject with an autonomous adenoma (hot nodule) becomes hyperthyroid if given iodide.

Uses

Iodide (large dose) is *used* for *thyroid crisis (storm)* and *in preparation for thyroidectomy* because it rapidly benefits the patient by reducing hormone release and renders surgery easier and safer (above).

Potassium iodide in doses of 60 mg orally 8-hourly (longer intervals allow some escape from the iodide effect) produces some effect in 1–2 days, maximal after 10–14 days, after which the benefit declines as the thyroid adapts. A traditional formulation is Aqueous Iodine Oral Solution (Lugol's Iodine) (5% iodine + 10% potassium iodide in water: 130 mg iodine/ml: 0.1–0.3 ml 8-hourly). The iodine is rapidly converted into iodide in the liver.

Such therapy maximises iodide stores in the thyroid, which delays response to thionamides.

Prophylactic iodide (1 part in 100 000 parts) may be added to the salt, water or bread where goitre is endemic.

In economically underdeveloped communities a method of prophylaxis is to inject iodised oil i.m. every 3–5 years; given early enough to women, this prevents endemic cretinism; but occasional hyperthyroidism occurs (see autonomous adenoma above).

As an antiseptic for use on the skin, Weak Iodine Solution (90% alcoholic tincture) is very effective but is painful on broken skin; it is superseded by *povidone-iodine* (a complex of iodine with a sustained-release carrier, povidone or polyvinyl-pyrrolidone) which can be applied repeatedly and used as a surgical scrub, though less concentrated and therefore less effective than the solution.

Bronchial secretion. Iodide is concentrated in bronchial and salivary secretions. It acts as an expectorant (see cough).

Organic compounds containing iodine are used as contrast media in radiology. It is essential to ask patients specifically whether they are allergic to it before they are used. Some radiographical preparations do not contain iodine. An i.v. test dose ought to be given half an hour before the full i.v. dose if there is history of any allergy. If there is any reaction and it is essential to proceed with the investigation, repeated doses every half hour may be given, doubling the dose each time. A substantial dose of a corticosteroid may be given 60 min before the agent. Absence of a reaction to a test dose does not guarantee safety.

Adverse reactions

Patients vary enormously in their tolerance of iodine; some are intolerant or allergic to it both orally and when put on the skin. Symptoms of **iodism** include a metallic taste, excessive salivation with painful salivary glands running eyes and nose, sore mouth and throat, a productive cough, diarrhoea, and various rashes that may mimic chicken-pox. The Weak Iodine Solution (Tincture) used in antisepsis is caustic; it is sometimes drunk by suicidal patients: stomach washouts with solutions of starch are an antidote. Elimination can be enhanced by inducing a saline diuresis.

Goitre can occur (see above) with prolonged use of iodide-containing expectorants by bronchitics and asthmatics. Such therapy should therefore be intermittent, if it is used at all.

Topical application of iodine-containing antiseptics to neonates has caused hypothyroidism. Iodide intake above that in a normal diet will depress thyroid *uptake of administered radioiodine*, because the two forms will compete.

In the case of diet, medication and water-soluble radiodiagnostic agents, interference will cease 2–4 weeks after stopping the source, but with agents used for cholecystography it may last for 6 months or more (tissue binding).

Radioiodine (^{131}I)

^{131}I is treated by the body just like the ordinary non-radioactive isotope, so that when swallowed it is concentrated in the thyroid gland. It emits mainly β radiation (90%), which penetrates only 0.5 mm of tissue and thus allows therapeutic effect on the thyroid without damage to the surrounding structures, particularly the parathyroids. However, it also emits some γ rays, which are more penetrating and can be detected with a Geiger counter. ^{131}I has a physical (radioactive) $t_{\frac{1}{2}}$ of 8 days.

^{131}I is increasingly used as treatment of choice in hyperthyroidism at all ages, and in combination with surgery in some cases of thyroid carcinoma, especially those in which metastases are sufficiently differentiated to take up iodide selectively.

In hyperthyroidism the beneficial effects of a single dose may be felt in one month but its action is not maximal for 3 months. β-adrenoceptor block and, in severe cases, antithyroid drug (but see footnote 4), will be needed to render the patient comfortable whilst waiting. Very rarely the radiation damage to the thyroid causes a release of hormone and a thyroid storm. Repeated doses are sometimes needed.

In the event of inadvertent overdose, large doses of sodium or potassium iodide should be given to compete with the radioiodine for thyroid uptake and to hasten excretion by increasing iodide turnover (increased fluid intake and a diuretic are adjuvants).

Radioiodine offers the advantages that treatment is simple and in no way unpleasant (the patient just drinks it) and it carries no immediate mortality. However, it is slow in acting and it is difficult to judge the dose that will render the patient euthyroid.

In the first year after treatment 6–15% or even more (depending on the dose) of patients will become hypothyroid. After this 2–3% of patients become hypothyroid *annually* after treatment with radioiodine, perhaps because the capacity of thyroid cells to divide is permanently abolished so that cell renewal ceases. Patients must therefore be followed up *indefinitely* after radioiodine treatment, for all are likely to need treatment for hypothyroidism eventually.

Because such follow-up over years may fail and because the onset of hypothyroidism may be insidious and not easily recognised, some physicians prefer deliberately to render patients hypothyroid with the first dose and to educate them on the use of replacement therapy which is safe and effective.

Experience has eliminated the fear that radioiodine causes carcinoma of the thyroid, and it is now used in patients of all ages. But *pregnant women* should not be treated with radioiodine (^{131}I) because it crosses the placenta.

There is a theoretical risk of germ cell mutagenic effect and patients should not reproduce for a few (say, 6) months[5] after treatment. Larger doses of radioiodine are used for *thyroid carcinoma* than for hyperthyroidism, and there is an increased incidence of late leukaemia in these patients. The treatment of thyroid carcinoma is highly specialised.

Radioiodine uptake can be used to *test thyroid function*, but it has been largely superseded.

---

[5] Even today it can be embarrassing to offer such advice to an excited hyperthyroid unmarried woman or man. Yet to fail to do so could have grave consequences for a child. It is rumoured that some physicians have prescribed an oral contraceptive without telling the patient what it is; a procedure that is understandable if not ethically justifiable.

Preparation for surgery

Preparation of hyperthyroid patients for surgery can be satisfactorily achieved by making them euthyroid with one of the above drugs plus a β-adrenoceptor blocker for comfort (see below) and safety,[6] and *adding* iodide for 7–10 days before operation (not sooner) to reduce the surgically inconvenient vascularity of the gland. This procedure takes about 5 weeks.

An alternative is to prepare the patient with a β-adrenoceptor blocker (propranolol, 6-hourly) for 4 days (adjust dose to *eliminate*[6] tachycardia)

---

[6] No patient should be operated on with a resting pulse of 90/min or above, and no dose of β-adrenoceptor blocker, including the important postoperative dose, should be omitted. Toft A D et al. N Engl J Med 1978; 298: 643.

and to continue thus through the operation and for 7–10 days after.

The important differences with this second technique are that the gland is smaller and less friable, although the patient's *tissues* are still hyperthyroid, and it is essential, in order to avoid a hyperthyroid crisis or storm, that the β-adrenoceptor blocker be continued as above without the omission of even a single 6-hourly dose of propranolol; but erratic plasma concentrations can be a cause of failure.

Thyroid crisis or storm is rare with modern methods of preparing hyperthyroid patients for surgery. It is probably due to liberation of large amounts of hormone into the circulation. Treatment is urgently required to save life. Propranolol should be given immediately (i.v. *slowly*, 1 mg/min to max of 10 mg, in severe cases, preceded by atropine 1–2 mg i.v. to prevent excessive bradycardia); iodide to inhibit further hormone release from the gland (say 600 mg–1.0 g iodide orally or i.v. in the first 24 h) (see iodide), and hydrocortisone i.v. Mental disturbance may be treated by chlorpromazine; hyperthermia by cooling and aspirin; heart failure in the ordinary way.

Exophthalmos of hyperthyroidism

The cause may be related to an immunoglobulin that attacks the external ocular muscles and retrobulbar tissue. Antithyroid drugs do not help. TSH secretion is not responsible (it is high in primary thyroid gland failure in which exophthalmos does not occur). The patient should be rendered euthyroid. High systemic doses of prednisolone or less with another immuno-suppressive (cyclosporin) may help, but in urgent cases surgery is necessary, i.e. orbital decompression. Artificial tears (hypromellose) are useful when natural tears and blinking are inadequate to maintain corneal lubrication.

DRUGS THAT CAUSE UNWANTED HYPOTHYROIDISM

In addition to drugs used for their antithyroid effects, the following substances can cause hypothyroidism: PAS (for tuberculosis), phenyl-butazone (antirheumatic), iodide (see above), cobalt salts (for anaemia), sulphonylureas (for diabetes), resorcinol (for leg ulcers), lithium (for mania/depression), amiodarone (cardiac an-tidysrhythmic). Effects are generally reversible on withdrawal. Hepatic enzyme induction may rarely cause hypothyroidism.

CALCITONIN: see Chapter 39.

GUIDE TO FURTHER READING

Burrow G N 1985 The management of thyrotoxicosis in pregnancy. New England Journal of Medicine 313: 562

Franklyn J A et al 1990 Thyroxine replacement treatment and osteoporosis. British Medical Journal 300: 693

Frey, F J 1988 Altered metabolism and decreased efficacy of prednisolone in patients with hyperthyroidism. Clinical Pharmacology and Therapeutics 44: 510

Hamolsky M W 1982 Truth is stranger than factitious. [The physiology and diagnosis of deliberate self-administration of thyroid hormone]. New England Journal of Medicine 307: 436

Hedberg C W et al 1987 An outbreak of thyrotoxicosis caused by the consumption of bovine thyroid gland in ground beef. New England Journal of Medicine 316: 993

International Agranulocytosis and Aplastic Anaemia Study 1988 Risk of agranulocytosis and aplastic anaemia in relation to use of antithyroid drugs. British Medical Journal 297: 262

Kendall-Taylor P et al 1984 Ablative radioiodine therapy for hyperthyroidism: long-term follow up study. British Medical Journal 299: 361

Ladenson P W 1991 Treatments for Graves disease: letting the thyroid rest. New England Journal of Medicine 324: 989

Mandel S J et al 1990 Increased need for thyroxine during pregnancy in women with primary hypothyroidism. New England Journal of Medicine 323: 91

Utiger R D 1984 Beta-adrenergic antagonist therapy for hyperthyroid Graves' disease. New England Journal of Medicine 310: 1597

Utiger R D 1989 Treatment of Graves' ophthalmopathy. New England Journal of Medicine 321: 1403

Utiger R D 1990 Therapy of hypothyroidism: What changes are needed? New England Journal of Medicine 323: 126

Velkeniers B et al 1988 Treatment of hyperthyroidism with radioiodine: adjunctive therapy with antithyroid drugs reconsidered. Lancet 1: 1988

36

Endocrinology IV: hypothalamic and pituitary hormones, sex hormones, contraception, uterus

HORMONES, ANALOGUES AND ANTAGONISTS

Once the structure of natural hormones, local or systemic (including hormone-releasing hormones), is defined it becomes possible to synthesise not only the hormones themselves[1] but also *analogues* and *antagonists*. Thus, increasingly, there become available substances differing in selectivity and duration of action, and active by various routes of administration.

These hormones, analogues (agonists) and antagonists can be used:

- to analyse the functional integrity of endocrine control systems
- as replacement in hormone deficiency states
- to modify malfunction of endocrine systems
- to alter normal function where this is inconvenient, e.g. contraception.

The scope of the specialist endocrinologist continues to increase in amount and in complexity and only an outline is appropriate here.

HYPOTHALAMIC AND PITUITARY HORMONES

Hypothalamus: hormone-releasing hormones, hormone-release inhibiting hormones, gonadorelin.

[1] Hormones can be synthesised directly in the chemical laboratory or by inserting mammalian genes into microbes, e.g. *Escherichia coli*, recombinant DNA technology.

Anterior pituitary: growth hormone, gonadotrophic hormones, corticotrophin, thyrotrophin, prolactin.

Posterior pituitary: vasopressin, oxytocin.

HYPOTHALAMUS AND ANTERIOR PITUITARY

Some agents have restricted commercial availability. The $t_{\frac{1}{2}}$ of the polypeptide and glycoprotein hormones listed below is 5–30 min; they are digested if swallowed.

- **Corticotrophin releasing hormone (CRH), corticoliberin**, is a hypothalamic polypeptide that has diagnostic use; it is not generally available.
- **Corticotrophin, adrenocorticotrophic hormone (ACTH)**, see p. 561.
- **Thyroid stimulating hormone (TSH), thyrotrophin**, a glycoprotein of the anterior pituitary, controls the release of thyroid hormone from the gland, and also the uptake of iodide by the thyroid gland. **TSH** secretion is inhibited (via the hypothalamus and **TRH**, below) by a high level of thyroid hormone in the blood and stimulated by a low concentration, i.e. there is a negative feedback mechanism of control.

A stimulation test using TSH is no longer useful now that TSH blood concentration and free T_4 and T_3 can be measured.

Antithyroid drugs, by reducing thyroid hormone production, cause increased formation of TSH which is the cause of the thyroid enlargement that sometimes occurs during antithyroid drug therapy.

- **Thyrotrophin-releasing hormone (TRH), protirelin**, is a tripeptide formed in the hypothalamus and controlled by free plasma T_4, T_3 concentration. It has been synthesised and can be used in diagnosis to test the capacity of the pituitary to release thyroid-stimulating hormone (TSH), e.g. to determine whether hypothyroidism is due to primary thyroid gland failure or is secondary to pituitary disease or to a hypothalamic lesion.
- **Somatostatin, growth hormone release inhibiting hormone**, occurs in other parts of the brain as well as in the hypothalamus, and also in some peripheral tissues, e.g. pancreas, stomach. In addition to the action implied by its name, it inhibits secretion of thyrotrophin, insulin, gastrin and serotonin.

Octreotide is a synthetic analogue of somatostatin having a longer action ($t_{\frac{1}{2}}$ 1.5 h). Uses include acromegaly, carcinoid (serotonin secreting) tumours and other rare tumours of the alimentary tract.

- **Somatropin, growth hormone** (Genotropin), is a biosynthetic form (191 amino acids). It acts on many organs to produce a peptide (somatomedin) which causes muscle, bone and other tissues to increase growth, i.e. protein synthesis, and the size and number of cells.

It is used in childhood pituitary insufficiency (the bone epiphyses must be open) to prevent dwarfism and provide normal growth. Use simply to avoid low height for social reasons is controversial.

About 50% of the elderly have growth hormone secretion below the norm for people in their twenties. The bodily changes of age are not simply due to growth hormone deficiency. Administration of growth hormone to the elderly for 6 months induces modest increase in lean body mass, in skin fold thickness, in vertebral bone density, and reduction in adipose tissue; also a small increase in isometric strength. In excess (as in acromegaly) growth hormone causes diabetes, hypertension and arthritis. There is a need for large, prolonged and detailed clinical studies before growth hormone can be considered for use to improve the quality of life of otherwise healthy elderly people.

Possibilities of *abuse* have also arisen, e.g. creation of 'super' sportspeople.

Acromegaly. Growth hormone secretion is reduced by octreotide and by bromocriptine (see index).

- **Gonadorelin: gonadotrophin releasing hormone (GnRH)** releases luteinising hormone (LH) and follicle-stimulating hormone (FSH). Its full abbreviation is thus LH-FSH-RH, but it is commonly represented as LH-RH for brevity, or GnRH. It has use in assessment of pituitary function. Intermittent *pulsatile* administration evokes secretion of gonadotrophins (LH and FSH) and is used to treat infertility. But *continuous* use evokes tachyphylaxis due to down-regulation of its receptors, i.e. gonadotrophin release and therefore gonadal secretions, are reduced. Longer-acting analogues, e.g. buserelin, goserelin, nafarelin, deslorelin and leuprorelin are used to suppress androgen secretion in prostatic carcinoma. Other uses may include endometriosis, precocious puberty and contraception.

- **Follicle-stimulating hormone (FSH)** stimulates development of ova and of spermatozoa. It is prepared from the urine of postmenopausal women; *menotrophin* (Pergonal) also contains a small amount of LH, and *urofollotrophin* (Metrodin) is FSH alone. They are used in female and male hypopituitary infertility.

- **Chorionic gonadotrophin** (human chorionic gonadotrophin: HCG) is secreted by the placenta and is obtained from the urine of pregnant women. Its predominant action is that of luteinising hormone (LH) (interstitial cell stimulating hormone) which induces progesterone production by the corpus luteum, and, in the male, gonadal testosterone production. It is used in hypopituitary anovular and other infertility in both sexes (for LH effect is not confined to females despite its name). It is also used for cryptochidism in prepubertal boys (about 6 years; if it fails to induce testicular descent, there is time for surgery before puberty to provide maximal possibility of a full functional testis). It may also precipitate puberty in males where this is delayed.

- **Prolactin** is secreted in both women and men, and, despite its name, it influences numerous biological functions (as many as 80), though not all of physiological importance. Prolactin secretion is controlled by an inhibitory dopaminergic path. Thus, dopamine *agonists*, e.g. bromocriptine, reduce prolactin secretion and dopamine *antagonists* increase secretion. This explains the use of bromocriptine for suppression of lactation (p. 611) and in hyperprolactinaemia from other causes, e.g. pituitary tumours; also the occurrence of hyperprolactinaemia (causing galactorrhoea) during therapy with neuroleptic dopamine antagonist drugs, and with metoclopramide and methyldopa.

Hypopituitarism

In hypopituitarism there is a deficiency of all the hormones secreted by the anterior lobe of the pituitary. The posterior lobe hormones (below) may also be deficient in a few cases (e.g. when a tumour has destroyed the pituitary). Patients suffering from hypopituitarism may present in coma, in which case treatment is as for a severe acute adrenal insufficiency. Maintenance therapy is required, using adrenocortical and thyroid hormones. Sex hormones are not usually required, although androgens will help to establish a positive nitrogen balance in wasted patients.

Infertility: see p. 601.

POSTERIOR PITUITARY HORMONES AND ANALOGUES

Vasopressin: antidiuretic hormone

Vasopressin is the antidiuretic hormone (polypeptide) ($t_\frac{1}{2}$ 20 min). Its official name is unfortunate, for only in high doses does it affect the vascular system and its chief function is to provide renal antidiuresis.

Vasopressin increases membrane permeability and so water reabsorption in the distal tubule and collecting duct (V_1 receptors). In its absence free water, i.e. water without electrolyte, excretion is increased.

Secretion of the antidiuretic hormone is stimulated by any increase in the osmotic pressure of the blood supplying the hypothalamus and by a variety of drugs, notably *nicotine*. Secretion is inhibited by a fall in blood osmotic pressure and by *alcohol*.

In large non-physiological doses (pharmacotherapy) vasopressin causes *contraction of all smooth muscle* (V_2 receptors), raising the blood pressure and causing intestinal colic. The smooth-muscle stimulant effect provides an example of tachyphylaxis (frequently repeated doses give progressively less effect). It is not only inefficient when used to raise the blood pressure, but is also dangerous, since it causes constriction of the coronary arteries and sudden death has occurred following its use.

For replacement therapy of *pituitary diabetes insipidus* the longer acting desmopressin is preferred.

Desmopressin

Desmopressin (DDAVP) (des-amino-D-arginine vasopressin) has two major advantages: the vasoconstrictor effect has been reduced to near insignificance and the duration of action with nasal instillation, spray on or s.c. injection, is 8–20 h ($t_{\frac{1}{2}}$ 75 min) so that, using it 2–3 times a day, patients are not inconvenienced by frequent recurrence of polyuria during their waking hours and can also expect to spend the night continuously in bed. Duration of action of the alternative, *lypressin*, is 3–4 h. The dose for children is about half that for adults.

Nephrogenic diabetes insipidus, as is to be expected, does not respond to antidiuretic hormone.

Nocturnal enuresis: see p. 283.

In *bleeding oesophageal varices* in hepatic cirrhosis, use is sometimes made of the vasoconstrictor effect of vasopressin (as terlipressin, a vasopressin prodrug): see p. 544.

In *haemophilia* desmopressin can enhance blood concentration of factor VIII.

Felypressin is used as a vasoconstrictor with local anaesthetics.

Diabetes insipidus

Desmopressin replacement therapy is the first choice. *Thiazide diuretics* (and chlorthalidone) also have paradoxical antidiuretic effect in diabetes insipidus. That this is not due to Na depletion is suggested by the fact that the non-diuretic thiazide, diazoxide (see index), also has this effect. It is probable that changes in the proximal renal tubule result in increased reabsorption and in delivery of less Na and water to the distal tubule, but the mechanism remains incompletely elucidated. Some cases of the *nephrogenic* form, which is not helped by antidiuretic hormone, may be benefited.

Drugs, e.g. lithium and demeclocycline, may cause nephrogenic diabetes insipidus.

Chlorpropamide. A patient with diabetes *insipidus*, wrongly believing himself to suffer from diabetes mellitus, 'at his own discretion' took chlorpropamide.[2] His physician was surprised at the apparent therapeutic effect and tried the drug on other patients, confirming it.

Chlorpropamide (but not other sulphonylureas) and *carbamazepine* are effective in *partial* pituitary diabetes insipidus, i.e. some natural hormone production remains, because they act on the kidney potentiating the effect of vasopressin on the renal tubule. Hypoglycaemia may occur with chlorpropamide.

Evidently all these drugs may cause difficulty due to their other actions that are not desired, and none is drug of first choice for this disease.

Syndrome of inappropriate antidiuretic hormone secretion (SIADH)

A variety of tumours, e.g. oat-cell lung cancer, can make vasopressin, and of course they are not subject to normal homeostatic mechanisms. Dilutional hyponatraemia may occur, and fludrocortisone may be needed along with fluid restriction (soon becomes intolerable) and infusion of hypertonic saline (in acute cases only). Demeclocycline, which inhibits the renal action of vasopressin, can be useful. Chemotherapy to the causative tumour is likely to be the most effective treatment.

Oxytocin: see p. 612.

SEX (GONADAL) HORMONES AND ANTAGONISTS: STEROID HORMONES

Steroid hormone receptors (for gonadal steroids and adrenocortical steroids) are complex proteins inside the target cell. The steroid penetrates, is bound and translocates into the cell

[2] Arduino F et al. J Clin Endocrinol 1966; 26: 1325.

nucleus, which is the principal site of action and where RNA/protein synthesis occurs. Compounds that occupy the receptor without causing translocation into the nucleus or the replenishment of receptors act as antagonists, e.g. spironolactone to aldosterone, cyproterone to androgens, clomiphene to oestrogens.

Selectivity. Many synthetic analogues, although classed as, e.g. androgen, anabolic steroid, progestogen, are *unselective* and bind to several types of receptor as agonist, partial agonist, antagonist. The result is that their effects are complex, as will be seen in the following account.

Pharmacokinetics

Steroid sex hormones are well absorbed through the skin (factory workers need protective clothing) and the gut. Most are subject to extensive hepatic metabolic inactivation (some so much that oral administration is ineffective or requires very large doses if a useful amount is to pass through the liver and reach the systemic circulation). There is some enterohepatic recirculation, especially of oestrogen, and this may be interrupted by severe diarrhoea to cause loss of efficacy. There are some nonsteroid analogues that are more slowly metabolised. Sustained-release (depot) preparations are used. The hormones are carried in the blood extensively bound to sex-hormone-binding globulin. In general the plasma $t^{\frac{1}{2}}$ relates to the duration of cellular action. Duration of action is implied in the recommended dosage schedules.

ANDROGENS

Testosterone is the natural androgen secreted by the interstitial cells of the testis; it is necessary for normal spermatogenesis, for the development of the male secondary sex characteristics, and for the growth, at puberty, of the sexual apparatus. It is probably converted by hydroxylation to the active dihydrotesterone.

Protein *anabolism* is increased by androgens, i.e., androgens increase the proportion of protein laid down as tissue, especially muscle. Growth of bone is promoted, but the rate of closure of the epiphyses is also hastened, causing short stature in cases of precocious puberty or of androgen overdose in the course of treating hypogonadal children.

Pharmacokinetics: see above.

Indications for androgen therapy

The prime indication is *testicular failure* which may be primary or secondary (due to lack of pituitary gonadotrophins). In either case *replacement* with androgens is often necessary. Unfortunately, sterility is not remedied, although loss of libido and of secondary sex characteristics can be greatly improved. Impotence is helped if it is hypogonadal, but not if it has a psychological cause (which is often the case).

For *male contraception* androgens are under trial; they inhibit pituitary gonadotrophin production and have a direct testicular action.

If androgen is given to a boy with delayed puberty, a growth spurt and sexual development will occur. Such treatment is not usually indicated until the age of 16 years since up to that age natural delay in pituitary secretion may be responsible and normal development may yet occur. In *hepatic cirrhosis* degradation of oestrogens in the liver may be impaired, leading to raised blood concentrations of oestrogen with feminisation; androgens may help such patients. They may also stop the *itching* of *biliary obstruction*. Relatively small amounts of androgens can be used to increase the *formation of new tissue*, e.g. in osteoporosis in androgen deficient men (see below). Androgens may also help in some cases of *anaemia* due to bone marrow failure. Androgens are now little used in *metastatic breast cancer* because of their virilising effects.

Preparations and choice of androgens

- *Testosterone* given orally is subject to extensive hepatic first-pass metabolism and is therefore best given as an implant. Testosterone esters, e.g. enanthate, may be given orally or as depot injections 2–3 weekly; these esters do not injure the liver (see below).

• *Mesterolone* provides oral therapy; its molecular structure is such that its hypothalamic feedback inhibition of pituitary gonadotrophin secretion is less and it does not cause liver injury (see below).

See also: anabolic steroids, danazol.

Adverse effects

Adverse effects are mainly those to be expected of a male sex hormone (including hypothalamic-pituitary suppression of gonadotrophin production); increased libido may lead to undesirable sexual activity, especially in mentally unstable patients, and virilisation is obviously undesired by most women. Androgens have a weak *salt and water retaining activity*, which is not often clinically important. Liver injury (cholestatic) can occur, particularly with 17 α-alkyl derivatives (methyltestosterone, ethyloestrenol, stanozolol, danazol, oxymetholone); it is reversible; these agents should be avoided in hepatic disease.

Effects on *blood lipids* are complex and variable, and the balance may be to disadvantage.

In patients with malignant disease of bone androgen administration may be followed by hypercalcaemia. The less virilising androgens are used to promote anabolism and are discussed below.

ANTIANDROGENS (androgen antagonists)

Plainly oestrogens and progestogens are physiological antagonists to androgens. But compounds which compete selectively for androgen receptors have been made.

Cyproterone

Cyproterone is a derivative of progesterone; its combination of structural similarities and differences results in the following:

• Competition with testosterone for receptors in target *peripheral organs* (but not causing feminisation as do oestrogens); it reduces spermatogenesis even to the level of azoospermia (reverses over about 4 months after the drug is stopped); abnormal sperm occur during treatment.
• Competition with testosterone in the central nervous system, reducing sexual drive and thoughts, and causing impotence.
• Some agonist progestogenic activity on hypothalamic receptors, inhibiting gonadotrophin secretion, which also inhibits testicular androgen production.

Uses

Cyproterone is used for reducing male hypersexuality and in prostatic cancer and severe female hirsutism. A formulation of cyproterone plus ethinyloestradiol (Dianette) is offered for this latter purpose as well as for severe acne in women; this preparation acts as an oral contraceptive but should not be used primarily for this purpose. Plainly long-term use of the drug poses both medical and ethical problems. It is even advised that for management of male hypersexuality formally witnessed written consent be obtained.

Cyproterone causes hepatomas in rats.

Cyproterone is plainly unsuitable for male contraception (see actions above).

Flutamide is similar to cyproterone.

Spironolactone (p. 464) also has antiandrogen activity and may help hirsutism in women.

Androgen secretion may be diminished by continued use of a gonadorelin (LH-RH) analogue (see p. 592).

Ketoconazole (antifungal) interferes with androgen and corticosteroid synthesis and may be used in prostatic carcinoma.

ANABOLIC STEROIDS

Androgens are effective protein anabolic agents, but their clinical use for this purpose is limited by the amount of virilisation that women will tolerate. Attempts made to separate anabolic from androgenic action have been only partially successful and *all anabolic steroids also have androgenic effects*. They have little use in male osteoporosis. They can also prevent the calcium and nitrogen loss in the urine that occurs in patients bedridden for a long time and they have therefore been recommended in the treatment of some severe fractures.

The use of anabolic steroids in conditions of *general wasting* is justifiable in extreme debilitating disease, such as severe ulcerative colitis, after major surgery; in the later stages of malignant disease they may make the patient feel and look less wretched. Their general use as tonics is scandalous as is their use in sport (see index). They may be tried in *aplastic anaemia.*

The *itching of biliary obstruction* may be relieved and these drugs are perhaps preferable to testosterone for the purpose. There remains, however, a risk of increasing the degree of jaundice (see p. 542).

Anabolic steroids do not usefully counter the unwanted catabolic effects of adrenocortical hormones.

Hereditary angioedema (lack of inhibition of the C1 complement component) may be prevented by androgens (stanozolol and danazol are used).

None of these agents is free from virilising properties in high doses; acne and greasy skin may be the early manifestation of virilisation. See also, Adverse effects of androgens (p. 596); and Drugs and sport.

Oestrogens have only modest anabolic effect.

Administration should generally be intermittent in courses of 3–12 weeks with similar intervals, to reduce the occurrence of unwanted effects, especially liver injury.

There is little to choose between the principal available drugs nandrolone (Durabolin) (i.m. once a week) and stanozolol (Stromba) (orally) except that the latter is contraindicated in liver disease.

OESTROGENS AND ANTIOESTROGENS

Oestrone and oestradiol are both natural oestrogens secreted by the ovary. Oestrogens are responsible for the normal development of the female genital tract, of the breast and of the female secondary sex characteristics. The pubertal growth spurt is less marked in females than in males, probably because oestrogens have less protein anabolic action than do androgens, although they are as effective in promoting closure of epiphyses. Blood oestrogen concentrations must be above a critical level for the maintenance of both proliferative and (together with progesterone) secretory phases of the uterine endothelium. If the oestrogen level falls too low then the endothelium can no longer be maintained and uterine bleeding follows. Thus uterine bleeding may be stopped temporarily by giving large doses of oestrogens, or started by abrupt withdrawal (oestrogen-withdrawal bleeding). Bleeding may occur despite a high blood oestrogen concentration if large doses are given for a long time, due to infarctions in the greatly hypertrophied endometrium. Oestrogens are necessary for the maintenance of normal pregnancy and for the accompanying breast hyperplasia. The vagina is more sensitive to oestrogens than is the endometrium.

Pharmacokinetics: see p. 595.

Preparations of oestrogens

Innumerable oestrogen preparations are available, but the following selection should cover all needs. The dose varies greatly according to whether replacement of physiological deficiencies is being carried out (*replacement therapy*) or whether *pharmacotherapy* is being used.

- *Ethinyloestradiol* ($t_{\frac{1}{2}}$ 13 h) is a synthetic agent of first choice; it is effective by mouth.
- *Oestradiol* and *oestriol* are orally active mixed natural oestrogens.
- *Conjugated oestrogens* (Premarin) are orally active mixed natural oestrogens obtained from the urine of pregnant mares.
- *Estropipate* (piperazine oestrone sulphate) is an orally active synthetic conjugate.
- *Stilboestrol* is the first synthetic oestrogen: its use is confined to androgen dependent cancers (breast, prostate).
- *Centchroman* is a *nonsteroid* (benzopyran) with partial agonist oestrogenic activity; it has been introduced for oral contraception.

Choice of oestrogen

Ethinyloestradiol is a satisfactory first choice. However, individual patients may be intolerant of any one agent, when it is worth trying the others. It remains uncertain whether all oestrogens have exactly similar hormonal and non-hormonal effects, including adverse effects.

Transdermal formulations are available.

Indications for oestrogen therapy

Replacement therapy in hypo-ovarian conditions. Ethinyloestradiol (up to 50 μg orally daily for 21 days) followed by a progestogen (norethisterone or medroxyprogesterone 5 mg orally) for 7–10 days per monthly cycle is generally acceptable.

Unless the cause of the hypo-ovarian state is primary ovarian failure, treatment should be stopped after every third cycle to see if spontaneous menstruation will occur.

For menopausal symptoms (flushes, dry vagina) severe enough to demand treatment combined oestrogen-progestogen formulations are used for one year or more. The oestrogen may be cyclical or continuous and the progestogen cyclical. Most women will experience intermittent withdrawal bleeding.

Special calendar packs of various regimens are available under a range of proprietary names, e.g. Menophase, Prempak. Oestrogens used include ethinyloestradiol, oestradiol and conjugated oestrogens; progestogens include norgestrel and norethisterone.

Vasomotor menopausal symptoms may occasionally be helped by low doses of clonidine (Dixarit).

The oestrogen-progestogen formulations do not provide adequate contraception and non-hormonal methods should be used until it is quite certain that the menopause is fully accomplished (45–55 years).

But increasingly hormone therapy is prolonged, as follows:

Postmenopausal hormone replacement therapy (HRT) has been practised for many years (in the 1970s more than 30% of post-menopausal women in some rich countries were taking prescribed oestrogen) for its benefits on general well being including a hoped-for reduction in facial wrinkles, to prevent osteoporosis (certainly) and to prevent cardiovascular disease (probably).

'Unopposed' oestrogen therapy, if prolonged for years, is associated with an increased incidence of endometrial carcinoma. This may obtain whether administration is continuous or cyclical. Addition of a progestogen ('opposed' oestrogen therapy) reduces the risk; but it is unnecessary in the absence of a uterus. Breast cancer may increase, but if it does, the effect is (very) small. Women should conduct careful self-examination.

Duration of therapy may be 10 years on present knowledge, perhaps longer. Currently used formulations, e.g. Menophase, Cyclo-Progynova, Trisequens, do not provide reliable contraception. Women requiring surgery should be treated as those using the combined contraceptive pill.

Pharmacotherapy

- **Contraception**: see below.
- **Menstrual disorders**: see below.
- **Vaginitis**. Senile vaginitis usually responds to daily use of an oestrogen pessary or cream which can also be used in small girls with vaginitis. Absorption can occur sufficiently to cause systemic effects.
- **Inhibition of lactation**. Oestrogen, alone and in combination with a progestogen or androgen, has been used for 50 years. But it causes thromboembolism as well as stimulating the endometrium at a time when it should be undergoing involution. Such use is obsolete; see Bromocriptine, p. 611.
- **Androgen-dependent carcinoma**. High doses of oestrogens are used in prostatic carcinoma, which is an androgen-dependent neoplasm. Feminisation is inevitable and the gynaecomastia is often painful. Prevention of thrombosis is sought by concurrent use of aspirin for its antiplatelet effect.

● **To reduce sexual urge** in men whose activities are qualitatively or quantitatively unacceptable to the community and/or to themselves is an occasional indication for oestrogens: 1 mg of stilboestrol daily should be enough. See also antiandrogen (cyproterone) and benperidol.

● **Epistaxis**: as a last resort in recurrent cases, e.g. telangiectasia.

● **Atrophic rhinitis** may benefit, as also may **acne**.

Adverse effects

Adverse effects consist largely of overdose causing excess of the physiological actions. Withdrawal uterine bleeding is common but seldom prolonged; and bleeding occurs with prolonged high dose. In men, reduced libido, impotence and gynaecomastia (which may be painful) occur. In both sexes *oedema* due to salt and water retention, and *thromboembolism* occur. Natural oestrogens may cause less thromboembolism than do synthetic oestrogens (due to increased clotting factors and increased platelet adhesiveness).

● *Oral administration* is liable to cause nausea, vomiting and diarrhoea.

● Long-term unopposed oestrogen replacement therapy in postmenopausal women is associated with increased incidence of *gallbladder disease* and *endometrial carcinoma*.

● Stilboestrol (obsolete except in prostatic cancer) has been incriminated as a *transplacental carcinogen*, i.e. administered to the mother in the first 18 weeks of pregnancy (in an attempt to prevent miscarriage) it has caused vaginal adenocarcinoma in the offspring (peak age 18 years).

● *Blood lipids*: the effect of oestrogens is on balance favourable, but the addition of a progestogen (unless gestodene or desogestrel) reverses the balance.

● Oestrogens added to *cosmetics* (skin and hair creams) can cause precocious puberty in children and postmenopausal bleeding and gynaecomastia in adults. Cosmetics are not subject to the same official controls as are medicines.

Contraindications to oestrogen therapy include women who may have an oestrogen-dependent neoplasm, e.g. breast cancer, who may be pregnant, or have a disposition to thromboembolism. Hypertension, liver disease or gallstones, migraine, diabetes, uterine fibroids or endometriosis may all be made worse by oestrogen.

ANTIOESTROGENS

Obviously the virilising effects of androgens and progestogens antagonise physiologically many of the effects of oestrogens. But selective competitive agents blocking the oestrogen receptor are more likely to be clinically useful.

Clomiphene is structurally related to stilboestrol; it is a weak oestrogen having less activity than natural oestrogens, so that its occupation of receptors results in antagonism, i.e. it is a partial agonist. Such partial agonists are sometimes referred to as 'impeded' oestrogens. Clomiphene blocks hypothalamic oestrogen receptors so that the negative feedback of natural oestrogens is prevented and the pituitary responds by increased secretion of gonadotrophins, which may induce ovulation. Clomiphene is used to treat anovulatory infertility. Multiple ovulation with multiple pregnancy may occur and this is its principal adverse effect. **Cyclofenil** acts similarly. **Tamoxifen** is a nonsteroid competitive oestrogen antagonist on target organs; it is used for anovulatory infertility and for treatment of oestrogen-dependent *breast cancer;* it is under trial for the prevention of breast cancer in high risk groups.

PROGESTERONE AND PROGESTOGENS

Progesterone ($t_{\frac{1}{2}}$ 5 min) is produced by the corpus luteum and converts the uterine epithelium from the proliferative to the secretory phase. It is thus necessary for successful implantation of the ovum, and is essential throughout pregnancy, in the last two-thirds of which it is secreted in large amounts by the placenta. It acts particularly on tissues that are sensitised by oestrogens. Some synthetic progestogens are less selective, having varying oestrogenic and androgenic activity, and these may inhibit ovulation, though not very reliably.

Progestogens are of two principal kinds:

- *progesterone and its derivatives*: allyloestrenol, dydrogesterone, hydroxyprogesterone, medroxyprogesterone ($t_{\frac{1}{2}}$ 28 h);
- *testosterone derivative*: norethisterone and its prodrug ethynodiol ($t_{\frac{1}{2}}$ 10 h), levonorgestrel, desogestrel, gestodene, gestronol, norgestimate.

All can virilise directly or via metabolites (except progesterone and dydrogesterone) and fetal virilisation to the point of sexual ambiguity has occurred with vigorous use during pregnancy. See also contraception (p. 606).

Megestrol is used only in cancer; it causes tumours in the breasts of beagle dogs.

Pharmacokinetics: see p. 595.

Uses

The clinical uses of progestational agents are ill-defined, apart from contraception (see below), the menopause and postmenopausal hormone replacement therapy (see above).

Other possible uses include *menstrual disorders* e.g. menorrhagia, endometriosis, dysmenorrhoea and premenstrual syndrome (doubtful efficacy); also *breast* and *endometrial cancer*.

Preparations

Available progestogens (some used only in combined formulations) include:

- *oral*: allyloestrenol, norethisterone, dydrogesterone, gestodene, desogestrel, levonorgestrel, megestrol, medroxyprogesterone
- *suppositories or pessaries*: progesterone
- *injectable*: progesterone, hydroxyprogesterone, medroxyprogesterone.

Adverse effects of prolonged use include raised blood pressure and adverse trend in blood lipids. Gestogene, norgestimate and desogestrel may have less affinity for androgen receptors and therefore less unfavourable effect on blood lipids.

ANTIPROGESTOGENS

Menstruation (in its luteal phase) is dependent on progesterone, and uterine bleeding follows antagonism of progesterone. Pregnancy is dependent on progesterone (for implantation, endometrial stimulation, suppression of uterine contractions and placenta formation), and abortion follows progesterone antagonism in early pregnancy.

Mifepristone is a pure competitive antagonist at progesterone and glucocorticoid receptors. Clinical trials of oral use in hospital outpatients have shown it to be safe and effective in terminating pregnancy (used up to 3 weeks from the first missed period). Efficacy is enhanced if its use is followed by administration of a prostaglandin (gemeprost) (vaginally) to produce uterine contractions (the success rate is raised from 85% to above 95%). Adverse effects of the combined treatment include nausea and vomiting, dizziness, asthenia, abdominal pain; uterine bleeding may be heavy.

The use of this (and other) methods of terminating pregnancy attracts antagonism, as well as enthusiasm, on moral, social and economic grounds; although of great importance, these issues are beyond the scope of this book.

The possible roles of antiprogestogens in cervical dilation during induction of labour, contraception, breast cancer and meningioma are being explored.

DANAZOL

Danazol (Danol) is a derivative of the progestogen, ethisterone. It has partial agonist androgen activity and is described as an 'impeded' androgen; it has little progestogen activity. It is a relatively selective inhibitor of pituitary gonadotrophin secretion (LH, FSH) affecting the surge in the mid-menstrual cycle more than basal secretion. This reduces ovarian function, which leads to atrophic changes in endometrium, both uterine and elsewhere (ectopic), i.e. endometriosis. In males it reduces spermatogenesis. Androgenic unwanted effects occur in women (acne, hirsutism and, rarely, enlargement of the clitoris).

It is chiefly used for: *endometriosis, fibrocystic mastitis, gynaecomastia*, precocious puberty, menorrhagia and hereditary angioedema (p. 486).

Gestrinone is similar.

FERTILITY REGULATION

INFERTILITY

The treatment of infertility in either sex is a highly specialised business, requiring a detailed understanding of reproductive physiology and analysis of the cause. *Depending on the cause*, the following agents, already described, are used:

For women: to procure ovulation

- Hypothalamic hormone: gonadorelin (p. 592)
- Anterior pituitary hormones: follicle stimulating hormone (p. 593); chorionic gonadotrophin (p. 593)
- Antioestrogens: clomiphene etc (p. 599)
- Bromocriptine for hyperprolactinaemia (p. 610).

For men: to enhance spermatogenesis: the
same agents as for ovulation are used; androgens are not useful unless there is hypogonadism.

CONTRACEPTION BY DRUGS AND HORMONES

The requirements of a successful hormonal contraceptive are stringent, for it will be used by millions of healthy people who wish to separate sexual relations from physical reproduction. It must therefore be *extremely safe* as well as *highly effective* and its action must be *quick in onset* and

quickly and completely reversible, even after years of continuous use. It must not affect libido. The fact that alternative methods are less reliable implies that their use will lead to more unwanted pregnancies with their attendant inconvenience, morbidity and mortality, and this must be taken into account in deciding what risks of hormonal contraception are acceptable.

Possible sites of action

1. *Direct inhibition of spermatogenesis*: this presents many problems including the lag in onset of effect due to storage of mature spermatozoa until they are ejaculated or die of old age.

2. *Indirect inhibition of spermatogenesis by suppression of hypothalamic/pituitary activity*, which controls it, e.g. by progestogen-androgen combinations; see gonadorelin.

3. *Immunological techniques* (vaccines), to induce antibodies to pituitary gonadotrophins, sperm, or other components of the reproductive process in either sex, are being developed.

4. *Inhibition of ovulation* presents a different and easier biological problem. There is no need to suppress continuous formation of the gametes, as in the male, but only to prevent their release from the ovary approximately 13 times a year.

Either the pituitary gonadotrophin may be inhibited or the ovary may be made unresponsive to it.

5. *Prevention of fertilisation*: the female genital tract may be made inhospitable to spermatozoa, e.g. by altering cervical mucus or fallopian tube function.

6. *Antizygotic drugs*: compounds effective in the rat have been developed.

7. *Inhibition of implantation*: implantation does not occur unless the endometrium is in the right state, and this depends on a delicate balance between oestrogen and progesterone. This balance can readily be disturbed.

Mice fail to become pregnant if, after mating, they are exposed to the smell of alien males (via a chemical communicator or pheromone). This approach does not yet seem to have been explored in humans and 'it would be rash indeed to suppose that a contraceptive perfume is on the way'.[3]

8. *Use of spermicides in the vagina.*

Hormonal and chemical contraception in women

- Oestrogen and progestogen (combined and phased administration)
- Progestogen alone

Mode of action of currently used oestrogen-progestogen combined contraceptives

Oral contraceptives have been extensively used since 1956. The principal mechanism is inhibition of ovulation (4, above) by action on the hypothalamus inhibiting the release of hormone-releasing hormones and pituitary. In addition the endometrium is altered, so that implantation is less likely (7, above) and cervical mucus becomes more viscous and impedes the passage of the spermatozoa (5, above).

Oestrogens alone can inhibit ovulation but, used alone, they are not completely reliable; they cause thromboembolism and endometrial cancer.

Progestogens used alone inhibit ovulation in up to 40% of cycles, render cervical mucus less easily penetrable by sperm and induce a premature secretory change in the endometrium so that implantation does not occur. There is liable to be break-through bleeding and some are a cause of raised blood pressure and an adverse trend in blood lipids and arterial disease.

An appropriate dose of oestrogen + progestogen gives complete reliability with good menstrual cycle control. The following account applies to these combined preparations.

The combination is conveniently started on the first day of the cycle (first day of menstruation) and continued for 21 days (this is immediately effective, inhibiting the first ovulation). Withdrawal bleeding usually begins 1–4 days after discontinuation. After an interval of 7 days,[4]

regardless of menstruation, a new 21-day course is begun, and so on, i.e. active tablets are taken daily for 3 weeks out of 4. But packaging of numbered tablets (21 active: 7 dummy) so that the woman takes one every day without interruption may be best for easy compliance. If the course is *not* started on the first day of menstruation, but on the fifth day (to give a full month between the menses at the outset), an alternative method of contraception should be used until the 14th 'pill'[5] has been taken, since the first ovulation may not have been suppressed in women who have short menstrual cycles.

The 'Pill'[5] should be taken at the same time every day and preferably not just before intercourse (for pharmacokinetic reasons).

The monthly bleeds that occur 1–2 days after the cessation of active hormone administration are hormone withdrawal bleeds not natural menstruation. They are not an essential feature of oral contraception (3-monthly bleed regimens, phased pills, are available), but women are accustomed to monthly bleeds and they provide monthly reassurance of the absence of pregnancy.

Numerous field trials have shown that progestogen-oestrogen mixtures, if taken precisely as directed, are the most reliable reversible contraceptives known. (The only close competitors are depot progestogens and progestogen-releasing intrauterine devices.)

Some important aspects of the combined oestrogen-progestogen pill

Subsequent fertility. After stopping the pill, fertility that is normal for the age the woman has now reached is restored in 99.9% of subjects, although conception may be delayed for a few months longer in younger and as much as a year in older users than if other methods had been used. Permanent damage to fertility is very rare.

Effect on an existing pregnancy. Although

---

[3] Parkes A S. Practitioner 1965; 194: 455.

[4] A 7-day interval may be too long, i.e. follicles may develop. A safer regimen may be 22 days' hormone administration with a 6-day interval, and this is available.
[5] The word *'pill'* has gained currency in both professional and popular usage to mean 'oral contraceptive', losing its original precise technical pharmaceutical meaning.

progestogens can masculinise the female fetus, the doses for contraception are so low that risk of harming an undiagnosed pregnancy is extremely low, probably less than 1 in 1000 (the background incidence of birth defects is 1–2%).

Carcinoma of the *breast* and *cervix* may be unaffected or very slightly increased; *hepatoma* (very rare) is increased. The risk to life seems to be less than that of moderate smoking (10 cigarettes/day). Carcinoma of the *ovary* and *endometrium* are substantially reduced. Total incidence of cancer is unaltered.

Effect on menstruation (it is not true menstruation, see above) is generally to regularise it, and often to diminish blood loss, but amenorrhoea can occur. In some women 'breakthrough' intermenstrual bleeding occurs, especially at the outset, but this seldom persists for more than a few cycles. *Premenstrual tension* and *dysmenorrhoea* are much reduced.

Libido is greatly subject to psychosocial influences, and removal of fear of pregnancy may permit enthusiasm for the first time. It is likely that direct pharmacological effect (reduction) is rare. There is evidence that the normal increase in female-initiated sexual activity at ovulation time is suppressed.[6]

Cardiovascular complications. Incidence of venous thromboembolism is increased in pill users. It is directly related to the amount of oestrogen in the preparation. The small increase in hypertension, cerebrovascular accident and acute myocardial infarction is principally confined to smokers.

Increased arterial disease also appears to be associated with the amount of progestogen in the combined pill. The progestogen-only pill does not affect coagulation.

Major surgery (in patients taking oestrogen-progestogen contraceptives and postmenopausal hormone replacement therapy). Because of the added risk of venous thromboembolism (surgery causes a fall in antithrombin III) it has been advised that these oral contraceptives should be withdrawn, if practicable, 4 weeks before all lower limb operations or any major elective surgery (and started again at the first menstruation to occur more than 2 weeks after surgery). But increases in clotting factors may persist for many weeks and there is also the risk of pregnancy to be considered (plainly, alternative contraception should be used). An alternative for emergencies is to use low-dose heparin (though this may not reverse all the oestrogen effects on coagulation) and other means (mechanical stimulation of venous return) to prevent postoperative thrombosis. A similar problem arises with *prolonged immobilisation* from other causes.

Hepatic function may be impaired as may drug-metabolising capacity ($t_{\frac{1}{2}}$ antipyrine, a general indicator of drug-metabolising capacity, may increase by 30%). Gallbladder disease is more common, and highly vascular hepatocellular adenomas occur (rare).

Cervical erosion incidence is doubled (it is a harmless condition). *Crohn's disease* may be more frequent.

Decreased glucose tolerance occurs, perhaps due to a peripheral effect reducing the action of insulin.

Plasma lipoproteins may be adversely affected; least where the progestogen is desogestrel or low-dose norethisterone.

Plasma proteins. Oestrogens cause an increase in proteins, particularly globulins that bind hydrocortisone, thyroxine and iron. As a result, the *total* plasma concentration of the bound substances is increased, though the concentration of *free* and active substance remains normal. This can be misleading in diagnostic tests, e.g. of thyroid function. This effect on plasma proteins passes off about 6 weeks after cessation of the oestrogen.

Other adverse effects

Often more prominent at the outset and largely due to oestrogen, these include: nausea and, rarely, vomiting; breast discomfort, fluid retention, headache (increase in migraine), lethargy, abdominal discomfort, vaginal discharge or dryness. Depression may occur (and some patients have low blood concentration of pyridoxine); it may be benefited by pyridoxine (try 25 mg orally/day

[6] Adams D B et al. N Engl J Med 1978; 299: 1145.

and stop after 4 weeks if there is no benefit). Most depression in pill users is not pill caused.

Benefits additional to contraception

Side-effects are commonly assumed always to be unpleasant aspects of drug action, but they can sometimes also be pleasant.

The oestrogen-progestogen pill is associated with *reduced* risk of functional ovarian cysts and cancer, of endometrial cancer, and of benign breast disease; there is a reduced risk of uterine fibroids and they bleed less; there is perhaps less risk of autoimmune thyroid disease; menses are regular and blood loss is not excessive; menses are accompanied by less premenstrual tension and dysmenorrhoea; and there may even be less ear wax.

Contraindications

Carcinoma of the breast or of the genital tract, past or present, is regarded as an absolute contraindication, as is a history of thromboembolic disease. In patients with a history of liver disease, they should only be used if liver function tests are normal. Diabetes may become more difficult to control or may be precipitated. Lactation may be reduced by combinations but not by progestogens alone. Migraine may be precipitated. Hypertension will be worsened.

Smoking (15 cigarettes/day) *greatly* enhances (× 3) the risks of circulatory disease, and constitutes a contraindication for women over 35 years. Other risk factors for circulatory disease are hyperlipidaemia, hypertension, obesity and age.

Duration of use does not enhance risks of itself. The increase in risk with increased duration of use is due to increasing age. The approaching menopause presents an obvious problem. Because cyclic bleeding will continue to occur under the influence of the drugs even after the natural menopause, the only way of deciding whether contraception can be permanently abandoned is by abandoning it (and using another technique) for 3 months annually to see if natural menstruation is resumed; or stop the combined pill for

one month and measure LH/FSH concentration in the blood, which indicates the state of pituitary function.

Ex-users. There may be persistence of cardiovascular risk for a few years after stopping in those with cardiovascular risk factors.

Conclusions

- Pregnancy carries risk.
- *Serious* adverse effects of the combined pill are rare and 'several times a rare event is still a rare event.'[7]
- Precise figures on risk with current low-dose formulations are not available. The major studies, involving, e.g. 23 000 women, used higher dose formulations and cannot be replicated (cost, logistics) to keep up with developments.
- *Overall* mortality amongst users (having low risk factors) is either unaffected or only slightly increased.

Preparations of oestrogen-progestogen combination

The *oestrogen* is ethinyloestradiol or mestranol.

The *progestogen* is levonorgestrel, norethisterone, ethynodiol, gestodene, desogestrel or lynoestrenol.

The most important variable is the dose of oestrogen, which is usually between 20 and 50 µg. The incidence of thromboembolism has been found higher with high-dose oestrogen preparations, e.g. 100 µg, but it is not known if there is any difference between doses below 50 µg.

It is now appreciated that the earlier preparations had much more oestrogen than was necessary for efficacy. It seems probable that 20 µg is about the limit below which serious loss of efficacy can be expected. Indeed in hepatic enzyme-induced patients, e.g. using antiepileptics, some antirheumatics, it is advisable to use a preparation containing 50 µg oestrogen or more to avoid loss of efficacy due

---

[7] Guillebaud J 1989 The pill. Oxford University Press. A general reference for all practical aspects of use.

to increased oestrogen metabolism (elimination of breakthrough bleeding is a guide to adequacy of dose).

Common problems

Missed pill. Inadvertent omission of a dose is less serious on the higher dose preparations, e.g. if one active tablet is omitted the woman remains protected for 24 h if she has been taking a 50 µg oestrogen preparation, but for only 12 h if using a 30 µg oestrogen preparation.

- If an omitted dose is remembered *within 12 hours* it should be taken at once and the next dose at the usual time, and all should be well (unless it is the *first or last* active pill in the packet, in which case follow the advice in the next paragraph).
- If *more than 12 hours* has elapsed the same procedure should be followed *but* an alternative barrier method of contraception should be used for 7[8] days (or abstinence).

Plainly a regimen in which a pill is taken every day (dummy pills) may confuse the subject who will then need advice.

Intercurrent gut upset. Obviously a patient may *vomit* the dose; if vomiting occurs <3 h after a pill, behave as under *missed pill*, above. The hormones are rapidly absorbed and only severe diarrhoea would interfere significantly with efficacy.[9] But if there is doubt, it would be prudent to use a barrier method during and for 14 days after the episode.

Changing of preparation. If a woman is uncomfortable on one preparation she should be changed to another containing a different dose of oestrogen and/or progestogen. The new preparation should start *the day after* she has finished a cycle on the previous preparation. If this is done no extra risk of pregnancy occurs.

Breakthrough bleeding (bleeding on days of active pill taking) can mean a higher dose of oestrogen or progestogen is required.

Choice of oestrogen-progestogen combination

There is a wide choice of formulations:

1. *low oestrogen (20–35 µg)* plus *low progestogen*, e.g. Marvelon, Minulet, Femodene.
2. *low oestrogen* plus *high progestogen*, e.g. Ovran 30, Eugynon 30.
3. *high oestrogen (50 µg plus low or high progestogen*, e.g. Ovran, Norinyl-1.

In general users should employ the lowest total hormone dose that suits them (good cycle control and minimal side-effects) and should make a start with a preparation from 1 above.

Postcoital contraception ('morning after pill'),[10] emergency contraception

Overall probability of pregnancy following unprotected intercourse is 1:25 to 1:50 (higher in mid cycle, lower at end cycle); it may be prevented before implantation by disrupting the normal hormonal arrangements; mode of action is probably by delaying or preventing ovulation or by preventing implantation of the fertilised ovum, though there may also be a post-implantation action.

Postcoital contraception may be successful *up to 72 hours* after the exposure. A usual technique is to take 2 tablets of an oestrogen-progestogen combined formulation (containing 50 µg of oestrogen and 250 µg of levonorgestrel) (Schering PC4) at the earliest opportunity, followed by a further 2 tablets exactly 12 hours later. Vomiting may occur and must be taken into account as a cause of failure (if tablets are vomited, repeat the dose with an antiemetic). The failure rate is hard to estimate (controlled trials are not practicable, but studies on rape and volunteer cases have been made) and may be about 1:200 (but

---

[8] If these 7 unprotected days run beyond the beginning of the routine intended pill-free days, the next cycle (packet) should follow without a gap, thus postponing the menses by a month (Family Planning Assoc).

[9] Otme M et al. Unintended pregnancies and contraceptive use. Brit Med J 1991; 302: 79.

[10] A popular term that misleads women (see text below).

higher in mid cycle); ectopic pregnancy may perhaps be promoted. If pregnancy is present the procedure will not cause abortion. It is not known if injury to a pregnancy may occur. If it can, the risk is probably less than 1:1000; some people will consider abortion. The procedure should not be used more than once in a cycle; nor where absolute contraindications for oestrogen exist.

Phased-formulation contraceptives

Phased pills employ low doses and variable ratios between oestrogen and progestogen, in 2 (*biphasic*) or 3 (*triphasic*) periods within the menstrual cycle. The dose of progestogen is low at the beginning and higher at the end, the oestrogen remaining either constant or rising slightly in mid cycle. The objective is to achieve effective contraception with minimal distortion of natural hormonal rhythms.

The advantages claimed for these techniques are diminished adverse metabolic changes, e.g. blood lipids, and a particularly reliable monthly bleeding pattern without loss of contraceptive efficacy. But against these (potential) advantages, there is even less latitude of safety if a dose is forgotten. Preparations include BiNovum, TriNovum, Logynon.

Progestogen-only contraception

Progestogen-only contraception (Mini-Pill): the oral formulation is taken every day throughout the 28 day cycle; a 3-month depot i.m. injection is an alternative. *Subcutaneous implants* that release hormone for several years are in use; they can be removed surgically, e.g. Norplant, if adverse effects develop or pregnancy is desired.

Oral progestogen-only contraception is less effective but safer (no effect on blood coagulation) than combined formulations. Intramuscular progestogen is equal in efficacy to the combined pill. It works by inhibiting ovulation, though much less effectively than the combined pill, but principally by rendering the cervical mucus inhospitable (thick and scanty) to spermatozoa maximally 5 hours after a daily dose (so time the oral dose appropriately where sexual practice is regular).

Progestogen-only contraception is particularly appropriate to women having an absolute contraindication for oestrogen, e.g. history of thromboembolism, smokers (who refuse to give it up), and for diabetics; it is used for *lactating women* as it interferes with the milk less than the combined pill. *A missed oral dose allows even less latitude than the combined pill*. If a dose is more than *3 hours* late it should be taken at once and a barrier method used for 2 days (this short interval can be a great nuisance). Behave similarly in the presence of vomiting and severe diarrhoea.

A significant limitation to the use of the progestogen-only pill is erratic uterine bleeding which many women understandably dislike. There may be no bleeding for months or there may be frequent and irregular bleeding. Ectopic pregnancy may be more frequent due to a fertilised ovum being held up in a functionally depressed fallopian tube. Other adverse effects are generally less than the combined pill (blood coagulation is unaffected); data on breast cancer are conflicting but are largely reassuring.

The progestogens used orally include norgestrel, levonorgestrel, ethynodiol, desogestrel, norethisterone (e.g. Noriday, Micronor, Femulen); medroxyprogesterone (Depo-Provera) ($t_{\frac{1}{2}}$ 28 h) is a sustained-release (aqueous suspension) i.m. injection given 3-monthly.

The use of i.m *medroxyprogesterone* has been much criticised ('ban the jab') on ethical and social grounds, e.g. consent, and there are real ethical issues, especially with mentally retarded women. But it is important that criticism be properly directed (which it has not been) at the *way* the drug is used, not at the (safe) drug itself. Much has also been made of 'menstrual chaos' by the critics, but the tolerance of bleeding irregularities will be a matter of personality and counselling, and some patients will prefer the infrequent (and private) injection according to their own social situation. It is essential that a drug, useful to some, be not banned because some prescribers have used it wrongly or too casually, reprehensible though that may be.

Drug interactions with steroid contraceptives

Particularly now that the lowest effective doses are in use there is little latitude between success and failure if the absorption, distribution and metabolism are disturbed. Any additional drug taking must be looked at critically lest it reduces efficacy.

The classic example of interference with the combined pill is the increase of breakthrough bleeding and pregnancy in young women being treated with rifampicin for tuberculosis (1971). Rifampicin is a potent inducer of hepatic drug-metabolising enzymes. Enhanced metabolism of the steroids caused failure. Antiepileptics (phenytoin and carbamazepine but not sodium valproate) create a similar risk.

All drugs that induce metabolising enzymes (see p. 97) whether prescribed or self-administered (alcohol, tobacco smoking) constitute a risk to contraceptive efficacy and prescribing should be specifically reviewed for this effect. Pregnancies have occurred in women taking a contraceptive who commence an antiepileptic drug and doctors have been sued (for negligence) successfully in a court of law.

Hypothalamic/pituitary hormone approach to contraception: see gonadorelin.

Other methods of contraception

Intrauterine devices that are also sustained-release formulations of a progestogen or copper to enhance their efficacy by local action on the endometrium have been developed.

Vaginal preparations, to immobilise or kill (spermicide) spermatozoa, are used to add safety to various mechanical contraceptives. They are very unreliable and should be used alone only in an emergency. Substances used include nonoxinols (surfactants that alter the permeability of the sperm lipoprotein membrane) as pessary, gel or foam.

Oil-based lubricants cause condom failure; many 'lubricants', e.g. hand or baby creams wash off readily, but are oil-based.

Risks of contraception in relation to benefit

Whether a drug should be prescribed involves an assessment of benefit to the patient versus risk to the patient. Even when there is a defined disease the decision can be difficult. It is even more so when the subject is healthy, as is the case with most contraception, and perception of benefit will vary widely between individuals.

It has been pointed out that a woman having regular sexual intercourse faces a finite chance of death from pregnancy, childbirth or from measures to avoid or interrupt pregnancy.

But as well as the risks of unwanted pregnancy, the risk of oral contraceptives (see above) should be viewed in the context of the risks of everyday life, which are substantial.

The death rate from taking oral contraceptives is probably about the same magnitude as deaths from cricket and football (in Britain) and much less than those from swimming (750 men, 250 women per annum in Britain). A car driver may expect, on average, to be admitted to hospital once in 20 years due to a road accident. A woman would have to use oral contraceptives for 2000 years for a similar chance due to a thrombotic episode. It has been calculated that a death in a family that has acquired an outboard motor boat is 10 times more likely than death where the mother is taking an oral contraceptive.[11]

Any danger oral contraceptives may have for the individual must also be seen in relation to their benefits, not only to the individual, but to the community, e.g. fewer self-induced and criminal abortions, fewer unwanted children, slowing down of the speed of increase of world population with less hunger and misery.

The debate will continue, and so will technical advances which will require to be tested on willing subjects (see Ethics of research, Ch. 4).

That research in this field has major ethical implications is illustrated by the now notorious San Antonio study[12] as follows.

[11] Potts D M Br Med Bull 1970; 26: No 1, 27.
[12] Quoted from Levine R J 1986 Ethics and regulation of clinical research. Urban and Schwarzenburg: recommended reading.

In order to distinguish between genuine pharmacodynamic side-effects of an oral contraceptive and the symptoms of everyday life, women seeking contraception were entered into a randomised, placebo controlled, double blind, crossover study; they were not told of the placebo but were advised to use a spermicidal vaginal cream. Of the 76 subjects 11 became pregnant, 10 whilst taking placebo. With the development of research ethics review committees, such studies, it is to be hoped, are now impossible. Indeed, such a study has never been ethically acceptable.

Male contraception (systemic)

Suppression of spermatogenesis may be achieved by interfering with:

- extra-gonadal endocrine control, i.e. the hypothalamic/pituitary/gonadal axis
- direct action on gonadal spermatogenesis
- vaccines to produce antibodies to sperm.

Approaches include androgen or combinations of androgen with danazol, or progestogen, or oestrogen, also gonadorelin. Gossypol, a phenol from the cotton plant, has been under evaluation in China since about 1974[13] but it appears to have unacceptable adverse effects, e.g. hypokalaemia. In one study of injected testosterone enanthate, men became azoospermic in 120 days.

Natural regulators of mitosis (chalones) are tissue specific, and their identification should allow synthesis of analogues that might provide the necessary specificity and reversibility to deserve trial as male contraceptives. Whether a risk of genetic damage is inherent in drugs acting on spermatogenesis is unknown. The obvious biological problems of male contraception, need for continuous effect as opposed to elimination of a single regular event (ovulation) plus the ready availability of female contraception, plus the fact that men do not get pregnant, reduce

the commercial incentives to seek and to use contraceptives for men.

DEVELOPMENT OF NEW CONTRACEPTIVES

Extension of the range of contraceptives (hormonal or non-hormonal) to include new mechanisms of action, and especially to include men, has been the subject of social and political demand. This is partly because current contraceptives are still imperfect, not only with regard to safety, efficacy and convenience, but also with regard to cultural, socioeconomic and religious aspects. The first combined oestrogen-progestogen pill was developed over 5 years. Development of a new agent that is not just a variant of existing agents is now likely to require 15–20 years and the cost will be enormous. Regulatory requirements will be rigorous and extensive (see Ch. 3, 5).

For the female contraceptive, regulatory bodies generally require that the preparation be used in at least 20 000 cycles with a quarter of the data derived from long-term use. New drugs or methods will be subject to close scrutiny as to whether they truly prevent conception or induce abortion, a distinction that raises moral issues.

For a male systemic contraceptive the regulatory requirements remain undefined, but they will be strict.

Claims that pharmaceutical developers should compensate sufferers of adverse reactions also may deter all but the boldest and richest companies from making the necessary investment in research unless society, i.e. governments, accept at least some of the liability for injury where there is no fault on the part of the developer.

MENSTRUAL DISORDERS

HORMONES IN MENSTRUAL DISORDERS

Only a note on the simpler uses is appropriate here.

---

[13] Attention was drawn to gossypol by the high prevalence of male infertility in rural areas where food was cooked in cotton-seed oil.

Amenorrhoea, primary or secondary, requires specialist endocrinological diagnosis. Where the cause is failure of hormone production, cyclical replacement therapy is indicated.

Severe dysfunctional uterine bleeding (often due to oestrogen excess) can be controlled *during bleeding*, generally within 48 hours, by a *progestogen* (norethisterone) 5 mg/day for 10 days (a withdrawal bleed follows in 2–4 days). To prevent an *anticipated* excessive bleed: give 10 mg/day from 19th–26th days of the cycle (for 2–3 cycles). There will be withdrawal bleeding. This may be followed, if appropriate, by cycle control with an oestrogen-progestogen combination (particularly one with high progestogen content) (an oral contraceptive will serve).

Danazol continuously can also be effective. Other agents that may help resistant cases of dysfunctional uterine bleeding include antifibrinolytic agent (tranexamic acid), indomethacin or mefenamic acid (to inhibit prostaglandin synthesis given just before and during menstruation) and ethamsylate (by inhibiting prostaglandin synthesis and capillary fragility); but none of these is treatment of first choice. These treatments may be effective in the presence of an intrauterine contraceptive device; but not in the presence of fibroids.

Less severe cases, moderately heavy periods, are likely to respond to prostaglandin synthase inhibition, e.g. mefenamic acid 500 mg when the blood loss becomes heavy followed by 250 mg × 3/day for 3 days if necessary. Aspirin and paracetamol are ineffective.

The timing of menstruation

Sometimes there are pressing reasons to prevent menstruation at the normal time, but obviously this cannot be done at the last moment.

Menstruation can be postponed by giving norethisterone 5 mg × 3/day, starting 3 days before the expected onset; bleeding occurs 2–3 days after withdrawal. Users of the combined oral contraceptive pill (having a 7-day break) can simply continue with active pills when they would normally stop for 7 days.

Although there is no evidence that harm follows such manoeuvres, it is obviously imprudent to practise them frequently.

Note. These uses of progestogen should *not* be undertaken if there is any possibility of pregnancy.

Endometriosis. It has been observed that endometriosis is benefited by pregnancy and so a 'pseudopregnancy treatment' has been practised, by giving an oestrogen-progestogen oral contraceptive for about 9 months; marked improvement and even cure may result. But danazol, taken continuously, or norethisterone can be effective; as can analogues of gonadorelin, e.g. goserelin; adverse reactions are troublesome.

Dysmenorrhoea is due to uterine contractions resulting from excess prostaglandins in the uterus during ovulatory cycles. It can be treated by suppressing ovulation (using the combined pill or norethisterone); also by using inhibitors of prostaglandin synthesis, e.g. aspirin, indomethacin, naproxen, or by inducing anovulatory cycles (oral contraception). The analgesic prostaglandin synthase inhibitor (NSAID) may need to be given for several days before menstruation or only at the time of the pain.

Premenstrual tension syndrome may be due to an imbalance of natural oestrogen and progesterone secretion, but knowledge of the syndrome remains imprecise. Psychosocial factors can be important. Placebo effects are strong. Drugs are not necessarily the preferred treatment.

There is evidence for and against:

- *Restriction of salt and fluid plus a thiazide diuretic* in the second half of the menstrual cycle where symptoms suggest fluid retention.
- *Pyridoxine* (vitamin B_6, a coenzyme): try 100 mg/day orally (not more) for 3 months and abandon if there is no benefit. It may help depression and irritability particularly.
- *Oestrogen-progestogen* oral contraceptive combination.
- *Bromocriptine*, especially where there is breast pain.
- *Prostaglandin synthase inhibition*. e.g. mefenamic acid.

Cyclical breast pain or mastalgia, when severe, may respond to continuous use of gamolenic acid (orally); it is an essential unsaturated fatty acid for cell membranes (patients have low concentrations); it may act by reducing cellular uptake of prolactin and ovarian hormones. Danazol and bromocriptine also help.

MYOMETRIUM

He gently prevails on his patient to try
The magic effects of the ergot of rye.
(attributed to Alfred, Lord Tennyson, 1809–1892)

ERGOT AND DERIVATIVES

Ergot is a fungus which preys on grasses, especially rye, bread made from which has caused epidemics of, particularly, painful peripheral gangrene and abortion due to its smooth muscle stimulant actions. For medicinal production the plant is artificially infected.

Ergotism is now very rare but an epidemic was reported in England in 1928[14] and in France in 1951[15] although the genuineness of both these has been questioned.

The uterine effects of ergot have been known for at least 400 years and active alkaloids were isolated at the beginning of the 20th century. But the identification of what is clinically the most important (ergometrine, ergonovine) had to wait until 1932 when a clinical obstetrician[16] was asked to investigate why extracts of ergot seemed to be active on the uterus when pharmacologist said they ought not to be.

Fortunately, the study was published in a journal that has a correspondence column so that the subsequent clash of opinion between clinician and pharmacologist could take place in public.

Aspects of the curiously complex pharmacology of ergot[17]

Ergot alkaloids are related to lysergic acid and are based on ergoline which bears structural resemblance to the biogenic amines, noradrenaline, dopamine and serotonin (5-HT). Therefore it is no surprise that ergot derivatives can act as agonists, antagonists or both simultaneously (partial agonists) at these amine receptors. Indeed, it is combinations of these actions on the receptors by these amines that largely account for the multifarious actions of *ergot derivatives*; none is completely receptor specific:

- Co-dergocrine (Hydergine) is the most active α-adrenoceptor antagonist.
- Ergotamine is the most active α-adrenoceptor agonist.
- Methysergide is the most active serotonin (5-HT) antagonist.
- Bromocriptine, lysuride and pergolide are the most active dopamine receptor agonists.
- Methylergometrine is the most active uterine α-adrenoceptor agonist. (But selectivity alters with changing drug concentrations and specificity may only be attained at carefully adjusted concentrations.)
- Lysergide (LSD) is the most active hallucinogen (mechanism uncertain). But all supply of and research on LSD was stopped by the pharmaceutical firm that invented it following the surge of hallucinogen abuse in the early 1960s.

Metabolism: ergot alkaloids are metabolised in the liver.

Bromocriptine

Bromocriptine provides an example of the exploitation of the extraordinarily wide spectrum of activities of ergot derivatives. Ergotoxine has oxytocic and cardiovascular effects. It also prevents, by a *dopamine receptor agonist* action on the anterior pituitary, the release of prolactin. Bromocriptine (t $\frac{1}{2}$ 6 h) was the product of a research programme aimed at eliminating the oxytocic and cardiovascular effects whilst retaining the prolactin release inhibiting effect. The result has been a useful dopamine receptor agonist which *suppresses lactation* and *prolactinomas, benefits cyclic mastalgia*, and suppresses types of *hypogonadism* associated with hyperprolactinaemia (which reduces gonadotrophin

[14] Robertson J et al. Br Med J 1928; 1: 302.
[15] Gabbai et al. Br Med J 1951; 2: 650, editorial, ibid., 596.
[16] Moir C. Br Med J 1932; 1: 1119, 1189; 2: 75.
[17] Berde B, Schild H O, eds. Ergot alkaloids and related compounds. Berlin: Springer, 1978.

secretion); it also has some efficacy in parkinsonism (unrelated to prolactin) (see p. 312). It increases growth hormone release in healthy people and suppresses it in acromegaly (see also index).

Carbergoline is also a dopamine receptor agonist.

Suppression of lactation

Inhibition of lactation is sometimes necessary, e.g. dead child, sick mother.

One alternative which is not considered often enough is . . . A tight binder, sympathy, and occasional sedatives (which) will carry many women through the initial discomfort of engorged breasts. Without the stimulus of suckling, the high prolactin concentrations at delivery fall to normal within a week and lactation soon peters out. Fluid restriction is unnecessary.[18]

The procedure is safe and cheap.

Pituitary secretion of prolactin is normally under inhibitory tone from the hypothalamus via prolactin release-inhibiting factor (PIF), which may be dopamine.

Dopamine receptor agonists activate or mimic hypothalamic prolactin-inhibiting factor, the plasma prolactin concentration falls and lactation stops. *Bromocriptine* is used to *prevent* lactation (oral dose 2.5 mg on day of birth, then 2.5 mg twice a day for 14 days); for *suppression* of lactation (2.5 mg daily for 3 days, then 2.5 mg twice a day for 14 days); since prolactin suppresses ovulation during lactation, use of a contraceptive will be appropriate; galactorrhoea from other causes may require higher doses.

Oestrogens are effective but can cause thrombosis.

Ergotamine (see Migraine)

Ergotamine causes vasoconstriction (arteries and veins), which may be sufficient to cause hypertension, by an α-adrenoceptor agonist action and also by sensitising to endogenously released noradrenaline. The degree of vasoconstriction is determined by the pre-existing vascular tone. The $t_{\frac{1}{2}}$ of ergotamine is 2 h, but tissue storage allows

---

[18] Editorial. Br Med J 1977; 1: 189.

prolonged action, so that if it is being given several times a day for migraine there is short-term accumulation that can be dangerous, causing peripheral gangrene, for which sodium nitroprusside i.v. may be used.

Dihydroergotamine constricts veins particularly and has efficacy in prophylaxis of deep vein thrombosis in the legs after surgery (the blood flow faster in the constricted large veins).

Ergometrine

Ergometrine (ergonovine) ($t_{\frac{1}{2}}$ 2 h) is now the only ergot alkaloid used for stimulating uterine activity (α-adrenoceptor and dopamine receptor agonist), as ergotamine is slow in acting even after i.v. injection, whereas ergometrine acts almost immediately when injected i.v. Serious circulatory side-effects are also less frequent (see below). The uterus is stimulated at all times, but is much more sensitive in late pregnancy.

Ergometrine and oxytocin (see below) differ in their actions on the uterus. In moderate doses oxytocin produces slow generalised contractions with full relaxation in between; ergometrine produces faster contractions superimposed on a tonic contraction. High doses of both substances produce sustained tonic contraction. It will be seen, therefore, that oxytocin is more suited to induction of labour and ergometrine to the prevention and treatment of post-partum haemorrhage, the incidence of which is reduced by its routine prophylactic use (generally i.m.).

Dosage

Ergometrine may be given:

- *Orally*: 0.5–1 mg, when action begins in about 8 min and lasts about 1 hour.
- *i.v.*: 100–500 µg; onset of action about 1 min; used as treatment of established post-partum haemorrhage.
- *i.m.*: 200–500 µg; action begins in about 6 min; the onset is speeded by mixing hyaluronidase, which enhances tissue permeation and so speeds absorption (1500 units) with the injection, and is about as quick as i.v. injection.

This combination is appropriate for use by birth attendants who are not permitted to give an i.v. injection.

Oxytocin i.m. is an alternative for quick (but brief) action. Plainly speed of onset can be vital if the woman is bleeding profusely. *Oxytocin has therefore been mixed with ergometrine* (Syntometrine: ergometrine 500 µg plus oxytocin 5 IU) to obtain the advantages of quick (2 min) onset of action and prolonged effect.

When given during labour the timing of the injection is the subject of disagreement. It is commonly given when the anterior shoulder of the child is delivered, but some give it earlier at the crowning of the head (never before this) or later when the placenta has separated or has been delivered. Ergometrine tablets may be given orally (0.5 mg/ × 3/day) for 3 days in the early puerperium or in incomplete abortion.

Hypertension, lasting hours or even days after ergometrine, occurs occasionally. It seems that in some patients ergometrine is capable of inducing vascular effects of a magnitude similar to those of ergotamine. It is most likely to occur in toxaemic patients[19] and in cases where sympathomimetic vasoconstrictors have been used, e.g. with a local anaesthetic. It can be severe and complaints of headache post-partum should be taken seriously. The blood pressure can be reduced by chlorpromazine (10–15 mg) i.v. or i.m. and then larger doses orally, or by any other α-adrenoceptor blocking drug. Ergometrine can also cause hypotension.

Methysergide: see Migraine and above.

Co-dergocrine (Hydergine) is a mixture of hydrogenated alkaloids, dihydroergocryptine-cristine, -cornine. There is weak evidence for a modest beneficial effect on impaired mental function in the aged. It is probably without efficacy. *Nicergoline* is similar.

Adverse effects

Adverse effects of ergot derivatives are mostly predictable from the various receptor actions mentioned above.

CNS: vomiting due to dopaminergic effect on the chemoreceptor trigger zone; hypotension, especially postural, due to depression of the vasomotor centre, which is enhanced by peripheral α-adrenoceptor block (hydrogenated alkaloids).

Overdose causes: confusion, depression, convulsions and a variety of neurological syndromes, probably vascular in origin.

Peripheral vessels: constriction even to gangrene (ergotamine) occurs and this alkaloid is dangerous in patients with peripheral vascular or ischaemic cardiac disease.

Blood pressure may rise or fall according to the varying central and peripheral adrenoceptor agonist and antagonist effects.

OXYTOCIN

Oxytocin is a peptide hormone of the posterior pituitary gland. It stimulates the contractions of the pregnant uterus, which becomes much more sensitive to it at term. However, patients with posterior pituitary disease (diabetes insipidus) can go into labour normally.

Oxytocin is reflexly released from the pituitary following suckling (and manual stimulation) and causes almost immediate contraction of the myoepithelium of the breast; it can be used to enhance milk ejection (nasal spray). The only other clinically important effect is on the blood pressure, which may fall if an overdose is given.

Synthetic oxytocin (Syntocinon) is pure and is not contaminated with vasopressin as is the natural product. It is therefore safer if high doses must be given.

Oxytocin in management of labour

Oxytocin is used i.v. in the *induction of labour* and sometimes for uterine inertia, haemorrhage or during abortion. It produces, almost immediately, rhythmic contractions with relaxion between, i.e. it mimics normal uterine activity. The association of oxytocin with neonatal jaundice appears to be due to increased erythrocyte fragility causing haemolysis.

The decision to use oxytocin requires special skill. It has a t $\frac{1}{2}$ of 6 min and is given by i.v.

---

[19] Synthetic oxytocin (Syntocinon) is preferable in such patients.

infusion at 1–3 milliunits per min; it *must* be closely supervised; the dose is adjusted by results; overdose can cause uterine tetany and even rupture. The dose may be increased every 10 min until contractions commence and then at intervals of at least 20 min. The utmost care is required.

Oxytocin is structurally close to vasopressin and it is no surprise that it also has antidiuretic activity. Serious water intoxication can occur with prolonged i.v. infusions, especially where accompanied by large volumes of fluid.

Oxytocin has been supplanted by ergometrine as prime treatment of post-partum haemorrhage except when, as occasionally happens, there is no response to ergometrine. There are advantages in a mixture of oxytocin and ergometrine (Syntometrine, see above).

UTERINE RELAXANTS

β_2-adrenoceptor agonists relax the uterus and are employed by obstetricians to inhibit *premature labour*, e.g. isoxsuprine, orciprenaline, terbutaline, ritodrine, salbutamol; their use is complicated by the expected cardiovascular effects, including tachycardia, hypotension.

PROSTAGLANDINS

(For a general account of prostaglandins see p. 212.)

Prostaglandins that soften the uterine cervix (by an action on collagen) and have a powerful oxytocic effect include:

Dinoprost (prostaglandin $F_{2\alpha}$, $PGF_{2\alpha}$) (Prostin F2 alpha) and **dinoprostone** (prostaglandin E_2; PGE_2) (Prostin E2). They are used to induce labour and to terminate pregnancy, including missed or partial abortion and in the treatment of hydatidiform mole; they are given by intra- or extra-amniotic injection, by vaginal tablet, or intracervical gel, by i.v. infusion or by mouth. Their safe and effective use (including choice of route) requires special skill.

Adverse effects include vomiting, diarrhoea, headache, pyrexia and local tissue reaction.

Gemeprost (prostaglandin E_1 analogue) (Cervagem) is used to soften the cervix before operative procedures in the first trimester of pregnancy and for abortion, alone and in combination with an antiprogestogen (mifepristone, p. 600). It is administered intravaginally.

Carboprost (prostaglandin $F_{2\alpha}$ analogue) is used for postpartum haemorrhage (resistant to ergometrine and oxytocin) for its oxytocic action. It is highly effective. Adverse effects include hypertension, asthma and pulmonary oedema.

USE OF DRUGS AND MORALITY

Increasingly, drug use is a cause of moral and social, as well as of technical, problems and this is particularly so in the field of reproduction (contraception and abortion).

Some doctors regard these uses as impermissible under any circumstances, some as permissible under certain circumstances, others see no moral issue. In any case it is desirable that all doctors should be technically informed if they are likely to meet patients who may be taking or seeking such treatment. Since pharmacological considerations are not fundamental to moral decisions, these contentious issues will not be discussed here.

GUIDE TO FURTHER READING

Belchetz P 1989 Hormone replacement treatment: deserves wider use. British Medical Journal 298: 1467

Conn P M et al 1991 Gonadotrophin-releasing hormone and its analogues. New England Journal of Medicine 324: 93

Gath D et al 1988 Treating the premenstrual syndrome. British Medical Journal 297: 237

Hartog M et al 1988 Hyperprolactinaemia: common and treatable. British Medical Journal 297: 701

Jones W R et al 1988 Phase I clinical trial of a World Health Organization birth control vaccine. Lancet 1: 1296

Magos A L 1990 Management of menorrhagia. British Medical Journal 300: 1537

Mastroanni L et al 1990 Development of contraceptives — obstacles and opportunities. New England Journal of Medicine 322: 482

Mishell D R 1989 Contraception. New England Journal of Medicine 320: 777

Robinson G E et al 1991 Changes in haemostasis after stopping the combined pill. British Medical Journal 302: 269

Salomon F et al 1989 The effects of treatment with recombinant human growth hormone on body composition and metabolism in adults with growth hormone deficiency. New England Journal of Medicine 321: 1797

Silvestre L et al 1990 Voluntary interruption of pregnancy with mifepristone and a prostaglandin analogue. New England Journal of Medicine 322: 6451; editorial p 691

Szarewski A, Guillebaud J 1991 Contraception: current state of the art. British Medical Journal 302: 1224

Vance M 1990 Growth hormone for the elderly? New England Journal of Medicine 323: 52

Vandenbroucke J P 1991 Postmenopausal oestrogen and cardioprotection. Lancet 337: 833, and subsequent correspondence, including the view that

women . . . will not want to wait for the results of colossal trials advocated by a well androgenised male (p. 1161)

Vessey M P et al 1989 Mortality among oral contraceptive users: 20 year follow-up of women in a cohort study. British Medical Journal 299: 1487

Wingfield M 1991 The daughters of stilboestrol: grown up but still at risk. British Medical Journal 302: 1414 — an account of the management of women (aged 20–35 years) injured by stilboestrol given to their mothers during pregnancy

World Health Organization 1990 Contraceptive efficacy of testosterone-induced azoospermia in normal men. Lancet 336: 955

Neoplastic disease and immunosuppression

MALIGNANT DISEASE: PREVENTION AND CURE

Malignant disease is of immense variety.

Prevention, by drugs, of the genetic change, whether spontaneous or induced by chemicals or viruses, that converts a normal cell to an invasive malignant cell has only now begun to be attained (p. 630). However, some cancers can be prevented, wholly or in part, by protecting people or inviting them to protect themselves from exposure to known carcinogens (industrial cancers, bronchial cancer).

Attempts to cure or palliate cancer employ five principal modes:

1. surgery, including lasers
2. radiotherapy
3. chemotherapy[1]
4. endocrine therapy
5. immunotherapy, including cytokines.

Details of the exploitation of all of these techniques, whether alone, sequentially or concurrently is beyond the scope of a book on clinical pharmacology. This account will be substantially confined to drugs.

---

[1] Although not in strict accord with the definition of Ch. 10, the word chemotherapy is in general use in this connection and it would be pedantic to avoid it. It arose because some malignant cells can be cultured and the disease transmitted by inoculation, as with bacteria. Some prefer to call it anticytotic or cytotoxic therapy.

Endocrine influence on cancer

The possibility of interfering with cancer other than by surgery, e.g. by *endocrine* manipulation was first tested in 1895 when a Scottish surgeon faced with a woman aged 33 years with advanced breast cancer 'put it to her husband and herself as to whether she should have performed the operation of removal of the [fallopian] tubes and ovaries. Its nature was fully explained to them both, and also that it was a purely experimental one . . . She readily consented . . . as she knew and felt her case was hopeless.'[2] Eight months after operation 'all vestiges of her previous cancerous disease had disappeared'. The surgeon concluded, after treating two further cases, that there may be ovarian influences in breast cancer and added that 'whether [this is] accepted or not, I am sure I shall be acquitted of having acted thoughtlessly or recklessly.'

The treatment had indeed been based on reason. The author, 20 years previously, had agreed to take charge of a Scottish landowner 'whose mind was affected'. His duties 'were at times exciting, but never onerous', and, having the time and the interest to observe the weaning of lambs on a local farm, he observed a similarity 'up to a point' between the proliferation of epithelial cells of the milk ducts in lactation and in cancer; he learned that some farmers practised oophorectomy to prolong lactation in cows; and he had the idea that cancer of the breast might be due to an abnormal ovarian stimulus and that removal of the ovaries might have therapeutic effect on cancer of the genital tract.

In 1941[3] it was shown that prostatic cancer with metastases was made worse by androgen and made better by oestrogen (stilboestrol). Activity of this cancer was particularly readily observable since the plasma acid phosphatase concentration provides a reliable *marker. Indeed the availability of some means of reliably measuring effect is crucial to the use of drugs in cancer.*

Cytotoxic drugs

Cytotoxic chemotherapy began with sulphur mustards (oily vesicant liquids) which had been developed and used as chemical weapons in World War I (1914–18). Amongst their actions depression of haemopoiesis and of lymphoid tissues were observed.

Preparations for World War II (1939–45) included research to increase the potency and toxicity ('efficacy') of these odious substances. It was found that substitution of a nitrogen atom for the sulphur atom, i.e. making nitrogen mustards, had the desired result. The disappearance of lymphocytes and granulocytes from the blood of rabbits was a useful marker of toxicity and gave rise to the idea of possible efficacy in lymphoid cancer. '*The problem was fundamental and simple: could one destroy a tumour with this group of cytotoxic agents before destroying the host?*'[4]

Nitrogen mustards, as anticancer agents, were first tested on experimental lymphoma in mice and the results were sufficiently encouraging to warrant a therapeutic trial in man. 'The response of the first patient was as dramatic as that of the first mouse', following 10 days treatment. *But* severe bone marrow depression occurred and, disappointingly, as the bone marrow recovered so did the tumour; in addition, with further courses, it rapidly became resistant. 'Twenty years later (1963) we can appreciate how accurately this first patient reflected the future trials and tribulations of therapy with alkylating agents'.[4]

The development of other classes of agents, e.g. antimetabolites, soon followed.

> **Chemotherapy** depends on developing drugs that *kill* malignant cells and leave those of the host unharmed or at least recoverable.

The comparative success of antimicrobial chemotherapy is due to the fact that the metabolism of the parasite differs qualitatively from that of host cells. But cancer cells are host cells that differ from normal cells quantitatively rather than

[2] Beatson G T. Lancet 1896; 2: 104, 162.
[3] Huggins C et al. Cancer Res 1941; 1: 293.

[4] Gilman A. Am J Surg 1963; 105: 574.

qualitatively, and *to attain adequate selectivity it is necessary to take into account and exploit every possible factor* that may improve the therapeutic index:

- the sensitivity of the malignant cell to drugs
- its endocrine environment
- the number of cells dividing at any one time
- the total number of cells (size of the tumour)
- the kinetics of the drugs
- the rate of recovery of normal tissues from the unavoidable toxic effects of the drugs (most important).

Infection with micro-organisms normally causes an *immune response* and antibacterial drugs that are merely cytostatic can be used: the host defence mechanisms of the body eliminating the bacteria whose replication has been arrested. But there is less immune response to cancer (attempts are being made to strengthen such response as there is) and cure can only be achieved by killing or otherwise removing cancer cells.

Thus in cancer the neoplastic cells are relatively closely allied to the normal cells and must be killed by treatment. Whereas in bacterial infections the cells are markedly different from the normal host cells and generally a treatment that arrests growth is sufficient.

Drug therapy cannot be conducted rationally without some understanding of the disease as well as of the drugs. Since cancer is not a single disease but many, although they share certain characteristics (see below), the following notes must be confined to what is usually true.

REFERENCE TABLES

The text that follows is supported by two large Tables (37.1 and 37.2) which provide reference data that would clog the main text but to which it is useful to have easy access. The tables provide details on:

1. *Drugs commonly used for different types of cancer,* arranged according to level of

benefit, i.e. major, moderate or minor (Table 37.1);
2. *Cytotoxic chemotherapeutic agents and their toxicities,* indicating, by emphasis, the effects that limit therapeutic dose (Table 37.2).

We think that these authoritative tables will provide useful background for reference.

CYTOTOXIC CHEMOTHERAPY

Tumour characteristics[5]

1. **Cancers,** despite their variability, share some common characteristics:

- Growth that is not subject to normal restrictions for that tissue
- Local invasiveness
- Tendency to spread to other parts of the body (metastasis)
- Less differentiated cell morphology
- Tendency to retain some characteristics of the tissue of origin.

2. **Survival**. In, for example, experimental leukaemia, it has been shown that:

- survival time is inversely related to the initial number of leukaemia cells, or to the number remaining after treatment;
- a single leukaemia cell is capable of multiplying and eventually killing the host.

3. **Cell kinetics and mode of action of drugs**. Cytotoxic drugs act against all cells that are multiplying. Bone marrow, mucosal surfaces (gut), hair follicles, reticuloendothelial system, germ cells, are all dividing more rapidly than many cancers and so are also targets for cytotoxic drugs, as is shown by the occurrence of adverse effects on these tissues during chemotherapy. Most solid tumours in man divide slowly and recovery from cytotoxic agents is slow but normal marrow and gut recover rapidly. This *rapid recovery of normal tissues is exploited in devising intermittent courses of chemotherapy.*

---

[5] WHO Tech. Rep. 605 (1977). Chemotherapy of solid tumours. Geneva.

Table 37.1 Reference data: Drugs commonly used for different types of cancer

Cancer type	Principal options: Drugs most often used
Diseases in which chemotherapy has major activity	
Acute lymphocytic leukaemia (ALL)	*Induction*: vincristine + prednisone + asparaginase ± doxorubicin CNS prophylaxis: intrathecal methotrexate + systemic high-dose methotrexate with leucovorin rescue *Maintenance*: methotrexate + mercaptopurine Bone marrow transplant for chemotherapy failures
Acute myelogenous leukaemia (AML)	Cytarabine + daunorubicin or idarubicin Bone marrow transplant with cyclophosphamide plus either total body irradiation or busulfan
Breast cancer* (see also text)	Tamoxifen Cyclophosphamide + methotrexate + fluorouracil ± prednisone (CMF or CMFP) For adjuvant treatment tamoxifen is generally preferred for postmenopausal patients and combinations of other drugs for premenopausal node-positive patients
Choriocarcinoma	Methotrexate ± leucovorin ± dactinomycin
Ewing's sarcoma*	Cyclophosphamide + doxorubicin + vincristine (CAV) A = Adriamycin = doxorubicin
Hodgkin's disease	Doxorubicin + bleomycin + vinblastine + dacarbazine (ABVD) ABVD alternated with MOPP Mechlorethamine + vincristine + procarbazine ± prednisone (MOPP) Marrow transplantation with carmustine, cyclophosphamide, etoposide
Lung, small cell (oat-cell)	Cisplatin + etoposide (PE) Cyclophosphamide + doxorubicin + vincristine (CAV) PE alternated with CAV
Non-Hodgkin's lymphoma Burkitt's lymphoma	Cyclophosphamide + vincristine + methotrexate
Diffuse large-cell lymphoma	Cyclophosphamide + doxorubicin + vincristine + prednisone (CHOP) ± methotrexate with leucovorin rescue Bleomycin + doxorubicin + cyclophosphamide + vincristine + prednisone (BACOP)
Osteogenic sarcoma*	Doxorubicin and high-dose methotrexate with leucovorin rescue ± cisplatin ± bleomycin
Testicular	Cisplatin + etoposide ± bleomycin (PEB) Autologous marrow transplantation with carboplatin + etoposide
Wilms' tumour* (nephroblastoma)	Dactinomycin + vincristine ± doxorubicin ± cyclophosphamide

Table 37.1 *(Cont'd)*

Cancer type	Principal options: Drugs most often used
Diseases in which chemotherapy has moderate activity	
Adrenocortical carcinoma	Mitotane Cisplatin
Bladder (urinary)	Cisplatin and/or doxorubicin ± methotrexate ± vinblastine
Brain glioblastoma	Carmustine or lomustine
Cervix uteri	Cisplatin + bleomycin ± methotrexate Bleomycin + mitomycin + vincristine ± cisplatin
Chronic lymphocytic leukaemia	Chlorambucil ± prednisone
Chronic myelogenous leukaemia (CML) Chronic phase	Busulfan Hydroxyurea, interferon Bone marrow transplantation with cyclophosphamide and total body irradiation or busulfan
Acute phase	Daunorubicin + cytarabine + vincristine + prednisone ± thioguanine
Colorectal	Fluorouracil + leucovorin Intra-arterial floxuridine (hepatic metastases)
Endometrial	Megestrol or medroxyprogesterone Doxorubicin ± cyclophosphamide ± cisplatin
Gastric	Fluorouracil
Head and neck, squamous cell	Cisplatin + fluorouracil ± leucovorin Bleomycin + cisplatin ± methotrexate
Islet cell: pancreas	Streptozocin ± fluorouracil ± doxorubicin
Kaposi's sarcoma (AIDS-related)	Etoposide or interferon or vinblastine
Mycosis fungoides	Combination chemotherapy as in Hodgkin's disease or non-Hodgkin's lymphoma Mechlorethamine (topical)
Myeloma	Melphalan (or cyclophosphamide) + prednisone
Non-Hodgkin's lymphoma Follicular lymphoma	Cyclophosphamide or chlorambucil, ± vincristine and prednisone, ± etoposide (combinations not demonstrably superior to single agents)
Ovary	Cisplatin + cyclophosphamide ± doxorubicin
Prostate (see also text)	Leuprolide (or goserelin) ± flutamide Diethylstilbestrol Cisplatin ± cyclophosphamide ± doxorubicin
Sarcomas (soft tissue, adult)	Doxorubicin + dacarbazine, ± cyclophosphamide (or ifosfamide with mesna)

Table 37.1 *(Cont'd)*

Cancer type	Principal options: Drugs most often used
Diseases in which chemotherapy has minor activity	
Liver	Doxorubicin Fluorouracil
Lung (non-small cell)	Vinblastine + cisplatin + mitomycin Cisplatin + etoposide
Melanoma	Interleukin-2 ± lymphokine activated killer (LAK) cells Dacarbazine
Pancreatic adenocarcinoma	Fluorouracil
Renal	Interleukin-2 Interferon

* Drugs have major activity only when combined with surgical resection, radiotherapy or both.
Note. Prednisolone may be preferred to prednisone.
Reproduced by courtesy of the Medical Letter on
Drugs and Therapeutics, New York (abbreviated; numerous regimens omitted).

In cancer, the normal feedback mechanism, perhaps from faulty cell contact signalling processes (transduction defects) that mediate cell growth, is defective. Cell multiplication, when it has reached its optimum, does not stop. These signalling processes offer multiple targets for developers of new anticancer drugs. In cancer, cells continue to multiply, at first exponentially, i.e. faster and faster as the numbers increase; until later there is a slowing down and the volume-doubling time becomes prolonged due to several factors, most of which conspire to render the *ageing cancer less susceptible to drugs:*

- increased cell cycle (division) time
- decrease in the number of cells actively dividing, with more in the resting state
- increased cell death within the tumour as it ages
- overcrowding of cells leading to defective nutrition (poor vascular supply) with defective access of drugs.

All cells, normal and malignant, engaged in division (cycling) go through a series of phases of synthesis of DNA, RNA, mitosis and rest. Cytotoxic drugs interfere with cell division at various points, e.g: synthesis of nucleotides from purines and pyrimidines, of DNA and RNA; also interference with mitosis; they are also mutagenic.

In general *drugs are most active against actively cycling cells (normal and malignant) and least active against resting cells.* These latter are particularly sinister in that, athough inactive, they retain the capacity to proliferate and may start cycling again after a completed course of chemotherapy. In order to eliminate them it is necessary to develop drugs that are active against the resting phase, to prolong chemotherapy to catch them when they become active, or to induce synchronous activity so that they may all be simultaneously vulnerable to cycle or phase-specific drugs (below).[6]

Plainly all this has important implications for the practice of chemotherapy.

---

[6] There are *circadian rhythms* in cell metabolism and proliferation and those of leukaemic cells differ from those of normal leucocytes. There is evidence that maintenance chemotherapy of some leukaemias is more effective if given in the evening (Rivard G E et al. Lancet 1985; 2: 1264).

Table 37.2 Reference data: Some anticancer drugs (non-hormone) and their toxicity

Drug	Dose-limiting effects are in **bold** type	
	Acute toxicity	Delayed toxicity*
Amsacrine	**Nausea and vomiting**; diarrhoea; pain or phlebitis on infusion; anaphylaxis	**Bone marrow depression**; hepatic injury; convulsions; stomatitis; ventricular fibrillation; alopecia
Asparaginase	**Nausea and vomiting**; fever; chills; headache; hypersensitivity, anaphylaxis; abdominal pain; hyperglycaemia leading to coma	CNS depression or hyperexcitability; acute haemorrhagic pancreatitis; coagulation defects; thrombosis; renal damage; hepatic damage
Bleomycin	Nausea and vomiting; fever; anaphylaxis and other allergic reactions	**Pneumonitis and pulmonary fibrosis; rash and hyperpigmentation**; stomatitis; alopecia; Raynaud's phenomenon; cavitating granulomas
Busulfan	Nausea and vomiting; rare diarrhoea	Bone marrow depression; pulmonary infiltrates and fibrosis; alopecia; gynecomastia; ovarian failure; hyperpigmentation; azoospermia; leukaemia; chromosome aberrations; cataracts; hepatitis
Carboplatin	Nausea and vomiting	**Bone marrow depression**; peripheral neuropathy (uncommon); hearing loss
Carmustine	**Nausea and vomiting**; local phlebitis	**Delayed leukopenia and thrombocytopenia** (may be prolonged); pulmonary fibrosis (may be irreversible); delayed renal damage; gynecomastia; reversible liver damage; veno-occlusive disease (hepatic or pulmonary) with high doses; leukaemia
Chlorambucil	Seizures; nausea and vomiting	**Bone marrow depression**; pulmonary infiltrates and fibrosis; leukaemia; hepatic toxicity; sterility
Cisplatin	**Nausea and vomiting**; anaphylactic reactions; fever; haemolytic-uraemic syndrome	**Renal damage**; ototoxicity; bone marrow depression; haemolysis; hypomagnesaemia; peripheral neuropathy; hypocalcaemia; hypokalaemia; Raynaud's disease; sterility; teratogenesis
Crisantaspase: see asparaginase		
Cyclophosphamide	**Nausea and vomiting**; Type 1 (anaphylactoid) hypersensitivity; facial burning with i.v. administration; visual blurring	**Bone marrow depression**; alopecia; haemorrhagic cystitis; sterility (may be temporary); pulmonary infiltrates and fibrosis; hyponatremia; leukaemia; bladder cancer; inappropriate ADH secretion; teratogenesis
Cytarabine	**Nausea and vomiting**; diarrhoea; anaphylaxis	**Bone marrow depression**; conjunctivitis; megaloblastosis; oral ulceration; hepatic damage; fever; pulmonary oedema and central and peripheral neurotoxicity with high doses; rhabdomyolysis
Dacarbazine	**Nausea and vomiting**; diarrhoea; anaphylaxis; pain on administration	**Bone marrow depression**; alopecia; flu-like syndrome; renal impairment; hepatic necrosis; facial flushing; paraesthesiae; photosensitivity; urticarial rash
Dactinomycin (actinomycin D)	**Nausea and vomiting**; diarrhoea; local reaction and phlebitis; anaphylactoid reaction	**Stomatitis; oral ulceration; bone marrow depression**; alopecia; folliculitis; dermatitis in previously irradiated areas
Daunorubicin	**Nausea and vomiting**; diarrhoea; red urine (not haematuria); severe local tissue damage and necrosis on extravasation; transient ECG changes; anaphylactoid reaction	**Bone marrow depression; cardiotoxicity**; alopecia; stomatitis; anorexia; diarrhoea; fever and chills; dermatitis in previously irradiated areas

Table 37.2 *(Cont'd)*

Drug	Dose-limiting effects are in bold type	
	Acute toxicity	Delayed toxicity*
Doxorubicin	**Nausea and vomiting**; red urine (not haematuria); severe local tissue damage and necrosis on extravasation; diarrhoea; fever; transient ECG changes; ventricular arrhythmia; anaphylactoid reaction	**Bone marrow depression; cardiotoxicity**; alopecia; stomatitis; anorexia; conjunctivitis; acral pigmentation; dermatitis in previously irradiated areas
Estramustine	Nausea and vomiting; diarrhoea	Mild gynecomastia; increased frequency of vascular accidents; myelosuppression (uncommon); oedema; dyspnoea; pulmonary infiltrates and fibrosis; leukaemia
Etoposide	**Nausea and vomiting**; diarrhoea; fever; hypotension; allergic reactions	**Bone marrow depression**; alopecia; peripheral neuropathy; mucositis and hepatic damage with high doses
Fluorouracil	**Nausea and vomiting**; diarrhoea; hypersensitivity reaction	**Oral and GI ulcers; bone marrow depression**; diarrhoea (especially with fluorouracil-leucovorin); neurological defects, usually cerebellar; cardiac arrhythmias; angina pectoris; alopecia; hyperpigmentation; palmar-plantar erythrodysaesthesia; conjunctivitis; heart failure
Hydroxyurea	Nausea and vomiting; allergic reactions to tartrazine dye	**Bone marrow depression**; stomatitis; dysuria; alopecia; rare neurological disturbances
Ifosfamide	Nausea and vomiting; confusion; nephrotoxicity; metabolic acidosis	**Bone marrow depression; haemorrhagic cystitis** (prevented by concurrent mesna); alopecia; inappropriate ADH secretion; neurotoxicity (somnolence, hallucinations, blurring of vision, coma); teratogenesis
Interferon Alfa-2a, Alfa-2b	Fever; chills; myalgias; fatigue; headache; arthralgias; hypotension	Bone marrow depression; anorexia; renal damage; hepatic damage
Interleukin-2	**Fever; fluid retention; hypotension**; rash, anaemia, thrombocytopenia; nausea and vomiting; diarrhoea, capillary leak syndrome, nephrotoxicity; myocardial toxicity, hepatotoxicity; erythema nodosum	Neuropsychiatric disorders; hypothyroidism
Lomustine	**Nausea and vomiting**	**Delayed (4–6 weeks) leukopenia and thrombocytopenia** (may be prolonged); transient elevation of transaminase activity; neurological reactions; pulmonary fibrosis; renal damage; leukaemia
Mechlorethamine	**Nausea and vomiting**; local reaction and phlebitis	**Bone marrow depression**; alopecia; diarrhoea; oral ulcers; leukaemia; amenorrhoea; sterility
Melphalan	Mild nausea; hypersensitivity reactions	**Bone marrow depression** (especially platelets); pulmonary infiltrates and fibrosis; amenorrhoea; sterility; leukaemia; inappropriate ADH secretion
Mercaptopurine	Nausea and vomiting; diarrhoea	**Bone marrow depression; cholestasis and rarely hepatic necrosis; oral and intestinal ulcers; pancreatitis**; allopurinol and azathioprine increase overall toxicity
Mesna	Nausea and vomiting; diarrhoea,	

Table 37.2 *(Cont'd)*

Drug	Acute toxicity	Delayed toxicity*
	Dose-limiting effects are in bold type	
Methotrexate	**Nausea and vomiting**; diarrhoea; fever; anaphylaxis; hepatic necrosis	**Oral and gastrointestinal ulceration**, perforation may occur; **bone marrow depression**; hepatic toxicity including cirrhosis; renal toxicity; **pulmonary infiltrates and fibrosis**; osteoporosis; conjunctivitis; alopecia; depigmentation; menstrual dysfunction
Mitomycin	**Nausea and vomiting**; local reaction; fever	**Bone marrow depression** (cumulative); stomatitis; alopecia; acute pulmonary toxicity; pulmonary fibrosis; hepatotoxicity; renal toxicity; amenorrhoea; sterility; haemolytic-uraemic syndrome; bladder calcification
Mitozantrone	Blue-green pigment in urine; blue-green sclerae; nausea and vomiting; stomatitis	**Bone marrow depression**; cardiotoxicity; alopecia; white hair; skin lesions; hepatic damage; renal failure
Mustine (see mechlorethamine)		
Plicamycin	**Nausea and vomiting**; diarrhoea; fever	**Haemorrhagic diathesis; bone marrow depression** (thrombocytopenia); coagulation abnormalities; hepatic damage; hypocalcaemia and hypokalaemia; stomatitis; renal damage
Procarbazine	**Nausea and vomiting**; CNS depression; disulfiram-like effect with alcohol	**Bone marrow depression**; stomatitis; peripheral neuropathy; pneumonitis; leukaemia
Thioguanine	Occasional nausea and vomiting	**Bone marrow depression**; hepatic damage; stomatitis
Thiotepa	**Nausea and vomiting**; local pain	**Bone marrow depression**; menstrual dysfunction; interference with spermatogenesis; leukemia
Vinblastine	**Nausea and vomiting**; local reaction and phlebitis with extravasation	**Bone marrow depression**; alopecia; stomatitis; loss of deep tendon reflexes; jaw pain; muscle pain; paralytic ileus; inappropriate ADH secretion
Vincristine	Local reaction with extravasation	**Peripheral neuropathy**; alopecia; mild bone marrow depression; constipation; paralytic ileus; jaw pain; inappropriate ADH secretion
Vindesine	Local reaction with extravasation; fever; nausea and vomiting; diarrhoea	Bone marrow depression; alopecia, peripheral neuropathy; jaw pain

* Cutaneous reactions (sometimes severe), hyperpigmentation, and ocular toxicity have been reported with virtually all nonhormonal anticancer drugs.
Reproduced (abbreviated) by courtesy of the Medical Letter on Drugs and Therapeutics, New York.

Principles of chemotherapy

1. Determine that there is no better (more effective and safe) treatment available.
2. Decide whether expected benefit (cure, palliation and the expected quality of life) justifies the risk.
3. Determine the marker (symptom, sign, laboratory measure) that will allow progress to be assessed.
4. With sensitive tumours *treat early* in the course of the disease to increase likelihood of total cell kill.

5. Choose drugs that are cycle non-specific or cycle specific, as appropriate; or that have been shown empirically to be effective.
6. Use combinations of drugs.
7. Repeat courses of high dose chemotherapy with intervals for recovery of normal tissues; this is ordinarily more effective than continuous low dose therapy.
8. Use adjuvant therapy to eliminate micrometastases.
9. Contraindications: very advanced disease, existing bone marrow depression, presence of active infection.

Objectives. Whether there is realistic expectation of cure or major life prolongation of acceptable (to the patient) quality, then it is appropriate to risk severe drug toxicity.

Where expectation is confined to palliation or modest life prolongation (but of poor quality) then less toxic drug regimens should be devised.

Plainly patients should understand the issues with the aid of appropriate counselling.

Whilst **selectivity** of drugs for the cancer cell is generally low compared with selectivity of drugs against bacteria, in some tumours it can be substantial, as in lymphoma, in which the tumour cell kill with some drugs is 10 000 times as great as that of marrow cells. Techniques for targeting drugs to cancer cells are greatly needed.

Cell destruction by drugs follows first-order kinetics, i.e. a given dose of drug kills a constant *fraction* of cells (not a constant *number*) regardless of the number of cells present, i.e. a treatment reducing a cell population from 1 000 000 to 10 000 will reduce a cell population of 100 to one. Therefore, where there are many cells (late presentation, macroscopic disease) it is necessary to repeat the dose, to use several drugs, and to repeat administration to the limit of patient (host) tolerance.[7] With some cancers final complete cell kill can be unattainable without unacceptable risk; therefore adjuvant chemotherapy is used (see below).

But cells remaining after initial doses are likely to be more resistant to drugs since cell sensitivity is not homogeneous at the outset due to random mutations as the tumour grows.

Drug action and cell resistance. Drugs that kill cancer cells may be:

- *Cycle non-specific:* kill cells whether resting or actively cycling (low growth fraction solid tumours, e.g. alkylating agents).
- *Cycle-specific:* kill only cells that are actively cycling (high growth fraction cancer such as leukaemia, e.g. antimetabolites).

These considerations are relevant to the choice of drugs in combination chemotherapy, and to the desirability of attaining synchronisation of cell cycling to achieve maximum cell kill.

However well-chosen the drug, it will be ineffective if it does not reach the malignant cells at a high enough concentration for a long enough time at the right stage of the cell cycle, for the cells are not like receptors, to be acted upon at any time. Considerations of pharmacokinetics in relation to cell kinetics are of the first importance, as drug treatment modifies the activity of both malignant and normal cells. Large solid tumours are better removed by surgery (the proportion of cells multiplying is often small) even if this is incomplete and what remains treated by cytotoxic drugs.

Cell resistance to single drugs is both frequently present at the outset (*primary* resistance), and develops readily with repeated exposure (*acquired* resistance). Increased dosage is limited by toxicity, e.g. to bone marrow, which does not become tolerant. Therefore combination therapy is now the routine. But *multiple drug resistance* is now a major problem. It appears to be due to activation of an ATP-dependent membrane efflux pump acting via a glycoprotein (developed as a protective mechanism against environmental toxins). The genetic expression of this glycoprotein is being unravelled and the possibility exists of interfering with it pharmacologically.

Well-designed treatment at the outset lessens this problem. In those tumours where cures can be achieved by chemotherapy (acute lymphoblastic leukaemia in childhood, Hodgkin's

---

[7] And even beyond, e.g. methotrexate with folinic acid 'rescue' (p. 629) and bone marrow transplant following remission induced by aggressive chemotherapy in leukaemia.

lymphoma, choriocarcinoma) *adequate initial chemotherapy is of the first importance*. If inadequate therapy is used, drug-resistant cells emerge and subsequent cure with intensive chemotherapy becomes difficult or even impossible.

Intermittent combination chemotherapy. Combinations of drugs are commonly used to obtain maximum cell kill; and they are repeated (scheduling, or pulsed courses) according to the following considerations:

1. having differing biochemical sites of action in the cell and used at full therapeutic doses
2. attacking cells at differing phases of the growth cycle
3. to synchronise the active cell cycles
4. using drugs that do not suppress bone marrow in between courses of those that do
5. empirically

The logical basis of 1 and 2 (above) is obvious. But synchronisation (3 above) represents a refinement; cells are killed or are arrested in mitosis by *vincristine*, which is then withdrawn so that the cells enter a new reproductive cycle more or less synchronously; and when the majority are judged to be in a phase sensitive to a particular phase-specific drug, then that drug is given; an example is vincristine followed by methotrexate or cytarabine.

In spite of the important kinetic considerations discussed above it remains true that the majority of chemotherapy regimens have been devised by using a *commonsense empiricism*, and do not rely on detailed knowledge of tumour kinetics (which is at best meagre).

The *drugs have been chosen* because:

- they are known to be effective as single agents,
- the toxicities do not overlap greatly,
- in trial and error (empirical) use, the margins of safety of the combination have been determined, and
- it is reasonably hoped that by mixing differing classes of agents with differing effects in the cell cycle a spectrum of activity against both dividing and non-dividing cells can be achieved, e.g. cycle

non-specific agents first to reduce tumour cell mass, and cycle-specific drugs second.

After an attempt to get maximum malignant cell-kill using drugs to the limit of normal host tolerance, including exploitation of special routes of administration (intrathecal, arterial perfusion), an interval must be left for sufficient recovery of the normal cells, including the recovery of immunological mechanisms that have been suppressed. An interval between courses of 2–3 weeks is usually enough.

The aggressive pursuit of cure by total cell kill is conducted with repeated courses of combinations of drugs known by their acronyms, see Table 37.1.

But *single drug therapy* is adequate in some cancers (Burkitt's lymphoma, choriocarcinoma, although two or more drugs are often used, see Table 37.1)

Adjuvant chemotherapy is therapy given after the initial surgery or radiation to eliminate any persisting micrometastases; it is chiefly used for tumours known for their propensity to such spread, e.g. breast cancer. The term includes therapy undertaken after relapses. It may be cytotoxic or endocrine. The objective is to hit tumour cells that may be present but undetectable at the early stage of growth when the cells of a tumour are more rapidly dividing and more sensitive to drugs. Over-liberal use of adjuvant therapy carries the risk of treating patients who in fact have been cured by the initial therapy and so exposing them needlessly to the risk of a second, drug-induced, tumour.

Adverse effects (see Table 37.2)

Principal adverse effects include:

1. *Nausea and vomiting* (see below)
2. *Bone marrow and lymphoreticular system:* pancytopenia and immunosuppression (depression of both antibody and cell-mediated immunity), leading to infections (see below)
3. *Gut lining* and other *mucosal surfaces:* diarrhoea, mouth ulcers
4. *Hair:* alopecia due to effect on hair bulb

(recovers 2–6 months after ceasing treatment). Prevention by scalp hypothermia may be tried

5. *Delayed wound healing*
6. *General immunosuppression*
7. *Germ cells:* sterility, teratogenesis, mutagenicity
8. *Various organ damage* (see Table 37.2)
9. *Secondary cancers* (see below)
10. *Local toxicity* if extravasation occurs.

Items 1 to 6 occur *immediately or in the short term* and are liable to be troublesome with any vigorously pursued regimen.

Nausea and vomiting. This is common, can be extremely severe and prolonged and cause patients to refuse treatment. Management is of the first importance (see also p. 524).

Vomiting commonly begins in 1–5 h and lasts from 6–48 h, depending on the agent.

Drugs most likely to cause nausea and vomiting, and its severity are shown in Table 37.2 (p. 621). Since emesis is largely predictable, preventive action can be taken.

The most effective drugs are competitive antagonists at serotoin (5-HT₃) receptors (ondansetron) (Zofran) and at the dopamine receptor (metoclopramide). They are used in combination with a benzodiazepine (anxiety is a major factor in promoting emesis when the patient *knows* that it will occur, as with cisplatin), and dexamethasone which benefits by an unknown mechanism. Other effective agents include prochlorperazine, domperidone and nabilone.

Combinations, e.g. benzodiazepine plus dexamethasone, plus a 5-HT₃ or dopamine receptor blocker (ondansetron, metoclopramide) are more effective than a single drug.

Routes of administration are chosen as commonsense counsels, e.g. prophylaxis may be oral, but when vomiting occurs injections and suppositories are available.

Bone marrow suppression is the single most important dose-limiting factor. Repeated blood counts are essential and transfusion of all formed elements of the blood may be needed, e.g. platelet transfusion for thrombocytopenic bleeding or where the platelet count falls below

$25\ 000 \times 10^9/l$. Cell growth factors, e.g. the natural granulocyte colony stimulating factor (filgrastim) has been shown effective in neutropenia.

Septicaemia occurs (often opportunistic infection by Gram-negative bacteria from the patient's own flora, e.g. from the gut, which has been injured by the drugs) and vigorous antimicrobial prophylaxis and therapy, often in combination, is used. Granulocyte transfusions are also helpful. Opportunistic infections with virus (herpes zoster), fungus (candida) and protozoa (pneumocystis) are also prominent. *Fever* in a patient under this treatment requires collection of samples for microbiological studies and urgent treatment.

Immune responses. There is evidence that vigorous and prolonged chemotherapy can impair the immune responsiveness of patients for as long as 3 years after ceasing therapy.

Effects on gonadal cells can lead to reduced sexual drive and to sterility, and the mutagenic effects of anticancer drugs mean that reproduction should be avoided during and for several months after therapy. But both men and women have reproduced successfully (normally) whilst undergoing chemotherapy. It has been recommended that when the long-term outlook for life is good and treatment may cause permanent sterility, e.g. in Hodgkin's lymphoma, men should be offered the facility for storage of sperm before undergoing treatment.

Urate nephropathy. Rapid *destruction of large numbers of malignant cells* results in substantial release of purines and pyrimidines, which are converted to uric acid, which may crystallise in the renal tubule (urate nephropathy). This can be avoided by high fluid intake, alkalinisation of the urine and use of allopurinol during the early stages of chemotherapy. In practice this only occurs when there is a large cell mass and the tumour is very sensitive to drugs, e.g. acute lymphocytic leukaemia and lymphomas.

Carcinogenicity (second tumours). Many cytotoxic drugs are carcinogenic, and a patient may be cured of the primary disease only to succumb to a second, treatment-induced, cancer 5 years later. Alkylating agents are particularly incriminated and also some antimetabolites (mercaptopurine) and antibiotics (doxorubicin). The risk can be as high as 10–20 times that of unexposed people and the cancers include leukaemia, lymphoma and squamous carcinoma.

In Hodgkin's lymphoma life is greatly prolonged by chemotherapy, but in ovarian cancer it is not; these aspects are plainly relevant to acceptance of risk of second tumours. Use of radiation concurrently does not increase risk of leukaemia.

Quality of life. There is growing concern that over-enthusiastic and aggressive use of cytotoxic drug therapy has done more harm than good to many patients, destroying the quality of the brief time remaining to them in exchange for little or no benefit. This state of affairs is contributed to by our present inability to target the drugs to the cells where they may do good, e.g. monoclonal antibodies used as drug carriers may in the future improve our ability to hit selected targets.

Hazards to staff handling cytotoxic agents. The urine of some nurses and of pharmacists who prepare infusions and injections of anticancer drugs has been found to contain drugs even to the extent of being sometimes mutagenic to bacteria. When they stopped handling the drugs the contamination ceased. It cannot be assumed that absorption of these small amounts (compared with therapeutic doses) of drugs is harmless (mutagenesis, carcinogenesis), especially when it occurs repeatedly over long periods.

Contamination occurs from spilt drugs, carelessly handled syringes (there should be a swab on the tip of the needle when expelling air), and even opening an ampoule can create an aerosol. Used ampoules, syringes, absorbent swabs constitute a hazard, as may body wastes of treated patients.

Precautions[8] appropriate to different drugs range from simply avoiding spillage, through

---

[8] The Royal Pharmaceutical Society of Great Britain has published useful guidelines. Pharmaceutical Journal Feb 26 (1983) p. 230. See also Williams C J. Handling cytotoxics. Br Med J 1985 291: 1299; also Martindale: The extra Pharmacopoeia: 29th edn. 1989: p 583.

gloves, surgical masks, goggles and aprons, to use of laminar flow cabinets. Special training of nominated drug handlers is essential. Pregnant staff should not handle these drugs.

ENDOCRINE THERAPY: hormones and antihormones

Some cancers are hormone dependent and growth can be inhibited by surgical removal of gonads, adrenals and pituitary. But administration of hormones, or antihormones, of oestrogens, androgens or progestogens is increasingly preferred (see Ch. 36). *Prostatic cancer* is androgen dependent, see also p. 593, 619.

[*Benign prostatic hypertrophy* is also androgen dependent. Drug therapy includes use of anti-androgen, inhibition of the enzyme (5α-reductase) that activates testosterone. Also reduction of smooth muscle tone of the prostate capsule and bladder neck by α-adrenoceptor block, e.g. prazosin, reducing urinary obstruction.]

Breast cancers may have receptors for oestrogen, progesterone and androgen, and tumours that have receptors for both oestrogen and progesterone are far more likely to respond to endocrine manipulation than are those that lack them. Receptor analysis of cells from tumours is used as a guide to the most effective therapy, choice of which is a specialised matter. In general, endocrine therapy with an antioestrogen (tamoxifen) for up to 2 years benefits older women; cytotoxic chemotherapy is more useful in younger women. Advanced metastatic disease may be palliated by more intensive endocrine therapy where steroid receptors are present (e.g. a progestogen or adrenalectomy). Androgens are seldom used because of their virilising effects.

Adrenocortical steroids are used for their action on the cancer itself and also to treat some of the complications of cancer (hypercalcaemia, raised intracranial pressure, see index).

Their principal use is in cancer of the lymphoid tissues and blood. In leukaemias they may also reduce the incidence of haematological complications such as haemolytic anaemia and thrombocytopenia. A glucocorticoid is preferred, e.g. prednisolone, as mineralocorticoid actions are not needed and cause fluid retention. High doses, e.g. 200 mg prednisolone per day, are used. Table 37.1 lists prednisone according to practice in USA whence this Table is taken.

General. Endocrine therapy carries much less serious consequences for normal tissues than do the cytotoxic agents.

IMMUNOTHERAPY

Immunotherapy derives from an observation in the 19th century that cancer sometimes regressed after acute bacterial infections, i.e. there may be non-specific immunostimulant effect.

Anticancer drugs are notable as being immunosuppressive and so are likely to diminish what little natural immune resistance to a tumour that there may be.

Exploration of immunotherapy has involved:

• Non-specific stimulation of active immunity with *vaccines*, e.g. BCG and *Corynebacterium parvum* vaccine. These have efficacy in animals, but results in man are controversial. *C. parvum* vaccine is used in the pleural cavity for malignant effusions but its benefit seems to be due to a local vigorous inflammatory effect rather than to immunostimulation.

• Use of specific vaccines prepared from the cells of the patient's tumour or from tumours in other people.

• Non-specific stimulation of active immunity with *drugs*, e.g. *levamisole* (an anthelminthic), which appears to enhance function of phagocytes and T-lymphocytes when this is subnormal. It has also been tried in immune deficiency states and autoimmune disease, e.g. rheumatoid arthritis.

• Use of *cytokines* (below), *monoclonal antibodies.*

Whilst none of these approaches has found a *major* role in therapeutics, they may do so in the future.

• **Cytokines** are natural substances that are produced in response to a variety of stimuli, including specific antigens, e.g. virus, cancer; but they are not antibodies. They regulate cell growth and activity, including immune responses. They can now be synthesised by recombinant DNA technology, and are increasingly available for clinical use. They may be expected to play an important role in therapeutics. They include:

Interferons: p. 198.
Haemopoietic growth factors (p. 500), cell colony-stimulating factors and interleukins.
Interleukin-2 (IL-2) stimulates proliferation of T-lymphocytes (it is called a *lymphokine*) and activates natural killer cells; its use in cancer is being explored. Other *interleukins*, e.g. 1,3,4, are also being explored.
Tumour necrosis factor (TNF) which, as its name implies, is toxic to abnormal, e.g. cancer, cells.

CLASSES OF CYTOTOXIC AGENTS

Drugs used (practical details of administration are of the utmost importance and the manufacturer's Data Sheet should be consulted), see below and Table 37.1; Table 37.2 provides detail of toxicity of individual agents.

Alkylating agents

Alkylating agents (nitrogen mustards and ethyleneimines) act by transferring alkyl groups to DNA in the N-7 position of guanine during cell division. There follows either DNA strand breakage or cross-linking of the two strands so that normal synthesis is prevented.

Examples: busulphan, chlorambucil, cyclophosphamide, ifosfamide, estramustine (a combination of oestrogen and mustine), ethoglucid, melphalan, mustine (mechlorethamine), thiotepa, treosulfan; the nitrosoureas (carmustine, lomustine) have an additional mode of action.

Alkylating agents particularly cause nausea and vomiting and bone marrow depression (delayed with the nitrosoureas) and cystitis[9] (cyclophosphamide, ifosfamide) and pulmonary fibrosis (especially busulphan).

Male infertility and premature menopause occur.

Antimetabolites

Antimetabolites are analogues of normal metabolites and act by competition, i.e. they 'deceive' or 'defraud' bodily processes.

Folic acid antagonist, methotrexate, competitively inhibits dihydrofolate reductase, preventing the synthesis of tetrahydrofolic acid (the coenzyme important in synthesis of amino and nucleic acids).

A cogent illustration of the need to exploit every possible means of enhancing selectivity is provided by methotrexate. A heavy (potentially fatal) dose of methotrexate is given and is followed about 24 h later by a dose of tetrahydrofolic (folinic) acid (as Ca folinate, Ca leucovorin), to by-pass and terminate its action. This is called folinic acid or leucovorin 'rescue', since if it is not given the patient will die. The therapeutic justification for this manoeuvre is that high concentrations of methotrexate are obtained and that the bone marrow cells recover better than the tumour cells and some degree of useful selectivity is achieved (also effective with fluorouracil).

There are also *purine antagonists* (mercaptopurine, azathioprine, thioguanine), and *pyrimidine antagonists* (fluorouracil, cytarabine), which similarly deprive cells of essential metabolites.

Antimetabolites cause gastrointestinal upsets including ulceration and bone marrow depression; renal failure potentiates them, especially methotrexate. Active excretion of methotrexate by the renal tubule is blocked by salicylate, which also displaces it from plasma protein (as do sulphonamides), with increased toxicity.

Natural and semisynthetic agents

Alkaloids: vincristine, vinblastine and vindesine cause cell cycle arrest in mitosis. They particularly cause bone marrow depression, peripheral neuropathy (vincristine) and alopecia.

Glucoside: etoposide (derived from epipodophyllotoxin, from a plant) has antimitotic action.

Antibiotics include: actinomycins (dactinomycin, actinomycin D), bleomycin, daunorubicin doxorubicin, idarubicin, epirubicin and the related mitozantrone and amsacrine; plicamycin (mithramycin), mitomycin, streptozotocin (islet-cell pancreatic tumour) interfere with DNA/RNA synthesis. They depress the bone marrow, cause gut upsets and stomatitis, alopecia, cardiomyopathy (daunorubicin and doxorubicin) and pulmonary fibrosis and skin rashes (bleomycin). The effects of some are radiomimetic, and use of radiation causes additive toxicity.

Crisantaspase (asparaginase) starves tumour cells dependent upon a supply of the amino acid, asparagine (except those able to synthesise it for themselves); its use is almost confined to acute lymphoblastic leukaemia.

Interferons are described on p. 198, and in Table 37.2. They are used in hairy cell leukaemia and Kaposi's sarcoma.

Platinum derivatives cisplatin and carboplatin probably act similarly to alkylating agents.

Miscellaneous: procarbazine, dacarbazine, hydroxyurea, razoxane.

Interactions of cytotoxics with other drugs

Examples of *therapeutic* interactions are shown in Table 37.1. *Non-therapeutic* interactions can be serious, e.g. inhibition of metabolism of cytotoxic drugs can cause toxicity, e.g. cimetidine increases the toxicity of fluorouracil and allopurinol increases toxicity of mercaptopurine and cyclophosphamide.

---

[9] A metabolite, acrolein, of cyclophosphamide and ifosfamide causes haemorrhagic cystitis. A high urine volume plus use of *mesna* (sodium 2-*me*rcapto-ethane*s*ulphon*a*te) which provides free thiol groups that bind acrolein, are used to prevent this serious complication.

CHEMOPREVENTION OF CANCER[10]

There is evidence that some vitamins and derivatives and dietary micronutrients inhibit the development of cancers, e.g. beta-carotene, isotretinoin, folic acid, ascorbic acid, alpha-tocopherol. Large scale trials of these substances and derivatives are in progress. Isotretinoin prevents second primary squamous cell tumours of the head and neck. Tamoxifen (antioestrogen) is being studied in women at high risk of breast cancer.

Cancer 'cures': unproven remedies

'So long as conventional medicine cannot cure all patients with cancer some will be willing to try anything that they think might help'.[11] This is perfectly understandable and up to 50% of patients may use unproven methods, including medicines (see complementary medicine). Innumerable methods are and have been offered for cancer. A recent prominent remedy is laetrile, a preparation of apricot seeds (pits, pips), which contains amygdalin (a β-glucoside) which incorporates cyanide. It is claimed to relieve pain, prolong survival and even to induce complete remission of cancer. Benefit is reputed to result from release of cyanide in the body, which is claimed to kill cancer cells but not normal cells.

As has so often been the case in the past, and no doubt will continue to be in the future, the calm evaluation of such claims is obstructed by a mixture of emotionalism and exploitation. Scientific clinical investigation shows no benefit.

Although it is claimed that laetrile has no toxic effects, an 11-month-old girl has died after swallowing tablets (1–5) being used by her father. The toxicity is due to metabolic formation, in the intestine, of hydrocyanic acid. Deaths are also reported from eating material intended for injection.

Interestingly, despite criticism of over-permissive laxity of the drug regulatory authority

(FDA) in the USA, the public is unwilling to accept the opinion of the FDA when it advises against the use of laetrile.

There is a long and generally dishonourable history of the promotion of cancer 'cures', but as each new one appears the medical profession must yet again be willing to look dispassionately at the possibility that this time there really may be something in it, whilst avoiding the tragic raising of hopes that will not be realised — a sad and difficult task.

IMMUNOSUPPRESSION

Suppression of immune responses mediated via mononuclear cells (lymphocytes, plasma cells) is used in therapy of:

- autoimmune and collagen and connective tissue disease (see below)
- organ transplantation; to prevent immune rejection.

Cytotoxic cancer chemotherapeutic agents are immunosuppressive because they interfere with mononuclear cell multiplication and function. But they are generally too toxic for the above purposes and the following are principally used for intended immunosuppression:

- adrenocortical steroids
- azathioprine (below)
- cyclosporin (below)
- (somes alkylating agents: cyclophosphamide and chlorambucil: see p. 628 and Table 37.2)
- antilymphocyte immunoglobulin (below).

With the exception of *cyclosporin*, all the above cause non-specific immunosuppression so that the general defences of the body against infection are impaired.

Adrenal steroids destroy lymphocytes, reduce inflammation and impair phagocytosis (see Ch. 33).

Cytotoxic agents destroy immunologically competent cells. *Azathioprine*, a prodrug for the purine antagonist mercaptopurine, is used in autoimmune disease because it provides enhanced immunosuppressive activity. Cyclophos-

[10] Meyskens F L 1990 Coming of age — the chemoprevention of cancer. New Eng J Med 323 : 825.
[11] Editorial. Br Med J 1977 1 : 3.

phamide is a second choice. Bone marrow is depressed as is to be expected.

Cyclosporin(e) is a polypeptide obtained from a soil fungus. It is a highly effective immuno-suppressive and has important advantages over other agents; it acts selectively and reversibly on lymphocytes, inhibiting the functions (of T and B cells) that mediate specific recognition of alien molecules, whilst sparing non-specific functions of, e.g. granulocytes, that are responsible for phagocytosis and metabolism of foreign sub-stances; it does not depress bone marrow haemopoiesis. Such selectivity is lost when the drug is used in combination with other im-munosuppressives.

Cyclosporin is *used* to prevent rejection of organ transplants (kidney, liver, heart-lung) and to treat episodes of rejection in patients treated with other immunosuppressives. It is also useful in bone marrow transplants.

Cyclosporin ($t_{\frac{1}{2}}$ 7 h) is metabolised in the liver, and metabolism is inhibited (leading to increased plasma concentrations) by drugs utilising the same cytochrome oxidation path, e.g. keto-conazole, erythromycin, oral contraceptives, calcium channel antagonists. Hepatic enzyme in-duction, e.g. by phenytoin, reduces plasma concentration.

Cyclosporin is nephrotoxic and synergises with other nephrotoxic drugs, e.g. antimicrobials. Other adverse effects include hepatotoxicity, hypertension, hypertrichosis and hyperkalaemia. It is not teratogenic in animals and may not be so in man. Long-term use may cause lymphoma.

Use, which must continue indefinitely, requires careful monitoring, including measurement of plasma concentration where practicable.

Cyclosporin may be given orally or i.v.

Antilymphocyte immunoglobin is used in organ graft rejection, a process in which lymphocytes are involved; it is made by preparing antisera to human lymphocytes in animals (horses); allergic reactions are common. It largely spares the patient's response to infection.

Uses

Diseases in which immunosuppression may be useful include: tissue transplantations, inflam-matory bowel disease, rheumatoid arthritis, chronic active hepatitis, systemic lupus ery-thematosus, glomerulonephritis, nephrotic syn-drome, some haemolytic anaemias and throm-bocytopenias, uveitis, myasthenia gravis, polyarterities, polymyositis, systemic sclerosis, Behçet's syndrome.

Hazards of life on immunosuppressive drugs

Impaired immune responses render the subject more liable to *bacterial and viral* infections; Cyclosporin may be less liable to do this. Treat all infection early and vigorously (using bac-tericidal drugs where practicable); use human gamma globulin to protect if there is exposure to virus infections, e.g. measles, varicella.

Carcinogenicity is also a hazard, generally after 4–7 years of therapy. The cancers most likely to occur are those thought to have viral origin (leukemia, lymphoma, skin). Where cytotoxics are used there is the additional hazard of mutagenicity, which may induce cancer.

Hazards also include those of *long-term cor-ticosteroid therapy*, and of *cytotoxics* in general (bone marrow depression, infertility and teratogenesis).

Whilst the hazards are relatively acceptable for treating grave life-endangering disease, they give more cause for concern when immunosuppress-ive regimens are used in younger patients with less serious disease, e.g. rheumatoid arthritis, ulcerative colitis.

Active immunisation during immunosuppressive therapy

Response to non-living antigens (tetanus, typhoid, poliomyelitis) is diminished and 1 or 2 extra doses may be wise. With living vaccines (some polio) there is a risk of serious generalised disease; boosters are safer than primary vacci-nation. If vaccination *must* be performed (an unlikely event) reduce or stop the immuno-suppressive therapy and vaccinate lightly (6 months later); if a severe reaction occurs use an appropriate antiviral agent or a specific immuno globulin if available. See also adrenocorticosteroids.

Immunostimulation:

see Immunotherapy, p. 628.

GUIDE TO FURTHER READING

Carpenter C B 1990 Immunosuppression in organ transplantation. New England Journal of Medicine 322: 1224

Coltman C A et al 1990 Treatment-related leukaemia. New England Journal of Medicine 322: 52

Editorial 1989 Adjuvant systemic treatment for breast cancer meta-analysed. Lancet 1: 81

Editorial 1989 Multidrug resistance in cancer. Lancet 2: 1075

Editorial 1991 Growth factors and cancer chemotherapy. Lancet 338: 217

Ferrara J L M et al 1991 Graft-versus-host disease. New England Journal of Medicine 324: 667

Greenberg E R et al 1988 Social and economic factors in the choice of lung cancer treatment. New England Journal of Medicine 318: 612

Grunberg S M 1990 Making chemotherapy easier [control of nausea vomiting]. New England Journal of Medicine 322: 846

Hobbs J R 1989 Immunotherapy of human cancers. British Medical Journal 299: 1177

Jardin A et al 1991 Alfuzosin for treatment of benign prostatic hypertrophy. Lancet 337: 1457 (also Chapple C R 1991 Lancet 338: 182)

Macleod A M et al 1988 Cancer after transplantation. British Medical Journal 297: 4

Moertel G G et al 1982 A clinical trial of amygdalin (laetrile) in the treatment of human cancer. New England Journal of Medicine 306: 201 (also Editorial by Relman A S p. 236)

Mullan F 1985 Seasons of survival: reflections of a (32-year old) physician with cancer. New England Journal of Medicine 313: 270

Razavi D et al 1990 Psychosocial correlates of oestrogen and progesterone receptors in breast cancer. Lancet 335: 931

Rees G J 1991 Cancer treatment: deciding what we can afford. British Medical Journal 302: 799

Slevin M L et al 1990 Attitudes to chemotherapy: comparing views of patients with cancer with those of doctors. British Medical Journal 300: 1458

38

Drugs and the skin

SYNOPSIS

It is well-established that the skin may react to emotion, e.g. in eczema or psoriasis, and sedatives or tranquillisers may be useful adjuvant therapy of skin diseases.

To avoid repetition from earlier chapters, the following account is confined to therapy directed primarily at the skin.

- Dermal pharmacokinetics: Vehicles for delivering drugs to the skin; Miscellaneous substances — keratolytics, insect repellants
- Topical analgesia
- Antipruritics
- Adrenocortical steroids
- Sunscreens, sunburn and photosensitivity
- Dermal adverse drug reactions
- Treatment of individual skin disorders

It is easy to do more harm than good with potent drugs, and this is particularly true in skin diseases. Many skin lesions are in fact caused by systemic or local use of drugs. In patients prone to any allergy it is very easy to provoke skin reactions during treatment.

Local or *topical* treatment of skin lesions appears to offer a unique opportunity for the trial of different treatments on similar lesions in the same individual at the same time, but substances applied locally are sometimes absorbed and may exert effects on the body as a whole; also the healing of a lesion at one site, sometimes for no known reason, may be accompanied by improvement in similar lesions elsewhere. Conversely, to provoke a flare-up at one site may make all the other lesions worse as well. Thus a 'control' treatment may at first appear to have caused healing or exacerbation that is in fact due to the effects of a more active substance applied elsewhere.

DERMAL PHARMACOKINETICS

There is a greater variety in the presentation of drugs to the skin than to any other organ. Drugs are presented in *vehicles*, e.g. cream, ointment, which may contain substances intended to enhance penetration, e.g. squalane, by diffusion of the active agent into the stratum corneum (superficial keratin layer). Most modern dermatological formulations are washable hydrophilic oil-in-water emulsions.

The stratum corneum is both the principal barrier to penetration of drugs into the skin and a reservoir for drugs, e.g. corticosteroid may be detectable even 4 weeks after a single application.

Absorption through normal skin varies with site; as is to be expected, absorption from the sole of the foot and the palm of the hand is relatively low, and it increases progressively on the forearm, the scalp, the face until on the scrotum and vulva it is very high.

Where the skin is damaged by inflammation, burn or exfoliation, absorption is further increased.

Hydration of the stratum corneum enhances absorption of drugs, and if an *occlusive dressing* (impermeable plastic membrane) is used, absorption increases by as much as ×10 (plastic pants for babies are occlusive, and some ointments are partially occlusive). Hydration is promoted by oil-in-water creams (vanishing cream) to which active drug may be added.

Serious systemic toxicity can result from use of occlusive dressing over large areas.

Drug readily diffuses from the stratum corneum into the epidermis and then into the dermis, where it enters the capillary microcirculation of the skin, and thus the systemic circulation. There is some presystemic (first-pass) metabolism in the epidermis and dermis.

Transdermal delivery systems. These systems are used to administer drugs for systemic effect via the skin. They are discussed in Chapter 7, p. 93.

Vehicles for delivering drugs to the skin

As well as presenting a drug to the skin, the *vehicle* has actions of its own and it also determines the acceptability to the patient of the formulation.

Lotions or **wet dressings** are generally used to cleanse, cool and relieve pruritus in acutely inflamed lesions, especially where there is much exudation and on hairy areas. Water is the most important component. The initial application, and frequent reapplication, and the cooling effect of evaporation of the water reduces the inflammatory response by inducing superficial vasoconstriction. Sodium chloride solution 0.9%, or solutions of *astringent*[1] and weakly antimicrobial substances, e.g. Aluminium Acetate Lotion, are often used. Soaks of approximately 0.05% potassium permanganate are satisfactory if the lesion is on the limbs. Lotions containing more active ingredients are sometimes used on subacute lesions, but occasionally these irritate the skin further. The use of lotions or wet dressings over very large areas can reduce body temperature dangerously in the old or the very ill.

Shake lotions, e.g. Calamine Lotion, are essentially a convenient way of applying a powder to the skin with additional cooling due to evaporation of the water. They are contraindicated when there is much exudate because crusts form. They sometimes produce excessive drying of the skin, but this can be reduced if oils are included, as in Oily Calamine Lotion.

Creams are emulsions either of *oil-in-water* (washable; cosmetic vanishing creams) or *water-in-oil*. A cooling effect (cold creams) is obtained with both groups as the water evaporates.

Water-in-oil creams, e.g. Oily Cream, Zinc Cream, behave like oils in that they do not mix with serous discharges, but their chief advantage over ointment is that the water content makes them easier to spread, and they give a better cosmetic effect. They are specially useful as barrier preparations for protecting the skin, e.g. when it is chapped or dried, or on babies' buttocks, and can be used on hairy parts. They can be used as vehicles, particularly for fat-soluble substances. A dry skin is mainly short of water and oily substances are needed to provide a barrier that reduces evaporation of water; the presence of oils contributes in some measure to epidermal hydration.

Oil-in-water creams (e.g. Aqueous Cream; see Emulsifying Ointment, below) do mix with serous discharges and are especially useful as vehicles for water-soluble active drugs. They may contain a wetting (surface tension reducing) agent (cetomacrogol).

---

[1] Astringents are weak protein precipitants, e.g. tannins, salts of aluminium and zinc.

Aqueous Cream is also used as an *emollient*, i.e. as well as hydrating the skin, it soothes and smoothes scaly conditions. Various other ingredients, e.g. calamine, zinc, may be added to it.

Barrier preparations of many different kinds have been devised for use in industry and in medicine to reduce dermatitis. They rely on water-repellent substances, e.g. silicones (Dimethicone Cream), and on soaps, as well as on substances that form an impermeable deposit (titanium, zinc, calamine). They are not usually very effective, because it is impossible to maintain a complete barrier that is also easily removed by ordinary washing when no longer needed. If it is not readily removable, complications due to blockage of sweat glands and follicles and skin irritation follow. Allergic reactions occur.

Barrier creams may make the cleansing of the skin more easy after dirty work, but it is essential that they should be shown to be less harmful than the dirt itself before being used for this.

They are more effective in protecting skin from discharges and secretions (colostomies, napkin rash) than when used under industrial working conditions. *Silicone* sprays may be effective in preventing and treating pressure sores.

Masking creams (camouflaging preparations) for obscuring unpleasant blemishes from view are greatly valued by the victims. They may consist of the inert titanium oxide in an ointment base with colouring appropriate to the site and the patient. Best results are got by consulting a cosmetician.

Ointments are thicker than creams and are used in chronic dry conditions; they are of three kinds:

1. *Non-emulsifying*. These do not mix with water: they adhere to the skin and prevent evaporation and heat loss: they can be considered a form of occlusive dressing (with increased systemic absorption of active ingredients): skin maceration occurs: although they are helpful in chronic conditions to soften crusts, and as vehicles, they are not used in acute conditions in which free removal of exudate and cooling are needed: they are difficult to remove except with oil or detergents and are messy and inconvenient,

especially on hairy skin; Paraffin Ointment contains beeswax, paraffins and cetostearyl alcohol; Simple Ointment is similar.

2. *Emulsifying*. These allow evaporation as they mix with water and skin exudate: they are useful as vehicles for active drugs; Emulsifying Ointment is made from emulsifying wax (cetostearyl alcohol and sodium lauryl sulphate) and paraffins; Aqueous Cream is an oil-in-water emulsion of Emulsifying Ointment.

3. *Water soluble*. These are mixtures of macrogols and polyethylene glycols: the consistency can be varied readily; they are easily washed off and are used in burn dressings, as lubricants and as vehicles that readily allow passage of active drugs into the skin, e.g. hydrocortisone.

Pastes, e.g. Zinc Compound Paste, are stiff, semi-occlusive ointments containing insoluble powders. They are very adhesive and give good protection to circumscribed lesions. Their powder content enables them to absorb a moderate amount of discharge. They are also used as vehicles, e.g. Coal Tar Paste, which is Zinc Compound Paste with 7.5% coal tar.

Dusting powders, e.g. Zinc Starch and Talc.[2] Dusting-powder may cool by increasing the effective surface area of the skin and they reduce friction between skin surfaces by their lubricating action. Though usefully absorbent, they cause crusting if applied to exudative lesions. They may be used alone as well as a vehicle for, e.g. fungicides.

Gels or **jellies** are semisolid colloidal solutions or suspensions.

Some miscellaneous substances

Keratolytics are used to destroy unwanted tissue, including warts and corns. Great care is obviously necessary to avoid ulceration. They include trichloracetic acid, silver nitrate sticks, salicylic acid and many others. Resorcinol and sulphur are mild keratolytics used in acne.

---

[2] Talc is magnesium silicate. It must not be used for dusting surgical gloves as it causes granulomas if it gets into wounds or body cavities.

Squalane is a saturated hydrocarbon insoluble in water but soluble in sebum. It therefore penetrates the skin and can deliver active agents, and is water repellent (used for incontinence, prevention of bed sores). It appears in mixed formulations.

Tars are mildly antiseptic, antipruritic and they modify keratinisation in an ill understood way. They are safe in low concentrations. They are used in chronic conditions associated with parakeratosis, e.g. psoriasis. Photosensitivity occurs. There are very many preparations, which usually contain other substances, e.g. Calamine and Coal Tar Ointment, or Coal Tar and Salicylic Acid Ointment; it is sometimes useful to add an adrenal steroid. *Ichthammol* is a sulphurous tarry distillation product of fossilised fish (obtained in the Austrian Tyrol), it has a weaker effect than coal tar.

Zinc oxide provides mild astringent, barrier and occlusive actions.

Calamine is a basic zinc carbonate that owes its pink colour to added ferric oxide. It has a mild astringent action and is used as a dusting powder and in shake and oily lotions.

Urea is used topically to assist skin hydration, e.g. in ichthyosis.

Insect repellents, e.g. against mosquitoes, ticks, fleas, such as deet (diethyl toluamide), dimethyl phthalate. These are applied to the skin and repel insects principally by vaporisation. They must be applied to all exposed skin, and sometimes also to clothes if their objective is to be achieved (some damage plastic fabrics and spectacle frames). Their duration of effect is limited by the rate at which they vaporise (skin and ambient temperature), by washing off (sweat, rain, immersion) and by mechanical factors causing rubbing (physical activity). They can cause allergic and toxic effects, especially with prolonged use. About 10% is absorbed. Plainly the vehicle in which they are applied is also important in relation to all the factors, and an acceptable substance achieving persistence of effect beyond a few hours has yet to be developed. But the alternative of spreading insecticide in the environment causing general pollution with indiscriminate insect kill is largely unacceptable.

Selective environmental measures against some insects, e.g. mosquitoes, are sometimes feasible.

Benzyl benzoate may be used on clothes; it resists 1 or 2 washings.

TOPICAL ANALGESIA (Counter-irritants: rubefacients)

Counter-irritants are used to stimulate nerve endings in intact skin to relieve pain in viscera or muscle supplied by the same nerve root. All produce inflammation of the skin which becomes flushed, hence *rube*facients. They are often effective, and, though how they act is unknown, there is no lack of theories. The psychological effect is certainly important and other possibilities are:

● That vasodilatation at the site of the pain, produced by release of prostaglandins, may promote relief. This vasodilatation can be blocked by NSAIDs, e.g. aspirin, indomethacin.

● That the arrival in the CNS of numerous afferent impulses from the skin may alter the effect of impulses from other parts supplied by the same nerve root, e.g. via endorphins.

The best counter-irritants are physical agents, especially heat. Many drugs, however, have been used for this purpose and suitable liniments (e.g. Turpentine Liniment), ointments (e.g. Methyl Salicylate Ointment), and poultices (e.g. Kaolin Poultice) and preparations of menthol, camphor and capsicum, are also available to inflame. Histamine and various nicotinates are used in a wide variety of proprietary topical remedies for aches and pains.

Topical NSAIDs (numerous agents) may relieve local pain transiently.

Volatile aerosol sprays, beloved by sportspeople, produce analgesia by cooling and by placebo effect.

ANTIPRURITICS

Itch mechanisms are both peripheral and central. Impulses pass along the same nerve fibres as those of pain, but the sensation experienced differs qualitatively as well as quantitatively from pain. In the CNS endogenous opioid peptides are released and naloxone can relieve some cases of intractable itch. Local liberation of histamine and other autacoids in the skin also causes itch and may be responsible for much of the itch of urticarial allergic reactions. Many drugs, especially the morphine group, are known to be histamine liberators; bile salts also release histamine and this may explain some, but not all, of the itch of obstructive jaundice. It is likely that other chemical mediators, e.g. serotonin and prostaglandins, are involved.

Treatment of the underlying cause is obviously required, e.g. parasites, renal failure and reticuloses, but there remain those patients in whom the cause either cannot be removed or is not known. Scratching or rubbing seems to give relief by converting the intolerable persistent itch into a more bearable pain, and may even cure the itch at the cost of removing the epidermis. A vicious cycle can be set up in which itching provokes scratching and scratching leads to skin lesions which itch, as in *neurodermatitis*. Covering the lesion or enclosing it in plaster so as to prevent any further scratching or rubbing may help.

In *severe pruritus*, sedation is sometimes helpful during the day and a hypnotic is usually required at night. In chronic cases a sedative antidepressant may help.

Antihistamines (H_1-receptor) orally are used in pruritus, but except in urticarial conditions they probably act by their sedative effect; they should not be applied topically due to risk of allergy.

Any cooling application has some antipruritic effect, but a variety of substances, such as *phenol* menthol or camphor is often added because they have a reputation as antipruritics probably by weak local anaesthetic action. *Calamine* and astringents (aluminium acetate, tannic acid) may help, as may *coal tar*. *Local anaesthetics* do not offer any long-term solution and since they are liable to sensitise the skin they are best avoided; but lignocaine is least troublesome in this respect.

Chlorpromazine or a related drug, e.g. trimeprazine (Vallergan), sometimes helps, probably by altering the patient's attitude to the itching.

Crotamiton, an acaricide, is reputed to have a specific but unexplained antipruritic action,

although it may exacerbate an already inflamed skin; convenient proprietary preparations (Eurax) are available.

Topical *hydrocortisone* or fluorinated steroid preparations are probably the most effective antipruritics in local inflammatory conditions, e.g. eczema. Obviously they should not be used for generalised pruritus due to systemic disease (see below).

The itching of *obstructive jaundice* may be relieved by androgens but jaundice may increase. If obstruction is only partial, *cholestyramine* can be useful.

Pruritus ani is managed by meticulous hygiene and weak corticosteroid with antiseptic/anticandida application used as briefly as practicable (some cases are a form of neurodermatitis).

Local anaesthetics (of the *-caine* class) should be used briefly on a small area, if at all; contact allergy occurs.

ADRENOCORTICAL STEROIDS

So remarkable is the therapeutic effect of topical corticosteroids that professional dermatologists hardly expect to see a patient who has not already tried one and been disappointed.

Adrenal steroids topically are effective in suppressing inflammation in the skin (with vasoconstriction), particularly when there is an allergic factor; symptomatic relief can be dramatic. They also reduce epidermal cell division, which is useful in psoriasis. Since the cause of the lesion is not affected it is not surprising that relapse often follows when they are withdrawn. They must not be used in *infective* inflammation without effective accompanying chemotherapy because the infection will exacerbate and spread.

The difficulties and dangers of *systemic* adrenal steroid therapy are sufficient to restrict such use to serious conditions (such as pemphigus and generalised exfoliative dermatitis) not responsive to other forms of therapy.

Used with restraint topical corticosteroids are effective and safe.

Local applications of *fluorinated* steroids (particularly) can be absorbed from large areas (especially if occlusive dressings are used) in amounts sufficient to cause hypothalamic/pituitary/adrenal suppression and all the adverse effects of long-term use; they are teratogenic in animals and the risk for man is uncertain.

The most efficacious and potent steroids for use on the skin are the fluorinated compounds *clobetasol* and *halcinonide*. It is an excellent thing to have these highly potent substances, but their use carries particular responsibilities (above).

Guidelines for topical corticosteroids[3]

- Employ the weakest preparation that will control the disorder, especially if long-term use is likely.
- In cases likely to be resistant, use a high therapeutic potency preparation for 3 weeks to gain control, after which change to a less potent preparation.
- Advise the patient to apply the formulation very thinly, just enough to make the skin surface shine slightly.
- Prescribe in small amounts so that serious overuse is unlikely to occur without the doctor knowing, e.g. weekly quantity by group (Table 38.1): very potent 15 g; potent 30 g; others 50 g.
- Occlusive dressing should only be used briefly. NB. babies' plastic pants are an occlusive dressing as well as being a social amenity.

Choice

Corticosteroids are classified according to their *therapeutic potency (efficacy)* (according to drug and to % concentration). High potency preparations are commonly needed for lichen planus and discoid lupus erythematosus. Potent preparations for psoriasis, and weaker preparations (hydrocortisone 0.5–2.5%) are usually adequate for eczema.

When a skin disorder requiring a corticosteroid is already infected, a preparation containing an antimicrobial is used, e.g. neomycin, clotri-

mazole, nystatin, chlorquinaldol, clioquinol. When the infection is eliminated the corticosteroid may be continued alone.

It is inappropriate to use corticosteroid/antimicrobial preparations in the absence of initial infection.

Intralesional injections are occasionally used to provide high local concentrations without systemic effects in chronic dermatoses.

Adverse effects

Adverse effects are more likely with formulations ranked therapeutically as very potent or potent in Table 38.1.

Short-term use: spread of infection.

Long-term use: *skin atrophy* (which may or may not be fully reversible; can occur within 4 weeks); *striae* (irreversible); local hirsutism; *perioral dermatitis* (young women), which responds to steroid withdrawal and may be mitigated by a course of tetracycline (4–6 weeks); *depigmentation* (local); *acne* (local); potent corticosteroids should not be used on the face unless this is unavoidable; systemic absorption can lead to all the adverse effects of systemic corticosteroid use; enough absorption to suppress the hypothalamic/pituitary axis can occur with 20% of the body under an occlusive dressing with midly potent agents, but even without occlusion with the very potent agents.

Applications to the eye lids may get into the eye and cause glaucoma.

Rebound exacerbation of the disease can occur after abrupt cessation of therapy. This can lead the patient to reapply the steroid and so form a vicious cycle.

Occlusive dressings (see above) are particulary used with adrenal steroids in highly keratinised lesions, e.g. psoriasis. Dressings are generally kept in place for up to 2 days or only at night; *substantial absorption with systemic effects can occur*. Complications include infections (bacterial, monilial) and even heat stroke when large areas are occluded.

Allergy. Corticosteroids may cause contact dermatitis and the possibility of this should be considered where expected benefit fails to occur.

---

[3]Munro D D Prescriber's Journal 1977; 17: 84.

Table 38.1 Topical corticosteroid formulations conventionally ranked according to *therapeutic* potency, i.e. efficacy

Very potent	Clobetasol (0.05%) (also formulations of diflucortolone: halcinonide)
Potent	Beclomethasone (0.025%) (also formulations of betamethasone: budesonide, desonide, desoxymethasone, diflucortolone, fluclorolone, fluocinolone, fluocinonide)
Moderately potent	Clobetasone (0.05%) (also formulations of desoxymethasone: fluocinolone, fluocortolone, fluandrenolone, hydrocortisone plus urea)
Mildly potent	Hydrocortisone (0.1–2.5%) (also formulations of alclomethasone: fluocinolone, methylprednisolone)
Important note:	the ranking is based on agent *and* its concentration: the same drug appears in more than one rank.

SUNSCREENS, SUNBURN AND PHOTOSENSITIVITY

Ultraviolet (UV) solar radiation consists of:

- **UVA** (320–400 nanometres): causes skin cancer and skin ageing (damage to collagen)
- **UVB** (290–320 nm): causes sunburn and tanning, skin cancer and skin ageing
- **UVC** (200–290 nm) is prevented, at present, from reaching the earth at sea level by the stratospheric ozone layer, though it can cause skin injury at high mountain altitude.

Protection of the skin from UV radiation is effected by

- *absorbent sunscreens*: e.g. aminobenzoic acid and aminobenzoates (padimate O), benzophenones (mexenone, oxybenzone), cinnamates, dibenzoylmethanes.
- *reflectant sunscreens*: e.g. inert minerals such as titanium dioxide, zinc oxide, calamine: they are cosmetically unattractive.

The performance of a sunscreen is expressed as *sun protective factor* (SPF), which hitherto has referred mainly to UVB (UVA is more troublesome to measure); but the techniques are now being standardised and so the SPF is only a general guide. It is agreed that there should be protection against both UVB and UVA. Also, the washability of the preparation (including by sweat and swimming) is relevant to efficacy and to frequency of application; some penetrate the stratum corneum (padimate O) and are more persistent than others.

Despite the diversity the following guidance is offered:

Subjects who burn easily should use a preparation with SPF 15–20; it will reduce or prevent tanning as well as burn. If solar exposure is to be *prolonged* a sunscreen that, though it may be primarily effective against UVB, also offers protection against UVA should be chosen (benzophenones, dibenzoylmethanes, titanium dioxide). UVA protection is also needed by people having *photosensitivity* due to disease (photodermatoses) or to drugs (below).

Sunscreens can cause allergic dermatitis (but not titanium dioxide, though its vehicle may).

Numerous formulations are available (ingredients ought to be set out on the label).

Sunburn

Treatment of mild sunburn is usually with a lotion such as Oily Calamine Lotion. Severe cases are helped by Hydrocortisone Cream (1%). An NSAID can help if given early, by preventing the formation of prostaglandins, e.g. indomethacin.

Photosensitivity

Drug photosensitivity means that an adverse effect occurs as a result of drug plus light; sometimes even the amount of ultraviolet radiation from fluorescent tubes is sufficient. Drugs taken *systemically* that induce photosensitivity include: sulphonamides (including sulphonylurea hypoglycaemics, frusemide, thiazide diuretics), tetracyclines, griseofulvin, phenothiazines, nalidixic acid, oral contraceptives, chlordiazepoxide, amiodarone, piroxicam.

Substances that, applied *locally*, can produce photosensitivity include: various deodorant substances, halogenated salicylanilides, e.g. antimicrobials used in soaps, hexachlorophane, para-aminobenzoic acid and its esters (used as sunscreens), coal tar derivatives, juices of various plants.

There are two forms of photosensitivity:

- **Phototoxicity**: this is, like drug toxicity, a normal effect of too high a dose of UVB in a subject who has been exposed to the drug. The reaction is like severe sunburn. *The threshold returns to normal when the drug is stopped.*
- **Photoallergy**: is, like drug allergy, a cell-mediated immunological effect that occurs only in some people, and which may be severe with a small dose. Photoallergy due to drugs is the result of a photochemical reaction caused by UVA by which the drug combines with tissue protein to form an antigen. *Reactions may persist for years after the drug is withdrawn*; they are usually eczematous.

Systemic protection, as opposed to application of drug to exposed areas, should only be considered in the most severe cases of photosensitivity in which a patient is confined indoors. *Chloroquine* for short periods may be effective in polymorphic light eruptions.

Psoralens (obtained from citrus and other plants), e.g. methoxsalen, are used to induce photochemical reactions in the skin. After local or systemic administration of the psoralen and subsequent exposure to UVB there is an erythematous reaction that goes deeper than ordinary sunburn and that may only reach its maximum after 48 h (sunburn maximum: 12–24 h). Melanocytes are activated and pigmentation occurs over the following week. This action is used to repigment areas of disfiguring depigmentation. It is also used in some social suntan preparations (as oil of bergamot).

But in the presence of UVA the psoralen interacts with DNA and RNA and inhibits DNA synthesis. Psoralen plus UVA (PUVA) treatment is used in severe psoriasis (a disease characterised by increased epidermal proliferation), mycosis fungoides and some cases of lichen planus.

Severe adverse reactions can occur with psoralens and ultraviolet radiation, including increased risk of skin cancer (due to mutagenicity inherent in the action), cancer of the male genitalia, cataracts and accelerated skin ageing; the treatment is only used by specialists.

DERMAL ADVERSE DRUG REACTIONS

Drugs taken systemically or applied locally often cause rashes. These take many different forms and the same drug will produce different rashes in different people.

Contact dermatitis is commonly eczematous and is often caused by antimicrobials, local anaesthetics and antihistamines. It can also be due to the vehicle in which the active drug is applied.

Reactions to *systemically administered* drugs are commonly erythematous, like those of measles, scarlatina or erythema multiforme. They give no useful clue to the cause. They commonly occur during the first 2 weeks of therapy, but some immunological reactions may be delayed for months.

Though drugs may change, the clinical problems remain depressingly the same: a patient develops a rash; he is taking many different tablets; which, if any, of these caused his eruption, and what should be done about it? It is no answer simply to stop all drugs, though the fact that this can often be done casts some doubt on the patient's need for them in the first place. All too often potentially valuable drugs are excluded from further use on totally inadequate grounds. Clearly some guidelines are needed but no simple set of rules exists that can cover this complex subject . . .

The following questions should be asked in every case:[4]

- Can other skin diseases be excluded?
- Are the skin changes compatible with a drug cause?

---

[4] Hardie R A, Savin J A. Br Med J 1979; 1: 935, to whom we are grateful for this quotation and the following classification.

- Which drug is most likely to be responsible?
- Are any further tests worth while?
- Is any treatment needed?

These questions are deceptively simple but the answers are often difficult.

Drug-specific rashes

Despite great variability, some hints at drug-specific or characteristic rashes from drugs *taken systemically*, can be discerned, as follows:

Acne: e.g. corticosteroids, androgens.

Toxic erythema commonly occurs at about the 9th day of treatment (or day 2–3 in previously exposed patients); causes include antimicrobials especially ampicillin, sulphonamides and derivatives (sulphonylureas, frusemide and thiazide diuretics).

Erythema multiforme, including Stevens-Johnson syndrome: e.g. NSAIDs, sulphonamides, barbiturates, phenytoin.

Erythema nodosum: e.g. sulphonamides, oral contraceptives, prazosin.

Allergic vasculitis: e.g. sulphonamides, NSAIDs, thiazides, chlorpropamide, phenytoin.

Purpura: e.g. thiazides, sulphonamides, sulphonylures, phenylbutazone, quinine.

Eczema: e.g. penicillins, phenothiazines.

Exfoliative dermatitis and erythrodermia: gold, carbamazepine, allopurinol, penicillins, neuroleptics.

Photosensitivity: see above.

Lupus erythematosus: e.g. hydralazine, isoniazid, procainamide, phenytoin.

Lichenoid eruption: e.g. chloroquine, thiazides, frusemide, captopril, gold, phenothiazines.

Fixed eruptions are eruptions that recur at the same site, often circumoral, with each administration of the drug: e.g. phenolphthalein (laxative self-medication), sulphonamides, quinine, tetracycline, barbiturates, naproxen, nifedipine.

Toxic epidermal necrolysis: e.g. phenytoin, sulphonamides, penicillins, NSAIDs.

Urticaria, chronic: e.g. penicillins, enalapril, gold, NSAIDs, e.g. aspirin.

Pruritus unassociated with rash: e.g. oral contraceptives, phenothiazines, rifampicin (due to biliary stasis).

Hair loss: e.g. cytotoxic anticancer drugs, etretinate, oral contraceptives, heparin, androgenic steroids (women), sodium valproate, gold.

Pigmentation: e.g. oral contraceptives, phenothiazines, heavy metals, amiodarone, chloroquine (pigmentations of nails and palate, depigmentation of the hair).

Recovery after withdrawal of the causative drug generally begins in a few days, but lichenoid reactions may not improve until weeks have passed.

Diagnosis. Study of the patient's drug history may give clues. Reactions are commoner during early therapy (days) rather than after the drug has been given for months. Diagnosis by re-administration of the drug (challenge) is safe with fixed eruptions, but not with others, particulary those that may be part of a generalised effect, e.g. vasculitis.

Patch tests are useful in contact dermatitis, for they reproduce the causative process. Intradermal tests introduce all the problems of allergy to drugs, metabolism, combination with protein, risk of systemic reaction, etc. (see p. 127).

Treatment. Remove the cause; use cooling applications and antipruritics; adrenal steroid for severe cases; histamine H_1-receptor blocker systemically for acute urticaria.

TREATMENT OF INDIVIDUAL SKIN DISORDERS (SUMMARY)

The traditional advice, *if it's wet, dry it; if it's dry wet it*, contains enough truth to be worth repeating. One or two applications a day are all that is usually necessary unless common sense dictates otherwise.

Table 38.2 is not intended to give the complete treatment of even the commoner skin conditions but merely to indicate a reasonable approach.

Secondary infections of ordinarily uninfected lesions may require local or systemic antimicrobials in addition.

Analgesics, sedatives or tranquillisers may be needed in painful or uncomfortable conditions, or where the disease is intensified by emotion or anxiety. Antidepressants may be helpful even where clinical depression is not apparent, particularly in chronic diseases.

Table 38.2 Summary of treatment of skin disorders

Condition	Treatment	Remarks
Acne	see p. 645	
Alopecia: baldness: Alopecia areata	Topical minoxidil is worth trying if the patient is embarrassed by baldness. 'Cosmetically acceptable' results may occur in up to 50%, but the hair falls out if treatment stops	Most patients who take minoxidil orally for hypertension experience some increased hair growth. It may act by a mitogenic effect on hair follicles. The response occurs in 4–12 months: stop treatment if no result in 1 year
Dermatitis herpetiformis	Dapsone can be effective in 24 h, or sulphapyridine. Prolonged therapy necessary	Antipruritics locally as required. Not other sulphonamides; beneficial effect *not* due to antimicrobial action. Methaemoglobinaemia may complicate dapsone therapy
Eczema Acute weeping	Lotions (aluminium acetate, calamine), wet dressings or soaks (sodium chloride, potassium permanganate); topical corticosteroid with antimicrobial if infected	Remove the cause where possible. Often exacerbated by soap and water. Antipruritics (not antihistamines or local anaesthetics) may be added to lotions, creams or pastes
Subacute	Zinc oxide cream or paste, with mild keratolytic if skin thickening present (salicylic acid or coal tar added); topical corticosteroid	Gamolenic acid (Epogam, evening primrose oil) an essential fatty acid which is one of the cell wall precursors of immunomodulatory and anti-inflammatory prostaglandins. Taken
Chronic, with dry scaly lesions	Keratolytics and moisturising creams and emollients; topical corticosteroid	long-term, it may benefit atopic eczema, especially itch and scaling. Possibility of benefit in a variety of other diseases is being explored
Exfoliative dermatitis	Chelating agent if due to a heavy metal. Cooling creams and powders locally. Adrenal steroid systemically when severe	
Hirsutism in women	*In severe cases*: combined oestrogen/progestogen contraceptive pill: or cyproterone plus ethinyloestradiol (Dianette)	Local cosmetic approaches: *epilation* by wax or electrolysis: *depilation* (chemical), e.g. thioglycollic acid, barium sulphide
Hyperhidrosis	Astringents reduce sweat production, especially aluminium chloride hexahydrate (20%) in ethyl alcohol (95%). Antimuscarinics (topical) may help and high local concentrations can be obtained with iontophoresis. Surgery, cryotherapy or radiation in extreme cases	Treatment better in theory than in practice; the volume of sweat dilutes the application; the characteristic smell is produced by bacterial action, so cosmetic deodorants contain antibacterials rather than substances that reduce sweat production
Ichthyosis or xeroderma	Emollients to hydrate and smooth the skin, e.g. Emulsifying Ointment. Very severe variants may need tretinoin	Avoid degreasing skin, e.g. by domestic detergents
Infections	see p. 646	
Intertrigo	Cleansing lotions, powders	To cleanse, lubricate and reduce friction
Lichen planus	Antipruritics: topical corticosteroid (rarely systemic)	May be drug caused, e.g. a phenothiazine, antimalarial
Lichen simplex (neurodermatitis)	Antipruritics: topical corticosteroid; explain scratch-itch cycle to patient	Covering the lesion so as to prevent scratching sometimes breaks the vicious cycle

Table 38.2 Summary of treatment of skin disorders

Condition	Treatment	Remarks
Lupus erythematosus affecting the skin	Potent adrenal steroid topically or intralesionally. Chloroquine or hydroxychloroquine, but eye toxicity serious hazard	A systemic disease
Marginal blepharitis (various organisms)	Ointment containing adrenal steroid and an antimicrobial	Undue persistence can be due to allergy to treatment
Nappy rash	*Prevention*: rid nappies of soaps, detergents and ammonia by rinsing. Change frequently and use barrier cream to keep skin dry. *Cure*: mild: Zn cream or calamine lotion, plus above measures. Severe: adrenal steroid locally, plus antimicrobial	Costly disposable nappies are useful Absorption occurs from raw areas, especially under occulsive plastic pants
Pediculosis (lice) (head, body, genitals)	Malathion or carbaryl; (anticholinesterases; safety depends on more rapid metabolism in man than in insects, and low absorption)	Ritual of application important. Permethrin systhetic derivative of pyrethrum (genus *Chrysanthemum*) is an alternative
Pemphigus: pemphigoid	Adrenal steroids systemically: other immunosuppressives, e.g. azathioprine sometimes, gold	Oral hygiene and general nutrition very important
Photosensitivity see p. 639		
Pityriasis rosea	Antipruritics as appropriate	The disease is self-limiting
Pruritus see p. 637		
Psoriasis see p. 644		
Rosacea	Topical benzoyl peroxide. Tetracycline, metronidazole, orally: mechanism unknown	Corticosteroid exacerbates. Flushing makes it worse. Oestrogens for menopausal flushing
Scabies (*Sarcoptes scabiei*)	Benzyl Benzoate Applic. or monosulfiram or lindane to whole body below the neck. Alternative: crotamiton	Correct ritual is essential. Crotamiton is also antipruritic and is useful as a supplementary application, to reduce persistent itch
Scleroderma	No proved therapy	
Serborrhoeic dermatitis: dandruff (*Pityriasis capitis*)	*Acute*. Adrenal steroid lotions (Betnovate or Dermovate scalp applications) and frequent use of soapless shampoos (1% cetrimide (Cetavlon) shampoo) *Chronic*. Regular shampooing with detergent shampoo with or without pryrithione zinc or other antiseptic helps mild cases. More severe cases need a mild keratolytic, e.g. coal tar in a liquid application. Occasional corticosteroid application helps where there is much inflammation	Antimicrobials if badly infected. Sulphur in various forms helps the seborrhoeic state but the reason is not known. Selenium irritates the eye, is poisonous if swallowed, and offers no advantage. Lithium ointment may benefit
Sunburn see p. 639		
Urticaria see p. 645		
Vitiligo	No safe and reliable treatment. Methoxsalen or other psoralen, topically or systemically, plus daily exposure to UVA (PUVA) is toxic, troublesome and often fails. Use cover-up cosmetics	Probably an autoimmune disease

Table 38.2 Summary of treatment of skin disorders

Condition	Treatment	Remarks
Warts	All treatments are *destructive* and should be applied with precision. Cryotherapy (liquid nitrogen, solid CO_2). Salicylic acid 12% in collodion daily. Many other caustic (keratolytic) preparations. Salicylic and lactic acid paint or gel. For plantar warts formaldehyde or glutaraldehyde: podophyllin (antimitotic) for plantar or anogenital warts. Follow the manufacturer's instructions meticulously	Non-surgical remedies may act by disrupting the wart so that virus is absorbed, antibodies develop and the wart is rejected immunologically. Warts often disappear spontaneously
X-ray dermatitis	Adrenal steroid locally	

Preparations for use on the skin. At the time of writing there are in the UK about 280 preparations for medical prescription (excluding minor variants and many of those on direct sale to the public). It is not practicable to give other than general guidance on choice. Physicians will select a modest range of products and get to know these well.

Psoriasis

In psoriasis there is increased ($\times 10$) epidermal undifferentiated cell proliferation with consequent increased numbers of horn cells that contain abnormal keratin; no normal stratum corneum is formed. Drugs are used to *dissolve keratin* (keratolysis) and to *inhibit cell division*.

The proliferated cells may be removed by scrubbing followed by a *dithranol* (antimitotic) ointment applied accurately to the lesions (but not on the face) for 1 hour and removed beginning with 0.1% and increasing to 1%; it stains skin and fabrics; it is used daily until the lesions have disappeared; it is irritant to normal skin. *Tar* preparations are less effective alternatives, and are commonly used for psoriasis of the scalp.

Topical adrenal steroids reduce epidermal cell division and application, especially under occlusive dressings, can be very effective, but increasing doses (concentrations) become needed and rebound follows withdrawal. They should only be used if dithranol or tar-containing preparations have failed or produced complications. *Systemic* corticosteroid administration should be avoided if at all possible (except for very brief use in very severe exacerbations), for high doses are needed to suppress the disease, which is liable to recur when treatment is withdrawn, as it must be if complications of long-term steroid therapy are to be avoided.

Calcipotriol is an analogue of calcitriol, the most active natural form of vitamin D (p. 653). Used topically it appears to be about as effective as dithranol and corticosteroid. It inhibits cell proliferation and encourages cell differentiation. Although it has less effect on calcium metabolism than does calcitrol, excessive use can raise the plasma calcium concentration.

Vitamin A (retinols) plays a role in epithelial function and the retinoic acid derivative, **etretinate** (Tigason, orally), inhibits psoriatic hyperkeratosis over 4–6 weeks. It is a prodrug for the active acitretin. It should be used in courses (6–9 months) with intervals (3–4 months). It is *teratogenic*, like other vitamin A derivatives. Rigorous precautions for use in women of childbearing potential are laid down by the manufacturer and *must* be followed, including contraception for *2 years* after cessation, because the drug is stored in the liver and in fat and released over many months. It has a plasma $t_{\frac{1}{2}}$ of 3 months. It can cause other serious toxicity (see Vitamin A).

A *psoralen* followed by ultraviolet light (PUVA) is used in severe cases, see Psoralens above. It may be combined with UVB and methotrexate.

Folic acid antagonists, e.g. methotrexate, also suppress epidermal activity temporarily, as does *cyclosporin*, but they are too toxic for use unless the psoriasis is life-threatening or severely disabling, and preferably patients should be past their reproductive years.

It is plain from this brief outline that treatment of psoriasis requires considerable judgement, and it is no surprise that patients have formed a Psoriasis Association.

Acne

Acne results from disordered function of the pilosebaceous follicle whereby abnormal keratin, and sebum (the production of which is androgen driven), form debris which plugs the mouth of the follicle. *Propionibacterium acnes* colonises the debris. Bacterial action releases inflammatory fatty acids from the sebum.

The following measures are used progressively and selectively as the disease is more severe; they may need to be applied for up to 6 months:

• Frequent *skin cleansing* and *degreasing*, including weak antiseptics and detergents, e.g. soap and water (mere washing usefully interrupts the logarithmic microbial growth), cetrimide, weak alcoholic solutions.

• Mild *keratolytic* (exfoliating, peeling) formulations to unblock pilosebaceous ducts, e.g. benzoyl peroxide, sulphur, salicylic acid.

• *Systemic antimicrobial therapy* (a tetracycline, erythromycin, co-trimoxazole at low dose) is used over months (response begins after 2 months). Bacterial resistance is not a problem; benefit is due to suppression of bacterial lipolysis of sebum, which generates inflammatory fatty acids. Raised intracranial pressure with loss of vision has occurred with tetracycline used thus.

• A topical *adrenal steroid* reduces inflammation.

• *Vitamin A (retinoic acid) derivatives* reduce sebum production and keratinisation. Vitamin A is a teratogen.

Tretinoin (Retin-A) is applied topically (*not* in combination with other keratolytics). It may promote UV-induced skin cancer. It should be avoided in pregnancy. Benefit is seen in about 10 weeks.

Isotretinoin (Roaccutane) orally is highly effective (in courses of 12–16 weeks), but is known to be a serious teratogen; *its use should be confined to the most severe cystic and conglobate cases*, and requires the utmost informed care and supervision. Women of child-bearing potential should be carefully informed on this risk, should be pregnancy-tested before commencement and should use contraception for 4 weeks before, during and for 4 weeks after cessation.[5]

• *Hormone therapy*. The objective is to reduce androgen production or effect by using, (a) oestrogen, to suppress hypothalamic/pituitary gonadotrophin production, or (b) an antiandrogen (cyproterone). An oestrogen alone as initial therapy to get the acne under control or, in women, the cyclical use of an oral contraceptive containing 50 µg of oestrogen diminishes sebum secretion by 40%. A combination of ethinyloestradiol and cyproterone (Dianette) orally is also effective in women (it has contraceptive effect, which is desirable as the cyproterone may feminise a male fetus).

• *Topical corticosteroid* should *not* be used.

Urticaria

Acute urticaria (named after its similarity to the sting of a nettle, *Urtica*) and *angioedema* usually respond well to H_1-antihistamines, although severe cases are relieved more quickly by adrenaline (Adrenaline Inj., 1 mg/ml: 0.1–0.3 ml, s.c.). A systemic corticosteroid may be needed in severe cases.

Cold urticaria is due to release of autacoids on exposure to cold. It may respond to combined H_1- and H_2-receptor antagonists; the combination is needed fully to block the vascular effects

---

[5] The risk of serious birth defect in a child of a woman who has taken isotretinoin when pregnant is estimated at 25%. Thousands of abortions have been done in such women. It is probable that hundreds of damaged children have been born. There can be no doubt that there has been irresponsible prescribing of this drug, e.g. to less severe cases. The fact that a drug having such grave effect is yet permitted to be available is a tribute to its high efficacy.

of histamine, which cause flush and hypotension. Cyproheptadine is usually preferred as the H_1-antihistamine.

Chronic urticaria may respond to an H_1-antihistamine plus ephedrine or terbutaline, or to a H_1-plus a H_2-antihistamine.

Hereditary angioedema, with deficiency of Cl esterase (a complement inhibitor), does not respond to antihistamines or corticosteroid but only to *fresh frozen plasma*. Delay in initiating treatment may lead to death from laryngeal oedema (try adrenaline i.m. in severe cases). For long-term prophylaxis androgen (stanozolol, danazol) is effective.

Skin infections

Superficial bacterial infections e.g. impetigo, eczema, are commonly staphylococcal or streptococcal. They are treated by a topical antimicrobial for less than 2 weeks; applied twice daily after removal of crusts that prevent access of the drug, e.g. by a povidone iodine preparation. Very extensive cases need systemic treatment.

Neomycin and *mupirocin* are preferred (as they are not ordinarily used for systemic infections and therefore development of drug resistant strains is less likely to have serious consequences). *Absorption of neomycin from all topical preparations can have serious consequences for the eighth cranial nerve. Framycetin is similar.*

Fusidic acid may be used, but only outside hospital as it may be needed for systemic infection.

Where prolonged treatment is required topical antiseptics (hexachlorophane, povidone-iodine, cetrimide, chlorhexidine) are preferred and bacterial resistance is less of a problem. Combination of antimicrobial with a *corticosteriod* (to suppress inflammation) is not generally useful but, if used, there *must* be *effective* antimicrobial treatment or the infection may spread.

The disadvantages of antibiotics are *contact allergy* and developments of *resistant organisms* (which may cause systemic, as well as local, infection). Failure to respond may be due to development of contact allergy (which may be masked by corticosteroid).

Infected leg ulcers generally do not benefit from antimicrobials. An antiseptic (plus a protective dressing with compression) is preferred if antimicrobial therapy is needed.

Nasal carriers of staphylococci may be cured (often temporarily) by mupirocin or neomycin plus chlorhexidine.

Formulations of antibacterials with and without corticosteroid are numerous.

Deep bacterial infections, e.g. boils, generally do not require antimicrobial therapy; but if they do it should be systemic. Cellulitis requires systemic chemotherapy.

Infected burns are treated with a variety of antimicrobials, including silver sulphadiazine and mupirocin.

Topical antifungals include: amphotericin, benzoic acid, benzoyl peroxide, clotrimazole, econazole, ketoconazole, miconazole, natamycin, naftifine, nystatin, salicylic acid, tioconazole, tolnaftate, undecenoates, e.g. of zinc.

Systemic antifungals for skin infections: griseofulvin, ketoconazole, terbinafine.

Topical antivirals: acyclovir: idoxuridine

Topical parasiticides (best as lotions): benzyl benzoate, monosulfiram, malathion, carbaryl, crotamiton, lindane.

Disinfection and cleansing of the skin. Numerous substances are used according to circumstances: ethanol or isopropyl alcohol (70%), chlorhexidine, cationic surfactants (benzalkonium, cetrimide), povidone-iodine (iodine complexed with polyvinylpyrollidone), phenol derivatives (chloroxylenol, hexachlorophane, triclosan).

GUIDE TO FURTHER READING

Brown D G et al 1971 Psychiatric treatment of eczema: a contolled trial. British Medical Journal 2: 729

Editorial 1988 Are insect repellents safe? Lancet 2: 610

Editorial 1991 Protecting man from UV exposure. Lancet 337: 1258

Finch R 1988 Skin and soft tissue infections. Lancet 1: 164

Greaves M W 1990 The new dermatology. British Medical Journal 300: 413

Murphy G M et al 1988 Acne and psoriasis. British Medical Journal 296: 546

Newbold P C H 1988 Antidepressants and skin disease. British Medical Journal 296: 379

Shrand A B 1989 Treating young men with hair loss. British Medical Journal 298:847

Simpson N 1986 Unwanted hair. British Medical Journal 293: 348

Simpson N 1988 Treating hyperhidrosis. British Medical Journal 296: 1345

Stern R S et al 1990 Genital tumours among men with psoriasis exposed to psoralens and ultraviolet A radiation (PUVA) and ultraviolet B radiation. New England Journal of Medicine 322: 1093

39

Vitamins, calcium, bone

SYNOPSIS

The principally *pharmacological* aspects of vitamins are described here. The *nutritional* aspects, physiological function, sources, daily requirements and deficiency syndromes (primary and secondary) are to be found in any textbook of Medicine.

- Vitamin A: retinol
- Vitamin B: complex
- Vitamin C: ascorbic acid
- Vitamin D, calcium, parathyroid hormone, calcitonin, biphosphonates, bone
- Treatment of calcium and bone disorders
- Vitamin E: tocopherol
- Vitamin K, see Chapter 27

Vitamins are substances that are essential for normal metabolism and must be chiefly supplied in the diet.

Man cannot synthesise any vitamins in his body except some vitamin D in the skin and nicotinamide from tryptophan. Lack of a particular vitamin may lead to a specific deficiency syndrome. This may be *primary* (inadequate diet), or *secondary*, due to failure of absorption (intestinal abnormality or chronic diarrhoea), or to increased metabolic need (growth, pregnancy, lactation, hyperthyroidism, fever).

Vitamin deficiencies are commonly multiple, and complex clinical pictures occur. There are numerous single and multivitamin preparations to provide prophylaxis and therapy.

It has often been suggested, but never proved, that subclinical vitamin deficiencies are a cause of much chronic ill-health and liability to infections. This idea has led to enormous consumption of vitamin preparations, which, for most consumers, probably have no more than placebo value. Fortunately most of the vitamins are comparatively non-toxic, but *prolonged administration of vitamins A and D can have serious ill-effects.*

A controversy has erupted over the validity of studies that purport to show that multivitamin supplements enhance intelligence in children. On present evidence the association, if any, could well be due to chance (see reference in Guide to Further Reading).

Vitamins fall into two groups:

- **water-soluble vitamins**: the B group and C
- **fat-soluble vitamins**: A, D, K and E.

VITAMIN A: RETINOL

Vitamin A is a generic term embracing substances having the biological actions of *retinol* and related substances (which are called *retinoids*). The principal functions of retinol are to sustain normal epithelia to form retinal (eye) photochemicals, to enhance immune functions and to protect against infections and probably some cancers. Deficiency of retinol leads to metaplasia and hyperkeratosis throughout the body. This metaplasia is reminiscent of the early stage of transformation of normal tissue to cancer.

Retinol and derivatives are used in doses above those needed in nutrition, i.e. pharmacotherapy, in dyskeratotic skin diseases (psoriasis, acne) and are being explored, with some success, in the prevention of cancers and infections.

Tretinoin is retinoic acid. It is used in *acne* by topical application, see p. 645.

Isotretinoin is a retinoic acid derivative ($t_\frac{1}{2}$ 20 h). It is used orally in *acne*, see p. 645. It is effective in preventing second primary tumours in patients who have been treated for squamous-cell carcinoma of the head and neck.

Etretinate is a retinoic acid derivative ($t_\frac{1}{2}$ 90 d). It is used orally for *psoriasis*, see p. 644.

Retinol itself is used in prevention and treatment of deficiency.

Measles. There is evidence that vitamin A deficiency, whether primary in malnourished children, or secondary to the infection, occurs in severe measles and increases the morbidity and mortality (pneumonia, diarrhoea) by enhancing the liability of vitamin deficient epithelia to infection. A randomised controlled trial in 189 children suggests that 'all children with severe measles should be given vitamin A supplements'.[1] The dose used in children was 200 000 IU orally on each of the first 2 days: 2 died in the treated group; 10 died in the placebo group.

Adverse effects

Toxic effects occur with prolonged high intake (in children 25 000 to 500 000 IU daily). A diagnostic sign of *chronic poisoning* is the presence of painful tender swellings on the long bones. Anorexia, skin lesions, hair loss, hepatosplenomegaly, papilloedema, bleeding and general malaise also occur. Vitamin A is very cumulative (it is stored in liver and fat) and effects take weeks to wear off. Most cases of vitamin A poisoning have been due to mothers administering large amounts of fish-liver oils to their children in the belief that it was good for them.

Chronic overdose also causes an increased liability of biological membranes and of the outer layer of the skin to peel off. An extreme example of this is the case of the hungry Antarctic explorer who in 1913 ate the liver of his husky sledge dogs. His feet felt sore and

the sight of my feet gave me quite a shock, for the thickened skin of the soles had separated in each case as a complete layer. . . .I did what appeared to be the best thing under the circumstances: smeared the new skin with lanoline. . .and with bandages bound the skin soles back in place.[2]

Vitamin A and its derivatives are teratogenic at above physiological doses, i.e. with pharmacotherapy. See use in *acne* and *psoriasis* for precautions. Misguided pregnant health enthusiasts may take enough self-prescribed supplements to hazard a fetus. The Teratology Society advises that supplements should not exceed 8000 IU (2400 μg) per day.

Acute overdose: travellers have been made ill by eating the livers of Arctic carnivores.

Eskimos never eat polar-bear liver, knowing it to be toxic, and husky dogs, with instinctive wisdom, also avoid it. . .Those who pooh-pooh the Eskimos' fears or the husky dogs' instincts and are tempted to enjoy a man's portion of polar-bear liver — appetites get sharp near the North Pole — will consume anything up to 10 000 000 IU of vitamin A (normal daily requirement is 5000 IU). This is too much of a good thing, and the diner will

[1] Hussey G D et al. New Eng J Med 1990; 323: 160.

[2] Shearman J C, Vitamin A and Sir Douglas Mawson. Br Med J 1978; 1: 283.

probably soon find himself drowsy, then overcome by headache and vomiting, and finally losing the outer layer of his skin.[3]

VITAMIN B COMPLEX

A number of widely differing substances are now, for convenience, classed the 'vitamin B complex'. Those used for pharmacotherapy include:

Thiamine (B_1) is used orally for nutritional purposes, but is given i.v. in serious emergencies, e.g. Wernicke–Korsakoff syndrome, when it can cause anaphylactic shock; the injection should be given over 10 min (or i.m.).

Cobalamins (B_{12}): see Ch. 28.

Folic acid: see Ch. 28.

Methylfolate may be deficient in some psychiatric patients and daily oral administration (in addition to standard drug therapy) in depression and schizophrenia may promote clinical and social recovery.[4]

Folate supplements (periconceptional) prevent neural tube defects (spina bifida), in second pregnancies in women who have already given birth to a defective child, see p. 500.

Pyridoxine (B_6) is a coenzyme (including decarboxylases) for transamination and is concerned with many metabolic processes. Heavy overdose causes peripheral neuropathy.

Pyridoxine may sometimes benefit premenstrual tension (see p. 609), vomiting of pregnancy and radiation sickness.

Isoniazid interferes with pyridoxine (there are structural resemblances) and causes a pyridoxine-deficiency peripheral neuritis that can be prevented by adding pyridoxine, without antagonising the antibacterial effect.

Pyridoxine, even in small doses, can block the therapeutic effect of *levodopa* in parkinsonism, by enhancing its decarboxylation to dopamine, which does not enter the brain. It does not interfere with the combined levodopa/ decarboxylase preparations because of the presence of the decarboxylase inhibitor.

Homocystinuria: some cases benefit.

Niacin (nicotinic acid, nicotinamide) (B_7) is an essential part of co-dehydrogenases I and II, and so it is present in every living cell.

Adverse effects do not occur with standard doses of *nicotinamide*. *Nicotinic acid*, which is converted into nicotinamide, causes peripheral vasodilation accompanied by an unpleasant flushing and itching, and the patient may faint.

Nicotinic acid is used in some hyperlipidaemias, see p. 455.

VITAMIN C: ASCORBIC ACID

Deficiency of ascorbic acid leads to *scurvy*,[5] which is characterised by petechial haemorrhages, haematomas, bleeding gums (if teeth are present) and anaemia. It has a memorable place in the history of therapeutic measurement.

Scurvy had been a scourge for thousands of years, particularly amongst sailors on long voyages. In 1753, Dr. James Lind performed a simple *controlled therapeutic trial* on 12 sailors with advanced scurvy. They were all on the same basic diet and were living in the same quarters on board ship at sea. He divided them into pairs and dosed each pair differently. The respective daily treatments were:

- cider
- sulphuric acid
- sea-water
- vinegar
- a concoction of garlic, mustard, balsam and myrrh
- two oranges and a lemon.

The pair receiving the oranges and lemon recovered and were back on duty within a week; of the others, only the pair taking cider was slightly improved. The efficacy of oranges and lemons in the prevention and cure of scurvy was repeatedly confirmed; but 40 years were to pass before any official attention was paid and a regular daily allowances of lemon juice provided in

---

[3] Editorial. Br Med J 1962; 1: 855.
[4] Godfrey PSA et al. Lancet 1990; 336: 392.

[5] Only man (and other primates), guinea-pigs, the Indian fruit bat and the red-vented bulbul (a bird) get scurvy; other animals are able to synthesise ascorbic acid for themselves.

the Navy. Unfortunately lime juice[6] was soon substituted for lemon juice because it could be had cheaply in the West Indian colonies. Lime juice contains only about a third as much ascorbic acid as lemon juice and failed to prevent scurvy completely. Synthetic ascorbic acid has been available since the 1930s.

Function

Ascorbic acid is required for the synthesis of collagen. It is also a powerful reducing agent (antioxidant) and plays a part in intracellular oxidation-reduction systems, and in mopping up oxidants (free radicals) produced endogenously or in the environment, e.g. cigarette smoke (see vitamin E).

Indications for ascorbic acid

- The prevention and cure of scurvy.
- Urinary acidification (rarely appropriate).
- Methaemoglobinaemia, for its properties as a reducing agent (see below).
- Coryza: it is possible that 'megadoses', large daily doses (1 g or more/day) of ascorbic acid (daily requirement 60 mg) may reduce the incidence and severity of coryza. Reliable trials in this disease are difficult and the results are inconclusive. To justify use of such doses in populations, benefit must be shown to be clinically, as well as statistically, significant; and harm insignificant. This has not been achieved.
- Persistent claims that ascorbic acid is effective treatment in advanced cancer (historical controls were used), receive no support from a double-blind random controlled therapeutic trial (see Guide to Futher Reading).

Adverse effects

Ill-effects do not occur at ordinary doses; it is eliminated in the urine unchanged and metab-

olised to oxalate. High doses may cause sleep disturbances, headaches and gut upsets.

Doses above 4 g/day, which have been taken over long periods in the hope of preventing coryza, increase urinary oxalate concentration sufficiently to form oxalate stones. Intravenous ascorbic acid may precipitate a haemolytic attack in subjects with glucose-6-phosphate dehydrogenase deficiency.

Methaemoglobinaemia

A reducing substance is needed to convert the methaemoglobin (ferric iron) back to oxyhaemoglobin (ferrous iron) whenever enough has formed seriously to impair the oxygen carrying capacity of the blood. Ascorbic acid is non-toxic (it acts by direct reduction) but is less effective than methylene blue. Both can be given orally, i.v. or i.m. Excessive doses of methylene blue can *cause* methaemoglobinaemia (it acts by stimulating NADPH-dependent enzymes).

Methaemoglobinaemia may be *drug-induced* by: phenacetin,[7] sulphonamides, nitrites, nitrates (may occur in drinking water), primaquine, sulfones, -caine local anaesthetics, dapsone, nitrofurantoin, nitroprusside, vitamin K analogues, chlorates, aniline and nitrobenzene. In the rare instance of there being urgency, methylene blue 1 mg/kg slowly i.v. benefits within 30 min. (Ascorbic acid competes directly with the chemical cause and is inadequate in severe cases, which are the only ones that need treatment.)

In the *congenital form* oral methylene blue with or without ascorbic acid gives benefit in days to weeks.

Methylene blue turns the urine blue and high concentrations can irritate the urinary tract, so that fluid intake should be high when big doses are used.

Sulphaemoglobinaemia cannot be treated by drugs. It can be caused by phenacetin, sulphonamides, nitrites or nitrates.

---

[6] Hence the term 'limey' for British sailors; generally now used pejoratively, principally by Australians.

[7] Phenacetin has been withdrawn in the UK and in many other countries.

VITAMIN D, CALCIUM, PARATHYROID HORMONE, CALCITONIN, BIPHOSPHONATES, BONE

The agents are closely interrelated and will be discussed together.

Vitamin D

Vitamin D comprises a number of structurally related sterol compounds having similar biological properties in that they prevent or cure the vitamin D deficiency disease, rickets:

- **D₂ or ergocalciferol** (calciferol) made by ultraviolet irradiation of ergosterol
- **D₃ or cholecalciferol**, made by ultraviolet irradiation of 7-dehydrocholesterol; it is the form that occurs in natural foods and is formed in the skin.

The above, D₂, D₃, are *25-hydroxylated* into more active forms in the *liver*, which are then 1α-hydroxylated in the *kidney* (under the control of parathormone) into the most active form. Thus the most active natural form of vitamin D is 1α-25-dihydroxycholecalciferol and this is available as **calcitriol**. In renal disease this final rate-limited renal α-hydroxylation is inadequate, and administration of the less biologically active precursors is therefore liable to lack efficacy.

But in 1978 there was introduced a 1α-hydoxylated form (1α-hydroxycholecalciferol) **alfacalcidol** (One-Alpha), that only requires hepatic 25-hydroxylation to become the highly active 1α-25-dihydroxycholecalciferol (calcitriol). Alfacalcidol (and of course calcitriol) is therefore effective in the presence of renal failure since the defective renal hydroxylation stage has been by-passed. Its extraordinary potency and efficacy is indicated by the adult dose, often only 1–2 µg/day.

In addition there is a structural variant of vitamins D₂ and D₃, **dihydrotachysterol** (AT10, Tachyrol), which is also biologically activated by *hepatic* 25-hydroxylation.

The advantages of *alfacalcidol* and *dihydro-tachysterol* include a faster onset (below) and shorter duration of *clinical* effect (days) than vitamins D₂ and D₃ (weeks). But these factors are not relevant to the ordinary management of vitamin D deficiency.

Actions are complex. Vitamin D promotes the active transport (absorption) of calcium and therefore of phosphate from the gut, to control, with parathormone, the mineralisation of bone and to promote the renal tubular reabsorption of calcium and phosphate. The plasma calcium concentration rises. After a dose of D₂ or D₃ there is a lag of about 21 h before the intestinal effect begins and this is probably due to the time needed for its metabolic conversion to the more active forms. But after the biologically active calcitriol the lag is only 2 h.

A large single dose of vitamin D has biological effects for as long as 6 months (because of metabolism and storage, knowledge of the plasma $t_{\frac{1}{2}}$ is of no practical importance). Thus the drug is cumulative and overdose by a mother anxious that her child shall have strong bones can cause serious toxicity.

Epileptic patients on long-term anticonvulsant therapy may develop osteomalacia (adults) or rickets (children). This may be due to enzyme induction increasing vitamin D metabolism and causing deficiency, or there may be inhibition of one of the hydroxylations that increase biological activity or an effect on calcium metabolism.

Indications for vitamin D are the prevention and cure of rickets of all kinds and osteomalacia and the symptomatic treatment of some cases of hypoparathyroidism; also psoriasis (see p. 644).

In osteomalacia secondary to steatorrhoea or renal disease there is defective absorption of calcium from the gut and large amounts of vitamin D are often needed to enhance absorption.

Dosage (1.0 µg = 40 IU). The therapeutic dose for primary, diet-deficiency rickets is 3000–4000 IU per day, but much more may be needed daily in malabsorption syndromes, e.g. 40 000 IU, or renal osteodystrophy (200 000 IU), and dosage must then be carefully controlled by measuring plasma calcium concentrations (a rise in total calcium above 2.75 mmol/l (11 mg/100 ml) is dangerous).

Prophylactic dose in diet-deficient people is about 1000 IU/day for a few months, then adequate diet.

The maximum antirachitic effect of vitamin D is delayed for 1–2 months and the plasma calcium concentration reflects the dosage given days or weeks before. Frequent changes of dose are thus pointless and confuse the picture.

Preparations are many and the choice is not critical, though the elderly with nutritional osteomalacia due to malabsorption are often best managed by Calciferol Inj. i.m., 6–12 monthly (eliminating problems or patient compliance and gut malabsorption) with biochemical monitoring.

It is important to recognise that, because of the need for very big doses in certain vitamin D-resistant cases, there is an *unusually wide range of dosage in single tablets* available, e.g. Calcium and Ergocalciferol Tabs contain 10 µg (400 IU) ergocalciferol. Special high dose Tabs (informally termed Strong or High Strength, but misleadingly named Calciferol Tabs BP) contain *enormous* doses: 10 000 IU (250 µg) and 50 000 IU (1250 µg). They are only for use in exceptional circumstances, e.g. hypoparathyroidism or metabolic rickets; their inadvertent administration to children can lead to disaster.

Alfacalcidol is an alternative to calciferol that may be used for some forms of metabolic rickets; it acts more quickly, i.e. in days rather than in weeks (see above). *Calcipotriol* is an analogue used for psoriasis (p. 644).

Symptoms of overdose are due mainly to excessive rise in plasma calcium. General effects include: malaise, drowsiness, nausea, abdominal pain, thirst, constipation and loss of appetite. Other long-term effects include ectopic calcification almost anywhere in the body, renal damage and an increased calcium output in the urine; renal calculi may be formed. It is dangerous to exceed 10 000 IU daily of vitamin D in an adult for more than about 12 weeks.

Much vitamin D toxicity is due to well-meaning, but needless, administration by parents. The US Food and Drug Administration warn that intake of fortified diet supplements should not exceed 400 IU a day.

Patients with *sarcoidosis* are intolerant of vitamin D possibly even to the tiny amount present in a normal diet, and to that synthesised in their skin by sunlight. The intolerance may be due to over production of calcitriol (see above) by macrophages activated by interferon; the overproduction is reversed by corticosteroid.

Adrenal steroids antagonise vitamin D by an uncertain mechanism and are used in the treatment of hypercalcaemic sarcoidosis and of severe hypervitaminosis D.

TREATMENT OF CALCIUM AND BONE DISORDERS

Tetany

In acute hypocalcaemia requiring systemic therapy *calcium gluconate* is given slowly i.v.; dihydrotachysterol is also used to increase Ca absorption; it acts quicker than vitamin D_2 or D_3.

Dietary calcium is increased by giving calcium gluconate (an effervescent tablet is available) or lactate, and this and vitamin D (in high dose) may be needed long-term for chronic cases, e.g. of hypoparathyroidism. *Aluminium hydroxide* binds phosphate in the gut causing hypophosphataemia, which stimulates renal formation of the most active vitamin D metabolite and so enhances calcium absorption.

Calcium Gluconate Inj. is given i.v. as a 10% solution, 10–20 ml being given at the rate of about 2 ml per min and repeated as necessary (every few hours). It must not be given i.m. as it is painful and causes necrosis. *Calcium glubionate* (Calcium Sandoz) can be given by deep i.m. injection in adults.

Adverse effects of intravenous calcium may be very dangerous. An early sign is tingling in the mouth and a feeling of warmth spreading over the body. Serious effects are those on the heart, which mimic and synergise with digitalis; fatal cardiac arrest may occur in digitalised animals and it would seem advisable to avoid i.v. calcium in any patient on a digitalis glycoside (except in severe symptomatic hypocalcaemia); indeed, reduction of ionised calcium by a chelating agent has been successful in treating digitalis dysrhythmia. The effect of calcium on the heart is antagonised by potassium and similarly the toxic effects of a high serum potassium in acute renal failure may be to some extent counteracted with calcium.

Hypercalcaemia

Treatment of severe acute hypercalcaemia causing symptoms is needed whether or not the cause can be removed; generally a plasma concentration of 3.0 mmol/l (12 mg/100 ml) needs urgent treatment if there is also clinical evidence of toxicity (individual tolerance varies greatly).

Temporary measures

After taking account of the patient's cardiac and renal function, the following measures may be employed selectively:

- First, correct *dehydration* and even *force fluid* to enhance renal calcium elimination; consider adding a high-efficacy *loop diuretic* (frusemide) for further effect (not a thiazide which increases renal reabsorption of calcium); careful attention to fluid balance and plasma electrolytes, including potassium, is essential.
- An *adrenocortical steroid*, e.g. prednisolone 20–40 mg/d orally, reduces intestinal absorption of calcium and may inhibit osteolytic cancer but it takes several days to work and has no effect in hyperparathyroidism. It is most effective in vitamin D intoxication and sarcoid.
- Hypercalcaemia due to cancer or hyperparathyroidism may be reduced by a single dose of *plicamycin* (p. 656); maximum effect is in 4 days.
- *Biphosphonates* (p. 656). Pamidronate is preferred; it is given i.v. in hypercalcaemia of malignant disease; it acts in 1–2 days and a dose lasts 3–4 weeks. Clodronate is an alternative (oral or i.v.).

Phosphate i.v. is quickly effective, but rarely used as it is hazardous, precipitating calcium in soft tissues including the kidney. When the hypercalcaemia is at least partly due to mobilisation from bone, *calcitonin* can be used to inhibit bone resorption, and it may enhance urinary excretion of calcium; the effect develops in a few hours, and responsiveness may be lost over a few days (and may sometimes be restored by an adrenal steroid).

- *Trisodium edetate* (therapeutically equivalent to disodium edetate) i.v. can be used; it chelates calcium and the inert complex is excreted by glomerular filtration; it is rapidly effective.
- *Gallium nitrate* is a reserve drug for hypercalcaemia due to cancer; it inhibits osteoclastic bone resorption; it is nephrotoxic.
- *Dialysis* is quick and effective and is likely to be needed in severe cases or with renal failure.

The above measures are temporary only, to give time to tackle the cause.

For long-term use

To bind dietary calcium in the gut sodium *cellulose phosphate* (Calcisorb) is an oral ion exchange substance with a particular affinity for calcium. Bound calcium is eliminated in the faeces. It is used particularly for patients who overabsorb dietary calcium and who develop hypercalciuria and renal stones.

Inorganic phosphate, e.g. sodium acid phosphate (Phosphate Sandoz) taken orally also binds calcium in the gut.

Hypercalciuria

In renal stone formers, in addition to general measures (low Ca diet, high fluid intake), urinary calcium may be diminished by a thiazide diuretic (with or without citrate to bind calcium) and oral phosphate (see above).

Parathyroid hormone

Parathyroid hormone acts chiefly on bone and kidney, regulating calcium and phosphate passage; its effects on the gut are indirect due to alteration of renal synthesis of 1α-25-dihydroxycholecalciferol (see vitamin D). It increases the rate of bone remodelling (mineral and collagen) and osteocyte activity, with, at high doses, an overall balance in favour of resorption (osteoclast activity) with a rise in plasmal calcium concentration (and fall in phosphate); but, at low doses, the balance favours bone formation (osteoblast activity). It increases the gut absorption of calcium (probably via its effect on vitamin D metabolism).

Natural (animal) and synthetic forms (of the first and active 34 amino acids of the 84 amino acid peptide hormone) are available. Endocrinologists use them for diagnosis in parathyroid disorder. The possibility of use of low doses for osteoporosis has been raised.

Calcitonin

Calcitonin is a peptide hormone produced by the C-cells of the thyroid gland (in mammals). It acts on bone (inhibits osteoclasts) to reduce the rate of bone turnover, and on the kidney to reduce reabsorption of calcium and phosphorus. It is obtained from natural sources (pork, salmon, eel), or synthesised. The $t_\frac{1}{2}$ varies according to source; $t_\frac{1}{2}$ human is 10 min. Antibodies develop particularly to pork calcitonin and neutralise its effect; salmon calcitonin is therefore preferred for prolonged use; loss of effect may also be due to down-regulation of receptors. Calcitonin is used (s.c. or i.m.) (intranasal use can be effective) to control hypercalcaemia (rapid effect), Paget's disease (relief of pain), and to relieve compression of nerves, e.g. auditory 8th cranial, metastatic bone cancer pain, and postmenopausal osteoporosis.

Adverse effects include allergy, nausea, flushing and tingling of the face and hands.

Biphosphonates (diphosphonates)

The biphosphonates, *disodium-etidronate, -pamidronate, -clodronate*, become absorbed onto bone crystals (hydroxyapatite) conferring resistance to hydrolysis and prolongation of $t_\frac{1}{2}$ in the skeleton. Also, when the complex is phagocytosed by an osteoclast that cell is inhibited and cannot resorb more bone. However, actions are more complex than this and biphosphonates find use in treatment of Paget's disease, osteoporosis, and hyper-

calcaemia due to cancer (pamidronate or clodronate). They may be given orally or i.v. and are eliminated unchanged by the kidney. Adverse effects include pyrexia, diarrhoea, increased bone pain (as well as relief), fractures (high dose, prolonged use only) due to demineralisation of bone.

Plicamycin (mithramycin)

Plicamycin is a cytotoxic antibiotic (made by a Streptomyces), now used only in *Paget's disease* and *acute hypercalcaemia*; it is relatively selective for osteoclasts and a single dose may give benefit for days. Its use should not exceed a few days because it depresses bone marrow.

Osteoporosis

One in 4 women in their 60s and one in 2 in their 70s experience an osteoporotic fracture. Yet 20% of family doctors (UK) claim never to have seen a case of the disease, although they are ideally placed to identify women likely to need preventive treatment and to prescribe it.[8]

Osteoporosis is an abnormal decrease in amount of bone, but what there is, is of normal quality.

Postmenopausal osteoporosis is due to gonadal deficiency; it can be prevented.

Oestrogen arrests the process by reducing bone resorption. *Progestogen arrests the process* by increasing bone formation, but therapeutic benefit is less than oestrogen. A combination of the 2 may achieve some overall reversal of the osteoporotic process over the first 2 years, though the bones are unlikely to become fully normal. Unopposed oestrogen has been widely used and it is effective, but it carries a risk of endometrial cancer, which is diminished by added progestogen; therefore combinations of oestrogen and progestogen are used (see Postmenopausal hormone replacement therapy). Such combinations are the mainstay of treatment of postmenopausal osteoporosis; they inhibit the rapid bone loss that occurs immediately after the menopause

---

[8] Anon Lancet 1990; 335: 219.

and should be continued for 5 years; perhaps even as long as 10 years. Prolonged oestrogen use reduces sensitivity of bone to natural resorbing agents and this results in compensatory stimulation of parathyroid hormone secretion. If the oestrogen is suddenly stopped there is a period (as long as 3 years) of enhanced bone loss due to the excess of parathyroid hormone.

Calcium dietary supplementation (Ca gluconate, carbonate, hydroxyapatite, citrate, maleate) reduces bone loss where intake may be inadequate, i.e. below 800 mg/d. Calcium is a weak inhibitor of bone resorption; it is not a substitute for hormones; they should be used together.

Calcitonin (see above) inhibits bone resorption.

The above treatments *arrest progress* of the disease, increasing bone mass a little or not at all.

Fluoride and biphosphonates may reverse osteoporosis.

Sodium fluoride increases bone mass by stimulating osteoblasts, but there is doubt about the quality of bone formed, e.g. there may be increased fragility. Its use remains controversial.

Biphosphonate, e.g. disodium etidronate (Didronel) (see above), used *cyclically* has been shown to decrease the incidence of vertebral fractures; plus calcium supplement.

Vitamin D analogues are under trial.

Parathyroid hormone (see above).

Secondary osteoporosis, e.g. due to intestinal malabsorption, corticosteroid therapy, hypoparathyroidism or alcoholism, may benefit from the above treatments.

Osteomalacia

Osteomalacia is due to *primary* or *secondary* vitamin D deficiency. In secondary cases, e.g. malabsorption or renal disease, high doses of vitamin D are sometimes needed. Long-term therapy with *antiepilepsy drugs* sometimes causes osteomalacia (p. 309).

Paget's disease of bone

This disease is characterised by bone resorption and formation (bone turnover) increased as much as 50 times normal, the results of which are large, vascular, deformed, painful bones. Some therapeutic success has been found with *calcitonin* (which inhibits bone resorption), with *cytotoxic agents* that inhibit osteoclasts (plicamycin, actinomycin D), and with *biphosphonates* (e.g. disodium etidronate), which inhibit crystal formation, growth and dissolution, such as must occur in bone mineralisation and demineralisation (bone turnover). The overall effects on the disease are modest, but pain, which is the chief indication for treatment, may be alleviated. The therapeutic effects may long outlast the period of administration of therapy.

VITAMINE E: TOCOPHEROL

The functions of vitamin E may be to take up (scavenge) the free radicals generated by normal metabolic process and by substances in the environment, e.g. hydrocarbons, and so to prevent them attacking polyunsaturated fats in cell membranes with resultant cellular injury. A deficiency syndrome is now recognised, including peripheral neuropathy with spinocerebellar degeneration; and a haemolytic anaemia in premature infants.

Alphatocopheryl acetate (Ephynal) pharmacotherapy may benefit the neuromuscular complications of congenital cholestasis and abetalipoproteinaemia. Studies in a wide variety of diseases, particularly cardiovascular, have been inconclusive.

VITAMIN K: see p. 475.

GUIDE TO FURTHER READING

Blinkhorn S 1991 A dose of vitamins and a pinch of salt [vitamins and IQ]. Nature 350: 13 (also p. 2, 5), and subsequent correspondence

Editorial 1962 Arctic offal. British Medical Journal 1:855

Editorial 1988 Retinoids and control of cutaneous malignancy. Lancet 2: 545

Heath D A 1987 Treating Paget's disease. British Medical Journal 294: 1048

Heath D A 1989 Hypercalcaemia in malignancy. British Medical Journal 298:1468

Hussey G D 1990 A randomized, controlled trial of vitamin A in children with severe measles. New England Journal of Medicine 323: 160

Lindsay R et al 1990 Fluoride and bone — quantity versus quality. New England Journal of Medicine 322: 845

Moertel C G et al 1985 High-dose vitamin C versus placebo in the treatment of patients with advanced cancer who have had no prior chemotherapy: A randomized double-blind comparison. New England Journal of Medicine 312: 137. Also Editorial, Wittes R E, p. 178

Munk-Jensen N et al 1988 Reversal of postmenopausal vertebral bone loss by oestrogen and progestogen: a double blind placebo contolled study. British Medical Journal 296: 1150

Reichel H et al 1989 The role of the vitamin D endocrine system in health and disease. New England Journal of Medicine 320: 980

Riggs B L 1990 A new option for treating osteoporosis. New England Journal of Medicine 323: 124

Rudman d 1983 Megadose vitamins: use and misuse. New England Journal of Medicine 309: 488

Truswell S 1990 Who should take vitamin supplements? British Medical Journal 301: 135

Appendix

Weights and measures: The prescription: Abbreviations: General references

WEIGHTS AND MEASURES

In this book doses are given in the metric system, or in international units (IU) when metric doses are impracticable.

Equivalents: 1 litre (1) = 1.76 pints
1 kilogram (kg) = 2.2 pounds (lb)

Abbreviations: 1 gram (g)
1 milligram (mg) $(1 \times 10^{-3}$ g)
1 microgram (μg)
   $(1 \times 10^{-6}$ g)
1 nanogram (ng) $(1 \times 10^{-9}$ g)
1 decilitre (dl) $(1 \times 10^{-1}$ 1)
1 millilitre (ml) $(1 \times 10^{-3}$ 1)
1 micrometre (μm)
   $(1 \times 10^{-6}$ metres)

Domestic measures. A standard 5 ml spoon is available. Otherwise the following approximations will serve:

1 tablespoonful = 14 ml
1 dessertspoonful = 7 ml
1 teaspoonful = 5 ml

PRESCRIBING

Prescriptions of pure drugs or of formulations from the British National Formulary (BNF) are satisfactory for almost all purposes. The composition of many of the preparations in the BNF is laid down in either the British Pharmacopoeia (BP) or British Pharmaceutical Codex (BPC).

Hence there is nowadays seldom any need to write a traditional prescription comprising base, adjuvant, corrective, flavouring and vehicle and the skill is virtually lost.

It is both unnecessary and unwise to try to continue the use of traditional forms of prescription writing in Latin, for facility in their use can only be attained by frequent practice. To try to use these old-fashioned terms when they do not come naturally to the mind is to court the embarrassment of issuing an incomprehensible, or worse, an inaccurate, prescription.

It is both easier and safer to state the requirements in English. However, entire consistency is seldom to be achieved in any such matter, and there is little doubt that certain convenient Latin abbreviations will survive for lack of English substitutes. These are chiefly used in hospital prescribing where instructions are given to nurses and not to patients for whom such abbreviations would be meaningless. They are listed, without approval or disapproval, at the end of this Appendix.

The elementary requirements of a prescription are that is should state **what** is to be given **to whom** and **by whom prescribed**, and give instructions on **how much** should be taken **how often, by what route** and sometimes for **how long**, thus:

1. **Date.**
2. **Address of doctor.**
3. **Name and address of patient.**

4. ℞. This is a traditional esoteric symbol[1] for the word '*Recipe*' — 'take thou!', which is addressed to the pharmacist. It is pointless; but since many doctors gain a harmless pleasure from writing ℞ with a flourish before the name of a proprietary preparation of whose exact nature they are ignorant, it is likely to survive as a sentimental link with the past.

5. **The name and dose of the medicine.**

6. **Directions to the pharmacist**, if any: 'mix', 'make a solution'. Write the total quantity to be dispensed if this is not stated in 5 above.

7. **Instruction for the patient**, to be written on container by the pharmacist. Here brevity, clarity and accuracy are especially important. It is dangerous to rely on the patient remembering verbal instructions. The BNF provides a list of recommended 'cautionary and advisory labels for dispensed medicines' representing a balance between 'the unintelligibly short and the inconveniently long'.

Pharmacists nowadays use their own initiative in giving advice to patients.

8. **Signature of doctor**.

It is now considered exceptional to conceal from patients the nature of their treatment and the name of the preparation should be written on the label unless there is a positive reason for not doing so.

Example of a prescription for a patient with an annoying unproductive cough.

1, 2, 3, as above.
4. ℞.
5. Codeine Linctus, BNF, 5 ml.
6. Send 60 ml.
7. Label: Codeine Linctus (or NP). Take 5 ml twice a day and on retiring.
8. Signature of doctor.

Legal aspects of prescribing are given in the BNF[2] which is supplied free to doctors practising

ABBREVIATIONS (see also Weights and measures, above)	
ac: ante cibum	before food.
bd: bis in die	twice a day (bid is also used).
BNF	British National Formulary.
BP	British Pharmacopoeia.
BPC	British Pharmaceutical Codex.
i.m: intramuscular	by intramuscular injection.
IU	International Unit.
iv: intravenous	by intravenous injection.
NP: nomen proprium	proper name.
od: omni die	every day.
om: omni mane	every morning.
on: omni nocte	every night.
pc: post cibum	after food.
po: per os	by mouth.
prn: pro re nata	as required. It is best to add the maximum frequency of repetition, e.g. Aspirin and Codeine Tablets, 1 or 2 prn, 4-hourly.
qds: quarter die sumendus	four times a day (qid is also used).
q or qq: quaque	every, e.g. qq6h = every 6 h.
q s: quantum sufficiat	a sufficiency, enough.
rep: repetatur	let it be repeated, as in rep. mist(ura), repeat the mixture.
sc: subcutaneous	by subcutaneous injection.
sos: si opus sit	if necessary. It is useful to confine sos to prescriptions to be repeated once only and to use prn where many repetitions are intended.
stat: statim	immediately.
tds: terdie sumendus	3 times a day (tid is also used).

---

[1]Derived from the eye of Horus, ancient Egyptian sun god.

[2] For example, *Controlled Drugs* (CD) (drugs liable to cause dependence or misuse) where *prescribers have 3 main responsibilities*: (1) to ensure they do not create dependence, (2) to ensure the patient does not increase the dose and create dependence, and (3) to ensure that they are not used as an unwitting source of supply to addicts.

in the National Health Service and to medical students, and also contains much **general guidance**.

Original pack dispensing. Increasingly medicines are dispensed in standard sealed packs provided by the manufacturer with, inside, printed information for the patient — *the patient package insert* (PPI). This is an expensive mode of dispensing but it may save money in the end by increased efficiency of medicine taking.

GENERAL REFERENCES

The following are sources of further information on any chapter:

Bernard C. *An introduction to the study of experimental medicine*, 1865. Various editions in English. This book should be read by anyone interested in or hoping to practise scientific medicine or research. It is beautifully written and reasoned and it remains the best and most readable short book on the subject.

Dollery C *Therapeutic drugs*. 1991 Edinburgh: Churchill Livingstone, 2 vols. An authoritative multi-author encyclopaedia.

Goodman and Gilman's, The pharmacological basis of therapeutics Gilman A G et al. eds. New York: Pergamon Press, current edition. A multi-author classic, specially valuable to clinicians.

The United States Pharmacopoeia Dispensing Information: current edition.

Martindale: The extra pharmacopoeia, current edition, London: Pharmaceutical Press. An encyclopaedia; invaluable for out-of-the-way information.

Meyler's Side-effects of drugs. Dukes M N G, ed. Amsterdam: Elsevier, current edition.

Side-effects of drugs annual: a worldwide survey of new data and trends, Dukes M N G. Amsterdam: Elsevier.

Drug and Therapeutics Bulletin (UK). Medical Letter on Drugs and Therapeutics (USA). Both these are short fortnightly publications that ruthlessly review evidence for and against drugs. The British publication was founded by the American and has since become independent (owned by the Consumers' Association). They are useful sources of up-to-date facts and opinions (a condensation of the views of numerous advisers).

Clinical Pharmacology and Therapeutics is the monthly publication of the American Therapeutics Society. Original papers and reviews.

European Journal of Clinical Pharmacology: monthly.

British Journal of Clinical Pharmacology: monthly publication of the British Pharmacological Society.

Annual Review of Pharmacology: George R et al. eds. Annual Reviews, California: Palo Alto. Specialised, largely animal work.

Drugs: Clinical review articles: monthly.

Clinical Pharmacokinetics: monthly.

Trends in Pharmacological Sciences (TIPS) monthly: short reviews. Sponsored by the International Union of Pharmacology (IUPHAR).

Index

Proprietary names (an incomplete list, inevitably) are in *italic type*, followed by the non-proprietary name.